Stan Brein
9/78

D1508286

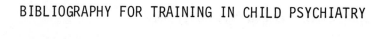

BIBLIOGRAPHY FOR TRAINING IN CHILD PSYCHIATRY

Child Psychiatry and Psychology Series

BIBLIOGRAPHY OF CHILD PSYCHIATRY
AND CHILD MENTAL HEALTH
With a Selected List of Films

Edited by

IRVING N. BERLIN, M.D.

An Official Publication of
The Academy of Child Psychiatry

Monograph of the Journal of
The Academy of Child Psychiatry

Melvin Lewis, M.D., Editor

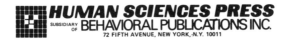

HUMAN SCIENCES PRESS
SUBSIDIARY OF BEHAVIORAL PUBLICATIONS INC.
72 FIFTH AVENUE, NEW YORK, N.Y. 10011

Library of Congress Cataloging in Publication Data

Berlin, Irving Norman, 1917-
   Bibliography for training in child psychiatry.

   First ed. published in 1963 under title: Bibliography of child psychiatry.
   Includes indexes.
   1. Child psychiatry—Bibliography. I. American Academy of Child
Psychiatry. Journal. II. Title. [DNLM: ZWS350 B515b]
Z6671.5.B4   1975   016.6189'28'9   74-11813
ISBN 0-87705-244-1

BIBLIOGRAPHY FOR TRAINING IN CHILD PSYCHIATRY

Published by

Human Sciences Press
72 Fifth Avenue, New York, N.Y., 10011

DEDICATION

Jeremiah A. O'Mara, Chief Librarian of the Western Psychiatric Institute Library and Clinic, died in June of 1974 at age 50. Jerry was my adviser, expert consultant, and reassuring friend. In the previous *Bibliography* Jerry and his staff, then at the American Psychiatric Association library, did the verification of all of the references. Prior to reorganizing the APA library Jerry had been the librarian for the Chicago Institute for Psychoanalysis.

In this *Bibliography* Jerry at once sensed the increasing complexity and problems presented by the vast increase in the number of references. He suggested methods of organization, of citing references, and finally of reducing the expense of publication and thus the cost to students. Throughout this process Jerry was constantly available to offer advice and suggestions whenever a problem occurred.

This renaissance man in psychiatric librarianship, Jerry O'Mara knew and could quote from, it seemed, all of the new books and references in all specialties of psychiatry; I would like to think with a special flair for child psychiatry. He would constantly remind me of references that should be considered. He had an uncanny nose for inaccurate references.

An extraordinary scholar, a fount of wisdom, an inexhaustible resource of bibliographic knowledge who warmly gave of himself to all of us who knew him and to all who needed his help--he is irreplaceable.

I would like to dedicate this *Bibliography* to his memory.

Irving N. Berlin, M.D.

CONTENTS

PART II

PSYCHOPATHOLOGY, DISEASE AND DISORDER
(0543-2377.19)

PART III

THERAPEUTICS
(2378 - 3234.2)

PART IV

COMMUNITY PSYCHIATRY
(3235-3641.1)

PART V

TRAINING IN ADMINISTRATION AND RESEARCH
(3642-4158.5)

PART VI

TEXTBOOKS OF CHILD PSYCHIATRY
(4159-4178)

PART VII

CREATIVITY
(4179 - 4257)

FILMS
(Sources, page 361)

CONTRIBUTORS

PAUL ADAMS, M.D.
   University of Miami
   Miami, Florida

ELISSA BENEDEK, M.D.
   University of Michigan Medical Center
   Ann Arbor, Michigan

CHARLES BINGER, M.D.
   Langley Porter Neuropsychiatric Institute
   San Francisco, California

GASTON E. BLOM, M.D.
   University of Colorado Medical Center
   Denver, Colorado

ELSIE R. BROUSSARD, M.D.
   University of Pittsburgh School of Medicine
   Pittsburgh, Pennsylvania

DONALD J. CAREK, M.D.
   Milwaukee, Wisconsin

*STELLA CHESS, M.D.
   New York University Medical Center
   New York, New York

MORTON CHETHIK, M.D.
   University of Michigan Medical Center
   Ann Arbor, Michigan

*RICHARD COHEN, M.D.
   University of Pittsburgh School of Medicine
   Pittsburgh, Pennsylvania

GORDON FARLEY, M.D.
   University of Colorado Medical Center
   Denver, Colorado

*BARBARA FISH, M.D.
    University of California Medical Center
    Los Angeles, California

*SAUL I. HARRISON, M.D.
    University of Michigan Medical Center
    Ann Arbor, Michigan

 JUERGEN HOMANN, M.D.
    University of Pittsburgh School of Medicine
    Pittsburgh, Pennsylvania

 JAMES G. KAVANAUGH, Jr., M.D.
    University of Virginia Medical Center
    Charlottesville, Virginia

 WILLIAM KIRK, M.D.
    Ypsilanti State Hospital
    Ypsilanti, Michigan

**ZANVEL KLEIN, Ph.D.
    University of Chicago
    Chicago, Illinois

*JOHN LANGDELL, M.D.
    Langley Porter Neuropsychiatric Institute
    San Francisco, California

 ROBERT L. LEON, M.D.
    University of Texas Medical School
    San Antonio, Texas

*CHARLES A. MANGHAM, M.D.
    Northwest Clinic of Psychiatry and Psychoanalysis
    Seattle, Washington

*EDWARD MASON, M.D.
    Harvard Medical School
    Boston, Massachusetts

*AKE MATTSON, M.D.
    University of Virginia Medical Center
    Charlottesville, Virginia

*TARLTON MORROW, M.D.
    The Menninger Clinic
    Topeka, Kansas

 EDWARD J. NUFFIELD, M.D.
    University of Pittsburgh School of Medicine
    Pittsburgh, Pennsylvania

JOHN O'MALLEY, M.D.
Madigan General Hospital
Tacoma, Washington

JEREMIAH O'MARA
University of Pittsburgh School of Medicine
Pittsburgh, Pennsylvania

*ELEANOR PAVENSTEDT, M.D.
Tufts University, Columbia Point Health Center
Dorchester, Massachusetts

GUILLERMO PEZZAROSSI, M.D.
Ypsilanti State Hospital
Ypsilanti, Michigan

CARL M. PFEIFER, M.D.
University of Texas Medical School
San Antonio, Texas

*IRVING PHILLIPS, M.D.
Langley Porter Neuropsychiatric Institute
San Francisco, California

*ROBERT PRALL, M.D.
Eastern Pennsylvania Psychiatric Institute
Philadelphia, Pennsylvania

*DANE PRUGH, M.D.
University of Colorado Medical Center
Denver, Colorado

NAOMI RAGINS, M.D.
University of Pittsburgh School of Medicine
Pittsburgh, Pennsylvania

JOHN B. REINHART, M.D.
University of Pittsburgh School of Medicine
Pittsburgh, Pennsylvania

*SAM RITVO, M.D.
Yale University School of Medicine, Child Study Center
New Haven, Connecticut

MICHAEL ROTHENBERG, M.D.
University of Washington School of Medicine
Seattle, Washington

DONALD RUEDINGER, M.D.
University of Michigan Medical Center
Ann Arbor, Michigan

MARSHALL D. SCHECHTER, M.D.
University of Oklahoma Medical Center
Oklahoma City, Oklahoma

ALBERTO C. SERRANO, M.D.
University of Texas Medical School
San Antonio, Texas

MOHAMMED SHAFII, M.D.
University of Michigan Medical Center
Ann Arbor, Michigan

*TED SHAPIRO, M.D.
New York University School of Medicine
New York, New York

*S. A. SZUREK, M.D.
Langley Porter Neuropsychiatric Institute
San Francisco, California

SAM WAGONFELD, M.D.
University of Colorado Medical Center
Denver, Colorado

SIDNEY WERKMAN, M.D.
University of Colorado Medical Center
Denver, Colorado

JACK WESTMAN, M.D.
Madison, Wisconsin

HERBERT C. WIMBERGER, M.D.
University of Washington School of Medicine
Seattle, Washington

JOEL P. ZRULL, M.D.
University of Michigan Medical Center
Ann Arbor, Michigan

* Special responsibility taken by a member of the editorial
board of the *Journal of the American Academy of Child Psychiatry* or a section editor.

** We are indebted to Zanvel Klein for his generosity in sharing
with us his Bibliography in Clinical Research in Child Psychiatry.

FOREWORD

From the earliest days of the child guidance clinics, child
psychiatrists invested heavily in the training of their colleagues
in children's work and they soon added special preparation for
the social workers and clinical psychologists who joined them on
clinic staffs. As the child psychiatric facilities have moved
into hospitals and medical communities in larger numbers, their
leaders have continued the investment in specialty training so
characteristic of the community clinic.

The child psychiatry community itself is and has always been
a tightly-knit group. During these nearly sixty years, ideas,
problems and goals have been freely shared among colleagues with
a deep interest in child psychiatric education. Seminar lists
and reading lists have been exchanged and a few papers written to
put some order into the varied and variable training formats and
formulations.

It was not until 1963, however, when the Langley-Porter group
under the leadership of Irving Berlin and Stanislaus Szurek put
together a bibliography for career training in child psychiatry
that we had available a list of readings which could be widely
used. Published for a modest price by the American Psychiatric
Association, this *Bibliography* soon became the property of every
training director and most fellows over the country.

When the copies of the first edition began to run out, the
American Psychiatric Association graciously consented to the
proposition that the *Journal of the American Academy of Child
Psychiatry* take over the task of preparing a new edition under
Dr. Berlin's leadership.

The differences between this second edition and the first
reflect more than the energy of the editor and the generosity of
his collaborators, although these are significant: they represent

1

the range of conceptualizing, planning and programming in which
contemporary child psychiatrists are now involved. Much of what
currently goes on in the children's service of a mental health
center can resemble the activities of the child guidance clinic
of the 1930's which go alongside programs more common in the
1950's and '60's. Infant and child development research is far
more sophisticated and involves larger numbers of child psychiatrists: infant intervention programs are beginning to appear.
Many more child analysts play a part in the service, training
and research activities of child psychiatric facilities. Service
programs are often more complex and a wider range of paraprofessional and professional personnel are in training. Consultation
activities take in a large number of settings and new community
groupings create liaisons with child psychiatry. Close collaboration with adult psychiatry and with other medical services is a
preoccupation in many centers. And the return of an interest in
primary care brings the child psychiatrist closer to the medical
student and to the medical school.

Far more purposefully than a decade or two ago, child psychiatrists are resting their complicated and diverse activities
and hence their teaching upon the foundations of developmental
theory. Here is a schema directing our attention to growth, what
accelerates it, what retards it; to individual and group resources, how they can be used and misused; to the adaptive powers
of each individual as he progresses along the developmental pathway; and to the idiosyncratic struggles and weaknesses he brings
to the struggle with inner and outer strivings. The developmental point of view grounds us in biology and keeps us aware of
the milieu in which infant, child and adult lives and of its influence upon his adaptation. It helps us assess his strengths
and difficulties and to decide whether and how help may be given
to him in our programs.

Irving Berlin, who has contributed steadily to our literature since the mid-'40's, sketched an outline of what a comprehensive bibliography of the 1970's should subsume and invoked the
assistance of a number of colleagues, all members of the American Academy of Child Psychiatry. Once his total listing was complete, Berlin chose those papers he considered especially significant for the trainee in child psychiatry. This *Bibliography*
then offers a reading list for all training programs and a comprehensive set of references for those who want to go much further in detail or range into a specific topic. We do not claim
an all-inclusive quality for this *Bibliography*. Some references undoubtedly have been left out that others would enter
and vice versa. Child psychiatrists of senior status, as many
of the contributors undoubtedly are, tend to be opinionated:
many of "our favorites" are here.

It is an ambitious and even awe-inspiring volume which Irving Berlin has edited for the *Journal of the American Academy of Child Psychiatry*. In it, an intuitive person can discern the reaches of child psychiatrists today, often beyond us, alas; the accomplishments of child psychiatrists, considerable in the past and today; and the complexity of the task child psychiatrists set out to do.

On behalf of the *Journal* and of the American Academy of Child Psychiatry, I want to thank Irving Berlin and his colleagues. Training directors and trainees will keep remembering them for years to come. Obsolescence overtakes methods and materials rapidly these days; but this Second Edition of the *Bibliography for Training in Child Psychiatry* will remain an important historical document long after a third edition is in use. The meticulous care with which it was prepared tells us something significant about the respect and concern with which this group of child psychiatrists approaches the objects of our care, the boys and girls of our country.

Eveoleen N. Rexford, M. D.
Editor, *Journal of the American Academy of Child Psychiatry*

PREFACE

The *Bibliography* is meant to be used in the training of child psychiatrists and other mental health professionals specializing in work with children. It is also designed to help general psychiatrists and all mental health professionals who will have some orientation in work with children.

Each section and subsection is, wherever possible, developmentally oriented. Thus, references on infants and younger children appear first.

The starred references are chosen by the section editors as the most important ones to be read in that section. Additional references permit both more extensive reading as well as a wider choice of significant references which may be preferred by each literature seminar leader.

Efforts at dealing with the section editor's particular theoretical bias has resulted in requests for additional readings to other collaborators to broaden the base for each section.

The organization of the *Bibliography* which numbers each reference follows the example of Zanvel Klein's very useful bibliography. It permits a search of either author or subject index to lead to a precise reference.

A literature seminar which utilizes the starred references is designed to cover the two-year training period in Child Psychiatry. More selective use of the starred references will allow for one-year or six-month literature seminars.

The list of films is organized to follow the literature sections and encourages the use of films as part of the litera-

5

ture review. All of the films noted have been found useful in teaching by various of the collaborating editors.

It is the intent of the editor and the collaborating editors from the Editorial Board of the *Journal* to publish short updating versions of the *Bibliography* every three years to keep abreast of the burgeoning literature. Since the original *Bibliography* was published in 1963, the volume of literature has increased almost 100 fold. It is obviously not all represented in this volume which is only six times larger than the original one.

We are, however, convinced, despite inadvertent omissions, many of them perhaps major ones, that this version of the *Bibliography* should be a major aid in training of all child mental health professionals.

The editor, as in the previous *Bibliography*, would be grateful to its users for their ideas on how it could be more usefully organized and used. We would also appreciate receiving citations from the literature omitted in this *Bibliography* to be added to the next addendum to the *Bibliography*.

Irving N. Berlin, M.D.

ACKNOWLEDGEMENT

I wish to express my deep appreciation to Vicki Carney and Jeanette Ashby who have done such a careful, patient, and devoted job in typing, checking, and rechecking the references through many revisions. Their unflagging optimism and meticulous attention to detail have kept the project going through numerous adversities. And to the University of Washington Library's Reference and Serials Divisions, always willing to aid in our searches.

To my family and especially Roxie Berlin for their patience through what has seemed an endless process.

To my collaborators, the section editors, and the collaborators they turned to for help, my gratitude for their support and appreciation for the excellence of their work in putting the various sections together.

We are all indebted to our esteemed colleague Eveoleen Rexford, Editor of the *Journal* of the Academy and the Presidents of the Academy of Child Psychiatry, Sid Berman, Al Solnit, and Joe Noshpitz, for their unfailing support and financial backing of this enterprise of the *Journal*.

Finally, our deep appreciation to the hundreds of colleagues in child psychiatry, psychology, social work, and nursing who as gadflies constantly reminded me and the *Journal* Editorial Board that they were still eagerly awaiting this *Bibliography*.

Irving N. Berlin, M.D.

PART I

HISTORICAL, DEVELOPMENTAL, CULTURAL AND PSYCHOANALYTIC BASES

I. HISTORY OF CHILD PSYCHIATRY

EARLY HISTORY

0001   Marx, O. M. What is the history of psychiatry? *American Journal of Orthopsychiatry*, 1970, *40*, 593-605.

0002   Ridenour, N. A. *Mental health in the United States: A fifty-year history.* Cambridge: Harvard University Press, 1961. Pp. 35-44.

0003   Watson, R. I. History of the study of the child. In *Psychology of the child*. New York: Wiley, 1959. Pp. 3-37.

0004   *Crutcher, R. Child psychiatry: A history of its development. *Psychiatry*, 1943, *6*, 191-201.

0005   *Lowrey, L. G. Psychiatry for children. A brief history of developments. *American Journal of Psychiatry*, 1944, *101*, 375-388.

0006   *MacMillan, M. B. Extra-scientific influences in the history of childhood psychopathology. *American Journal of Psychiatry*, 1960, *116*, 1091-1096.

0007   *Levy, D. M. Beginnings of the child guidance movement. *American Journal of Orthopsychiatry*, 1968, *38*, 799-804.

0008   *Lowrey, L. G. The birth of orthopsychiatry. In *Orthopsychiatry 1923-1948: Retrospect and prospect.* New York: American Orthopsychiatric Association, 1948. Pp. 190-208.

0009   *Shakow, D. The development of orthopsychiatry: The contributions of Levy, Menninger, and Stevenson. *American Journal of Orthopsychiatry*, 1968, *38*, 804-809.

0010   Healy, W. & Bronner, A. F. The child guidance clinic: Birth and growth of an idea. In L. G. Lowrey (Ed.), *Orthopsychiatry 1923-1948: Retrospect and prospect.* New York: American Orthopsychiatric Association, 1948. Pp. 14-49.

0011   Liss, E. From the founders of child psychiatry: The vicissitudes of a hybrid. *Journal of the American Academy of Child Psychiatry*, 1964, *3*, 762-768.

0012   Selesnick, S. T. Historical perspectives in the development of child psychiatry. *International Journal of Psychiatry*, 1967, *3*, 368-382.

0013   Coleman, J. V. Appraising the contribution of the mental hygiene clinic to its community. 2. In the promotion of mental health. *American Journal of Orthopsychiatry*, 1951, *21*, 83-93.

11

mental health. *American Journal of Orthopsychiatry,* 1951, *21,* 83-93.

0014   Barhash, A. Z., et al. Appraising the contribution of the mental hygiene clinic to its community. 3. Discussion. *American Journal of Orthopsychiatry,* 1951, *21,* 94-104.

0015   Lowrey, L. G. The contribution of orthopsychiatry to psychiatry: Brief historical note. *American Journal of Orthopsychiatry,* 1955, *25,* 475-478.

0016   Gardner, G. E. Appraising the contribution of the mental hygiene clinic to its community. 1. In psychiatric treatment, training and research. *American Journal of Orthopsychiatry,* 1951, *21,* 74-82.

0017   Witmer, H. L. *Psychiatric clinics for children.* New York: Commonwealth Fund, 1940.

0018   Lazure, D. La psychiatrie infantile au Canada. *Canadian Psychiatric Association Journal,* 1969, *14,* 601-606.

0018.1   Hunt, D. *Parents and children in history.* New York: Basic Books, 1970.

0018.2   Aries, P. *Centuries of childhood.* New York: Alfred A. Knopf, 1962.

FOUNDERS OF CHILD PSYCHIATRY

0019   *Eisenberg, L. Child psychiatry: The past quarter century. *American Journal of Orthopsychiatry,* 1969, *39,* 389-401.

0020   Allen, F. H. Symposium, 1955: Progress in orthopsychiatry. Psychiatry. *American Journal of Orthopsychiatry,* 1955, *25,* 479-491.

0021   *Kanner, L. Arnold Gesell's place in the history of developmental psychology and psychiatry. In C. Shagass & B. Pasamanick (Eds.), *Child development and child psychiatry.* Washington: American Psychiatric Association, 1960. Pp. 1-9. (*Psychiatric research reports, no. 13*)

0022   *Allen, F. H. From the founders of child psychiatry: Child psychiatry comes of age. *Journal of the American Academy of Child Psychiatry,* 1963, *2,* 187-198.

0023   *Kanner, L. Child psychiatry: Retrospect and prospect. *American Journal of Psychiatry,* 1960, *117,* 15-22.

0024   Adamson, W. C. History of child psychiatry. I: Frederick H. Allen, M.D., child psychiatrist. *Transactions and Studies of the College of Physicians of Philadelphia,* 1968, *36,* 96-103.

0025   Senn, M. J. E. The bequest of Frederick H. Allen to child psychiatry. *Journal of the American Academy of Child Psychiatry,* 1971, *10,* 589-602.

0026   Gardner, G. E. William Healy (1869-1963). *Journal of the American Academy of Child Psychiatry,* 1972, *11,* 1-29.

0026.1 Kanner, L. The birth of early infantile autism. *Journal of Autism and Childhood Schizophrenia*, 1973, *3*, 93-95.

0026.2 Kanner, L. Historical perspective on developmental deviations. *Journal of Autism and Childhood Schizophrenia*, 1973, *3*, 187-198.

THE CHILD GUIDANCE TEAM

0027 Axelrad, S. Symposium, 1955: Progress in orthopsychiatry. Allied disciplines. *American Journal of Orthopsychiatry*, 1955, *25*, 524-538.

SOCIAL WORK-CONTRIBUTIONS

0028 *Ginsburg, E. L. Psychiatric social work. In L. G. Lowrey (Ed.), *Orthopsychiatry 1923-1948: Retrospect and prospect*. New York: American Orthopsychiatric Association, 1948. Pp. 471-483.

0029 *Moore, M. U. Contributions of orthopsychiatry to family casework. In L. G. Lowrey (Ed.), *Orthopsychiatry 1923-1948: Retrospect and prospect*. New York: American Orthopsychiatric Association, 1948. Pp. 310-322.

0030 Berkman, T. D. Symposium, 1955: Progress in orthopsychiatry. Psychiatric social work. *American Journal of Orthopsychiatry*, 1955, *25*, 511-524.

0031 Lurie, H. L. The development of social welfare programs in the United States. *Social Work Year Book*, 1957, *13*, 19-44.

0034 French, L. A. M. *Psychiatric social work*. New York: Commonwealth Fund, 1940.

CLINICAL PSYCHOLOGY-CONTRIBUTIONS

0035 *Watson, R. I. A brief history of clinical psychology. *Psychological Bulletin*, 1953, *50*, 321-346.

0036 *Shakow, D. Clinical psychology: An evaluation. In L. G. Lowrey (Ed.), *Orthopsychiatry 1923-1948: Retrospect and prospect*. New York: American Orthopsychiatric Association, 1948. Pp. 231-247.

0037 Beck, S. J. Clinical psychology: A discipline--quantitative and humanist. In S. J. Beck & H. B. Molish (Eds.), *Reflexes to intelligence*. Glencoe, Ill.: Free Press, 1959. Pp. 482-495.

0038   Watson, R. I.   Symposium, 1955:   Progress in orthopsychi-
       atry. Psychology. *American Journal of Orthopsychia-
       try,* 1955, *25,* 491-510.
0039   Chaplin, J. P. & Krawiec, T. S.   *Systems and theories of
       psychology.* New York: Holt, Reinhart, and Winston,
       1960.
0040   Murphy, G.   *An historical introduction to modern psychol-
       ogy.* (Rev. ed.) New York: Harcourt, Brace, 1930.

PRESENT STATUS OF CHILD PSYCHIATRY

0041   *Group for the Advancement of Psychiatry.   Committee on
       Child Psychiatry. *The diagnostic process in child.
       psychiatry.* GAP report, no. 38.   New York: Group for
       the Advancement of Psychiatry, 1957.
0042   *Group for the Advancement of Psychiatry.   Committee on
       Child Psychiatry. *Basic concepts in child psychiatry.*
       GAP report, no. 12.   Topeka, Kan.: Group for the Ad-
       vancement of Psychiatry, 1950.
0043   Cameron, K.   Past and present trends in child psychia-
       try. *Journal of Mental Science,* 1956, *102,* 599-603.
0044   Rae-Grant, Q. A. F.   Symposium: Child psychiatry. Adult
       and child psychiatry--One or two nations? *Canadian
       Psychiatric Association Journal,* 1970, *15,* 247-251.
0045   *Rexford, E. N.   Children, child psychiatry, and our
       brave new world. *Archives of General Psychiatry,* 1969,
       20, 25-37.
0046   Richmond, J. B.   Future projections of orthopsychiatry.
       American Journal of Orthopsychiatry, 1968, *38,* 809-813.
0047   *Solnit, A. J.   Who deserves child psychiatry?   A study in
       priorities. *Journal of the American Academy of Child
       Psychiatry,* 1966, *5,* 1-16.
0048   *Anthony, E. J.   The emergence of child psychiatry as an
       academic discipline. *Child Psychiatry and Human Devel-
       opment,* 1970, *1,* 4-15.
0049   *Rexford, E. N.   Child psychiatry and child analysis in
       the United States today. *Journal of the American Acad-
       emy of Child Psychiatry,* 1962, *1,* 365-384.
0050   *Freud, A.   A short history of child analysis. *Psycho-
       analytic Study of the Child,* 1966, *21,* 7-14. (*Writ-
       ings,* vol. 7, p. 48-58.)
0051   Freud, S. (1909) Analysis of a phobia in a five-year-old
       boy.   In *Standard Edition, 10:* 5-149. London: Hogarth
       Press, 1955.
0052   *Levine, M. & Levine, A.   *A social history of helping
       services: Clinic, court, school and community.* New
       York: Appleton/Century/Crofts, 1970.
0052.1 Anthony, E. J.   The state of the art and science in child
       psychiatry. *Archives of General Psychiatry,* 1973, *29,*
       299-305.

0052.2 Rexford, E. Children, child psychiatry, and our brave new world. *Archives of General Psychiatry*, 1969, *20*, 25-37.
0052.3 Edwards, L. The rights of children. *Federal Probation*, 1973, *37(2)*, 34-41.
0052.4 McDermott, J. F. Jr., Bolman, W. M., Arensdorf, A. M. & Markoff, R. A. The concept of child advocacy. *American Journal of Psychiatry*, 1973, *130*, 1203-1206.
0052.5 Kanner, L. Approaches: Retrospect and prospect. *Journal of Autism and Childhood Schizophrenia*, 1971, *1*, 453-459.

II. CHILD DEVELOPMENT

GENERAL SECTION/Primary References/*SYNOPTIC ACCOUNTS OF SEVERAL DEVELOPMENTAL THEORIES*

0053 *Baldwin, A. L. Toward an integrated theory of child development. In *Theories of child development*. New York: Wiley, 1966. Pp. 579-599.
0054 *Emmerich, W. Personality development and concepts of structure. *Child Development*, 1968, *39*, 671-690.
0055 *Wolff, P. H. *The developmental psychologies of Jean Piaget and psychoanalysis*. New York: International Universities Press, 1960.
0055.1 Sears, R. R. & Feldman, S. S. *The seven ages of man; a survey of human development, body, personality and abilities through life*. Los Altos, Calif.: Kaufmann, 1973.

GENERAL SECTION/Primary References/*SPECIFIC AREAS OF DEVELOPMENT/ Biological (including ethology)*

0056 Blizzard, R. M. Differentiation, morphogenesis and growth, with emphasis on the role of pituitary growth hormone. In D. B. Cheek (Ed.), *Human growth, body composition, cell growth, energy and intelligence*. Philadelphia: Lea & Febiger, 1968. Pp. 41-59.
0057 *Harlow, H. F. & Harlow, M. K. Social deprivation in monkeys. *Scientific American*, 1962, *207*, 136-146.
0058 *Hess, E. H. Imprinting in birds. *Science*, 1964, *146*, 1128-1139.
0059 Kraus, R. F. Implications of recent developments in primate research for psychiatry. *Comprehensive Psychiatry*, 1970, *11*, 328-335.
0060 *Krech, D., Rosenzweig, M. R. & Bennett, E. L. Environmental impoverishment, social isolation and changes in brain chemistry and anatomy. *Physiology and Behavior*, 1966, *1*, 99-104.

0061   Levine, S. Maternal and environmental influences on the
        adrenocortical response to stress in weanling rats.
        Science, 1967, *156*, 258-260.
0062   Petersen, I. et al. Paroxysmal activity of EEG of nor-
        mal children. In P. Kellaway & I. Petersen (Eds.),
        Clinical electroencephalography of children. Stock-
        holm: Almquist & Wiksell, 1968. Pp. 167-187.
0063   *Rheingold, H. L. A comparative psychology of develop-
        ment. In H. W. Stevenson, E. H. Hess & H. L. Rhein-
        gold (Eds.), *Early behavior: Comparative and develop-
        mental approaches*. New York: Wiley, 1967. Pp. 279-
        293.
0064   *Scott, J. P. Critical periods in behavioral development.
        Science, 1962, *138*, 949-958.
0065   *Thomson, A. M. The evaluation of human growth patterns.
        American Journal of Diseases of Children, 1970, *120*,
        398-403.
0066   *Walter, W. G. The development of electrocerebral activ-
        ity in children. In J. G. Howells (Ed.), *Modern per-
        spectives in international child psychiatry*. Edin-
        burgh: Oliver & Boyd, 1969. Pp. 391-417. (Modern
        perspectives in psychiatry, vol. 3)
0066.1 McCall, R. B., Appelbaum, M. I. & Hogarty, P. S. *Devel-
        opmental changes in mental performance*. Chicago:
        University of Chicago Press, 1973. (*Monographs of the
        Society for Research in Child Development*, serial no.
        150, v. 38, no. 3)
0066.2 Association for Research in Nervous and Mental Disease.
        *Biological and environmental determinants of early
        development*. [proceedings of the Association, Dec. 3
        and 4, 1971] Baltimore: Williams & Wilkins, 1973.
        (*Research publications. Association for Research in
        Nervous and Mental Disease*, v. 51)
0066.3 Birch, H. G. Malnutrition, learning, and intelligence.
        In S. Chess & A. Thomas (Eds.), *Annual progress in
        child psychiatry and child development: 1973*. New
        York: Brunner/Mazel, 1974. Pp. 321-346.
0066.4 Yuwiler, A., Ritvo, E. R., Bald, D., Kipper, D. & Koper,
        A. Examination of circadian rhythmicity of blood sero-
        tonin and platelets in autistic and non-autistic chil-
        dren. *Journal of Autism and Childhood Schizophrenia*,
        1971, *1*, 421-435.
0066.5 Werner, E. E. Infants around the world: Cross-cultural
        studies of psychomotor development from birth to two
        years. In S. Chess & A. Thomas (Eds.), *Annual progress
        in child psychiatry and child development: 1973*. New
        York: Brunner/Mazel, 1974. Pp. 84-112.

GENERAL SECTION/Primary References/*SPECIFIC AREAS OF DEVELOPMENT/*
Psychosexual and Psychosocial Development

0067   *Allen, F. H. The dilemma of growth. In *Positive aspects
of child psychiatry.* New York: Norton, 1963. Pp. 60-
71.
0068   Becker, W. C. & Krug, R. S. A circumplex model for
social behavior in children. *Child Development,* 1964,
35, 371-396.
0069   *Benedek, T. The family as a psychologic field. In E.
J. Anthony & T. Benedek (Eds.), *Parenthood: Its psychology and psychopathology.* Boston: Little, Brown,
1970. Pp. 109-136.
0070   *Bloom, B. S. *Stability and change in human characteristics.* New York: John Wiley, 1964.
0071   Bowlby, J. *Attachment and loss.* London: Hogarth Press,
1969-73. (2 v. Contents--v.1. *Attachment.* v.2. *Separation, anxiety and anger.*)
0072   *Bowlby, J. The nature of the child's tie to his mother.
International Journal of Psychoanalysis, 1958, *39,* 350-
373.
0073   *Emmerich, W. Continuity and stability in early social
development. *Child Development,* 1964, *35,* 311-332.
0074   *Erikson, E. H. Growth and crises of the healthy personality. In *Identity and the life cycle.* New York:
International Universities Press, 1959. Pp. 50-100.
0075   *Erikson, E. H. The theory of infantile sexuality. In
Childhood and society. New York: Norton, 1963.
Pp. 48-108.
0076   *Freud, A. The assessment of normality in childhood. In
Normality and pathology in childhood. London: Hogarth
Press, 1966. Pp. 54-107. (*Writings,* vol. 6, p. 54-
107)
0077   *Freud, S. (1933) "The dissection of the psychical personality." In *Standard Edition, 22:* 57-80. London:
Hogarth Press, 1964. [Note: *New Introductory Lec-
tures,* Lecture 21]
0078   Freud, S. (1915) Instincts and their vicissitudes. In
Standard Edition, 14: 117-140. London: Hogarth
Press, 1957.
0079   Freud, S. (1905) Three essays on the theory of sexuality. In *Standard Edition, 7:* 135-243. London: Hogarth
Press, 1953.
0080   *Gillespie, W. H. The psychoanalytic theory of child development. In E. Miller (Ed.), *Foundations of child
psychiatry.* Oxford: Pergamon, 1968. Pp. 51-69.
0081   *Gilmore, J. B. The role of anxiety and cognitive factors in children's play behavior. *Child Development,*
1966, *37,* 397-416.
0082   *Handel, G. (comp.) *The psychosocial interior of the
family: A sourcebook for the study of whole families.*
Chicago: Aldine, 1967.

0083   *Howells, J. G.   Fathering.   In *Modern perspectives in
       international child psychiatry*.   Edinburgh: Oliver &
       Boyd, 1969.   Pp. 125-156.   (Modern perspectives in
       psychiatry, vol. 3)
0084   *Josselyn, I. M.   Passivity.   *Journal of the American
       Academy of Child Psychiatry*, 1968, *7*, 569-588.
0085   *Kagan, J. & Moss, H. A.   The stability of passive and
       dependent behavior from childhood through adulthood.
       Child Development, 1960, *31*, 577-591.
0086   *Khan, M. M. R.   The concept of cumulative trauma.   *Psy-
       choanalytic Study of the Child*, 1963, *18*, 286-306.
0087   Klein, M.   The development of a child.   In *Contributions
       to psycho-analysis: 1921-1945*.   London: Hogarth
       Press, 1948.   Pp. 13-67.
0088   Marshall, H. H.   Behavior problems of normal children:
       A comparison between the lay literature and develop-
       mental research.   *Child Development*, 1964, *35*, 469-
       478.
0089   Meili, R.   A longitudinal study of personality develop-
       ment.   In L. Jessner & E. Pavenstedt (Eds.), *Dynamic
       psychopathology in childhood*.   New York: Grune &
       Stratton, 1959.   Pp. 106-123.
0090   Nash, J.   The father in contemporary culture and current
       psychological literature.   *Child Development*, 1965,
       36, 261-297.
0091   Parsons, T. & Bales, R. F.   *Family socialization and
       interaction process*.   Glencoe, Ill.: Free Press, 1954.
0092   *Phillips, R. H.   The nature and function of children's
       formal games.   *Psychoanalytic Quarterly*, 1960, *29*,
       200-207.
0093   *Rexford, E. N.   A developmental concept of the problems
       of acting out.   *Journal of the American Academy of
       Child Psychiatry*, 1963, *2*, 6-21.
0094   Ruesch, J. & Bateson, G.   *Communication, the social ma-
       trix of psychiatry*.   New York: Norton, 1951.
0095   *Rutter, M.   Normal psychosexual development.   *Journal of
       Child Psychology and Psychiatry and Allied Disciplines*,
       1971, *11*, 259-283.
0096   *Simmel, M. L.   Developmental aspects of the body scheme.
       Child Development, 1966, *37*, 83-95.
0097   *Szurek, S. A.   The child's needs for his emotional
       health.   In J. G. Howells (Ed.), *Modern perspectives
       in international child psychiatry*.   Edinburgh: Oliver
       & Boyd, 1969.   Pp. 157-199.   (Modern perspectives in
       psychiatry, vol. 3)
0098   Waelder, R.   The psychoanalytic theory of play.   *Psycho-
       analytic Quarterly*, 1933, *2*, 208-224.
0099   *Winnicott, D. W.   Growth and development in immaturity.
       In *The family and individual development*.   London:
       Tavistock, 1965.   Pp. 21-29.

0099.1   Spitz, R. A., Emde, R. N. and Metcalf, D. R. Further
          prototypes of ego formation: A working paper from a
          research project on early development. *Psychoanalytic
          Study of the Child*, 1970, *25*, 417-441.
0099.2   White, B. L. & Watts, J. C. *Experience and environment:
          Major influences on the development of the young child*.
          Vol. 1. Englewood Cliffs, N.J.: Prentice-Hall, 1973.

GENERAL SECTION/Primary References/*SPECIFIC AREAS OF DEVELOPMENT/
Cognitive Development*

0100   *Cravioto, J. Nutritional deficiencies and mental per-
          formance in childhood. In D. C. Glass (Ed.), *Environ-
          mental influences: Proceedings of a conference under
          the auspices of Russell Sage Foundation and the Rocke-
          feller University*. New York: Rockefeller University
          Press, 1968. Pp. 3-51.
0101   *DeHirsch, K. A review of early language development.
          Developmental Medicine and Child Neurology, 1970, *12*,
          87-97.
0102   *Dubin, R. & Dubin, E. R. Children's social perceptions:
          A review of research. *Child Development*, 1965, *36*,
          809-838.
0103   *Ervin-Tripp, S. Language development. *Review of Child
          Development Research*, 1966, *2*, 55-105.
0104   *Gesell, A. L. & Amatruda, C. S. *Developmental diagnosis;
          normal and abnormal child development, clinical meth-
          ods and pediatric applications.*(2nd ed.) New York:
          Hoeber, 1947.
0105   Huttenlocher, J. Development of formal reasoning on con-
          cept formation problems. *Child Development*, 1964, *35*,
          1233-1242.
0106   *Korner, A. F. & Grobstein, R. Visual alertness as re-
          lated to soothing in neonates: Implications for mater-
          nal stimulation and early deprivation. *Child Develop-
          ment*, 1966, *37*, 867-876.
0107   *Kreitler, H. & Kreitler, S. Children's concepts of
          sexuality and birth. *Child Development*, 1966, *37*, 363-
          378.
0108   *Langer, J. Werner's comparative organismic theory. In
          L. Carmichael, *Manual of child psychology*. Vol. 1.
          (3rd ed.) New York: Wiley, 1970. Pp. 733-771.
0109   Lipsitt, L. P. Learning in the human infant. In H. W.
          Stevenson, E. H. Hess & H. L. Rheingold (Eds.), *Early
          behavior: Comparative and developmental approaches*.
          New York: Wiley, 1967. Pp. 225-247.
0110   *Piaget, J. Piaget's theory. In L. Carmichael, *Manual
          of child psychology*. Vol. 1. (3rd ed.) New York:
          Wiley, 1970. Pp. 703-732.
0111   Piaget, J. & Inhelder, B. *The psychology of the child*.
          New York: Basic Books, 1969.

0112   *Rosenblith, J. F. Prognostic value of neonatal assessment. *Child Development,* 1966, *37,* 623-631.
0113   *Vernon, M. D. The development of perception. In J. G. Howells (Ed.), *Modern perspectives in child psychiatry.* London: Oliver & Boyd, 1965. Pp. 85-103. (Modern perspectives in psychiatry, vol. 1)
0114   *Walters, R. H. & Parke, R. D. The role of the distance receptors in the development of social responsiveness. In L. P. Lipsitt & C. C. Spiker (Eds.), *Advances in child development and behavior.* Vol. 2. New York: Academic Press, 1963. Pp. 59-96.
0115   Witkin, H. A. Heinz Werner: 1890-1964. *Child Development,* 1965, *36,* 307-328.
0115.1 Chomsky, N. Recent contributions to the theory of innate ideas. In S. G. Sapir & A. C. Nitzburg (Eds.), *Children with learning problems: Readings in a developmental-interaction approach.* New York: Brunner/ Mazel, 1973. Pp. 99-108.
0115.2 Kephart, N. C. Developmental sequences. In S. G. Sapir & A. C. Nitzburg (Eds.), *Children with learning problems: Readings in a developmental-interaction approach.* New York: Brunner/Mazel, 1973. Pp. 318-334.
0115.3 Kagan, J. Impulsive and reflective children: Significance of conceptual tempo. In S. G. Sapir & A. C. Nitzburg (Eds.), *Children with learning problems: Readings in a developmental-interaction approach.* New York: Brunner/Mazel, 1973. Pp. 308-317.
0115.4 Macnamara, J. Cognitive basis of language learning in infants. In S. Chess & A. Thomas (Eds.), *Annual progress in child psychiatry and child development: 1973.* New York: Brunner/Mazel, 1974. Pp. 265-284.

GENERAL SECTION/Primary References/*SPECIFIC AREAS OF DEVELOPMENT/ Sociocultural (Including "Moral" Development)*

0116   *Allen, F. H. Dynamics of roles as determined in the structure of the family. In *Positive aspects of child psychiatry.* New York: Norton, 1963. Pp. 83-94.
0117   Becker, W. C. & Krug, R. S. The parent attitude research instrument: A research review. *Child Development,* 1965, *36,* 329-365.
0118   *Bodin, A. M. Conjoint family assessment: An evolving field. In P. McReynolds (Ed.), *Advances in psychological assessment.* Vol. 1. Palo Alto, Calif.: Science & Behavior Books, 1968.
0119   *Clausen, J. A. Family structure, socialization, and personality. In *Review of Child Development Research,* 1966, *2,* 1-53.
0120   *Coles, R. The place of the child. In *Children of crisis: A study of courage and fear.* Vol. 1. Boston: Little, Brown, 1967. Pp. 319-332.

0121   *Coles, R.   The meaning of race.   In *Children of crisis: A study of courage and fear.* Vol. 1.   Boston: Little, Brown, 1967.   Pp. 333-350.

0122   *Coles, R.   The children.   In *Children of crisis: A study of courage and fear.* Vol. 2.   Boston: Little, Brown, 1967.   Pp. 45-272.

0123   *Emmerich, W.   Personality development and concepts of structure.   *Child Development,* 1968, *39,* 671-690.

0125   Gewirtz, H. B. & Gewirtz, J. L.   Caretaking settings, background events and behavior differences in four Israeli child-rearing environments: Some preliminary trends.   In B. M. Foss (Ed.), *Determinants of infant behaviour.* Vol. 4.   London: Methuen, 1967.   Pp. 229-252.

0126   *Hess, R. D.   Social class and ethnic influences upon socialization.   In L. Carmichael, *Manual of child psychology.* Vol. 2.   (3rd. ed.)   New York: Wiley, 1970.   Pp. 457-557.

0127   *Hoffman, M. L.   Moral development.   In L. Carmichael, *Manual of child psychology.* Vol. 2.   (3rd ed.)   New York: Wiley, 1970.   Pp. 261-359.

0128   Irvine, E. E.   Children in kibbutzim: Thirteen years after.   *Journal of Child Psychology and Psychiatry and Allied Disciplines,* 1966, *7,* 167-178.

0129   *Jones, H. G.   Research methodology and child psychiatry.   In J. G. Howells (Ed.), *Modern perspectives in child psychiatry.* London: Oliver & Boyd, 1965.   Pp. 3-19.   (Modern perspectives in psychiatry, vol. 1)

0130   *Kagan, J.   American longitudinal research on psychological development.   *Child Development,* 1964, *35,* 1-32.

0131   Kamii, C. K. & Radin, N. L.   Class differences in the socialization practices of Negro mothers.   *Journal of Marriage and the Family,* 1967, *29,* 302-310.

0132   Karr, C. & Wesley, F.   Comparison of German and U.S. child-rearing practices.   *Child Development,* 1966, *37,* 715-723.

0133   *LeVine, R. A.   Cross-cultural study in child psychology.   In L. Carmichael, *Manual of child psychology.* Vol. 2.   (3rd. ed.)   New York: Wiley, 1970.   Pp. 559-612.

0135   *Lytton, H.   Observation studies of parent-child interaction: A methodological review.   *Child Development,* 1971, *42,* 651-684.

0136   Miller, L.   Child rearing in the kibbutz.   In J. G. Howells (Ed.), *Modern perspectives in international child psychiatry.* Edinburgh: Oliver & Boyd, 1969.   Pp. 321-346.   (Modern perspectives in psychiatry, vol. 3)

0137   *Opler, M. K.   Culture and child rearing.   In J. G. Howells (Ed.), *Modern perspectives in international child psychiatry.* Edinburgh: Oliver & Boyd, 1969.   Pp. 292-320.   (Modern perspectives in psychiatry, vol. 3)

0138   Stout, I. W. & Langdon, G. A study of the home life of
        well adjusted children. *Journal of Educational Sociol-
        ogy*, 1950, *23*, 442-460.
0139   Walters, J., Connor, R., and Zunich, M. Interaction of
        mothers and children from lower-class families. *Child
        Development*, 1964, *35*, 433-440.
0140   *Whiteman, P. H. & Kosier, K. P. Development of chil-
        dren's moralistic judgments: Age, sex, IQ, and cer-
        tain personal-experimental variables. *Child Develop-
        ment*, 1964, *35*, 843-850.
0141   Yarrow, M. R. Problems of methods in parent-child re-
        search. *Child Development*, 1963, *34*, 215-226.
0141.1 Scrofani, P. J., Suziedelis, A. & Shore, M. F. Concep-
        tual ability in black and white children of different
        social classes: An experimental test of Jensen's
        hypothesis. *American Journal of Orthopsychiatry*, 1973,
        43, 541-553.
0141.2 Caldwell, B. M. & Ricciuti, H. N. (Eds.) *Review of child
        development research*. Vol. 3. *Child development and
        social policy*. Chicago: University of Chicago Press,
        1973.
0141.3 Mech, E. V. Adoption: A policy perspective. In B. M.
        Caldwell & H. N. Ricciuti (Eds.), *Review of child
        development research*. Vol. 3. *Child development and
        social policy*. Chicago: University of Chicago Press,
        1973. Pp. 467-508.
0141.4 Deutsch, C. P. Social class and child development. In
        B. M. Caldwell & H. N. Ricciuti (Eds.), *Review of child
        development research*. Vol. 3. *Child development and
        social policy*. Chicago: University of Chicago Press,
        1973. Pp. 233-282.
0141.5 Herzog, E. & Sudia, C. E. Children in fatherless fami-
        lies. In B. M. Caldwell & H. N. Ricciuti (Eds.),
        Review of child development research. Vol. 3. *Child
        development and social policy*. Chicago: University
        of Chicago Press, 1973. Pp. 141-232.
0141.6 Berkowitz, L. Control of aggression. In B. M. Caldwell
        & H. N. Ricciuti (Eds.), *Review of child development
        research*. Vol. 3. *Child development and social policy*.
        Chicago: University of Chicago Press, 1973. Pp. 95-
        140.

GENERAL SECTION/Additional References

0142   *Baldwin, A. L. The study of child behavior and develop-
        ment. In P. H. Mussen (Ed.), *Handbook of research
        methods in child development*. New York: Wiley, 1960.
        Pp. 3-35.
0143   *Baldwin, A. L. *Theories of child development*. New York:
        Wiley, 1966.

0144   Bandura, A. & Walters, R. H. *Social learning and per-*
        sonality development. New York: Holt, Rinehart, &
        Winston, 1963.
0145   *Birch, H. G. & Gussow, J. D. *Disadvantaged children:*
        Health, nutrition and school failure. New York: Grune
        & Stratton, 1970.
0146   *Bowlby, J. *Attachment and Loss.* Vol. 1. *Attachment.*
        New York: Basic Books, 1969.
0147   Bowlby, J. *Maternal care and mental health.* Geneva:
        World Health Organization, 1951. (Monograph series,
        no. 2)
0148   *Bronson, W. C. Central orientations: A study of behav-
        ior organization from childhood to adolescence. *Child*
        Development, 1966, *37,* 125-155.
0149   Bronson, W. C. Early antecedents of emotional expres-
        siveness and reactivity control. *Child Development,*
        1966, *37,* 793-810.
0150   *Cravioto, J. et al. *Nutrition, growth, and neurointe-*
        grative development: An experimental and ecologic
        study. Evanston, Ill.: American Academy of Pedia-
        trics, 1966.
0151   Darwin, C. R. *The expression of the emotions in man and*
        animals. Chicago: University of Chicago Press, 1965.
0152   Dubos, R. Environmental determinants of human life. In
        D. C. Glass (Ed.), *Environmental influences: Proceed-*
        ings of a conference under the auspices of Russell Sage
        Foundation and the Rockefeller University. New York:
        Rockefeller University Press, 1968. Pp. 138-154.
0153   Erikson, E. H. *Childhood and society.* (2nd ed.) New
        York: Norton, 1963.
0154   Erikson, E. H. *Identity and the life cycle.* New York:
        International Universities Press, 1959. (*Psychological*
        Issues, 1959, *1,* no. 1)
0155   Fanon, F. *Black skin, White masks.* New York: Grove
        Press, 1967.
0156   *Flavell, J. H. *The developmental psychology of Jean*
        Piaget. Princeton, N.J.: Van Nostrand, 1963.
0157   Freud, A. *The ego and the mechanisms of defense.* New
        York: International Universities Press, 1946. (*Writ-*
        ings, vol. 2)
0158   Freud, A. *Normality and pathology in childhood.* London:
        Hogarth Press, 1966. (*Writings,* vol. 6)
0159   Freud, S. (1923) The ego and the id. In *Standard Edi-*
        tion, 19, 12-66. London: Hogarth Press, 1961.
0160   Freud, S. (1940) [1938] An outline of psycho-analysis.
        In *Standard Edition, 23,* 144-207. London: Hogarth
        Press, 1964.
0161   Goodwin, R. B. *It's good to be black.* Garden City,
        N.Y.: Doubleday, 1953.
0162   Harlow, H. F., Harlow, M. K. & Hansen, E. W. The mater-
        nal affectional system of rhesus monkeys. In H. L.
        Rheingold (Ed.), *Maternal behavior in mammals.* New

York: Wiley, 1963. Pp. 254-281.

0163   Hartmann, H. *Ego psychology and the problem of adaptation.* New York: International Universities Press, 1958.

0164   Hatfield, J. S., Ferguson, L. R. & Alpert, R. Mother-child interaction and the socialization process. *Child Development,* 1967, *38,* 365-414.

0165   Hebb, D. O. *The organization of behavior: A neuropsychological theory.* New York: Wiley, 1949.

0166   Heilbrun, A. B. The measurement of identification. *Child Development,* 1965, *36,* 111-127.

0167   *Hess, E. H. Ethology and developmental psychology. In L. Carmichael, *Manual of child psychology.* Vol. 1. (3rd ed.) New York: Wiley, 1970. Pp. 1-38.

0168   *Kagan, J. & Moss, H. A. (Eds.) *Birth to maturity: A study in psychological development.* New York: Wiley, 1962.

0169   Kuhn, D. Z., Madsen, C. H., Jr. & Becker, W. C. Effects of exposure to an aggressive model and "frustration" on children's aggressive behavior. *Child Development,* 1967, *38,* 739-745.

0170   Lewis, M. *Clinical aspects of child development.* Philadelphia: Lea & Febiger, 1971.

0171   Maier, H. W. *Three theories of child development: The contributions of Erik H. Erikson, Jean Piaget, and Robert R. Sears, and their applications.* (Rev. ed.) New York: Harper & Row, 1969.

0172   Mittler, P. Genetic aspects of psycholinguistic abilities. *Journal of Child Psychology and Psychiatry and Allied Disciplines,* 1969, *10,* 165-176.

0173   Parsons, T. & Bales, R. F. *Family socialization and interaction process.* Glencoe, Ill.: Free Press, 1954.

0174   Peiper, A. *Cerebral function in infancy and childhood.* New York: Consultants Bureau, 1963.

0175   Piaget, J. *The language and thought of the child.* (3rd ed.) New York: Humanities Press, 1959.

0176   Piaget, J. *The origins of intelligence in children.* New York: International Universities Press, 1952.

0177   Sears, R. R., Rau, L. & Alpert, R. *Identification and child rearing.* Stanford, Calif.: Stanford University Press, 1965.

0178   Sears, R. R., Maccoby, E. E. & Levin, H. *Patterns of child rearing.* Evanston, Ill.: Row, Peterson, 1957.

0179   Stevenson, H. W., Hess, E. H. & Rheingold, H. L. (Eds.) *Early behavior: Comparative and developmental approaches.* New York: Wiley, 1967.

0180   Sullivan, H. S. *The interpersonal theory of psychiatry.* New York: Norton, 1953.

0181   Walter, W. G. *The living brain.* New York: Norton, 1953.

0182   *Whiting, B. B. (Ed.) *Six cultures: Studies of child
       rearing.* New York: Wiley, 1963.
0182.1 Dinnage, R. *The handicapped child; research review.*
       London: Longman [in association with] National Bureau
       for Co-operation in Child Care, (1970-7). (Studies
       in child development [v. 14, v. 18])
182.2 Seglow, J., Pringle, M. K. & Wedge, P. *Growing up adop-
       ted: A long-term national study of adopted children
       and their families.* Slough: National Foundation for
       Educational Research in England and Wales, 1972.
182.3 Piaget, J., Inhelder, B. & Sinclair-de Zwart, H. *Memory
       and intelligence.* London: Routledge & Kegan Paul,
       1973.
182.4 Joint Commission on Mental Health of Children. *Mental
       Health: From infancy through adolescence; reports of
       Task Forces I, II, and III and the Committees on Edu-
       cation and Religion.* New York: Harper & Row, 1973.
182.5 George, V. & Wilding, P. *Motherless families.* London:
       Routledge & Kegan Paul, 1972.
182.6 Jones, M. C., Bayley, N. et al. (Eds.) *The course of
       human development; selected papers from the longitudi-
       nal studies.* [Institute of Human Development, Univer-
       sity of California, Berkeley.] Waltham, Mass.: Xerox
       College Pub., 1971.
182.7 Piaget, J. *The child and reality; problems of genetic
       psychology.* New York: Grossman, 1973.

PREGNANCY AND THE NEONATAL PERIOD/Pregnancy/*PRIMARY REFERENCES/
General*

0183   *Benedek, T. The psychobiology of pregnancy. In E. J.
       Anthony & T. Benedek (Eds.), *Parenthood.* Boston:
       Little, Brown, 1970. Pp. 137-151.
0184   *Senay, E. C. Therapeutic abortion: Clinical aspects.
       Archives of General Psychiatry, 1970, *23,* 408-415.

PREGNANCY AND THE NEONATAL PERIOD/Pregnancy/*PRIMARY REFERENCES/
Constitutional (Including Ethologic Studies)*

0186   Baird, D. (Ed.) Physiology and nutrition in pregnancy
       and lactation. In J. M. M. Kerr, *Combined textbook of
       obstetrics and gynaecology for students and practition-
       ers.* (8th ed.) Edinburgh: Livingstone, 1969. Pp.
       95-119.

PREGNANCY AND THE NEONATAL PERIOD/Pregnancy/*PRIMARY REFERENCES/ Familial*

0187   Bibring, G. L.   Some considerations of the psychological processes in pregnancy. *Psychoanalytic Study of the Child,* 1959, *14,* 113-121.

0188   *Bibring, G. L., Dwyer, T. F., Huntington, D. S. & Valenstein, A. F.   A study of the psychological processes in pregnancy and of the earliest mother-child relationship. II. Methodological considerations. *Psychoanalytic Study of the Child,* 1961, *16,* 25-72.

0189   Colman, A. D.   Psychological state during first pregnancy. *American Journal of Orthopsychiatry,* 1969, *39,* 788-797.

0190   *Flapan, M.   A paradigm for the analysis of childbearing motivations of married women prior to birth of the first child. *American Journal of Orthopsychiatry,* 1969, *39,* 402-417.

0191   Grimm, E. & Venet, W. R.   The relationship of emotional adjustment and attitudes to the course and outcome of pregnancy. *Psychosomatic Medicine,* 1966, *28,* 34-49.

0192   *Jessner, L., Weigert, E. & Foy, J. L.   The development of parental attitudes during pregnancy. In E. J. Anthony & T. Benedek (Eds.), *Parenthood.* Boston: Little, Brown, 1970. Pp. 209-244.

0193   Kaij, L., Malmquist, A. & Nilsson, A.   Psychiatric aspects of spontaneous abortion. II. The importance of bereavement, attachment and neurosis in early life. *Journal of Psychosomatic Research,* 1969, *13,* 53-59.

0194   Kazzaz, D. S.   Attitude of expectant mothers in relation to onset of labor. *Obstetrics and Gynecology,* 1965, *26,* 585-591.

0195   Lerner, B., Raskin, R. & Davis, E. B.   On the need to be pregnant. *International Journal of Psychoanalysis,* 1967, *48,* 288-297.

0196   *Malmquist, A., Kaij, L. & Nilsson, A. I. A matched control study of women with living children. *Journal of Psychosomatic Research,* 1969, *13,* 45-51.

0197   McDonald, R. L.   Fantasy and the outcome of pregnancy. *Archives of General Psychiatry,* 1965, *12,* 602-606.

0197.1   Group for the Advancement of Psychiatry. Committee on Public Education. *The joys and sorrows of parenthood.* New York: GAP, 1973. (GAP report, no. 84)

0197.2   Greenbaum, H.   Marriage, family and parenthood. *American Journal of Psychiatry,* 1973, *130,* 1262-1265.

PREGNANCY AND THE NEONATAL PERIOD/Pregnancy/*PRIMARY REFERENCES/ Societal*

0198   Davids, A. & Rosengren, W.   Social stability and psychological adjustment during pregnancy. *Psychosomatic*

Medicine, 1962, *24*, 579-583.
0199 Greenberg, N. H., Loesch, J. G. & Lakin, M. Life situations associated with the onset of pregnancy. 1. The role of separation in a group of unmarried pregnant women. *Psychosomatic Medicine*, 1959, *21*, 296-310.
0200 *Loesch, J. G. & Greenberg, N. H. Some specific areas of conflicts observed during pregnancy: A comparative study of married and unmarried pregnant women. *American Journal of Orthopsychiatry*, 1962, *32*, 624-636.

PREGNANCY AND THE NEONATAL PERIOD/Neonate/*PRIMARY REFERENCES/*
General

0201 *Blauvelt, H. & McKenna, J. Mother-neonate interaction: Capacity of the human newborn for orientation. In B. M. Foss (Ed.), *Determinants of infant behaviour*. Vol. 1. New York: Wiley, 1961. Pp. 3-29.
0202 *Lidz, T. F. The neonate and the new mother. In *The person*. New York: Basic Books, 1968. Pp. 93-116.
0203 Wolff, P. H. Mother-infant relations at birth. In J. G. Howells (Ed.), *Modern perspectives in international child psychiatry*. Edinburgh: Oliver & Boyd, 1969. Pp. 80-97. (Modern perspectives in psychiatry, vol. 3)
0204 Burns, P., et al. Distress in feeding: Short-term effects of caretaker environment of the first 10 days. *Journal of the American Academy of Child Psychiatry*, 1972, *11*, 427-439.
0204.1 Bowlby, J. *Attachment and loss*. Vol. 2. *Separation, anxiety and anger*. London: Hogarth Press, 1973.
0204.2 Gaensbauer, T. J. & Emde, R. N. Wakefulness and feeding in human newborns. *Archives of General Psychiatry*, 1973, *28*, 894-897.
0204.3 Hutt, S. J. & Hutt, C. *Early human development*. London: Oxford University Press, 1973.

PREGNANCY AND THE NEONATAL PERIOD/Neonate/*PRIMARY REFERENCES/*
Constitutional

0205 *Bowlby, J. Ontogeny of human attachment. In *Attachment and loss*. Vol. 1. New York: Basic Books, 1969. Pp. 264-358.
0206 *Call, J. D. Newborn approach behaviour and early ego development. *International Journal of Psychoanalysis*, 1964, *45*, 286-294.
0207 *Korner, A. F. & Grobstein, R. Individual differences at birth: Implications for mother-infant relationship and later development. *Journal of the American Academy of Child Psychiatry*, 1967, *6*, 676-690.
0208 Richmond, J. B. & Lustman, S. L. Autonomic function in the neonate: I. Implications for psychosomatic theory.

Psychosomatic Medicine, 1955, *17,* 269-275.

0209 *Richmond, J. B. & Lipton, E. L. Some aspects of the neurophysiology of the newborn and their implications for child development. In L. Jessner & E. Pavenstedt (Eds.), *Dynamic psychopathology in childhood.* New York: Grune & Stratton, 1959. Pp. 78-105.

0210 Rosenblatt, J. S. Turkewitz, G. & Schneirla, T. C. Development of suckling and related behavior in neonate kittens. In E. L. Bliss (Ed.), *Roots of behavior.* New York: Hoeber, 1962. Pp. 198-210.

0211 *Scheibel, M. E. & Scheibel, A. B. Some neural substrates of postnatal development. In M. L. Hoffman & L. W. Hoffman (Eds.), *Review of child development research.* Vol. 1. New York: Russell Sage Foundation, 1964. Pp. 481-519.

0211.1 Hebb, D. O. Drive and the C.N.S. (Conceptual Nervous System). In S. G. Sapir & A. C. Nitzburg (Eds.), *Children with learning problems: Readings in a developmental-interaction approach.* New York: Brunner/ Mazel, 1973. Pp. 131-147.

0211.2 Korner, A. F. & Thoman, E. B. The relative efficacy of contact and vestibular-proprioceptive stimulation in soothing neonates. In S. Chess & A. Thomas (Eds.), *Annual progress in child psychiatry and child development: 1973.* New York: Brunner/Mazel, 1974. Pp. 30-41.

PREGNANCY AND THE NEONATAL PERIOD/Neonate/*PRIMARY REFERENCES/ Familial*

0212 Barnett, C. R., Leiderman, P.H., Grobstein, R. & Klaus, M. Neonatal separation: The maternal side of interactional deprivation. *Pediatrics,* 1970, *45,* 197-205.

0214 *Klaus, M. H., Kennell, J. H., Plumb, N. & Zuehlke, S. Human maternal behavior at the first contact with her young. *Pediatrics,* 1970, *46,* 187-192.

0214.1 Ainsworth, M. D. S. The development of infant-mother attachment. In B. M. Caldwell & H. N. Ricciuti, (Eds.), *Review of child development research.* Vol. 3. *Child development and social policy.* Chicago: University of Chicago Press, 1973. Pp. 1-94.

0214.2 Greenberg, M., Rosenberg, I. & Lind, J. First mothers rooming-in with their newborns: Its impact upon the mother. *American Journal of Orthopsychiatry,* 1973, *43,* 783-788.

0215 *Klaus, M. H. & Kennell, J. H. Mothers separated from their newborn infants. *Pediatric Clinics of North America,* 1970, *17*(4), 1015-1037.

0216 Levine, S. Maternal and environmental influences on the adrenocortical response to stress in weanling rats. *Science,* 1967, *156,* 258-260.

0218   *Yalom, I. D., Lunde, D. T., Moos, R. H. & Hamburg, D. A.
"Postpartum blues" syndrome: A description and related variables. *Archives of General Psychiatry*, 1968,
18, 16-27.
0219   Cohen, D. J. et al. Personality development in twins:
Competence in the newborn and preschool periods. *Journal of the American Academy of Child Psychiatry*, 1972,
11, 625-644.

INFANCY/Primary References/*GENERAL*

0220   *Bayley, N. and Schaefer, E. S. *Correlations of maternal
and child behaviors with the development of mental
abilities: Data from the Berkeley growth study.*
Chicago: Child Development Publications, Society for
Research in Child Development, 1964. *(Monographs of
the Society for Research in Child Development*, v. 29,
no. 6, serial no. 97)
0221   *Bell, R. Q. Retrospective and prospective views of early personality development. *Merrill-Palmer Quarterly*,
1960, *6*, 131-144.
0222   *Brody, S. & Axelrad, S. *Anxiety and ego formation in
infancy.* New York: International Universities Press,
1970. Pp. 10-26.
0223   *Caldwell, B. M. What is the optimal learning environment for the young child? *American Journal of Orthopsychiatry*, 1967, *37*, 8-21.
0224   *Caplan, H., Bibace, R. & Rabinovitch, M. S. Paranatal
stress, cognitive organization and ego function: A
controlled follow-up study of children born prematurely. *Journal of the American Academy of Child Psychiatry*, 1963, *2*, 434-450.
0225   *Carmichael, L. The onset and early development of behavior. In *Manual of child psychology*. Vol. 1. (3rd
ed.) New York: Wiley, 1970. Pp. 447-563.
0226   *Erikson, E. H. The theory of infantile sexuality. In
Childhood and society. New York: Norton, 1963.
Pp. 48-108.
0227   *Geschwind, N. The organization of language and the
brain. *Science*, 1970, *170*, 940-952.
0228   Kessen, W., Haith, M. M. & Salapatek, P. H. Human infancy. In L. Carmichael, *Manual of child psychology*.
Vol. 1. (3rd ed.) New York: Wiley, 1970. Pp. 287-
445.
0229   Lewis, M. *Clinical aspects of child development*. Philadelphia: Lea & Febiger, 1971.
0230   Paine, R. S. The contribution of developmental neurology
to child psychiatry. *Journal of the American Academy
of Child Psychiatry*, 1965, *4*, 353-386.
0231   *Richmond, J. B. & Caldwell, B. M. Child-rearing practices and their consequences. In A. J. Solnit & S. A.

Provence (Eds.), *Modern perspectives in child development.* New York: International Universities Press, 1963. Pp. 627-654.

0232   Spitz, R. A. *The first year of life.* New York: International Universities Press, 1965.

0233   *Thompson, W. R. & Grusec, J. E. Studies of early experience. In L. Carmichael, *Manual of child psychology.* Vol. 1. (3rd ed.) New York: Wiley, 1970. Pp. 565-654.

0233.1 Stone, L. J., Smith, H. T. & Murphy, L. B. (Eds.) *The competent infant; research and commentary.* New York: Basic Books, 1973.

0233.2 Fraiberg, S. The clinical dimension of baby games. *Journal of the American Academy of Child Psychiatry,* 1974, *13,* 202-220.

0233.3 Yarrow, L. J., Rubenstein, J. L., Pedersen, F. A. & Jankowski, J. J. Dimensions of early stimulation and their differential effects on infant development. In S. Chess & A. Thomas (Eds.), *Annual progress in child psychiatry and child development: 1973.* New York: Brunner/Mazel, 1974. Pp. 3-17.

0233.4 Lewis, M. & McGurk, H. Evaluation of infant intelligence: Infant intelligence scores--true or false? In S. Chess & A. Thomas (Eds.), *Annual progress in child psychiatry and child development: 1973.* New York: Brunner/Mazel, 1974. Pp. 42-49.

0233.5 Connolly, K. Learning and the concept of critical periods in infancy. In S. Chess & A. Thomas (Eds.), *Annual progress in child psychiatry and child development: 1973.* New York: Brunner/Mazel, 1974. Pp. 115-127.

INFANCY/Primary References/*CONSTITUTIONAL*

0234   Brazelton, T. B. Crying in infancy. *Pediatrics,* 1962, *29,* 579-588.

0235   *Brazelton, T. B., Scholl, M. L. & Robey, J. S. Visual responses in the newborn. *Pediatrics,* 1966, *37,* 284-290.

0236   *Bronson, G. W. The development of fear in man and other animals. *Child Development,* 1968, *39,* 409-431.

0237   *Emde, R. N. & Metcalf, D. R. An electroencephalographic study of behavioral rapid eye movement states in the human newborn. *Journal of Nervous and Mental Disease,* 1970, *150,* 376-386.

0238   *Evans, J. Rocking at night. *Journal of Child Psychology and Psychiatry and Allied Disciplines,* 1961, *2,* 71-85.

0239   Hagne, I. Development of the waking EEG in normal infants during the first year of life. In P. Kellaway & I. Petersen (Eds.), *Clinical electroencephalography of children.* Stockholm: Almquist & Wiksell, 1968. Pp. 97-118.

0240   Harris, L. E., Corbin, H. P. F. & Hill, J. R.   Anorectal
        rings in infancy: incidence and significance.   *Pediat-
        rics*, 1954, *13*, 59-63.

0241   Illingworth, R. S.   The predictive value of developmental
        assessment.   In *The development of the infant and young
        child: normal and abnormal*.   (4th ed.)   Edinburgh:
        Livingstone, 1970.   Pp. 5-25.

0242   Illingworth, R. S.   Normal development.   In *The develop-
        ment of the infant and young child: normal and abnor-
        mal*.   (4th ed.)   Edinburgh: Livingstone, 1970.
        Pp. 169-207.

0243   *Illingworth, R. S. & Lister, J.   The critical or sensi-
        tive period, with special reference to certain feeding
        problems in infants and children.   *Journal of Pediat-
        rics*, 1964, *65*, 839-848.

0244   McIntosh, R. et al.   The incidence of congenital malfor-
        mations: A study of 5,964 pregnancies.   *Pediatrics*,
        1954, *14*, 505-522.

0245   Parmelee, A. H., Jr., et al.   The electroencephalogram
        in active and quiet sleep in infants.   In P. Kellaway
        & I. Petersen (Eds.), *Clinical electroencephalography
        of children*.   Stockholm: Almquist & Wiksell, 1968.
        Pp. 77-88.

0246   Parmelee, A. H., Wenner, W. H. & Schulz, H. R.   Infant
        sleep patterns: From birth to 16 weeks of age.   *Jour-
        nal of Pediatrics*, 1964, *65*, 576-582.

0247   *Rutter, M., Birch, H. G., Thomas, A. & Chess, S.   Tem-
        peramental characteristics in infancy and the later
        development of behavioural disorders.   *British Journal
        of Psychiatry*, 1964, *110*, 651-661.

0248   Rutter, M., Korn, S. & Birch, H. G.   Genetic and environ-
        mental factors in the development of 'primary reaction
        patterns.'   *British Journal of Social and Clinical
        Psychology*, 1963, *2*, 161-173.

0249   *Silberstein, R. M., Blackman, S. & Mandell, W.   Auto-
        erotic head banging: A reflection on the opportunism
        of infants.   *Journal of the American Academy of Child
        Psychiatry*, 1966, *5*, 235-242.

0250   Spock, B.   Innate inhibition of aggressiveness in infan-
        cy.   *Psychoanalytic Study of the Child*, 1965, *20*,
        340-343.

0251   *Spock, B. & Bergen, M.   Parents' fear of conflict in
        toilet training.   *Pediatrics*, 1964, *34*, 112-116.

0252   *Spock, B.   The striving for autonomy and regressive ob-
        ject relationships.   *Psychoanalytic Study of the Child*,
        1963, *18*, 361-364.

0253   *Stern, E. et al.   Sleep cycle characteristics in infants.
        Pediatrics, 1969, *43*, 65-70.

0254   Stevenson, O.   The first treasured possession: A study
        of the part played by specially loved objects and toys
        in the lives of certain children.   *Psychoanalytic Study
        of the Child*, 1954, *9*, 199-217.

0255 *Thomas, A., Birch, H. G., Chess, S. & Robbins, L. C. Individuality in responses of children to similar environmental situations. *American Journal of Psychiatry*, 1961, *117*, 798-803.

0256 *Traisman, A. S. & Traisman, H. S. Thumb- and finger-sucking: A study of 2,650 infants and children. *Journal of Pediatrics*, 1958, *53*, 566-572.

0257 *White, R. W. Competence and the psychosexual stages of development. *Nebraska Symposium on Motivation*, 1960, *8*, 97-141.

0258 *Winnicott, D. W. Transitional objects and transitional phenomena: A study of the first not-me possession. *International Journal of Psychoanalysis*, 1953, *34*, 89-97.

0259 *Wolff, P. H. 'Critical periods' in human cognitive development. *Hospital Practice*, 1970, *5*(11), 77-87.

0259.1 Cohen, D. J., Allen, M. G., Pollin, W., Inoff, G., Werner, M. & Dibble, E. Personality development in twins: Competence in the newborn and preschool periods. *Journal of the American Academy of Child Psychiatry*, 1972, *11*, 625-644.

0259.2 Chess, S. Temperament in the normal infant. In S. G. Sapir & A. C. Nitzburg (Eds.), *Children with learning problems: Readings in a developmental-interaction approach.* New York: Brunner/Mazel, 1973. Pp. 291-307.

0259.3 McCall, R. B., Hogarty, P. S. & Hurlburt, N. Transitions in infant sensorimotor development and the prediction of childhood IQ. In S. Chess and A. Thomas (Eds.), *Annual progress in child psychiatry and child development: 1973.* New York: Brunner/Mazel, 1974. Pp. 50-83.

INFANCY/Primary References/*FAMILIAL*

0260 *Brazelton, T. B. A child-oriented approach to toilet training. *Pediatrics*, 1962, *29*, 121-128.

0261 *Caplan, G., Mason, E. A. & Kaplan, D. M. Four studies of crisis in parents of prematures. *Community Mental Health Journal*, 1965, *1*, 149-161.

0262 *Formby, D. Maternal recognition of infant's cry. *Developmental Medicine and Child Neurology*, 1967, *9*, 293-298.

0263 *Josselyn, I. M. Concepts related to child development: 1. The oral stage. *Journal of the American Academy of Child Psychiatry*, 1962, *1*, 209-224.

0264 *Josselyn, I. M. Concepts related to child development: 2. Weaning. *Journal of the American Academy of Child Psychiatry*, 1963, *2*, 357-369.

0265   *Kaplan, D. M. & Mason, E. A. Maternal reactions to pre-
        mature birth viewed as an acute emotional disorder.
        American Journal of Orthopsychiatry, 1960, *30,* 539-547.
0266   Kennell, J. H. & Bergen, M. E. Early childhood separa-
        tions. *Pediatrics,* 1966, *37,* 291-298.
0267   *Klaus, M. H. & Kennell, J. H. Mothers separated from
        their newborn infants. *Pediatric Clinics of North
        America,* 1970, *17*(4), 1015-1037.
0268   *Lourie, R. S. The first three years of life: An over-
        view of a new frontier of psychiatry. *American Jour-
        nal of Psychiatry,* 1971, *127,* 1457-1463.
0269   *Rheingold, H. L. & Eckerman, C. O. The infant separates
        himself from his mother. *Science,* 1970, *168,* 78-83.
0270   *Robson, K. S. The role of eye-to-eye contact in mater-
        nal-infant attachment. *Journal of Child Psychology
        and Psychiatry and Allied Disciplines,* 1967, *8,* 13-
        25.
0271   *Robson, K. S. & Moss, H. A. Patterns and determinants
        of maternal attachment. *Journal of Pediatrics,* 1970,
        77, 976-985.
0272   *Schaffer, H. R. & Emerson, P. E. Patterns of response
        to physical contact in early human development. *Jour-
        nal of Child Psychology and Psychiatry and Allied Dis-
        ciplines,* 1964, *5,* 1-13.
0272.1 Lewis, M. & Rosenblum, L. A. *The effect of the infant
        on its caregiver.* New York: Wiley, 1974.
0272.2 Junker, K. S. *Selective attention in infants and con-
        secutive communicative behavior.* Stockholm: Almqvist
        & Wiksell, 1972. (*Acta Paediatrica Scandinavica.* Sup-
        lement 231.)

INFANCY/Primary References/*SOCIETAL*

0273   Bernfeld, S. *The psychology of the infant.* New York:
        Brentano's, 1929.
0275   Mead, M. (Ed.) *Cultural patterns and technical change.*
        Paris: UNESCO, 1953.
0276   *Werner, E. E., Bierman, J. M. & French, F. E. *The chil-
        dren of Kauai.* Honolulu: University of Hawaii Press,
        1971.
0277   *Wortis, H. & Freedman, A. The contribution of social
        environment to the development of premature children.
        American Journal of Orthopsychiatry, 1965, *35,* 57-68.
0277.1 Bronson, G. W. *Infants' reactions to unfamiliar per-
        sons and novel objects.* Chicago: University of Chi-
        cago Press, 1972. (*Monographs of the Society for Re-
        search in Child Development,* serial no. 147, v. 37,
        no. 3)
0277.2 McFadden, D. N. (Ed.) *Early childhood development pro-
        grams and services: Planning for action.* Columbus,
        Ohio: Battelle Memorial Institute, 1972. (Battelle
        monograph, no. 2)

INFANCY/Additional References

0279   Ingersoll, H. L. A study of the transmission of author-
        ity patterns in the family. In *Genetic Psychology
        Monographs*, 1948, *38*, 225-302.
0279.1 Clarke-Stewart, K. A. Interactions between mothers and
        their young children; characteristics and consequences.
        *Monographs of the Society for Research in Child Devel-
        opment*, Ser. no. 152, *38*, no. 6-7.

PRESCHOOL PERIOD/Primary References/*GENERAL*

0280   *Biber, B. & Franklin, M. B. The relevance of develop-
        mental and psycho-dynamic concepts to the education of
        the preschool child. *Journal of the American Academy
        of Child Psychiatry*, 1967, *6*, 5-24.
0281   *Erikson, E. H. The growth of the ego. In *Childhood and
        society*. New York: Norton, 1963. Pp. 187-274.
0282   *Erikson, E. H. The theory of infantile sexuality. In
        Childhood and society. New York: Norton, 1963.
        Pp. 48-108.
0283   *Freud, A. The concept of developmental lines. *Psycho-
        analytic Study of the Child*, 1963, *18*, 245-265.
0284   Josselyn, I. M. *The happy child*. New York: Random
        House, 1955.
0285   Murphy, L. B. *The widening world of childhood, paths
        toward mastery*. New York: Basic Books, 1962. Pp.
        189-374.
0285.1 Decarie, T. G. *The infant's reaction to strangers*. New
        York: International Universities Press, 1974.
0285.2 Schwarz, J. C., Krolick, G. & Strickland, R. G. Effects
        of early day care experience on adjustment to a new
        environment. *American Journal of Orthopsychiatry*,
        1973, *43*, 340-346.

PRESCHOOL PERIOD/Primary References/*CONSTITUTIONAL*

0286   Flavell, J. H. *The developmental psychology of Jean
        Piaget*. Princeton, N.J.: Van Nostrand, 1963.
0287   *Fraiberg, S. Libidinal object constancy and mental
        representation. *Psychoanalytic Study of the Child*,
        1969, *24*, 9-47.
0288   *Freud, A. The role of bodily illness in the mental life
        of children. *Psychoanalytic Study of the Child*, 1952,
        7, 69-81. (*Writings*, vol. 4, p. 260-279)
0289   Hoffman, M. L. Moral development. In L. Carmichael,
        Manual of child psychology. Vol. 2. (3rd ed.) New
        York: Wiley, 1970. Pp. 261-359.
0290   Katan, A. Some thoughts about the role of verbalization
        in early childhood. *Psychoanalytic Study of the Child*,
        1961, *16*, 184-188.

0291   *Kleeman, J. A.   Genital self-discovery during a boy's
        second year. A follow-up. *Psychoanalytic Study of
        the Child*, 1966, *21*, 358-392.
0292   Kris, E.   Neutralization and sublimation: Observations
        on young children. *Psychoanalytic Study of the Child*,
        1955, *10*, 30-46.
0293   Mahler, M. S.   On human symbiosis and the vicissitudes
        of individuation. *Journal of the American Psychoana-
        lytic Association*, 1967, *15*, 740-763.
0294   *Mahler, M. S.   On the concepts of symbiosis and separa-
        tion-individuation. In *On human symbiosis and the
        vicissitudes of individuation*. Vol. 1. New York:
        International Universities Press, 1968. Pp. 7-31.
0295   *Mittelmann, B.   Motility in infants, children, and
        adults: Patterning and psychodynamics. *Psychoanalyt-
        ic Study of the Child*, 1954, *9*, 142-177.
0296   *Moore, T. & Ucko, L. E.   Four to six: Constructiveness
        and conflict in meeting doll play problems. *Journal
        of Child Psychology and Psychiatry and Allied Disci-
        plines*, 1961, *2*, 21-47.
0297   *Nagera, H.   Children's reactions to the death of impor-
        tant objects: A developmental approach. *Psychoana-
        lytic Study of the Child*, 1970, *25*, 360-400.
0298   *Nagera, H.   Sleep and its disturbances approached devel-
        opmentally. *Psychoanalytic Study of the Child*, 1966,
        21, 393-447.
0299   *Peller, L. E.   Language and development. In P. B.
        Neubauer (Ed.), *Concepts of development in early child-
        hood education*. Springfield, Ill.: Thomas, 1965.
        Pp. 53-83.
0300   Schur, H.   An observation and comments on the development
        of memory. *Psychoanalytic Study of the Child*, 1966,
        21, 468-479.
0301   *Shapiro, T. & Stine, J.   The figure drawings of three-
        year-old children: A contribution to the early devel-
        opment of body image. *Psychoanalytic Study of the
        Child*, 1965, *20*, 298-309.
0302   Sperling, O. E.   An imaginary companion, representing a
        prestage of the superego. *Psychoanalytic Study of the
        Child*, 1954, *9*, 252-258.
0302.1 Graham, P., Rutter, M. & George, S.   Temperamental char-
        acteristics as predictors of behavior disorders in
        children. *American Journal of Orthopsychiatry*, 1973,
        43, 328-339.

PRESCHOOL PERIOD/Primary References/*FAMILIAL*

0303   *Abelin, E. L.   The role of the father in the separation-
        individuation process. In J. B. McDevitt & C. F.
        Settlage (Eds.), *Separation-individuation: Essays in
        honor of Margaret S. Mahler*. New York: International

Universities Press, 1971. Pp. 229-252.
0304 *Anthony, E. J. The reactions of parents to the oedipal
child. In E. J. Anthony & T. Benedek (Eds.), *Parenthood*. Boston: Little, Brown, 1970. Pp. 275-288.
0305 *Barnes, M. J. Reactions to the death of a mother.
Psychoanalytic Study of the Child, 1964, *19*, 334-357.
0306 Despert, J. L. *Children of divorce*. Garden City, N.Y.:
Doubleday, 1953.
0307 Freud, A. & Burlingham, D. T. *Infants without families*.
New York: International Universities Press, 1973.
0308 *Furman, R. A. Death and the young child: Some preliminary considerations. *Psychoanalytic Study of the
Child*, 1964, *19*, 321-333.
0309 Kris, E. Decline and recovery in the life of a three-
year-old; or, Data in psychoanalytic perspective on
the mother-child relationship. *Psychoanalytic Study
of the Child*, 1962, *17*, 175-215.
0310 *Levenstein, P. Cognitive growth of preschoolers through
verbal interaction with mothers. *American Journal of
Orthopsychiatry*, 1970, *40*, 426-432.
0311 *Lewis, H. The psychiatric aspects of adoption. In J.
G. Howells (Ed.), *Modern perspectives in child psychiatry*. London: Oliver & Boyd, 1965. Pp. 428-451.
(Modern perspectives in psychiatry, vol. 1)
0311.1 Anthony, E. J. & Koupernik, C. (Eds.) *The child in his
family*. Vol. 2. *The impact of disease and death*.
New York: Wiley-Interscience, 1973. (International
Yearbook for Child Psychiatry and Allied Disciplines,
v. 2)
0312 *Lidz, T. F. The family as the developmental setting.
In E. J. Anthony & C. Koupernik (Eds.), *The child in
his family*. New York: Wiley-Interscience, 1970.
Pp. 19-39. (International Yearbook for Child Psychiatry and Allied Disciplines, vol. 1)
0313 *Mahler, M. S., Pine, F. & Bergman, A. The mother's
reaction to her toddler's drive for individuation. In
E. J. Anthony & T. Benedek (Eds.), *Parenthood*. Boston:
Little, Brown, 1970. Pp. 257-274.
0314 *Marans, A. E. & Lourie, R. Hypotheses regarding the effects of childrearing patterns on the disadvantaged
child. In J. Hellmuth (Ed.), *Disadvantaged child*.
Vol. 1. New York: Brunner/Mazel, 1967. Pp. 17-41.
0315 *Neubauer, P. B. The one-parent child and his oedipal
development. *Psychoanalytic Study of the Child*, 1960,
15, 286-309.
0316 *Robertson, J. Mothering as an influence on early development: A study of well-baby clinic records. *Psychoanalytic Study of the Child*, 1962, *17*, 245-264.
0317 *Sears, R. R., Maccoby, E. E. & Levin, H. *Patterns of
child rearing*. Evanston, Ill.: Row, Peterson, 1957.
Pp. 102-269 & 362-393.

0318   *Waldrop, M. F. & Bell, R. Q. Relation of preschool
        dependency behavior to family size and density. *Child
        Development*, 1964, *35*, 1187-1195.
0319   *Winnicott, D. W. *The maturational process and the facil-
        itating environment*. London: Hogarth, 1965. Pp. 56-
        93.
0320   van Leeuwen, K. & Tuma, J. M. Attachment and explora-
        tion: A systematic approach to the study of separa-
        tion-adaptation phenomena in response to nursery school
        entry. *Journal of the American Academy of Child Psy-
        chiatry*, 1972, *11*, 314-340.
0320.1 Shatz, M. & Gelman, R. *The development of communication
        skills; modifications in the speech of young children
        as a function of listener*. Chicago: University of
        Chicago Press, 1973. (*Monographs of the Society for
        Research in Child Development*, serial no. 152, v. 38,
        no. 5)

PRESCHOOL PERIOD/Primary References/*SOCIETAL*

0321   *Karnes, M. B., Teska, J. A. & Hodgins, A. S. The ef-
        fects of four programs of classroom intervention on
        the intellectual and language development of 4-year-
        old disadvantaged children. *American Journal of Ortho-
        psychiatry*, 1970, *40*, 58-76.
0322   Raph, J. B. et al. The influence of nursery school on
        social interactions. *American Journal of Orthopsychi-
        atry*, 1968, *38*, 144-152.
0323   *Spurlock, J. Problems of identification in young black
        children--Static or changing. *Journal of the National
        Medical Association*, 1969, *61*, 504-507.
0324   *Wender, P. H., Pedersen, F. A. & Waldrop, M. F. A lon-
        gitudinal study of early social behavior and cognitive
        development. *American Journal of Orthopsychiatry*,
        1967, *37*, 691-696.
0325   *Westman, J. C., Rice, D. L. & Bermann, E. Nursery
        school behavior and later school adjustment. *Ameri-
        can Journal of Orthopsychiatry*, 1967, *37*, 725-731.
0326   *Whiteman, M. & Deutsch, M. Social disadvantage as re-
        lated to intellective and language development. In
        M. Deutsch, I. Katz, & A. Jensen (Eds.), *Social class,
        race, and psychological development*. New York: Holt,
        1968.
0327   *Wolins, M. Group care: Friends or foe? In S. Chess
        & A. Thomas (Eds.), *Annual progress in child psychia-
        try and child development*. New York: Brunner/Mazel,
        1970. Pp. 218-245.
0327.1 Kraus, P. E. *Yesterday's children: a longitudinal study
        of children from kindergarten into the adult years*.
        New York: Wiley, 1973.

0327.2   Briggs, J. L.   The issues of autonomy and aggression in
the three-year-old: The Utku Eskimo case.   In S. Chess
& A. Thomas (Eds.), *Annual progress in child psychiatry and child development: 1973.*   New York: Brunner/
Mazel, 1974.   Pp. 139-155.

LATER CHILDHOOD (LATENCY)/Primary References/*GENERAL*

0328   Bayley, N. & Schaefer, E. S.   *Correlations of maternal
and child behaviors with the development of mental
abilities: Data from the Berkeley growth study.*
Chicago: Child Development Publications, 1964.
(*Monographs of the Society for Research in Child Development,* v.29, no.6, serial no.97)

0329   *Buxbaum, E.   A contribution to the psychoanalytic knowledge of the latency period.   Workshop, 1950.   *American
Journal of Orthopsychiatry,* 1951, *21,* 182-198.

0330   Deutsch, H.   *The psychology of women.*   Vol. 1   New York:
Grune & Stratton, 1944.   Pp. 1-23.

0331   *Kaplan, E. B.   Reflections regarding psychomotor activities during the latency period.   *Psychoanalytic Study
of the Child,* 1965, *20,* 220-238.

0332   Lapouse, R. & Monk, M. A.   An epidemiologic study of
behavior characteristics in children.   *American Journal of Public Health,* 1958, *48,* 1134-1144.

0333   *Lapouse, R. & Monk, M. A.   Fears and worries in a representative sample of children.   *American Journal of
Orthopsychiatry,* 1959, *29,* 803-818.

0334   *Peller, L.   Reading and daydreams in latency, Boy-girl
differences.   *Journal of the American Psychoanalytic
Association,* 1958, *6,* 57-70.

0334.1   Thomas, A. & Chess, S. Development in middle childhood.
In *Annual progress in child psychiatry and child development: 1973.*   New York: Brunner/Mazel, 1974.   Pp.
172-186.

LATER CHILDHOOD (LATENCY)/Primary References/*CONSTITUTIONAL*

0335   *Blos, P.   Preadolescent drive organization.   *Journal of
the American Psychoanalytic Association,* 1958, *6,*
47-56.

0336   Bornstein, B.   Masturbation in the latency period.   *Psychoanalytic Study of the Child,* 1953, *8,* 65-78.

0337   *Bornstein, B.   On latency.   *Psychoanalytic Study of the
Child,* 1951, *6,* 279-285.

0338   *Erikson, E. H.   Genital modes and spatial modalities.
In *Childhood and society.*   New York: Norton, 1963.
Pp. 97-108.

0339   *Erikson, E. H.   Problems of ego identity.   In S. Klein
(Ed.), *Psychological issues.*   Part I.   *Identity and the*

life cycle. New York: International Universities Press, 1959. Pp. 101-164.

0340   *Flavell, J. H. Concrete operations. In *The developmental psychology of Jean Piaget.* Princeton, N. J.: Van Nostrand, 1963. Pp. 164-201.

0341   Freud, A. *Normality and pathology in childhood: Assessments of development.* New York: International Universities Press, 1965. Pp. 62-66, 163-164, 188-189, & 195. (*Writings,* v.6)

0342   Freud, S. (1924) The dissolution of the Oedipus complex. In *Standard Edition, 19,* 173-179. London: Hogarth Press, 1961.

0343   Freud, S. (1905) The period of sexual latency in childhood and its interruptions. In *Standard Edition, 7,* 176-179. London: Hogarth Press, 1953.

0344   *Fries, M. E. Review of the literature on the latency period, with special emphasis on the so-called "normal case". *Journal of the Hillside Hospital,* 1958, *7,* 3-16.

0345   *Grinder, R. E. Relations between behavioral and cognitive dimensions of conscience in middle childhood. *Child Development,* 1964, *35,* 881-891.

0346   Kaplan, S. Scientific proceedings. Panel reports: The latency period. *Journal of the American Psychoanalytic Association,* 1957, *5,* 525-538.

0347   Peller, L. E. Libidinal phases, ego development, and play. *Psychoanalytic Study of the Child,* 1954, *9,* 178-198.

0348   *Sandler, J. et al. The classification of superego material in the Hampstead Index. *Psychoanalytic Study of the Child,* 1962, *17,* 107-127.

0349   *Sarnoff, C. A. Ego structure in latency. *Psychoanalytic Quarterly,* 1971, *40,* 387-414.

0350   Wolfenstein, M. Development of the joke facade. In *Children's humor; a psychological analysis.* Glencoe, Ill.: Free Press, 1954. Pp. 159-191.

LATER CHILDHOOD (LATENCY)/Primary References/*FAMILIAL*

0351   Crandall, V., Dewey, R., Katkovsky, W. & Preston, A. Parents' attitudes and behaviors and grade-school children's academic achievements. *Journal of Genetic Psychology,* 1964, *104,* 53-66.

0352   Gildea, M., Glidewell, J. & Kantor, M. Maternal attitudes and general adjustment in school children. In J. Glidewell (Ed.), *Parental attitudes and the child behavior.* Springfield, Ill.: C. C. Thomas, 1961. Pp. 42-89.

0353   *Kestenberg, J. S. The effect on parents of the child's transition into and out of latency. In E. J. Anthony & T. Benedek (Eds.), *Parenthood.* Boston: Little, Brown, 1970. Pp. 289-306.

0353.1 Stierlin, H. Shame and guilt in family relations. *Archives of General Psychiatry*, 1974, *30*, 381-389.

LATER CHILDHOOD (LATENCY)/Primary References/*SOCIETAL*

0354 Barker, R. G. & Wright, H. F. *One boy's day*. Hamden, Conn.: Archon Books, 1966. [1951]
0355 Biber, B. et al. Language and thinking in their social context. In *Child life in school*. New York: Dutton, 1942. Pp. 109-177.
0356 Biber, B. et al. Conclusions and implications for education. In *Child life in school*. New York: Dutton, 1942. Pp. 562-591.
0357 *Clark, K. B. Fifteen years of deliberate speed. In S. Chess & A. Thomas (Eds.), *Annual progress in child psychiatry and child development*. New York: Brunner/Mazel, 1970. Pp. 279-287.
0358 Deutsch, M. The role of social class in language development and cognition. *American Journal of Orthopsychiatry*, 1965, *35*, 78-88.
0359 Pringle, M. L. *11,000 seven-year-olds*. London: Longmans, 1966. (Studies in child development, vol. 2)
0360 *Spurlock, J. Problems of identification in young black children--Static or changing. In S. Chess & A. Thomas (Eds.), *Annual progress in child psychiatry and child development*. New York: Brunner/Mazel, 1970. Pp. 299-306.
0360.1 Konopka, G. Formation of values in the developing person. *American Journal of Orthopsychiatry*, 1973, *43*, 86-96.

LATER CHILDHOOD (LATENCY)/Additional References

0361 Hartley, R. E. & Goldenson, R. M. *The complete book of children's play*. (Rev. ed.) New York: Crowell, 1963.
0362 *Koppitz, E. M. *Psychological evaluation of children's human figure drawings*. New York: Grune & Stratton, 1968.
0363 *Minuchin, P. P., Biber, B. et al. *The psychological impact of school experience*. New York: Basic Books, 1969.
0363.1 Harris, D. B. & Roberts, J. *Intellectual maturity of children; demographic and socioeconomic factors, United States*. Rockville, Md.: U.S. Health Services and Mental Health Administration, 1972. (*Vital and Health Statistics*. Ser. 11: no. 116) [DHEW pub. no. (HSM) 72-1059]

ADOLESCENCE/Primary References/*GENERAL*

0364   Baittle, B. & Offer, D. On the nature of male adoles-
        cent rebellion. *Annals of the American Society for
        Adolescent Psychiatry*, 1971, *1*, 139-160.
0365   *Bakan, D. Adolescence in America: From idea to social
        fact. *Daedalus*, 1971, *100*, 979-995,
0366   *Erikson, E. H. Toward contemporary issues: Youth. In
        Identity, youth & crisis. New York: Norton, 1968.
        Pp. 232-260.
0367   *Gordon, C. Social characteristics of early adolescence.
        Daedalus, 1971, *100*, 931-960.
0368   Greenacre, P. Youth, growth, and violence. *Psychoana-
        lytic Study of the Child*, 1970, *25*, 340-359.
0369   Johnson, K. G. et al. Survey of adolescent drug use.
        I--Sex and grade distribution. *American Journal of
        Public Health*, 1971, *61*, 2418-2432.
0370   Keniston, K. Youth as a stage of life. *Annals of the
        American Society for Adolescent Psychiatry*, 1971, *1*,
        161-175.
0371   Noshpitz, J. D. Certain cultural and familial factors
        contributing to adolescent alienation. *Journal of the
        American Academy of Child Psychiatry*, 1970, *9*, 216-
        223.
0372   *Offer, D. & Offer, J. Four issues in the developmental
        psychology of adolescents. In J. G. Howells (Ed.),
        Modern perspectives in adolescent psychiatry. Edin-
        burgh: Oliver & Boyd, 1971. Pp. 28-44. (Modern
        perspectives in psychiatry, vol. 4)
0373   *Wieder, H. & Kaplan, E. H. Drug use in adolescents:
        psychodynamic meaning and pharmacogenic effect. *Psy-
        choanalytic Study of the Child*, 1969, *24*, 399-431.

ADOLESCENCE/Primary References/*CONSTITUTIONAL*

0374   *Berman, S. Alienation: An essential process of the
        psychology of adolescence. *Journal of the American
        Academy of Child Psychiatry*, 1970, *9*, 233-250.
0375   *Blos, P. The child analyst looks at the young adoles-
        cent. *Daedalus*, 1971, *100*, 961-978.
0376   *Blos, P. *On adolescence: A psychoanalytic interpreta-
        tion*. New York: Free Press, 1962. Pp. 1-216.
0377   *Erikson, E. H. Identity vs. role confusion. In *Child-
        hood and society*. New York: Norton, 1963. Pp. 261-
        263.
0378   *Erikson, E. H. The life cycle: Epigenesis of identity.
        In *Identity, youth and crisis*. New York: Norton,
        1968. Pp. 91-141.
0379   *Freud, A. Adolescence as a developmental disturbance.
        In G. Caplan & S. Lebovici (Eds.), *Adolescence: Psy-
        chosocial perspectives*. New York: Basic Books, 1969.
        Pp. 5-10.

0380   *Laufer, M. Object loss and mourning during adolescence.
       Psychoanalytic Study of the Child, 1966, *21*, 269-293.
0381   Lickorish, J. R. The significance of intelligence rat-
       ings in adolescence. In J. G. Howells (Ed.), *Modern
       perspectives in adolescent psychiatry.* Edinburgh:
       Oliver & Boyd, 1971. Pp. 66-99. (Modern perspectives
       in psychiatry, vol. 4)
0382   *Piaget, J. The intellectual development of the adoles-
       cent. In G. Caplan & S. Lebovici (Eds.), *Adolescence:
       Psychosocial perspectives.* New York: Basic Books,
       1969. Pp. 22-26.
0383   *Schofield, M. Normal sexuality in adolescence. In J.
       G. Howells (Ed.), *Modern perspectives in adolescent
       psychiatry.* Edinburgh: Oliver & Boyd, 1971. Pp. 45-
       65. (Modern perspectives in psychiatry, vol. 4)
0384   *Schonfeld, W. A. The body and the body-image in adoles-
       cents. In G. Caplan & S. Lebovici (Eds.), *Adolescence:
       Psychosocial perspectives.* New York: Basic Books,
       1969. Pp. 27-53.
0385   *Tanner, J. M. Sequence, tempo, and individual variation
       in the growth and development of boys and girls aged
       twelve to sixteen. *Daedalus*, 1971, *100*, 907-930.
0386   *Young, H. B. The physiology of adolescence. In J. G.
       Howells (Ed.), *Modern perspectives in adolescent psy-
       chiatry.* Edinburgh: Oliver & Boyd, 1971. Pp. 3-27.
       (Modern perspectives in psychiatry, vol. 4)
0387   Hart, M. & Sarnoff, C. A. The impact of the menarche:
       A study of two stages of organization. *Journal of the
       American Academy of Child Psychiatry*, 1971, *10*, 257-
       271.

ADOLESCENCE/Primary References/*FAMILIAL*

0388   *Biller, H. B. A note on father absence and masculine
       development in lower-class Negro and white boys.
       Child Development, 1968, *39*, 1003-1006.
0389   *Lidz, T. F. The adolescent and his family. In G. Cap-
       lan & S. Lebovici (Eds.), *Adolescence: Psychosocial
       perspectives.* New York: Basic Books, 1969. Pp. 105-
       112.
0390   *McWhinnie, A. M. The adopted child in adolescence. In
       G. Caplan & S. Lebovici (Eds.), *Adolescence: Psycho-
       social perspectives.* New York: Basic Books, 1969.
       Pp. 133-142.
0391   *Shapiro, R. L. Adolescent ego autonomy and the family.
       In G. Caplan & S. Lebovici (Eds.), *Adolescence: Psy-
       chosocial perspectives.* New York: Basic Books, 1969.
       Pp. 113-121.

ADOLESCENCE/Primary References/*SOCIETAL*

0392   Anthony, E. J. The reactions of adults to adolescents
        and their behavior. In G. Caplan & S. Lebovici (Eds.),
        Adolescence: Psychosocial perspectives. New York:
        Basic Books, 1969. Pp. 54-78.
0393   Freeman, D. M. A. Adolescent crises of the Kiowa-Apache
        Indian male. In E. B. Brody (Ed.), *Minority group
        adolescents in the United States.* Baltimore: Wil-
        liams & Wilkins, 1968. Pp. 157-204.
0394   *Hollingshead, A. B. *Elmtown's youth.* New York: Science
        Editions, 1961. Pp. 439-454.
0395   *Marcus, I. M. From school to work: Certain aspects of
        psychosocial interaction. In G. Caplan & S. Lebovici
        (Eds.), *Adolescence: Psychosocial perspectives.* New
        York: Basic Books, 1969. Pp. 157-164.
0396   *Mays, J. B. The adolescent as a social being. In J. G.
        Howells (Ed.), *Modern perspectives in adolescent psy-
        chiatry.* Edinburgh: Oliver & Boyd, 1971. Pp. 126-
        151. (Modern perspectives in psychiatry, vol. 4)
0397   *Mead, M. *From the south seas: Studies of adolescence
        and sex in primitive societies.* New York: Morrow,
        1939.
0398   *Pierce, C. M. Problems of the Negro adolescent in the
        next decade. In E. B. Brody (Ed.), *Minority group
        adolescents in the United States.* Baltimore: Wil-
        liams & Wilkins, 1968. Pp. 17-47.
0399   Preble, E. The Puerto Rican-American teen-ager in New
        York City. In E. B. Brody (Ed.), *Minority group ado-
        lescents in the United States.* Baltimore: Williams
        & Wilkins, 1968. Pp. 48-72.
0400   Schaffer, C. & Pine, F. Pregnancy, abortion, and the
        developmental tasks of adolescence. *Journal of the
        American Academy of Child Psychiatry,* 1972, *11,* 511-
        536.
0400.1 Eron, L. D., Heusmann, L. R., Lefkowitz, M. M. & Walder,
        L. O. How learning conditions in early childhood--
        Including mass media--relate to aggression in late
        adolescence. *American Journal of Orthopsychiatry,*
        1974, *44,* 412-423.

ADOLESCENCE/Additional References

0401   Erikson, E. H. *Identity, youth and crisis.* New York:
        Norton, 1968.
0402   *Goodman, P. *Growing up absurd.* New York: Random
        House, 1960.
0403   Hollingshead, A. B. *Elmtown's youth.* New York: Science
        Editions, 1961.
0404   *Keniston, K. *Young radicals.* New York: Harcourt,
        Brace & World, 1968.

0405   *Keniston, K. *Youth and dissent.* New York: Harcourt, Brace, Jovanovich, 1971.
0405.1   Grinder, R. E. *Adolescence.* New York: Wiley, 1973.

III. CULTURAL ASPECTS OF CHILD PSYCHIATRY

ANIMAL STUDIES AND IMPLICATIONS FOR MAN

0406   *Hayes, K. J. & Hayes, C. The cultural capacity of chimpanzee. In J. A. Gavan (Ed.), *The Non-human primates and human evolution.* Detroit: Wayne University Press, 1955. Pp. 110-125.
0407   *Scott, J. P. Animal and human children. *Children,* 1957, *4,* 163-168.
0408   *LaBarre, W. *The human animal.* Chicago: University of Chicago Press, 1954.
0409   *Ford, C. S. & Beach, F. A. *Patterns of sexual behavior.* New York: Harper, 1951.
0410   *Harlow, H. F. The nature of love. *American Psychologist,* 1958, *13,* 673-685.
0411   Harlow, H. F. & Zimmermann, R. R. Affectional responses in the infant monkey. *Science,* 1959, *130,* 421-432.
0411.1   Harlow, H. F. & Suomi, S. J. Production of depressive behaviors in young monkeys. *Journal of Autism and Childhood Schizophrenia,* 1971, *1,* 246-255.
0411.2   Hess, E. H. *Imprinting; early experience and the developmental psychobiology of attachment.* New York: Van Nostrand, Reinhold, 1973.
0411.3   van Lawick-Goodall, J. The behavior of chimpanzees in their natural habitat. *American Journal of Psychiatry,* 1973, *130,* 1-12.

CULTURE AND PERSONALITY

0412   *Mead, M. The implications of culture change for personality development. In D. G. Haring (Ed.), *Personal character and cultural milieu.* (3rd ed.) Syracuse, N.Y.: Syracuse University Press, 1956. Pp. 623-636.
0413   *Bateson, G. Cultural determinants of personality. In J. McV. Hunt (Ed.), *Personality and behavior disorders.* Vol. 2. New York: Ronald Press, 1944. Pp. 714-735.
0414   *Leighton, A. H. *My name is legion: Foundations for a theory of man in relation to culture.* New York: Basic Books, 1959. (Stirling County study of psychiatric disorder and sociocultural environment, Vol. 1)
0415   *Henry, J. Cultural change and mental health. *Mental Hygiene,* 1957, *41,* 323-326.

0416   *Watson, R. I. Socialization, behavior tendencies, and
        personality. In *Psychology of the child*. (2nd ed.)
        New York: Wiley, 1965. Pp. 74-96.
0417   *Sarason, S. B. & Gladwin, T. Psychological and cultural
        problems in mental subnormality: A review of re-
        search. *Genetic Psychology Monographs*, 1958, *57*, 3-
        290.
0418   *Halliday, J. L. *Psychosocial medicine: A study of the
        sick society*. New York: Norton, 1948.
0419   Murphy, J. M. & Leighton, A. H. (Eds.) *Approaches to
        cross-cultural psychiatry*. Ithaca, N.Y.: Cornell
        University Press, 1965.
0420   Caudill, W. A. & Doi, L. T. Interrelations of psychia-
        try, culture and emotion in Japan. In I. Galdston
        (Ed.), *Man's image in medicine and anthropology*. New
        York: International Universities Press, 1963. Pp.
        374-421.
0421   *Kardiner, A. *The psychological frontiers of society*.
        New York: Columbia University Press, 1945.
0421.1 Nicholi, A. M. II. A new dimension of the youth cul-
        ture. *American Journal of Psychiatry*, 1974, *131*, 396-
        401.

ADAPTATION TO CULTURAL CHANGE

0422   *Leighton, A. H. Cultural change and psychiatric dis-
        order. In A. V. S. DeReuck & R. Porter (Eds.),
        Transcultural psychiatry. London: Churchill, 1965.
        Pp. 216-228. (CIBA Foundation Symposium)
0423   *Chen, E. & Cobb, S. Family structure in relation to
        health and disease: A review of the literature.
        Journal of Chronic Diseases, 1960, *12*, 544-567.
0424   *Spiro, M. E. Religious systems as culturally consti-
        tuted defense mechanisms. In *Context and meaning in
        cultural anthropology*. New York: Free Press, 1965.
        Pp. 100-113.
0425   *Meggitt, M. J. Male-female relationships in the high-
        lands of Australian New Guinea. *American Anthropolo-
        gist Special Publication*, 1964, *66*, 204-224.
0426   *Hitson, H. M. & Funkenstein, D. H. Family patterns and
        paranoidal personality structure in Boston and Burma.
        International Journal of Social Psychiatry, 1959, *5*,
        182-190.
0427   *Whittaker, J. O. Alcohol and the Standing Rock Sioux
        Tribe. *Quarterly Journal of Studies on Alcohol*, 1962,
        23, 468-479.
0428   Pittman, D. J. & Snyder, C. R. (Eds.) *Society, cul-
        ture, and drinking patterns*. New York: Wiley, 1962.
0429   *Parker, S. Eskimo psychopathology in the context of
        Eskimo personality and culture. *American Anthropolo-
        gist*, 1962, *64*, 76-96.

0431   Wallace, A. F. C. Dreams and the wishes of the soul:
        A type of psychoanalytic theory among the seventeenth
        century Iroquois. *American Anthropologist*, 1958, *60*,
        234-248.
0432   Valentine, C. A. Men of anger and men of shame: Laka-
        lai ethnopsychology and its implications for socio-
        psychological theory. *Ethnology*, 1963, *2*, 441-447.
0433   Spiro, M. E. Social systems, personality, and function-
        al analysis. In B. Kaplan (Ed.), *Studying personality
        cross-culturally*. Evanston, Ill.: Row, Peterson,
        1961. Pp. 93-127.
0434   Weinstein, E. A. *Cultural aspects of delusion: A
        psychiatric study of the Virgin Islands*. New York:
        Free Press of Glencoe, 1962.
0435   Field, M. J. *Search for security: An ethno-psychiatric
        study of rural Ghana*. Evanston, Ill.: Northwestern
        University Press, 1960.
0436   *Bandura, A. Social-learning theory of identificatory
        processes. In D. A. Goslin (Ed.), *Handbook of social-
        ization theory and research*. Chicago: Rand McNally,
        1969. Pp. 213-262.
0437   *Clark, C. Race, identification, and television vio-
        lence. In G. A. Comstock, E. A. Rubinstein & J. P.
        Murray (Eds.), *Television and social behavior*. Vol.
        5. *Television's effects: Further explorations*.
        Washington, D.C.: U.S. Govt. Print. Off., 1972.
        Pp. 120-184.
0438   *Ekman, P. et al. Facial expressions of emotion while
        watching televised violence as predictors of subse-
        quent aggression. In G. A. Comstock, E. A. Rubin-
        stein & J. P. Murray (Eds.), *Television and social
        behavior*. Vol. 5. *Television's effects: Further
        explorations*. Washington, D.C.: U.S. Govt. Print.
        Off., 1972. Pp. 22-43.
0439   U.S. Surgeon General's Scientific Advisory Committee on
        Television and Social Behavior. *Television and
        growing up: The impact of televised violence*. Rock-
        ville, Md.: U.S. National Institute of Mental Health,
        1972.
0440   Weiss, W. Effects of the mass media of communication.
        In G. Lindzey & E. Aronson (Eds.), *Handbook of social
        psychology*. Vol. 5. (2nd ed.) Reading, Mass.:
        Addison-Wesley, 1969. Pp. 77-195.

CULTURAL CHANGE AND PSYCHIATRIC DISORDER

0441   Leighton, D. C., Harding, J. S., Macklin, D. B., Mac-
        millan, A. M. & Leighton, A. H. *The character of
        danger*. New York: Basic Books, 1963. (Stirling
        County study of psychiatric disorder and sociocultur-
        al environment, vol. 3)

0442   *Murphy, J. M. & Leighton, A. H.   Native conceptions of
        psychiatric disorder. In *Approaches to cross-cultur-
        al psychiatry*. Ithaca, N.Y.:   Cornell University
        Press, 1965. Pp. 64-107.
0443   Kinsey, A. C., Pomeroy, W. B. & Martin, C. E. *Sexual
        behavior in the human male*. Philadelphia: Saunders,
        1948.
0444   *Benedict, P. K. & Jacks, I.   Mental illness in primitive
        societies. *Psychiatry*, 1954, *17*, 377-389.
0444.1 Halleck, S. L.   Legal and ethical aspects of behavior
        control. *American Journal of Psychiatry*, 1974, *131*,
        381-385.

PSYCHOSIS AS SEEN IN VARIOUS CULTURES

0445   *Rubel, A. J.   Concepts of disease in Mexican-American
        culture. *American Anthropologist*, 1960, *62*, 795-
        814.
0446   *Parker, S.   The wiitiko psychosis in the context of
        Ojibwa personality and culture. *American Anthropolo-
        gist*, 1962, *62*, 603-623.
0447   *Paul, B. D.   Mental disorder and self-regulating proc-
        esses in culture: A Guatemalan illustration.   In D.
        G. Haring (Ed.), *Personal character and cultural
        milieu*. (3rd ed.) Syracuse, N.Y.:   Syracuse Univer-
        sity Press, 1956.   Pp. 689-701.
0448   *Yap, P. M.   Phenomenology of affective disorder in
        Chinese and other cultures.   In A. V. S. DeReuck &
        R. Porter (Eds.), *Transcultural psychiatry*.   London:
        Churchill, 1965.   Pp. 84-108.   (CIBA Foundation Sym-
        posium)
0449   Aberle, D. F.   "Arctic hysteria" and latah in Mongolia.
        Transactions of the New York Academy of Sciences,
        1952, *14*, 291-297.
0450   *Van Loon, F. H. G.   Amok and Lattah. *Journal of Abnor-
        mal and Social Psychology*, 1927, *21*, 434-444.
0451   Yap, P. M.   The Latah reaction: Its psychodynamics and
        nosological position. *Journal of Mental Science*,
        1952, *98*, 515-564.
0452   *Newman, P. L.   "Wild man" behavior in a New Guinea high-
        lands community. *American Anthropologist*, 1964, *66*,
        1-19.
0453   Teicher, M. I. *Windigo psychosis; a study of a rela-
        tionship between belief and behavior among the Indians
        of northeastern Canada*.   Seattle: American Ethnologi-
        cal Society, 1960 [i.e. 1961].   (Proceedings of the
        1960 annual meeting of the American Ethnological
        Society.)
0454   Lieban, R. W.   Sorcery, illness and social control in a
        Philippine municipality. *Southwest Journal of Anthro-
        pology*, 1960, *16*, 127-143.

0455   *Lieban, R. W. The dangerous Ingkantos: Illness and
        social control in a Philippine community. *American
        Anthropologist*, 1962, *64*, 306-312.
0456   Cannon, W. B. "Voodoo" death. *American Anthropologist*,
        1942, *44*, 169-181.
0456.1 Beiser, M., Burr, W. A., Ravel, J.-L. & Collomb, H.
        Illnesses of the spirit among the Serer of Senegal.
        American Journal of Psychiatry, 1973, *130*, 881-886.

CROSS CULTURAL STUDIES OF CHILDREN AND ADOLESCENTS

0457   *Brody, S. Maternal behavior: The literature. In
        Patterns of mothering. New York: International
        Universities Press, 1956. Pp. 28-72.
0458   Bowlby, J. *Maternal care and mental health*. Geneva:
        World Health Organization, 1951. (Monograph series,
        no. 2)
0459   *Mead, M. Technological change and child development.
        Understanding the Child, 1952, *21*, 109-112.
0460   *Sears, R. R., Maccoby, E. E. & Levin, H. *Patterns of
        child rearing*. Evanston, Ill.: Row, Peterson, 1957.
0461   *Malinowski, B. The form of the family and child behav-
        ior. In W. Dennis (Ed.), *Readings in child psychol-
        ogy*. Englewood Cliffs, N.J.: Prentice-Hall, 1951.
        Pp. 491-506.
0462   *Erikson, E. H. Reflections on the American identity.
        In *Childhood and society*. New York: Norton, 1963.
        Pp. 285-325.
0463   *Erikson, E. H. *Observations on the Yurok*. Berkeley:
        University of California Press, 1943. (*University of
        California Publications in American Archaeology and
        Ethnology*, 1943, *35*, 256-302)
0464   *Erikson, E. H. Childhood and tradition in two American
        Indian tribes. *Psychoanalytic Study of the Child*,
        1945, *1*, 319-350. (Also in E. H. Erikson, *Childhood
        and society*. New York: Norton, 1950. Pp. 93-160)
0465   *Lewis, O. *The children of Sanchez*. New York: Random
        House, 1961.
0466   *Mead, M. Changing patterns of parent-child relations in
        an urban culture. *International Journal of Psycho-
        analysis*, 1957, *38*, 369-378.
0467   *Erikson, E. H. The legend of Hitler's childhood. In
        Childhood and society. New York: Norton, 1963. Pp.
        326-358.
0468   *Erikson, E. H. The legend of Maxim Gorky's youth. In
        Childhood and society. New York: Norton, 1963. Pp.
        359-402.
0469   Brody, S. *Patterns of mothering*. New York: Interna-
        tional Universities Press, 1956.
0470   Darwin, C. R. *The expression of the emotions in man and
        animals*. Chicago: University of Chicago Press, 1965.
0471   *Mead, M. *From the South Seas: Studies of adolescence
        and sex in primitive societies*. New York: Morrow, 1939.

0472   *Ausubel, D. P.   Acculturative stress in modern Maori
        adolescence. *Child Development*, 1960, *31*, 617-631.
0473   *Linton, R.   Marquesan culture.   In A. Kardiner, *The
        individual and his society*.   New York: Columbia
        University Press, 1965.   Pp. 137-196.
0474   *Kardiner, A.   Analysis of Marquesan culture.   In *The
        individual and his society*.   New York: Columbia
        University Press, 1965.   Pp. 197-250.
0475   *Linton, R.   The Tanala of Madagascar.   In A. Kardiner,
        The individual and his society.   New York: Columbia
        University Press, 1965.   Pp. 251-290.
0476   *Kardiner, A.   The analysis of Tanala culture.   In *The
        individual and his society*.   New York: Columbia
        University Press, 1965.   Pp. 291-351.
0476.1 Rollins, N.   *Child psychiatry in the Soviet Union; pre-
        liminary observations*.   Cambridge: Harvard University
        Press, 1972.
0476.2 Kaffman, M.   Evaluation of emotional disturbance in 403
        Israeli kibbutz children.   *American Journal of Psychi-
        atry*, 1961, *117*, 732-738.
0476.3 Kaffman, M.   Toilet-training by multiple caretakers:
        Enuresis among kibbutz children.   *Israel Annals of
        Psychiatry and Related Disciplines*, 1972, *10*, 341-
        365.
0476.4 Chang, S. C. & Kim, K.   Psychiatry in South Korea.
        American Journal of Psychiatry, 1973, *130*, 667-669.
0476.5 Kline, C. L. & Lee, N.   A transcultural study of dys-
        lexia: Analysis of language disabilities in 277
        Chinese children simultaneously learning to read and
        write in English and in Chinese.   In S. Chess & A.
        Thomas (Eds.), *Annual progress in child psychiatry and
        child development: 1973*.   New York: Brunner/Mazel,
        1974.   Pp. 297-320.

HEALING AND PSYCHOTHERAPY--VARIOUS CULTURES

0477   *Wallace, A. F. C.   The institutionalization of cathartic
        and control strategies in Iroquois religious psycho-
        therapy.   In M. K. Opler (Ed.), *Culture and mental
        health*.   New York: Macmillan, 1959.   Pp. 63-96.
0478   Brown, J.   Some changes in Mexican village curing prac-
        tices induced by Western medicine.   *America Indigena*,
        1963, *23*, 93-120.
0479   *Adair, J.   Physicians, medicine men and their Navaho
        patients.   In I. Galdston (Ed.), *Man's image in medi-
        cine and anthropology*.   New York: International Uni-
        versities Press, 1963.   Pp. 237-257.
0480   Adair, J.   The Indian health worker in the Cornell-
        Navaho Project.   *Human Organization*, 1960, *19*, 59-63.
0481   *Murphy, J. M.   Psychotherapeutic aspects of shamanism
        on St. Lawrence Island, Alaska.   In A. Kiev (Ed.),
        *Magic, faith, and healing: Studies in primitive psy-
        chiatry today*.   New York: Free Press, 1964.   Pp. 53-83.

0482   *Kiev, A. *Magic, faith, and healing: Studies in primi-
        tive psychiatry today.* New York: Free Press, 1964.
0483   Jahoda, G. Traditional healers and other institutions
        concerned with mental illness in Ghana. *International
        Journal of Social Psychiatry,* 1961, *7,* 245-268.
0484   *Frank, J. D. *Persuasion and healing: A comparative
        study of psychotherapy.* (Rev. ed.) Baltimore: Johns
        Hopkins University Press, 1973.
0485   Bidney, D. So-called primitive medicine and religion.
        In I. Galdston (Ed.), *Man's image in medicine and
        anthropology.* New York: International Universities
        Press, 1963. Pp. 141-156.
0486   Fejos, P. Magic, witchcraft and medical theory in
        primitive cultures. In I. Galdston (Ed.), *Man's
        image in medicine and anthropology.* New York: Inter-
        national Universities Press, 1963. Pp. 43-61.
0487   Carstairs, G. M. Cultural elements in the response to
        treatment. In A. V. S. DeReuck & R. Porter (Eds.),
        Transcultural psychiatry. London: Churchill, 1965.
        Pp. 169-175. (CIBA Foundation Symposium)
0488   Devereux, G. *Reality and dream; psychotherapy of a
        Plains Indian.* (2nd ed.) New York: New York Univer-
        sity Press, 1969.
0488.1 Bergman, R. L. A school for medicine men. *American
        Journal of Psychiatry,* 1973, *130,* 663-666.
0488.2 Allen, M. G. Psychiatry in the United States and the
        USSR: A comparison. *American Journal of Psychiatry,*
        1973, *130,* 1333-1337.

IV. PSYCHOANALYTIC FRAMEWORK OF CHILD PSYCHIATRY

GENERAL THEORY

0489   *Freud, S. (1905) Three essays on the theory of sexual-
        ity. In *Standard Edition, 7,* 135-243. London:
        Hogarth Press, 1953.
0490   *Freud, S. The passing of the Oedipus complex. In *Col-
        lected papers.* Vol. 2. London: Hogarth Press, 1956.
        Pp. 269-276.
0491   Freud, S. (1909) [1908] Family romances. In *Standard
        Edition, 9,* 237-241. London: Hogarth Press, 1959.
0492   Freud, S. (1924) The dissolution of the Oedipus com-
        plex. In *Standard Edition, 19,* 173-179. London:
        Hogarth Press, 1961.
0493   Freud, S. (1900-1901) The psychology of the dream-
        processes. In *Standard Edition, 5,* 509-621. London:
        Hogarth Press, 1953.
0494   *Freud, S. (1940) [1938] An outline of psychoanalysis.
        In *Standard Edition, 23,* 144-207. London: Hogarth,
        1964.
0495   *Weigert, E. Human ego functions in the light of animal
        behavior. *Psychiatry,* 1956, *19,* 325-332.

0496   *Sandler, J. & Rosenblatt, B. The concept of the representational world. *Psychoanalytic Study of the Child,* 1962, *17,* 128-145.

0497   Hartmann, H., Kris, E. & Loewenstein, R. M. Comments on the formation of psychic structure. *Psychoanalytic Study of the Child,* 1946, *2,* 11-38.

0498   *Schafer, R. The loving and beloved superego in Freud's structural theory. *Psychoanalytic Study of the Child,* 1960, *15,* 163-188.

0499   *Sandler, J. On the concept of superego. *Psychoanalytic Study of the Child,* 1960, *15,* 128-162.

0500   Schafer, R. *Aspects of internalization.* New York: International Universities Press, 1968.

0501   *Weigert, E. Loneliness and trust--Basic factors of human existence. *Psychiatry,* 1960, *23,* 121-131.

0502   *Rapaport, D. A historical survey of psychoanalytic ego psychology. In E. H. Erikson (Ed.), *Identity and the life cycle.* New York: International Universities Press, 1959. Pp. 5-17.

0503   *Freud, A. *The ego and the mechanisms of defense.* New York: International Universities Press, 1946. (*Writings,* vol. 2)

0504   Hartmann, H. *Ego psychology and the problem of adaptation.* New York: International Universities Press, 1958.

0505   *Erikson, E. H. *Identity and the life cycle.* New York: International Universities Press, 1959. *Psychological Issues, 1*(1), 1959.

0506   Brenner, C. *An elementary textbook of psychoanalysis.* (Rev. ed.) New York: International Universities Press, 1973.

0507   Silverberg, W. V. *Childhood experience and personal destiny.* New York: Springer, 1952.

0508   Szurek, S. A. *The roots of psychoanalysis and psychotherapy.* Springfield, Ill.: Thomas, 1959.

0509   Waelder, R. *Basic theory of psychoanalysis.* New York: International Universities Press, 1960.

0510   Abraham, K. (1916) The first pregenital stage of the libido. In *Selected papers of Karl Abraham.* New York: Basic Books, 1953. Pp. 248-279.

0511   Abraham, K. (1921) Contributions to the theory of the anal character. In *Selected papers of Karl Abraham.* New York: Basic Books, 1953. Pp. 370-392.

0512   Abraham, K. (1924) The influence of oral erotism on character formation. In *Selected papers of Karl Abraham.* New York: Basic Books, 1953. Pp. 393-406.

0513   Abraham, K. (1924) A short study of the development of the libido, viewed in the light of mental disorders. In *Selected papers of Karl Abraham.* New York: Basic Books, 1953. Pp. 418-501.

THEORETICAL ISSUES IN INFANCY AND LATENCY

0514   *Spitz, R. A. *The first year of life*. New York: Inter-
        national Universities Press, 1965.
0515   *Mahler, M. S. On the concepts of symbiosis and separa-
        tion-individuation. In *On human symbiosis and the
        vicissitudes of individuation*. Vol. 1. New York:
        International Universities Press, 1968. Pp. 7-31.
0516   *Mahler, M. S. The symbiosis theory of infantile psy-
        chosis. In *On human symbiosis and the vicissitudes of
        individuation*. Vol. 1. New York: International
        Universities Press, 1968. Pp. 32-65.
0517   *Klein, M. Our adult world and its roots in infancy.
        Human Relations, 1959, *12*, 291-303.
0518   *Fraiberg, S. Libidinal object constancy and mental
        representation. *Psychoanalytic Study of the Child*,
        1969, *24*, 9-47.
0519   *Brody, S. Problems of ego formation. In *Patterns of
        mothering*. New York: International Universities
        Press, 1956. Pp. 325-342.
0520   Rubenfine, D. L. Maternal stimulation, psychic struc-
        ture, and early object relations: With special refer-
        ence to aggression and denial. *Psychoanalytic Study
        of the Child*, 1962, *17*, 265-282.
0521   *Winnicott, D. W. Transitional objects and transitional
        phenomena; a study of the first not-me possession.
        International Journal of Psycho-analysis, 1953, *34*,
        89-97. (Also in *Collected papers: Through pediatrics
        to psycho-analysis*. New York: Basic Books, 1958.
        Pp. 229-242.
0522   *Alpert, A., Neubauer, P. B. & Weil, A. P. Unusual var-
        iations in drive endowment. *Psychoanalytic Study of
        the Child*, 1956, *11*, 125-163.
0523   Brody, S. Ego differentiation. In *Patterns of mother-
        ing*. New York: International Universities Press,
        1956. Pp. 358-375.
0524   Fraiberg, S. & Freedman, D. A. Studies in the ego de-
        velopment of the congenitally blind child. *Psychoana-
        lytic Study of the Child*, 1964, *19*, 113-169.
0525   Fries, M. E. Review of the literature on the latency
        period, with special emphasis on the so-called "nor-
        mal case". *Journal of the Hillside Hospital*, 1958,
        7, 3-16.
0526   *Blos, P. Preadolescent drive organization. *Journal of
        the American Psychoanalytic Association*, 1958, *6*, 47-
        56.
0527   *Benedek, T. Parenthood as a developmental phase: A
        contribution to the libido theory. *Journal of the
        American Psychoanalytic Association*, 1959, *7*, 389-417.

THEORETICAL ISSUES IN ADOLESCENCE

0528   *Freud, A. Adolescence. *Psychoanalytic Study of the Child*, 1958, *13*, 255-278. (*Writings*, vol. 5, pp. 136-166)

0529   *Buxbaum, E. Scientific proceedings. Panel reports: The psychology of adolescence. *Journal of the American Psychoanalytic Association*, 1958, *6*, 111-120.

0530   *Blos, P. The second individuation process of adolescence. *Psychoanalytic Study of the Child*, 1967, *22*, 162-186.

0531   *Josselyn, I. M. The ego in adolescence. *American Journal of Orthopsychiatry*, 1954, *24*, 223-237.

0532   *Buxbaum, E. Transference and group formation in children and adolescents. *Psychoanalytic Study of the Child*, 1945, *1*, 351-365.

0533   Laufer, M. Assessment of adolescent disturbances: The application of Anna Freud's diagnostic profile. *Psychoanalytic Study of the Child*, 1965, *20*, 99-123.

0534   *Katan, A. The role of "displacement" in agoraphobia. *International Journal of Psychoanalysis*, 1951, *32*, 41-50.

0535   Fraiberg, S. Some considerations in the introduction to therapy in puberty. *Psychoanalytic Study of the Child*, 1955, *10*, 264-286.

EXAMPLES OF APPLICATIONS

0536   *Freud, S. (1909) Analysis of a phobia in a five-year-old boy. In *Standard Edition*, *10*, 5-149. London: Hogarth Press, 1955.

0537   *Freud, A. *Normality and pathology in childhood: Assessments of development*. London: Hogarth Press, 1966. (*Writings*, vol. 6)

0538   Nagera, H. The developmental profile: notes on some practical considerations regarding its use. *Psychoanalytic Study of the Child*, 1963, *18*, 511-540.

0539   *Johnson, A. M. & Szurek, S. A. The genesis of antisocial acting out in children and adults. *Psychoanalytic Quarterly*, 1952, *21*, 323-343.

0540   *Aichhorn, A. (1925) *Wayward youth*. New York: Viking Press, 1935.

0541   Geleerd, E. R. *The child analyst at work*. New York: International Universities Press, 1967.

0542   Kohut, H. *The analysis of the self*. New York: International Universities Press, 1971.

PART II

PSYCHOPATHOLOGY, DISEASE AND DISORDER

V. NEUROTIC DISORDERS IN CHILDHOOD

HEALTHY RESPONSES

0543 *Chess, S. Healthy responses, developmental disturbances and stress or reactive disorders. I: Infancy and childhood. In A. M. Freedman & H. I. Kaplan (Eds.), *Comprehensive textbook of psychiatry*. Baltimore: Williams & Wilkins, 1967. Pp. 1358-1366.

0544 Mittelmann, B. Motility in infants, children, and adults: Patterning and psychodynamics. *Psychoanalytic Study of the Child*, 1954, *9*, 142-177.

0545 *Caldwell, B. M. What is the optimal learning environment for the young child? *American Journal of Orthopsychiatry*, 1967, *37*, 8-21.

0546 Lapouse, R. & Monk, M. A. Behavior deviations in a representative sample of children: Variation by sex, age, race, social class and family size. *American Journal of Orthopsychiatry*, 1964, *34*, 436-446.

0547 *Neubauer, P. B. The one-parent child and his oedipal development. *Psychoanalytic Study of the Child*, 1960, *15*, 286-309.

0548 Westman, J. C., Rice, D. L. & Bermann, E. Nursery school behavior and later school adjustment. *American Journal of Orthopsychiatry*, 1967, *37*, 725-731.

0549 *Wolff, S. Symptomatology and outcome of pre-school children with behaviour disorders attending a child guidance clinic. *Journal of Child Psychology and Psychiatry and Allied Disciplines*, 1961, *2*, 269-276.

0550 Bornstein, B. Masturbation in the latency period. *Psychoanalytic Study of the Child*, 1953, *8*, 65-78.

REACTIVE DISORDERS

0551 *Spitz, R. A. The psychogenic diseases in infancy. An attempt at their etiologic classification. *Psychoanalytic Study of the Child*, 1951, *6*, 255-275.

0552 Brody, S. Signs of disturbance in the first year of life. *American Journal of Orthopsychiatry*, 1958, *28*, 362-367.

57

0553   *Freud, A.   The psychoanalytic study of infantile feeding
        disturbances.   *Psychoanalytic Study of the Child,*
        1946, *2,* 119-132.   (*Writings,* vol. 4, pp. 39-59)
0554   *Rank, B., Putnam, M. C. & Rochlin, G.   The significance
        of the "emotional climate" in early feeding difficul-
        ties.   *Psychosomatic Medicine,* 1948, *10,* 279-283.
0555   *Wortis, H., Rue, R., Heimer, C., Braine, M., Redlo, M.
        & Freedman, A. M.   Children who eat noxious sub-
        stances.   *Journal of the American Academy of Child
        Psychiatry,* 1962, *1,* 536-547.
0556   *Millican, F. K. & Lourie, R. S.   The child with pica and
        his family.   In E. J. Anthony & C. Koupernik (Eds.),
        The child in his family.   New York: Wiley, 1970.
        Pp. 333-348.   (International Yearbook for Child Psy-
        chiatry and Allied Disciplines, vol. 1)
0557   Millican, F. K., Layman, E. M., Lourie, R. S. & Taka-
        hashi, L. Y.   Study of an oral fixation: Pica.
        Journal of the American Academy of Child Psychiatry,
        1968, *7,* 79-107.
0558   *Delgado, R. A. & Mannino, F. V.   Some observations on
        trichotillomania in children.   *Journal of the American
        Academy of Child Psychiatry,* 1969, *8,* 229-246.
0559   *Stewart, A.   Excessive crying in infants--A family
        disease.   In M. J. E. Senn (Ed.), *Conference on prob-
        lems of infancy and childhood.*   New York: Josiah
        Macy, Jr. Foundation, 1950.   Pp. 138-160.
0560   *Evans, J.   Rocking at night.   *Journal of Child Psychol-
        ogy and Psychiatry and Allied Disciplines,* 1961, *2,*
        71-85.
0561   Sperling, M.   Pavor nocturnus.   *Journal of the American
        Psychoanalytic Association,* 1958, *6,* 79-94.
0562   *Sperling, M.   Etiology and treatment of sleep disturb-
        ances in children.   *Psychoanalytic Quarterly,* 1955,
        24, 358-368.
0563   Teplitz, Z.   The ego and motility in sleepwalking.
        Journal of the American Psychoanalytic Association,
        1958, *6,* 95-110.
0564   Hirschberg, J. C.   Parental anxieties accompanying
        sleep disturbance in young children.   *Bulletin of
        the Menninger Clinic,* 1957, *21,* 129-139.
0565   *Lewis, M. & Sarrel, P. M.   Some psychological aspects of
        seduction, incest, and rape in childhood.   *Journal of
        the American Academy of Child Psychiatry,* 1969, *8,*
        606-619.
0566   *Harrison, S. I.   Reared in the wrong sex.   *Journal of
        the American Academy of Child Psychiatry,* 1970, *9,*
        44-102.
0567   *Stoller, R. J.   Male childhood transsexualism.   *Journal
        of the American Academy of Child Psychiatry,* 1968, *7,*
        193-209.
0568   *Furman, R. A.   Death and the young child: Some prelim-
        inary considerations.   *Psychoanalytic Study of the
        Child,* 1964, *19,* 321-333.

0569   *Nagera, H. Children's reactions to the death of impor-
        tant objects: A developmental approach. *Psychoana-*
        lytic Study of the Child, 1970, *25,* 360-400.
0570   *Beres, D. Clinical notes on aggression in children.
        Psychoanalytic Study of the Child, 1952, *7,* 241-263.
0571   *Frankl, L. Self-preservation and the development of
        accident proneness in children and adolescents. *Psy-*
        choanalytic Study of the Child, 1963, *18,* 464-483.
0572   Newman, M. B. & San Martino, M. R. The child and the
        seriously disturbed parent: Patterns of adaptation to
        parental psychosis. *Journal of the American Academy*
        of Child Psychiatry, 1971, *10,* 358-374.

DEVELOPMENTAL DEVIATIONS

0573   *Clarke, A. D. B. & Clarke, A. M. Some recent advances
        in the study of early deprivation. *Journal of Child*
        Psychology and Psychiatry and Allied Disciplines,
        1960, *1,* 26-36.
0574   *Bowlby, J. Separation anxiety: A critical review of
        the literature. *Journal of Child Psychology and Psy-*
        chiatry and Allied Disciplines, 1961, *1,* 251-269.
0575   Bowlby, J. Separation anxiety. *International Journal*
        of Psychoanalysis, 1960, *41,* 89-113.
0576   *Bowlby, J., Ainsworth, M., Boston, M. & Rosenbluth, D.
        The effects of mother-child separation: A follow-up
        study. *British Journal of Medical Psychology,* 1956,
        29, 211-247.
0577   Lax, R. F. Infantile deprivation and arrested ego devel-
        opment. *Psychoanalytic Quarterly,* 1958, *27,* 501-517.
0578   Pringle, M. L. K. & Bossio, V. Early, prolonged separa-
        tion and emotional maladjustment. *Journal of Child*
        Psychology and Psychiatry and Allied Disciplines,
        1960, *1,* 37-48.
0579   Alpert, A. Reversibility of pathological fixations as-
        sociated with maternal deprivation in infancy. *Psy-*
        choanalytic Study of the Child, 1959, *14,* 169-185.
0580   *Spitz, R. A. & Wolf, K. M. Anaclitic depression. An
        inquiry into the genesis of psychiatric conditions in
        early childhood, II. *Psychoanalytic Study of the*
        Child, 1946, *2,* 313-342.
0581   Spitz, R. A. Hospitalism: An inquiry into the genesis
        of psychiatric conditions in early childhood. *Psycho-*
        analytic Study of the Child, 1945, *1,* 53-74.
0582   *Provence, S. A. & Lipton, R. C. *Infants in institutions.*
        New York: International Universities Press, 1963.
0583   *Bullard, M. D., et al. Failure to thrive in the "neg-
        lected" child. *American Journal of Orthopsychiatry,*
        1967, *37,* 680-690. (Also in S. Chess & A. Thomas
        (Eds.), *Annual progress in child psychiatry and child*
        development. New York: Brunner/Mazel, 1968. Pp.
        540-554.

0584   *Freud, A. & Burlingham, D. T. *Infants without families.*
        New York: International Universities Press, 1973.
        (*Writings,* vol. 3, pp. 543-664.)
0585   Sandler, A., Daunton, E. & Schnurmann, A. Inconsistency
        in the mother as a factor in character development:
        A comparative study of three cases. *Psychoanalytic
        Study of the Child,* 1957, *12,* 209-225.
0586   Fineman, J. B., Kuniholm, P. & Sheridan, S. Spasmus
        nutans: A syndrome of auto-arousal. *Journal of the
        American Academy of Child Psychiatry,* 1971, *10,* 136-155.
0587   Brazelton, T. B., Young, G. G. & Bullowa, M. Inception
        and resolution of early developmental pathology: A
        case history. *Journal of the American Academy of
        Child Psychiatry,* 1971, *10,* 124-135.
0587.1 Hertzig, M. E., Birch, H. G., Richardson, S. A. &
        Tizard, J. Intellectual levels of school children
        severely malnourished during the first two years of
        life. In S. Chess & A. Thomas (Eds.), *Annual progress
        in child psychiatry and child development: 1973.*
        New York: Brunner/Mazel, 1974. Pp. 156-171.
0587.2 Remschmidt, H. Observations on the role of anxiety in
        neurotic and psychotic disorders at an early age.
        Journal of Autism and Childhood Schizophrenia, 1973,
        3, 106-114.

PSYCHONEUROTIC DISORDERS

0588   *Freud, A. *Normality and pathology in childhood.* London:
        Hogarth Press, 1966. Pp. 149-164. (*Writings,* vol. 6)
0589   *Anthony, E. J. Psychoneurotic disorders. In A. M.
        Freedman & H. I. Kaplan (Eds.), *Comprehensive textbook
        of psychiatry.* Baltimore: Williams and Wilkins,
        1967. Pp. 1387-1406.
0590   Barcai, A. The emergence of neurotic conflict in some
        children after successful administration of dextro-
        amphetamine. *Journal of Child Psychology and Psychi-
        atry and Allied Disciplines,* 1969, *10,* 269-276.
0591   *Lo, W. H. Aetiological factors in childhood neurosis.
        British Journal of Psychiatry, 1969, *115,* 889-894.
0592   *Nagera, H. On arrest in development, fixation, and
        regression. *Psychoanalytic Study of the Child,* 1964,
        19, 222-239.
0593   Gerard, M. W. *The emotionally disturbed child.* New
        York: Child Welfare League of America, 1956.
0593.1 Tolpin, M. The infantile neurosis: A metapsychologi-
        cal concept and a paradigmatic case history. *Psycho-
        analytic Study of the Child,* 1970, *25,* 273-305.

HYSTERIA AND OBSESSIVE COMPULSIVE NEUROSIS

0594   *Proctor, J. T. Hysteria in childhood. *American Journal of Orthopsychiatry*, 1958, *28*, 394-407.

0595   *Kaufman, I. Conversion hysteria in latency. *Journal of the American Academy of Child Psychiatry*, 1962, *1*, 385-396.

0596   *Creak, M. Hysteria in childhood. *Acta Paedopsychiatrica*, 1969, *36*, 269-274.

0597   *Judd, L. L. Obsessive compulsive neurosis in children. *Archives of General Psychiatry*, 1965, *12*, 136-143.

0598   Rock, N. L. Conversion reactions in childhood: A clinical study on childhood neuroses. *Journal of the American Academy of Child Psychiatry*, 1971, *10*, 65-93.

PHOBIAS

0599   *Rachman, S. & Costello, C. G. The aetiology and treatment of children's phobias: A review. *American Journal of Psychiatry*, 1961, *118*, 97-105.

0600   *Colm, H. N. Phobias in children. *Psychoanalysis and the Psychoanalytic Review*, 1959, *46*(3), 65-84.

0601   Berecz, J. M. Phobias of childhood: Etiology and treatment. *Psychological Bulletin*, 1968, *70*, 694-720.

0602   *Bornstein, B. The analysis of a phobic child: Some problems of theory and technique in child analysis. *Psychoanalytic Study of the Child*, 1949, *3-4*, 181-226.

0603   *Freud, S. (1909) Analysis of a phobia in a five-year-old boy. In *Standard Edition*, *10*, 5-149. London: Hogarth Press, 1955.

0604   Kolansky, H. Treatment of a three-year-old girl's severe infantile neurosis: Stammering and insect phobia. *Psychoanalytic Study of the Child*, 1960, *15*, 261-285.

0605   *Sperling, M. Animal phobias in a two-year-old child. *Psychoanalytic Study of the Child*, 1952, *7*, 115-125.

0606   Halpern, W. I., Hammond, J. & Cohen, R. A therapeutic approach to speech phobia: Elective mutism reexamined. *Journal of the American Academy of Child Psychiatry*, 1971, *10*, 94-107.

0606.1   Poznanski, E. O. Children with excessive fears. *American Journal of Orthopsychiatry*, 1973, *43*, 428-438.

SCHOOL "PHOBIA"

0607   *Johnson, A. M., Falstein, E. I., Szurek, S. A. & Svendsen, M. School phobia. *American Journal of Orthopsychiatry*, 1941, *11*, 702-711.

0608   *Eisenberg, L. School phobia: A study in the communi-
        cation of anxiety. *American Journal of Psychiatry*,
        1958, *114*, 712-718.
0609   *Coolidge, J. C., Tessman, E., Waldfogel, S. & Willer,
        M. L. Patterns of aggression in school phobia. *Psy-
        choanalytic Study of the Child*, 1962, *17*, 319-333.
0610   Hersov, L. A. Persistent non-attendance at school.
        *Journal of Child Psychology and Psychiatry and Allied
        Disciplines*, 1960, *1*, 130-136.
0611   *Hersov, L. A. Refusal to go to school. *Journal of
        Child Psychology and Psychiatry and Allied Disciplines*,
        1960, *1*, 137-145.
0612   *Malmquist, C. P. School phobia. A problem in family
        neurosis. *Journal of the American Academy of Child
        Psychiatry*, 1965, *4*, 293-319.
0613   *Agras, S. The relationship of school phobia to child-
        hood depression. *American Journal of Psychiatry*,
        1959, *116*, 533-536.
0613.1 Shapiro, T. & Jegede, R. O. School phobia: A babel of
        tongues. *Journal of Autism and Childhood Schizophre-
        nia*, 1973, *3*, 168-186.
0613.2 Coolidge, J. C. & Brodie, R. D. Observations of mothers
        of 49 school phobic children: Evaluated in a 10-
        year follow-up study. *Journal of the American Academy
        of Child Psychiatry*, 1974, *13*, 275-285.

THUMB SUCKING AND ENURESIS

0614   *Kaplan, M. A note on the psychological implications of
        thumb-sucking. *Journal of Pediatrics*, 1950, *37*, 555-
        560.
0615   *Gerard, M. W. Enuresis: A study in etiology. In F.
        Alexander & T. M. French (Eds.), *Studies in psycho-
        somatic medicine*. New York: Ronald Press, 1948.
        Pp. 501-513.
0616   *Sperling, M. Dynamic considerations and treatment of
        enuresis. *Journal of the American Academy of Child
        Psychiatry*, 1965, *4*, 19-31.
0617   *Glicklich, L. B. An historical account of enuresis.
        Pediatrics, 1951, *8*, 859-876.
0618   Katan, A. Experiences with enuretics. *Psychoanalytic
        Study of the Child*, 1946, *2*, 241-255.
0619   *Ritvo, E. R., et al. Arousal and nonarousal enuretic
        events. *American Journal of Psychiatry*, 1969, *126*,
        77-84.

FETISHISM AND TICS

0620   *Buxbaum, E. Hair pulling and fetishism. *Psychoanalyt-
        ic Study of the Child*, 1960, *15*, 243-260.

0621   *Mahler, M. S. Tics and impulsions in children: A study
        in motility. *Psychoanalytic Quarterly*, 1944, *13*, 430-
        444.
0622   *Mahler, M. S., Luke, J. A. & Daltroff, W. Clinical and
        follow-up study of the tic syndrome in children. *American Journal of Orthopsychiatry*, 1945, *15*, 631-647.
0623   *Lucas, A. R., Kauffman, P. E. & Morris, E. M. Gilles
        de la Tourette's disease: A clinical study of fifteen
        cases. *Journal of the American Academy of Child Psychiatry*, 1967, *6*, 700-722.
0623.1 Shapiro, A. K., Shapiro, E. & Wayne, H. L. The symptomatology and diagnosis of Gilles de la Tourette's
        syndrome. *Journal of the American Academy of Child
        Psychiatry*, 1973, *12*, 702-723.

FIRE SETTING

0624   *Yarnell, H. Firesetting in children. *American Journal
        of Orthopsychiatry*, 1940, *10*, 272-286.
0625   *Vandersall, T. A. & Wiener, J. M. Children who set fires.
        Archives of General Psychiatry, 1970, *22*, 63-71.
0626   *Kaufman, I., Heims, L. W. & Reiser, D. E. A re-evaluation of the psychodynamics of firesetting. *American
        Journal of Orthopsychiatry*, 1961, *31*, 123-136.
0627   Siegel, L. Case study of a thirteen-year-old firesetter: A catalyst in the growing pains of a residential treatment unit. *American Journal of Orthopsychiatry*, 1957, *27*, 396-410.
0628   Lewis, N. D. C. & Yarnell, H. Pathological Firesetting
        (pyromania). *Nervous and Mental Disease Monographs*,
        1951, no. 82.

ELECTIVE MUTISM

0629   *Reed, G. F. Elective mutism in children: A re-appraisal. *Journal of Child Psychology and Psychiatry and
        Allied Disciplines*, 1963, *4*, 99-107.
0630   Browne, E., Wilson, V. & Laybourne, P. C. Diagnosis
        and treatment of elective mutism in children. *Journal
        of the American Academy of Child Psychiatry*, 1963, *2*,
        605-617.

PERSONALITY DISORDERS AND BORDERLINE STATES

0631   *Frijling-Schreuder, E. C. M. Borderline states in children. *Psychoanalytic Study of the Child*, 1969, *24*,
        307-327.

0632   *Marcus, J. Borderline states in childhood. *Journal of Child Psychology and Psychiatry and Allied Disciplines*, 1963, *4*, 207-218.
0633   *Rosenfeld, S. K. & Sprince, M. P. An attempt to formulate the meaning of the concept "borderline". *Psychoanalytic Study of the Child*, 1963, *18*, 603-635.
0634   Rosenfeld, S. K. & Sprince, M. P. Some thoughts on the technical handling of borderline children. *Psychoanalytic Study of the Child*, 1965, *20*, 495-517.
0635   Chethik, M. & Fast, I. A function of fantasy in the borderline child. *American Journal of Orthopsychiatry*, 1970, *40*, 756-765.
0636   *Makkay, E. S. & Schwaab, E. H. Some problems in the differential diagnosis of antisocial character disorders in early latency. *Journal of the American Academy of Child Psychiatry*, 1962, *1*, 414-430.
0637   Jacobson, E. The "exceptions": An elaboration of Freud's character study. *Psychoanalytic Study of the Child*, 1959, *14*, 135-154.

DEPRESSION

0638   Spitz, R. A. & Wolf, K. M. Anaclitic depression. An inquiry into the genesis of psychiatric conditions in early childhood, II. *Psychoanalytic Study of the Child*, 1946, *2*, 313-342.
0639   *Rie, H. E. Depression in childhood: A survey of some pertinent contributions. *Journal of the American Academy of Child Psychiatry*, 1966, *5*, 653-685.
0640   *Sperling, M. Equivalents of depression in children. *Journal of the Hillside Hospital*, 1959, *8*, 138-148.
0641   *Nagera, H. Children's reactions to the death of important objects: A developmental approach. *Psychoanalytic Study of the Child*, 1970, *25*, 360-400.
0642   Poznanski, E. & Zrull, J. P. Childhood depression: Clinical characteristics of overtly depressed children. *Archives of General Psychiatry*, 1970, *23*, 8-15.
0643   Sandler, J. & Joffe, W. G. Notes on childhood depression. *International Journal of Psychoanalysis*, 1965, *46*, 88-96.
0644   *Arthur, B. & Kemme, M. L. Bereavement in childhood. *Journal of Child Psychology and Psychiatry and Allied Disciplines*, 1964, *5*, 37-49.
0645   Dizmang, L. H. Loss, bereavement, and depression in childhood. *International Psychiatry Clinics*, 1969, *6*(2), 175-195.
0646   *Caplan, M. G. & Douglas, V. I. Incidence of parental loss in children with depressed mood. *Journal of Child Psychology and Psychiatry and Allied Disciplines*, 1969, *10*, 225-232.

0647 *Burks, H. L. & Harrison, S. I. Aggressive behavior as a means of avoiding depression. *American Journal of Orthopsychiatry*, 1962, *32*, 416-422.
0648 *Glaser, K. Masked depression in children and adolescents. *American Journal of Psychotherapy*, 1967, *21*, 565-574.
0649 Feinstein, S. C. & Wolpert, E. A. Juvenile manic-depressive illness: Clinical and therapeutic considerations. *Journal of the American Academy of Child Psychiatry*, 1973, *12*, 123-136.
0649.1 Taylor, R. W. Depression and recovery at 9 weeks of age: Introduction and Summary by Mollie S. Smart. *Journal of the American Academy of Child Psychiatry*, 1973, *12*, 506-510.
0649.2 Cytryn, L. & McKnew, D. H., Jr. Proposed classification of childhood depression. In S. Chess & A. Thomas (Eds.), *Annual progress in child psychiatry and child development: 1973.* New York: Brunner/Mazel, 1974. Pp. 419-432.

OBSESSIVE-COMPULSIVE NEUROSES/Etiology and Diagnosis

0650 *Wisdom, J. O. What is the explanatory theory of obsessional neurosis? *British Journal of Medical Psychology*, 1966, *39*, 335-348.
0651 *Woolley, L. F. Studies in obsessive ruminative tension states: III. The effect of erratic discipline in childhood on emotional tensions. *Psychiatric Quarterly*, 1937, *11*, 237-252.
0652 *Adorno, T. W., et al. *The authoritarian personality.* New York: Harper, 1950.
0653 Schilder, P. The organic background of obsessions and compulsions. *American Journal of Psychiatry*, 1930, *94*, 1397-1416.
0654 Sandler, J. & Joffe, W. G. Notes on obsessional manifestations in children. *Psychoanalytic Study of the Child*, 1965, *20*, 425-438.
0655 *Jessner, L. The genesis of a compulsive neurosis. *Journal of the Hillside Hospital*, 1963, *12*, 81-95.
0656 Ramzy, I. Factors and features of early compulsive formation. *International Journal of Psychoanalysis*, 1966, *47*, 169-176.
0657 *Despert, J. L. Differential diagnosis between obsessive-compulsive neurosis and schizophrenia in children. *Proceedings of the American Psychopathological Association*, 1955, *44*, 240-253.
0658 Dugas, M. The diagnosis of obsessive neurosis in children. *Medicine Infantile* (Paris), 1961, *68*, 5-11.
0659 *Chess, S., Thomas, A., Birch, H. G. & Hertzig, M. Implications of a longitudinal study of child development for child psychiatry. *American Journal of Psychiatry*, 1960, *117*, 434-441.

0660   *Coddington, R. D. & Offord, D. R.   Psychiatrists' reli-
        ability in judging ego function. *Archives of General
        Psychiatry*, 1967, *16*, 48-55.
0661   Clancy, J. & Norris, A.   Differentiating variables:
        Obsessive-compulsive neurosis and anorexia nervosa.
        American Journal of Psychiatry, 1961, *118*, 58-60.
0662   Bakwin, H. & Bakwin, R. M.   *Behavior disorders in chil-
        dren*. (4th ed.)   Philadelphia: Saunders, 1972.

OBSESSIVE-COMPULSIVE NEUROSES/Psychopathology

0663   *Judd, L. L.   Obsessive compulsive neurosis in children.
        Archives of General Psychiatry, 1965, *12*, 136-143.
0664   Berman, L.   The obsessive-compulsive neurosis in chil-
        dren. *Journal of Nervous and Mental Disease*, 1942,
        95, 26-39.
0665   *Barnett, J.   On cognitive disorders in the obsessional.
        Contemporary Psychoanalysis, 1966, *2*, 122-134.
0666   Barnett, J.   On aggression in the obsessional neuroses.
        Contemporary Psychoanalysis, 1969, *6*, 48-57.
0667   *Winnicott, D. W.   Comment on obsessional neurosis and
        'Frankie'. *International Journal of Psychoanalysis*,
        1966, *47*, 143-144.
0668   Finney, J. C.   Maternal influences on anal or compulsive
        character in children. *Journal of Genetic Psychology*,
        1963, *103*, 351-367.
0669   *Weisner, W. M. & Riffel, A.   Scrupulosity: Religion
        and obsessive compulsive behavior in children. *Amer-
        ican Journal of Psychiatry*, 1960, *117*, 314-318.
0670   *Weissman, P.   Characteristic superego identifications
        of obsessional neurosis. *Psychoanalytic Quarterly*,
        1959, *28*, 21-28.
0671   *Sullivan, H. S.   Obsessionalism.   In *Clinical studies in
        psychiatry*. New York: Norton, 1956. Pp. 229-283.
0672   Shapiro, D.   Aspects of obsessive-compulsive style.
        Psychiatry, 1962, *25*, 46-59.
0673   Khan, M. M.   Infantile neurosis as a false-self organiza-
        tion. *Psychoanalytic Quarterly*, 1971, *40*, 245-263.
0674   Reich, W.   *Character analysis*. (3rd enlarged ed.) New
        York: Farrar, Straus & Giroux, 1972.
0675   Fraiberg, S.   A critical neurosis in a two-and-a-half-
        year-old girl. *Psychoanalytic Study of the Child*,
        1952, *7*, 173-215.
0676   *Nagera, H.   *Early childhood disturbances, the infantile
        neurosis, and the adulthood disturbances: Problems
        of a developmental psychoanalytic psychology*. New
        York: International Universities Press, 1966.
0678   Mahler, M. S.   A psychoanalytic evaluation of tic in
        psychopathology of children. Symptomatic and tic
        syndrome. *Psychoanalytic Study of the Child*, 1949,
        3-4, 279-310.

0679   Abraham, K. (1921) Contributions to the theory of the
        anal character. In *Selected papers of Karl Abraham*.
        New York: Basic Books, 1953. Pp. 370-392.
0680   Adler, A. *Superiority and social interest: A collection
        of later writings*. Edited by H. L. Ansbacher & R. R.
        Ansbacher. Evanston, Ill.: Northwestern University
        Press, 1964.
0681   Greenacre, P. A study of the mechanism of obsessive-
        compulsive conditions. *American Journal of Psychia-
        try*, 1922-23, *79*, 527-538.
0682   Lewis, A. Problems of obsessional illness. *Proceedings
        of the Royal Society of Medicine*, 1935, *29*, 325-336.
0683   Kringlen, E. Obsessional neurotics: A long-term follow-
        up. *British Journal of Psychiatry*, 1965, *111*, 709-722.
0684   *Freud, A. Obsessional neurosis: A summary of psycho-
        analytic views as presented at the congress. *Inter-
        national Journal of Psychoanalysis*, 1966, *47*, 116-122.
0685   Freud, A. The analysis of children and their upbring-
        ing. In *The psycho-analytical treatment of children*.
        New York: Schocken Books, 1964. Pp. 38-52.
0686   Fernando, S. J. M. Gilles de la Tourette's syndrome:
        A report on four cases and a review of published case
        reports. *British Journal of Psychiatry*, 1967, *113*,
        607-617.
0687   Fenichel, O. *The psychoanalytic theory of neurosis*.
        New York: Norton, 1945.
0688   Buxbaum, E. *Troubled children in a troubled world*.
        New York: International Universities Press, 1970.
0689   Lucas, A. R., Kauffman, P. E. & Morris, E. M. Gilles
        de la Tourette's Disease: A clinical study of fif-
        teen cases. *Journal of the American Academy of Child
        Psychiatry*, 1967, *6*, 700-722.

OBSESSIVE-COMPULSIVE NEUROSES/Family

0690   *Adams, P. L., Schwab, J. J. & Aponte, J. Authoritarian
        parents and disturbed children. *American Journal of
        Psychiatry*, 1965, *121*, 1162-1167.
0691   *Adams, P. L. Family characteristics of obsessive chil-
        dren. *American Journal of Psychiatry*, 1972, *128*,
        1414-1417.
0692   *Rosenberg, C. M. Familial aspects of obsessional neuro-
        sis. *British Journal of Psychiatry*, 1967, *113*, 405-413.
0693   *Henry, J. & Warson, S. Family structure and psychic
        development. *American Journal of Orthopsychiatry*,
        1951, *21*, 59-73.
0694   Henry, J. Family structure and the transmission of
        neurotic behavior. *American Journal of Orthopsychia-
        try*, 1951, *21*, 800-818.

0695   *Fisher, S. & Mendell, D. The communication of neurotic
        patterns over two and three generations. *Psychiatry,*
        1956, *19,* 41-46.
0696   Ehrenwald, J. Neurosis in the family: A study of psy-
        chiatric epidemiology. *Archives of General Psychiatry,*
        1960, *3,* 232-242.

OBSESSIVE-COMPULSIVE NEUROSES/Socio-Psychiatric Views

0697   *Dai, B. Obsessive-compulsive disorders in Chinese cul-
        ture. *Social Problems,* 1957, *4,* 313-321.
0698   *Salzman, L. Therapy of obsessional states. *American
        Journal of Psychiatry,* 1966, *122,* 1139-1146.
0699   Erikson, E. H. Growth and crises of the healthy per-
        sonality. *Psychological Issues,* 1959, *1,* 50-100.

OBSESSIVE-COMPULSIVE NEUROSES/Treatment

0700   *Chethik, M. The therapy of an obsessive-compulsive boy:
        Some treatment considerations. *Journal of the American
        Academy of Child Psychiatry,* 1969, *8,* 465-484.
0701   Hall, M. B. Obsessive-compulsive states in childhood
        and their treatment. *Archives of Disease in Child-
        hood,* 1935, *10,* 49-59.
0702   *Llorens, L. A. & Bernstein, S. P. Fingerpainting: With
        an obsessive-compulsive organically-damaged child.
        American Journal of Occupational Therapy, 1963, *17,*
        120-121.
0703   *Jackson, L. & Todd, K. M. *Child treatment and the ther-
        apy of play.* London: Methuen, 1946.
0704   *Barnett, J. Cognitive repair in the treatment of the
        obsessional neuroses. In *Proceedings of the Fourth
        World Congress of Psychiatry.* Vol. 4. New York:
        Excerpta Medica Foundation, 1968. Pp. 752-757.
        (Excerpta Medica. International Congress Series,
        no. 150)
0705   *Bonnard, A. The mother as a therapist, in a case of
        obsessional neurosis. *Psychoanalytic Study of the
        Child,* 1950, *5,* 391-408.
0706   *Bornstein, B. Fragment of an analysis of an obsessional
        child: The first six months of analysis. *Psychoana-
        lytic Study of the Child,* 1953, *8,* 313-332.
0707   *Weiner, I. B. Behavior therapy in obsessive-compulsive
        neurosis: Treatment of an adolescent boy. *Psycho-
        therapy: Theory, Research, and Practice,* 1967, *4,*
        27-29.
0708   Taylor, J. G. A behavioural interpretation of obses-
        sive-compulsive neurosis. *Behaviour Research and
        Therapy,* 1963, *1,* 237-244.

0709   *Stolorow, R. D. Mythic consonance and dissonance in
        the vicissitudes of transference. *American Journal
        of Psychoanalysis*, 1970, *30*, 178-179.
0710   Shapiro, A. K. & Shapiro, E. Treatment of Gilles de la
        Tourette's syndrome with Haloperidol. *British Journal
        of Psychiatry*, 1968, *114*, 345-350.
0711   Ritvo, S. Correlation of a childhood and adult neuro-
        sis: Based on the adult analysis of a reported child-
        hood case. *International Journal of Psychoanalysis*,
        1966, *47*, 130-131.

OBSESSIVE-COMPULSIVE NEUROSES/Research

0712   *Adams, P. L. *Obsessive children. A socio-psychiatric
        study*. New York: Brunner/Mazel, 1973.
0714   *Kayton, L. & Borge, G. F. Birth order and the obses-
        sive-compulsive character. *Archives of General Psy-
        chiatry*, 1967, *17*, 751-754.
0715   *Goodwin, D. W., Guze, S. B. & Robins, E. Follow-up
        studies in obsessional neurosis. *Archives of General
        Psychiatry*, 1969, *20*, 182-187.
0716   Slater, E. Genetical factors in neurosis. *British
        Journal of Psychology*, 1964, *55*, 265-269.
0717   *Woodruff, R. & Pitts, F. N. Monozygotic twins with
        obsessional illness. *American Journal of Psychiatry*,
        1964, *120*, 1075-1080.
0718   *Marks, I. M., Crowe, M., Drewe, E., Young, J. & Dew-
        hurst, W. G. Obsessive compulsive neurosis in iden-
        tical twins. *British Journal of Psychiatry*, 1969,
        115, 991-998.
0719   *Parker, N. Close identification in twins discordant
        for obsessional neurosis. *British Journal of Psychi-
        atry*, 1964, *110*, 496-504.
0720   Inouye, E. Similar and dissimilar manifestations of
        obsessive-compulsive neurosis in monozygotic twins.
        American Journal of Psychiatry, 1965, *121*, 1171-1175.
0721   *Sikkema, M. Observations on Japanese early child train-
        ing. *Psychiatry*, 1947, *10*, 423-432.
0722   Milner, A. D., Beech, H. R. & Walker, V. J. Decision
        processes and obsessional behaviour. *British Journal
        of Social and Clinical Psychology*, 1971, *10*, 88-89.

PROBLEMS OF SEXUAL IDENTIFICATION IN CHILDREN

0723   *Green, R. & Money, J. Stage-acting, role-taking, and
        effeminate impersonation during boyhood. *Archives of
        General Psychiatry*, 1966, *15*, 535-538.

0724   *Bakwin, H.   Deviant gender-role behavior in children:
       Relation to homosexuality. *Pediatrics,* 1968, *41,*
       620-629.
0725   Green, R.   Childhood cross-gender identification. *Jour-
       nal of Nervous and Mental Disease,* 1968, *147,* 500-509.
0726   *Greenson, R. R.   A transvestite boy and a hypothesis.
       International Journal of Psychoanalysis, 1966, *47,*
       396-403.
0727   *Stoller, R. J.   The mother's contribution to infantile
       transvestic behaviour. *International Journal of Psy-
       choanalysis,* 1966, *47,* 384-395.
0728   *Newman, L. E. & Stoller, R. J.   The oedipal situation in
       male transsexualism. *British Journal of Medical Psy-
       chology,* 1971, *44,* 295-303.
0729   *Harrison, S. I.   Reared in the wrong sex. *Journal of
       the American Academy of Child Psychiatry,* 1970, *9,*
       44-102.
0730   *Holemon, R. E. & Winokur, G.   Effeminate homosexuality:
       A disease of childhood. *American Journal of Ortho-
       psychiatry,* 1965, *35,* 48-56.
0731   *Green, R., Newman, L. E. & Stoller, R. J.   Treatment of
       boyhood "transsexualism": An interim report of four
       years' experience. *Archives of General Psychiatry,*
       1972, *26,* 213-217.
0732   Green, R.   Diagnosis and treatment of gender identity
       disorders during childhood. *Archives of Sexual Be-
       havior,* 1971, *1,* 167-173.
0733   Stoller, R. J.   The treatment of transvestism and trans-
       sexualism. *Current Psychiatric Therapies,* 1966, *6,*
       92-104.
0734   *Zuger, B. & Taylor, P.   Effeminate behavior present in
       boys from early childhood. II. Comparison with simi-
       lar symptoms in non-effeminate boys. *Pediatrics,*
       1969, *44,* 375-380.
0735   *Harrison, S. I., Cain, A. C. & Benedek, E.   The child-
       hood of a transsexual. *Archives of General Psychia-
       try,* 1968, *19,* 28-37.
0736   *Lebovitz, P. S.   Feminine behavior in boys: Aspects of
       its outcome. *American Journal of Psychiatry,* 1972,
       128, 1283-1289.
0737   *Newman, L. E.   Transsexualism in adolescence: Problems
       in evaluation and treatment. *Archives of General Psy-
       chiatry,* 1970, *23,* 112-121.
0738   Money, J. W. & Ehrhardt, A. A.   *Man and woman, boy and
       girl.* Baltimore: Johns Hopkins University Press, 1972.
0739   Green, R. & Money, J. (Eds.) *Transsexualism and sex
       reassignment.* Baltimore: Johns Hopkins University
       Press, 1969.
0740   *Stoller, R. J.   *Sex and gender.* New York: Science
       House, 1968.

0740.1   Stoller, R. J.   Symbiosis anxiety and the development of
          masculinity. *Archives of General Psychiatry*, 1974, *30*,
          164-172.
0740.2   Zuger, B.   Effeminate behavior in boys. *Archives of
          General Psychiatry*, 1974, *30*, 173-177.
0740.3   Green, R.   *Sexual identity conflict in children and
          adults*. New York: Basic Books, 1974.
0740.4   Stoller, R. J.   *Splitting: A case of female masculin-
          ity*. New York: Quadrangle Books, 1973.
0740.5   Green, R. & Fuller, M.   Family doll play and female
          identity in pre-adolescent males. *American Journal
          of Orthopsychiatry*, 1973, *43*, 123-127.

SUICIDE

0741   *Ackerly, W. C.   Latency-age children who threaten or
         attempt to kill themselves. *Journal of the American
         Academy of Child Psychiatry*, 1967, *6*, 242-261.
0742   *Toolan, J. M.   Suicide and suicidal attempts in chil-
         dren and adolescents. *American Journal of Psychiatry*,
         1962, *118*, 719-724.
0743   Shaw, C. R. & Schelkun, R. F.   Suicidal behavior in
          children. *Psychiatry*, 1965, *28*, 157-168.
0744   *Mattsson, A., Seese, L. R. & Hawkins, J. W.   Suicidal
          behavior as a child psychiatric emergency: Clinical
          characteristics and follow-up results. *Archives of
          General Psychiatry*, 1969, *20*, 100-109.
0745   *Lourie, R. S.   Clinical studies of attempted suicide in
          childhood. *Clinical Proceedings of the Children's
          Hospital*, 1966, *22*, 163-173.
0746   Gould, R. E.   Suicide problems in children and adoles-
          cents. *American Journal of Psychotherapy*, 1965, *19*,
          228-246.

GENERAL REFERENCES REGARDING CHILDHOOD PSYCHOPATHOLOGY (THROUGH
LATENCY)

0747   *Thomas, A., Chess, S. & Birch, H. G.   *Temperament and
          behavior disorders in children*. New York: New York
          University Press, 1968.
0748   *Yarrow, L. J.   Maternal deprivation. In A. M. Freed-
          man & H. I. Kaplan (Eds.), *Comprehensive textbook of
          psychiatry*. Baltimore: Williams and Wilkins, 1967.
          Pp. 1489-1493.
0749   World Health Organization. *Deprivation of maternal
          care: A reassessment of its effects*. Geneva: World
          Health Organization, 1962. (Public health papers,
          no. 14.)

0750   *Wolff, S. The contribution of obstetric complications
        to the etiology of behaviour disorders in childhood.
        *Journal of Child Psychology and Psychiatry and Allied
        Disciplines*, 1967, *8*, 57-66.
0751   Bowlby, J. *Maternal care and mental health.* Geneva:
        World Health Organization, 1951. (Monograph series,
        no. 2)
0752   Brody, S. *Patterns of mothering.* New York: Inter-
        national Universities Press, 1956.
0753   *De Elejalde, F. Inadequate mothering: Patterns and
        treatment. *Bulletin of the Menninger Clinic*, 1971,
        35, 182-198.
0754   Sandler, A., Daunton, E. & Schnurmann, A. Inconsist-
        ency in the mother as a factor in character develop-
        ment: A comparative study of three cases. *Psychoan-
        alytic Study of the Child*, 1957, *12*, 209-225.
0755   *Poznanski, E., Maxey, A. & Marsden, G. Clinical impli-
        cations of maternal employment: A review of research.
        Journal of the American Academy of Child Psychiatry,
        1970, *9*, 741-761.
0756   *Berg, I., Stark, G. & Jameson, S. Measurement of a
        stranger's influence on the behaviour of young chil-
        dren with their mothers. *Journal of Child Psychology
        and Psychiatry and Allied Disciplines*, 1966, *7*, 243-
        250.
0757   Beres, D. Clinical notes on aggression in children.
        Psychoanalytic Study of the Child, 1952, *7*, 241-263.
0758   *Kirk, H. D., Jonassohn, K. & Fish, A. D. Are adopted
        children especially vulnerable to stress? *Archives
        of General Psychiatry*, 1966, *14*, 291-298.
0759   *Anthony, E. J. The mutative impact of serious mental
        and physical illness in a parent on family life. In
        E. J. Anthony & C. Koupernik (Eds.), *The child in
        his family.* New York: Wiley, 1970. Pp. 131-163.
        (International Yearbook for Child Psychiatry and
        Allied Disciplines, vol. 1)
0760   Coles, R. Violence in ghetto children. *Children*,
        1967, *14*, 101-104.
0761   Ames, L. B. *Sleep and dreams in childhood.* New York:
        Macmillan, 1964.
0762   Group for the Advancement of Psychiatry. Committee on
        Child Psychiatry. *Psychopathological disorders in
        childhood: Theoretical considerations and a proposed
        classification.* New York: Group for the Advancement
        of Psychiatry, 1966. (GAP report, no. 62.)
0763   Freud, A. & Burlingham, D. T. *Infants without families.*
        New York: International Universities Press, 1973.
        (*Writings*, vol. 3, pp. 543-664)
0764   Provence, S. A. & Lipton, R. C. *Infants in institutions.*
        New York: International Universities Press, 1963.

0765   Freud, S. (1926)   Inhibitions, symptoms and anxiety.
          In *Standard Edition, 20,* 87-174. London: Hogarth
          Press, 1959.
0766   Waelder, R. Anxiety. In *Basic theory of psychoanaly-
          sis.* New York: International Universities Press,
          1960. Pp. 154-166.
0766.1   Rutter, M. L. Relationships between child and adult
          psychiatric disorders. In S. Chess & A. Thomas
          (Eds.), *Annual progress in child psychiatry and child
          development: 1973.* New York: Brunner/Mazel, 1974.
          Pp. 669-688.

VI. PSYCHO-PHYSIOLOGICAL DISORDERS

THEORETICAL ASPECTS

0767 *Engel, G. L. *Psychological development in health and disease.* Philadelphia: Saunders, 1962.

0768 *Ostfeld, A. et al. Factors relative to the occurrence and distribution of illness in a homogeneous population of ostensibly healthy individuals. *Journal of Nervous and Mental Disease,* 1956, *124,* 405-412.

0769 *Giovacchini, P. L. The ego and the psychosomatic state: Report of two cases. *Psychosomatic Medicine,* 1959, *21,* 218-227.

0770 *Schur, M. Comments on the metapsychology of somatization. *Psychoanalytic Study of the Child,* 1955, *10,* 119-164.

0771 Schwab, J. J., McGinnis, N. H., Norris, L. B. & Schwab, R. B. Psychosomatic medicine and the contemporary social scene. *American Journal of Psychiatry,* 1970, *126,* 1632-1642.

0772 *Ruesch, J. The infantile personality: The core problem of psychosomatic medicine. *Psychosomatic Medicine,* 1948, *10,* 134-144.

0773 Kepecs, J. G. The oral triad applied to psychosomatic disorders. *Psychoanalytic Quarterly,* 1957, *26,* 461-475.

0774 *Mendelson, M., Hirsch, S. & Webber, C. S. A critical examination of some recent theoretical models in psychosomatic medicine. *Psychosomatic Medicine,* 1956, *18,* 363-373.

0775 Knapp, P. H. & Bahnson, C. B. The emotional field: A sequential study of mood and fantasy in 2 asthmatic patients. *Psychosomatic Medicine,* 1963, *25,* 460-483.

0776 *Benedek, T. The psychosomatic implications of the primary unit: mother-child. *American Journal of Orthopsychiatry,* 1949, *19,* 642-654.

0777 *Parens, H., McConville, B. J. & Kaplan, S. M. The prediction of frequency of illness from the response to separation: A preliminary study and replication attempt. *Psychosomatic Medicine,* 1966, *28,* 162-176.

0778 *Garner, A. M. & Wenar, C. *The mother-child interaction in psychosomatic disorders.* Urbana, Ill.: University of Illinois Press, 1959.

0779 Deutsch, F. *The psychosomatic concept in psychoanalysis.* New York: International Universities Press, 1953.

0780 Gitelson, M. A critique of current concept in psychosomatic medicine. *Bulletin of the Menninger Clinic,* 1959, *23,* 165-178.

0781 Sperling, M. Psychosis and psychosomatic illness. *International Journal of Psychoanalysis,* 1955, *36,* 320-327.

0782   *Grossman, H. J. & Greenberg, N. H. Psychosomatic dif-
        ferentiation in infancy. I. Autonomic activity in
        the newborn. *Psychosomatic Medicine*, 1957, *19*, 293-
        306.
0783   *Richmond, J. B. & Lustman, S. L. Autonomic function in
        the neonate. I. Implications for psychosomatic
        theory. *Psychosomatic Medicine*, 1955, *17*, 269-275.
0784   Gerard, M. W. Genesis of psychosomatic symptoms in in-
        fancy. In F. Deutsch (Ed.), *The psychosomatic con-
        cept in psychoanalysis*. New York: International
        Universities Press, 1953. Pp. 82-95. (Monograph
        Series of the Boston Psychoanalytic Society and In-
        stitute, no. 1)
0785   *Kulka, A., Fry, C. & Goldstein, F. J. Kinesthetic
        needs in infancy. *American Journal of Orthopsychia-
        try*, 1960, *30*, 562-571.
0786   *Koupernik, C. The roots of hypochondriasis in the
        child. In E. J. Anthony and C. Koupernik (Eds.),
        The child in his family. Vol. 2. *The impact of
        disease and death*. New York: Wiley, 1973. Pp. 85-
        95. (International Yearbook for Child Psychiatry and
        Allied Disciplines, vol. 2)
0787   *Mohr, G. J., Richmond, J. B., Garner, A. M. & Eddy,
        E. J. A program for the study of children with psy-
        chosomatic disorders. In G. Caplan (Ed.), *Emotional
        problems of early childhood*. New York: Basic Books,
        1966. Pp. 251-268.
0788   Mutter, A. Z. & Schleifer, M. J. The role of psycho-
        logical and social factors in the onset of somatic
        illness in children. *Psychosomatic Medicine*, 1966,
        28, 333-343.
0789   *Szurek, S. A. Comments on the psychopathology of chil-
        dren with somatic illness. *American Journal of Psy-
        chiatry*, 1951, *107*, 844-849.
0790   *Titchener, J. L., Riskin, J. & Emerson, R. The family
        in psychosomatic process: A case report illustrating
        a method of psychosomatic research. *Psychosomatic
        Medicine*, 1960, *22*, 127-142.
0791   Harris, H. I. The range of psychosomatic disorders in
        adolescence. In J. G. Howells (Ed.), *Modern per-
        spectives in adolescent psychiatry*. Edinburgh: Oli-
        ver & Boyd, 1971. Pp. 237-253. (Modern perspectives
        in psychiatry, vol. 4)
0792   *Rosenbaum, M. The role of psychological factors in
        delayed growth in adolescence: A case report. *Amer-
        ican Journal of Orthopsychiatry*, 1959, *29*, 762-771.
0793   *Hellersberg, E. F. Unevenness of growth in its rela-
        tion to vulnerability, anxiety, ego weakness and the
        schizophrenic patterns. *American Journal of Ortho-
        psychiatry*, 1957, *27*, 577-586.
0794   *Looff, D. H. Psychophysiologic and conversion reac-
        tions in children: Selective incidences in verbal

and nonverbal families. *Journal of the American Academy of Child Psychiatry*, 1970, *9*, 318-331.

0795   Barber, T. X. The effects of "hypnosis" on pain: A critical review of experimental and clinical findings. *Psychosomatic Medicine*, 1963, *25*, 303-333.

0796   Paul, G. L. The production of blisters by hypnotic suggestion: Another look. *Psychosomatic Medicine*, 1963, *25*, 233-244.

0797   Crisp, A. H. Some psychosomatic aspects of neoplasia. *British Journal of Medical Psychology*, 1970, *43*, 313-331.

0798   LaBarba, R. C. Experiential and environmental factors in cancer: A review of research with animals. *Psychosomatic Medicine*, 1970, *32*, 259-276.

0799   *Savitt, R. A. Transference, somatization, and symbiotic need. *Journal of the American Psychoanalytic Association*, 1969, *17*, 1030-1054.

0800   Vernick, J. The use of the life space interview on a medical ward. *Social Casework*, 1963, *44*, 465-469.

0800.1 Coddington, R. D. The significance of life events as etiologic factors in the diseases of children. I. A survey of professional workers. *Journal of Psychosomatic Research*, 1972, *16*, 7-18.

0800.2 Coddington, R. D. The significance of life events as etiologic factors in the diseases of children. II. A study of a normal population. *Journal of Psychosomatic Research*, 1972, *16*, 205-213.

0800.3 Sigal, J. J., Chagoya, L., Villeneuve, C. & Mayerovitch, J. Later psychosocial sequelae of early childhood illness (Severe croup). *American Journal of Psychiatry*, 1973, *130*, 786-789.

0800.4 Winsberg, B. G., Bialer, I., Kupietz, S. & Tobias, J. Impaired children. *American Journal of Psychiatry*, 1972, *128*, 1425-1431.

ALLERGY AND ECZEMA

0801   *Block, J., Jennings, P. H., Harvey, E. & Simpson, E. Interaction between allergic potential and psychopathology in childhood asthma. *Psychosomatic Medicine*, 1964, *26*, 307-320.

0802   *Freeman, E. H., Feingold, B. F., Schlesinger, K. & Gorman, F. J. Psychological variables in allergic disorders: A review. *Psychosomatic Medicine*, 1964, *26*, 543-575.

0803   Jacobs, M. A., Anderson, L. S., Eisman, H. D., Muller, J. J. & Friedman, S. Interaction of psychologic and biologic predisposing factors in allergic disorders. *Psychosomatic Medicine*, 1967, *29*, 572-585.

0804   Block, J. Further consideration of psychosomatic predisposing factors in allergy. *Psychosomatic Medicine*, 1968, *30*, 202-208.

0805   *Long, R. T., et al. A psychosomatic study of allergic and emotional factors in children with asthma. *American Journal of Psychiatry*, 1958, *114*, 890-899.
0806   *Mohr, G. J., Tausend, H., Selesnick, S. & Augenbraun, B. Studies of eczema and asthma in the preschool child. *Journal of the American Academy of Child Psychiatry*, 1963, *2*, 271-291.
0807   *Miller, H. & Baruch, D. W. A study of hostility in allergic children. *American Journal of Orthopsychiatry*, 1950, *20*, 506-519.
0808   Miller, H. & Baruch, D. W. Psychotherapy of parents of allergic children. *Annals of Allergy*, 1960, *18*, 990-997.
0808.1 Sultz, H. A., Schlesinger, E. R., Mosher, W. E. & Feldman, J. G. Asthma and Eczema. In *Long-term childhood illness*. Pittsburgh, Pa.: University of Pittsburgh Press, 1972. Pp. 177-222.

ANOREXIA

0809   *Rowland, C. V. Anorexia nervosa: A survey of the literature and review of 30 cases. *International Psychiatry Clinics*, 1970, *7*(1), 37-137.
0810   *Lesser, L. I., Ashenden, B. J. Debuskey, M. & Eisenberg, L. Anorexia nervosa in children. *American Journal of Orthopsychiatry*, 1960, *30*, 572-580.
0811   Dally, P. *Anorexia nervosa*. London: Heinemann, 1969.
0812   *Ushakov, G. K. Anorexia nervosa. In J. G. Howells (Ed.), *Modern perspectives in adolescent psychiatry*. Edinburgh: Oliver & Boyd, 1971. Pp. 274-289. (Modern perspectives in psychiatry, vol. 4)
0813   *Crisp, A. H. Anorexia nervosa 'feeding disorder', 'nervous malnutrition' or 'weight phobia'? *World Review of Nutrition and Dietetics*, 1970, *12*, 452-504.
0814   *Crisp, A. H. Reported birth weights and growth rates in a group of patients with primary anorexia nervosa (weight phobia). *Journal of Psychosomatic Research*, 1970, *14*, 23-50.
0815   Crisp, A. H. Premorbid factors in adult disorders of weight, with particular reference to primary anorexia nervosa (weight phobia). A literature review. *Journal of Psychosomatic Research*, 1970, *14*, 1-22.
0816   Kaufman, M. R. & Heiman, M. *Evolution of psychosomatic concepts - anorexia nervosa: A paradigm*. New York: International Universities Press, 1964.
0817   Bliss, E. L. & Branch, C. H. H. *Anorexia nervosa*. New York: Hoeber, 1960. (Psychosomatic medicine monograph)
0818   *Bruch, H. Changing approaches to anorexia nervosa. *International Psychiatry Clinics*, 1970, *7*(1), 3-24.

0819   Thoma, H. *Anorexia nervosa*. New York: International
        Universities Press, 1967.
0820   Bruch, H. Death in anorexia nervosa. *Psychosomatic
        Medicine*, 1971, *33*, 135-144.
0821   Bruch, H. The insignificant difference: Discordant
        incidence of anorexia nervosa in monozygotic twins.
        American Journal of Psychiatry, 1969, *126*, 85-90.
0822   *Bruch, H. Anorexia nervosa in the male. *Psychosomatic
        Medicine*, 1971, *33*, 31-47.
0823   *Warren, W. A study of anorexia nervosa in young girls.
        *Journal of Child Psychology and Psychiatry and Allied
        Disciplines*, 1968, *9*, 27-40.
0824   *Bruch, H. Psychotherapy in primary anorexia nervosa.
        Journal of Nervous and Mental Disease, 1970, *150*, 51-
        67.
0825   *Berlin, I. N., Boatman, M. J., Sheimo, S. L. & Szurek,
        S. A. Adolescent alternation of anorexia and obesity.
        Workshop, 1950. *American Journal of Orthopsychiatry*,
        1951, *21*, 387-419.
0826   *Rollins, M. & Blackwell, A. The treatment of anorexia
        nervosa in children and adolescents: Stage I. *Jour-
        nal of Child Psychology and Psychiatry and Allied
        Disciplines*, 1968, *9*, 81-91.
0827   *Reinhart, J. B., Kenna, M. D. & Succop, R. A. Anorexia
        nervosa in children: Outpatient management. *Journal
        of the American Academy of Child Psychiatry*, 1972,
        11, 114-131.
0828   Sylvester, E. Analysis of psychogenic anorexia and
        vomiting in a four-year old-child. *Psychoanalytic
        Study of the Child*, 1945, *1*, 167-187.
0829   *Barcai, A. Family therapy in the treatment of anorexia
        nervosa. *American Journal of Psychiatry*, 1971, *128*,
        286-290.
0829.1 Minuchin, S., Baker, L., Liebman, R., Milman, L., Ros-
        man, B. & Todd, T. Anorexia nervosa: Successful
        application of a family therapy approach. *Jouranl of
        Pediatrics*, 1974. In press.
0829.2 Liebman, R., Minuchin, S. & Baker, L. An integrated
        treatment program for anorexia nervosa. *American
        Journal of Psychiatry*, 1974, *131*, 432-436.
0829.3 Wold, P. Family structure in three cases of anorexia
        nervosa: The role of the father. *American Journal
        of Psychiatry*, 1973, *130*, 1394-1397.
0829.4 Agras, A. S., Barlow, D. H., Chapin, H. N., Abel, G. G.
        & Leitenberg, H. Behavior modification of anorexia
        nervosa. *Archives of General Psychiatry*, 1974, *30*,
        279-286.
0829.5 Selvini-Palazzoli, M. The families of patients with
        anorexia nervosa. In E. J. Anthony and C. Koupernik
        (Eds.), *The child in his family*. New York: Wiley,
        1970. Pp. 319-332.

0829.6   Galdston, R. Mind over matter: Observations on 50
         patients hospitalized with anorexia nervosa. *Jour-*
         nal of the American Academy of Child Psychiatry,
         1974, *13*, 246-263.

RHEUMATIC FEVER IN CHILDREN

0830   *Brazelton, T. B., Holder, R. & Talbot, B. Emotional
       aspects of rheumatic fever in children. *Journal of*
       Pediatrics, 1953, *43*, 339-358.
0831   *Josselyn, I. M., Simon, A. J. & Eells, E. Anxiety in
       children convalescing from rheumatic fever. *American*
       Journal of Orthopsychiatry, 1955, *25*, 109-119.
0832   Glaser, H. H., Lynn, D. B. & Harrison, G. S. Compre-
       hensive medical care for handicapped children. I.
       Patterns of anxiety in mothers of children with rheu-
       matic fever. *American Journal of Diseases of Chil-*
       dren, 1961, *102*, 344-354.
0833   Kennell, J. H., Soroker, E., Thomas, P. & Wasman, M.
       What parents of rheumatic fever patients don't under-
       stand about the disease and its prophylactic manage-
       ment. *Pediatrics,* 1969, *43*, 160-167.

CONGENITAL HEART DISEASE

0834   *Rausch de Traubenberg, N. Psychological aspects of
       congenital heart disease in the child. In E. J.
       Anthony and C. Koupernik (Eds.), *The child in his*
       family. Vol. 2. *The impact of disease and death.*
       New York: Wiley, 1973. Pp. 75-83. (International
       Yearbook for Child Psychiatry and Allied Disciplines,
       vol. 2)
0835   *Glaser, H. H., Harrison, G. S. & Lynn, D. B. Emotional
       implications of congenital heart disease in children.
       Pediatrics, 1964, *33*, 367-379.
0836   *Landtman, B., Valanne, E., Pentti, R. & Aukee, M. Psy-
       chosomatic behaviour of children with congenital
       heart disease. *Annales Paediatriae Fenniae,* 1960,
       6 (15, suppl.).
0837   *Green, M. & Levitt, E. E. Constriction of body image
       in children with congenital heart disease. *Pediat-*
       rics, 1962, *29*, 438-441.

RHEUMATOID ARTHRITIS

0838   *Blom, G. E. & Nicholls, G. Emotional factors in chil-
       dren with rheumatoid arthritis. *American Journal of*
       Orthopsychiatry, 1954, *24*, 588-601.

0839   Morse, J., Seglin, J., Burnside, M. & Glode, G. Team-
        work in a center for juvenile rheumatoid arthritis.
        Rehabilitation Literature, 1966, *27*, 258-265.
0840   Morse, J. Involving fathers in the treatment of pa-
        tients with juvenile rheumatoid arthritis. *Social
        Casework*, 1968, *49*, 281-287.
0841   *Wolff, S. *Children under stress*. London: Allen Lane,
        1969.
0841.1 Sultz, H. A., Schlesinger, E. R., Mosher, W. E. &
        Feldman, J. G. Juvenile rheumatoid arthritis. In
        Long-term childhood illness. Pittsburgh: University
        of Pittsburgh Press, 1972. Pp. 427-443.

CYSTIC FIBROSIS

0842   *Leiken, S. J. & Hassakis, P. Psychological study of
        parents of children with cystic fibrosis. In E. J.
        Anthony and C. Koupernik (Eds.), *The child in his
        family*. Vol. 2. *The impact of disease and death*.
        New York: Wiley, 1973. Pp. 49-57. (International
        Yearbook for Child Psychiatry and Allied Disciplines,
        vol. 2)
0843   *Cytryn, L., Moore, P. & Robinson, M. E. Psychological
        adjustment of children with cystic fibrosis. In E.
        J. Anthony and C. Koupernik (Eds.), *The child in his
        family*. Vol. 2. *The impact of disease and death*.
        New York: Wiley, 1973. Pp. 37-47. (International
        Yearbook for Child Psychiatry and Allied Disciplines,
        vol. 2)
0843.1 Sultz, H. A., Schlesinger, E. R., Mosher, W. E. &
        Feldman, J. G. Cystic fibrosis and celiac disease.
        In *Long-term childhood illness*. Pittsburgh: Univer-
        sity of Pittsburgh Press, 1972. Pp. 249-281.

ASTHMA

0844   Long, R. T., et al. A psychosomatic study of allergic
        and emotional factors in children with asthma. *Ameri-
        can Journal of Psychiatry*, 1958, *114*, 890-899.
0845   Harris, I. D., Rapoport, L., Rynerson, M. A. & Samter,
        M. Observations on asthmatic children. *American
        Journal of Orthopsychiatry*, 1950, *20*, 490-505.
0846   Hahn, W. W. & Clark, J. A. Psychophysiological reac-
        tivity of asthmatic children. *Psychosomatic Medi-
        cine*, 1967, *29*, 526-536.
0847   Purcell, K., Muser, J., Miklich, D. & Dietiker, K. E.
        A comparison of psychologic findings in variously
        defined asthmatic subgroups. *Journal of Psychosomatic
        Research*, 1969, *13*, 67-75.

0848   *Sperling, M. Asthma in children: An evaluation of
       concepts and therapies. *Journal of the American Acad-
       emy of Child Psychiatry*, 1968, *7*, 44-58.
0849   Ottenberg, P., Stein, M., Lewis, J. & Hamilton, C.
       Learned asthma in the guinea pig. *Psychosomatic
       Medicine*, 1958, *20*, 393-400.
0850   *McFadden, E. R., Luparello, T. J., Lyons, H. A. &
       Bleecker, E. The mechanism of action of suggestion
       in the induction of acute asthma attacks. *Psycho-
       somatic Medicine*, 1969, *31*, 134-143.
0851   Luparello, T. J., Lyons, H. A., Bleecker, E. R. &
       McFadden, E. R. Influences of suggestion on airway
       reactivity in asthmatic subjects. *Psychosomatic
       Medicine*, 1968, *30*, 819-825.
0852   Luparello, T. J., Leist, N., Lourie, C. H. & Sweet, P.
       The interaction of psychologic stimuli and pharmaco-
       logic agents on airway reactivity in asthmatic sub-
       jects. *Psychosomatic Medicine*, 1970, *32*, 509-513.
0853   *Knapp, P. H. & Nemetz, S. J. Personality variations in
       bronchial asthma. A study of forty patients: Notes
       on the relationship to psychosis and the problem of
       measuring maturity. *Psychosomatic Medicine*, 1957,
       19, 443-465.
0854   Miller, H. & Baruch, D. W. The emotional problems of
       childhood and their relation to asthma. *American
       Journal of Diseases of Children*, 1957, *93*, 242-245.
0855   Kripke, S. S. Psychologic aspects of bronchial asthma.
       American Journal of Diseases of Children, 1960, *100*,
       935-941.
0856   Weiss, J. H., Martin, C. & Riley, J. Effects of sug-
       gestion on respiration in asthmatic children. *Psycho-
       somatic Medicine*, 1970, *32*, 409-415.
0857   *Knapp, P. H., Mushatt, C. & Nemetz, S. J. Asthma,
       melancholia, and death. I. Psychoanalytic considera-
       tions. *Psychosomatic Medicine*, 1966, *28*, 114-133.
0858   *Knapp, P. H., Carr, H. E., Mushatt, C. & Nemetz, S. J.
       Asthma, melancholia, and death. II. Psychosomatic
       considerations. *Psychosomatic Medicine*, 1966, *28*,
       134-154.
0859   *Jessner, L., et al. Emotional impact of nearness and
       separation for the asthmatic child and his mother.
       Psychoanalytic Study of the Child, 1955, *10*, 353-375.
0860   *Purcell, K., Brady, K., Chai, H., Muser, J., Molk, L.,
       Gordon, N. & Means, J. The effect on asthma in chil-
       dren of experimental separation from the family.
       Psychosomatic Medicine, 1969, *31*, 144-164.
0861   Knapp, P. H. The asthmatic and his environment. *Jour-
       nal of Nervous and Mental Diseases*, 1969, *149*, 133-
       151.
0862   *Kluger, J. M. Childhood asthma and the social milieu.
       Journal of the American Academy of Child Psychiatry,
       1969, *8*, 353-366.

0863   Bacon, C. L. The role of aggression in the asthmatic
        attack. *Psychoanalytic Quarterly*, 1956, *25*, 309-
        324.
0864   *Coolidge, J. C. Asthma in mother and child as a spe-
        cial type of intercommunication. *American Journal of
        Orthopsychiatry*, 1956, *26*, 165-178.
0865   Maher-Loughnan, G. P., Mason, A. A., Macdonald, N. &
        Fry, L. Controlled trial of hypnosis in the sympto-
        matic treatment of asthma. *British Medical Journal*,
        1962, *2*, no. 5301, 371-376.
0866   Moore, N. Behaviour therapy in bronchial asthma: A
        controlled study. *Journal of Psychosomatic Research*,
        1965, *9*, 257-276.
0867   McLean, J. A. & Ching, A. Y. T. Follow-up study of
        relationships between family situation and bronchial
        asthma in children. *Journal of the American Academy
        of Child Psychiatry*, 1973, *12*, 142-161.
0867.1 Pinkerton, P. Correlating physiologic with psychody-
        namic data in the study and management of childhood
        asthma. *Journal of Psychosomatic Research*, 1967, *11*,
        11.
0867.2 Pinkerton, P. & Weaver, C. M. Childhood asthma. In O.
        Hill (Ed.), *Modern trends in psychosomatic medicine*.
        London: Butterworths, 1970.
0867.3 Sultz, H. A., Schlesinger, E. R., Mosher, W. E. & Feld-
        man, J. G. Asthma and eczema. In *Long-term child-
        hood illness*. Pittsburgh, Pa.: University of Pitts-
        burgh Press, 1972. Pp. 177-222.

DIABETES

0868   *Falstein, E. I. & Judas, I. Juvenile diabetes and its
        psychiatric implications. *American Journal of Ortho-
        psychiatry*, 1955, *25*, 330-342.
0869   Kimball, C. P. Emotional and psychosocial aspects of
        diabetes mellitus. *Medical Clinics of North America*,
        1971, *55*(4), 1007-1018.
0870   *Swift, C. R., Seidman, F. & Stein, H. Adjustment prob-
        lems in juvenile diabetes. *Psychosomatic Medicine*,
        1967, *29*, 555-571.
0871   Kaufman, R. V. & Hersher, B. Body image changes in
        teenage diabetics. *Pediatrics*, 1971, *48*, 123-128.
0872   *Zeidel, A. Problems of emotional adjustment in juve-
        nile diabetes. In E. J. Anthony and C. Koupernik
        (Eds.), *The child in his family*. Vol. 2. *The impact
        of disease and death*. New York: Wiley, 1973. Pp.
        59-64. (International Yearbook for Child Psychiatry
        and Allied Disciplines, vol. 2)
0872.1 Baker, L., Minuchin, S., Milman, L., Liebman, R. & Todd,
        T. Psychosomatic aspects of juvenile diabetes melli-
        tus: A progress report. *Israel Journal of Medical
        Sciences*, 1973, *8*.

0872.2   Sultz, H. A., Schlesinger, E. R., Mosher, W. E. & Feld-
         man, J. G. Childhood diabetes mellitus. In *Long-
         term childhood illness.* Pittsburgh: University of
         Pittsburgh Press, 1972. Pp. 223-248.
0872.3   Hong, K-E. M. & Holmes, T. H. Transient diabetes mel-
         litus associated with culture change. *Archives of
         General Psychiatry,* 1973, *29,* 683-687.

ENCOPRESIS

0873   *Achenbach, T. M. & Lewis, M. A proposed model for clin-
         ical research and its application to encopresis and
         enuresis. *Journal of the American Academy of Child
         Psychiatry,* 1971, *10,* 535-554.
0874   *Warson, S. R., Caldwell, M. R., Warinner, A. & Kirk, A.
         J. The dynamics of encopresis. Workshop, 1953.
         American Journal of Orthopsychiatry, 1954, *24,* 402-
         415.
0875   *Richmond, J. B., Eddy, E. J. & Garrard, S. D. The syn-
         drome of fecal soiling and megacolon. *American Jour-
         nal of Orthopsychiatry,* 1954, *24,* 391-401.
0876   *Bemporad, J. R., Pfeifer, C. M., Gibbs, L., Cortner,
         R. H. & Bloom, W. Characteristics of encopretic
         patients and their families. *Journal of the American
         Academy of Child Psychiatry,* 1971, *10,* 272-292.
0877   *Hoag, J. M., Norriss, N. G., Himeno, E. T. & Jacobs,
         J. The encopretic child and his family. *Journal of
         the American Academy of Child Psychiatry,* 1971, *10,*
         242-256.
0878   Mercer, R. D. Constipation. *Pediatric Clinics of North
         America,* 1967, *14*(1), 175-185.
0879   Lockhart, H. E. & Mummery, M. Megacolon and megarectum
         in older children and young adults. *Proceedings of
         the Royal Society of Medicine,* 1967, *60,* 799-807.

ENURESIS

0882   *Achenbach, T. M. & Lewis, M. A proposed model for clin-
         ical research and its application to encopresis and
         enuresis. *Journal of the American Academy of Child
         Psychiatry,* 1971, *10,* 535-554.
0883   *Sperling, M. Dynamic considerations and treatment of
         enuresis. *Journal of the American Academy of Child
         Psychiatry,* 1965, *4,* 19-31.
0884   *Breger, E. Etiologic factors in enuresis: A psycho-
         biologic approach. *Journal of the American Academy
         of Child Psychiatry,* 1963, *2,* 667-676.
0885   Wahl, C. W. & Golden, J. S. Psychogenic urinary reten-
         tion: Report of 6 cases. *Psychosomatic Medicine,*
         1963, *25,* 543-555.

0886   *Williams, G. E. & Johnson, A. M.   Recurrent urinary
       retention due to emotional factors: Report of a case.
       Psychosomatic Medicine, 1956, *18*, 77-80.
0887   *Martin, G. I.   Imipramine pamoate in the treatment of
       childhood enuresis: A double-blind study.   *American
       Journal of Diseases of Children*, 1971, *122*, 42-47.
0888   *Raimbault, G.   Psychological problems in the chronic
       nephropathies of childhood.   In E. J. Anthony and
       C. Koupernik (Eds.), *The child in his family*.   Vol.
       2.   *The impact of disease and death*.   New York:
       Wiley, 1973.   Pp. 65-74.   (International Yearbook for
       Child Psychiatry and Allied Disciplines, vol. 2)

FEEDING

0889   *Lehman, E.   Feeding problems of psychogenic origin: A
       survey of the literature.   *Psychoanalytic Study of
       the Child*, 1949, *3-4*, 461-488.
0890   *Wortis, H., Rue, R., Heimer, C., Braine, M., Redlo, M.
       & Freedman, A. M.   Children who eat noxious sub-
       stances.   *Journal of the American Academy of Child
       Psychiatry*, 1962, *1*, 536-547.
0891   *Lourie, R. S. & Millican, F. K.   Pica.   In J. G.
       Howells (Ed.), *Modern perspectives in international
       child psychiatry*.   Edinburgh: Oliver & Boyd, 1969.
       Pp. 455-470.   (Modern perspectives in psychiatry,
       vol. 3)
0892   *Lewis, M., Solnit, A. J., Stark, M. H., Gabrielson, I.
       W. & Klatskin, E. H.   An exploration study of acci-
       dental ingestion of poison in young children.   *Jour-
       nal of the American Academy of Child Psychiatry*,
       1966, *5*, 255-271.
0893   *Millican, F. K., Layman, E. M., Lourie, R. S. & Taka-
       hashi, L. Y.   Study of an oral fixation: Pica.   *Jour-
       nal of the American Academy of Child Psychiatry*, 1968,
       7, 79-107.
0893.1 de la Burde, B. & Reames, B.   Prevention of pica, the
       major cause of lead poisoning in children.   *American
       Journal of Public Health*, 1973, *63*, 737-743.
0894   *Stein, M. L., Rausen, A. R. & Blau, A.   Psychotherapy
       of an infant with rumination.   *Journal of the Ameri-
       can Medical Association*, 1959, *171*, 2309-2312.
0895   *Werkman, S. L., Shifman, L. & Skelly, T.   Psychosocial
       correlates of iron deficiency anemia in early child-
       hood.   *Psychosomatic Medicine*, 1964, *26*, 125-134.
0896   *Whitten, C. F., Pettit, M. G. & Fischhoff, J.   Evidence
       that growth failure from maternal deprivation is
       secondary to undereating.   *Journal of the American
       Medical Association*, 1969, *209*, 1675-1682.
0897   Davenport, C. W., Zrull, J. P., Kuhn, C. C. & Harrison,
       S. I.   Cyclic vomiting.   *Journal of the American Acad-
       emy of Child Psychiatry*, 1972, *11*, 66-87.

OBESITY

0898   *Crisp, A. H., Douglas, J. W. B., Ross, J. M. & Stone-
       hill, E.   Some developmental aspects of disorders of
       weight. *Journal of Psychosomatic Research,* 1970, *14,*
       313-320.
0899   *Eid, E. E.   Follow-up study of physical growth of chil-
       dren who had excessive weight gain in first six
       months of life. *British Medical Journal,* 1970, *2,*
       no. 5670, 74-76.
0900   *Stunkard, A. J. & Wolff, H. G.   Pathogenesis in human
       obesity: Function and disorder of a mechanism of
       satiety. *Psychosomatic Medicine,* 1958, *20,* 17-29.
0901   *Penick, S. B. & Stunkard, A. J.   Newer concepts of
       obesity. *Medical Clinics of North America,* 1970,
       54(3), 745-754.
0902   *Kahn, E. J.   Obesity in children: Identification of a
       group at risk in a New York ghetto. *Journal of
       Pediatrics,* 1970, *77,* 771-774.
0903   Coddington, R. D. & Bruch, H.   Gastric perceptivity in
       normal, obese and schizophrenic subjects. *Psycho-
       somatics,* 1970, *11,* 571-579.
0904   Knittle, J. L.   Childhood obesity. *Bulletin of the New
       York Academy of Medicine,* 1971, *47,* 579-589.
0905   Bruch, H.   Psychological aspects of obesity. *Psychia-
       try,* 1947, *10,* 373-381.
0906   *Bruch, H.   Juvenile obesity: Its course and outcome.
       International Psychiatry Clinics, 1970, *7*(1), 231-
       254.
0907   Werkman, S. L. & Greenberg, E. S.   Personality and
       interest patterns in obese adolescent girls. *Psycho-
       somatic Medicine,* 1967, *29,* 72-80.
0908   Nathan, S. & Pisula, D.   Psychological observations of
       obese adolescents during starvation treatment. *Jour-
       nal of the American Academy of Child Psychiatry,* 1970,
       9, 722-740.
0909   Bruch, H.   Obesity in adolescence. In J. G. Howells
       (Ed.), *Modern perspectives in adolescent psychiatry.*
       Edinburgh: Oliver & Boyd, 1971. Pp. 254-273. (Mod-
       ern perspectives in psychiatry, vol. 4)
0910   Berlin, I. N., Boatman, M. J., Sheimo, S. L. & Szurek,
       S. A.   Adolescent alternation of anorexia and obes-
       ity.   Workshop, 1950. *American Journal of Orthopsy-
       chiatry,* 1951, *21,* 387-419.
0911   *Penick, S. B., Filion, R., Fox, S., & Stunkard, A. J.
       Behavior modification in the treatment of obesity.
       Psychosomatic Medicine, 1971, *33,* 49-55.
0912   *Fromm, E.   Dynamics in a case of obesity. *Journal of
       Clinical and Experimental Psychopathology and Quarter-
       ly Review of Psychiatry and Neurology,* 1958, *19,* 292-
       302.

0912.1   Levitz, L. S. and Stunkard, A. J. A therapeutic coali-
          tion for obesity: Behavior modification and patient
          self-help. *American Journal of Psychiatry*, 1974, *131*,
          423-427.

PSYCHOSOMATIC RESPONSES TO INJURY AND DISEASE

0913   *Blau, A. The psychiatric approach to posttraumatic and
          postencephalitic syndromes. *Research Publications of
          the Association for Research in Nervous and Mental
          Disease*, 1954, *34*, 404-423.
0914   *Levy, S. Post-encephalitic behavior disorder - A for-
          gotten entity: A report of 100 cases. *American Jour-
          nal of Psychiatry*, 1959, *115*, 1062-1067.
0915   *Holden, R. H. A review of psychological studies in
          cerebral palsy: 1947 to 1952. *American Journal of
          Mental Deficiency*, 1952, *57*, 92-99.
0916   *Harrington, J. A. & Letemendia, F. J. J. Persistent
          psychiatric disorders after head injuries in children.
          Journal of Mental Science, 1958, *104*, 1205-1218.
0917   *Pechtel, C. & Masserman, J. H. Cerebral localization:
          Not where but in whom? *American Journal of Psychia-
          try*, 1959, *116*, 51-54.
0918   *Mei-tal, V., Meyerowitz, S. & Engel, G. L. The role of
          psychological process in a somatic disorder: Multi-
          ple sclerosis. 1. The emotional setting of illness
          onset and exacerbation. *Psychosomatic Medicine*, 1970,
          32, 67-86.
0919   *Hilgard, J. R. & Szurek, S. A. Successful psychother-
          apy of a choreic syndrome. *Psychosomatic Medicine*,
          1943, *5*, 293-300.
0920   *Galdston, R. & Gamble, W. J. On borrowed time: Obser-
          vations on children with implanted cardiac pacemakers
          and their families. *American Journal of Psychiatry*,
          1969, *126*, 104-108.
0921   Bergman, A. The morbidity of cardiac nondisease in
          schoolchildren. *New England Journal of Medicine*,
          1967, *276*, 1008-1013.
0922   *Stone, W. E. Utilization of a pediatrician in a mental
          health clinic. II. An affluent community. *Pediat-
          rics*, 1970, *46*, 807-809.
0923   Apley, J. The child with recurrent abdominal pain.
          Pediatric Clinics of North America, 1967, *14*(1), 63-
          72.
0924   *Thomas, L. A., Milman, D. H. & Rodriguez-Torres, R.
          Anxiety in children with rheumatic fever: Relation
          to route of prophylaxis. *Journal of the American
          Medical Association*, 1970, *212*, 2080-2085.
0925   Jessner, L. Some observations on children hospitalized
          during latency. In *Dynamic psychopathology in child-
          hood*. New York: Grune & Stratton, 1959. Pp. 257-
          268.

0926   Apley, J. & Naish, N. Recurrent abdominal pains: A
        field survey of 1,000 school children. *Archives of
        Disease in Childhood*, 1958, *33*, 165-170.
0927   *Bernabeu, E. P. The effects of severe crippling on the
        development of a group of children. *Psychiatry*, 1958,
        21, 169-194.
0928   Schechter, M. D. The orthopedically handicapped child:
        Emotional reactions. *Archives of General Psychiatry*,
        1961, *4*, 247-253.
0929   *Watson, E. J. & Johnson, A. M. The emotional signifi-
        cance of acquired physical disfigurement in children.
        American Journal of Orthopsychiatry, 1958, *28*, 85-97.
0929.1 Sultz, H. A., Schlesinger, E. R., Mosher, W. E., & Feld-
        man, J. G. *Long-term childhood illness*. Pittsburgh,
        Pa.: University of Pittsburgh Press, 1972.
0929.2 Galdston, R. The burning and the healing of children.
        In S. Chess & A. Thomas (Eds.), *Annual progress in
        child psychiatry and child development: 1973*. New
        York: Brunner/Mazel, 1974. Pp. 464-478.

SEIZURES

0930   *Aird, R. B. Clinical syndromes of the limbic system.
        International Journal of Neurology, 1967, *6*, 340-
        352.
0931   *Focher, L. Convulsivinism. *Journal of the American
        Academy of Child Psychiatry*, 1965, *4*, 513-520.
0932   Gibbs, F. A. Abnormal electrical activity in the
        temporal regions and its relationship to abnormalities
        of behavior. *Research Publications of the Association
        for Research in Nervous and Mental Disease*, 1956, *36*,
        278-294.
0933   Aaronson, B. S. The influence of seizure perception on
        seizure occurrence. *Journal of Nervous and Mental
        Disease*, 1957, *125*, 507-510.
0934   Blau, A. The psychiatric approach to posttraumatic and
        postencephalitic syndromes. *Research Publications of
        the Association for Research in Nervous and Mental
        Disease*, 1954, *34*, 404-423.
0935   *Pechtel, C. & Masserman, J. H. Cerebral localization:
        Not where but in whom? *American Journal of Psychia-
        try*, 1959, *116*, 51-54.
0936   *Berlin, I. N. & Yeager, C. L. Correlation of epileptic
        seizures, electroencephalograms and emotional state:
        Some preliminary observations in several children.
        American Journal of Diseases of Children, 1951, *81*,
        664-670.
0937   *Gooddy, W. The borderland of epilepsy today as illus-
        trated by fits in adolescence. *Practitioner*, 1971,
        206, 207-214.

0938   Gottschalk, L. A. Psychological conflict and electro-
        encephalographic patterns: Some notes on the problem
        of correlating changes in paroxysmal electroencephalo-
        graphic patterns with psychologic conflicts. *Archives
        of Neurology and Psychiatry*, 1955, *73*, 656-662.
0939   *Gottschalk, L. A. The relationship of psychologic state
        and epileptic activity. Psychoanalytic observations
        on an epileptic child. *Psychoanalytic Study of the
        Child*, 1956, *11*, 352-380.
0940   *Epstein, A. W. & Ervin, F. Psychodynamic significance
        of seizure content in psychomotor epilepsy. *Psycho-
        somatic Medicine*, 1956, *18*, 43-55.
0941   *Fuchs, L. L. A psychogenic approach to epilepsy.
        Journal of Child Psychiatry, 1947, *1*, 58-90.
0942   Freedman, D. A. & Adatto, C. P. On the precipitation
        of seizures in an adolescent boy. *Psychosomatic
        Medicine*, 1968, *30*, 437-447.
0943   Bernstein, N. R. Psychogenic seizures in adolescent
        girls. *Behavioral Neuropsychiatry*, 1969, *1*(1), 31-
        34.
0944   *Libo, S. S., Palmer, C. & Archibald, D. Family group
        therapy for children with self-induced seizures.
        American Journal of Orthopsychiatry, 1971, *41*, 506-
        509.
0945   Tippett, D. L. & Pine, I. Denial mechanisms in masked
        epilepsy. *Psychosomatic Medicine*, 1957, *19*, 326-
        331.
0946   Zegans, L. S., Kooi, K. A., Waggoner, R. W. & Kemph,
        J. P. Effects of psychiatric interview upon paroxys-
        mal cerebral activity and autonomic measures in a
        disturbed child with petit mal epilepsy. *Psychosoma-
        tic Medicine*, 1964, *26*, 151-161.
0947   Rothenberg, M. B. & Voeller, K. K. S. Psychosocial
        aspects of the management of seizures in children.
        Pediatrics, 1973, *51*, 1072-1082.
0948   *Kelman, D. H. Gilles de la Tourette's disease in chil-
        dren: A review of the literature. *Journal of Child
        Psychology and Psychiatry and Allied Disciplines*,
        1965, *6*, 219-226.
0949   Lucas, A. R., Kauffman, P. E. & Morris, E. M. Gilles
        de la Tourette's disease: A clinical study of fif-
        teen cases. *Journal of the American Academy of Child
        Psychiatry*, 1967, *6*, 700-722.
0950   *Monsour, K. J. Migraine: Dynamics and choice of symp-
        tom. *Psychoanalytic Quarterly*, 1957, *26*, 476-493.
0951   *Markowitz, I. Psychotherapy of narcolepsy in an adoles-
        cent boy: Case presentation. *Psychiatric Quarterly*,
        1957, *31*, 41-56.

SKIN

0952   *Meerloo, J. A. M. Human camouflage and identification
        with the environment: The contagious effect of ar-
        chaic skin signs. *Psychosomatic Medicine*, 1957, *19*,
        89-98.
0953   *Seitz, P. F. D. Psychocutaneous conditioning during
        the first two weeks of life. *Psychosomatic Medicine*,
        1950, *12*, 187-188.
0954   Rosenthal, M. J. Neuropsychiatric aspects of infantile
        eczema: Special reference to the role of cutaneous
        pain receptors. *Archives of Neurology and Psychiatry*,
        1953, *70*, 428-451.
0955   *Mohr, G. J., Tausend, H., Selesnick, S. & Augenbraun,
        B. Studies of eczema and asthma in the preschool
        child. *Journal of the American Academy of Child Psy-
        chiatry*, 1963, *2*, 271-291.
0956   Kepecs, J. G., Robin, M. & Munro, C. Responses to
        sensory stimulation in certain psychosomatic dis-
        orders. *Psychosomatic Medicine*, 1958, *20*, 351-365.
0957   Yeh, Eng-kung. Recurrent urticaria alternating with
        psychosis: Report of a case. *Psychosomatic Medicine*,
        1958, *20*, 373-378.
0957.1 Early, L. F. & Lifschutz, J. E. A case of stigmata.
        Archives of General Psychiatry, 1974, *30*, 197-200.
0957.2 Seligman, R. A psychiatric classification system for
        burned children. *American Journal of Psychiatry*,
        1974, *131*, 41-46.

SPEECH, HEARING AND DEAFNESS

0958   *Barbara, D. A. Stuttering. In S. Arieti (Ed.), *Amer-
        ican handbook of psychiatry*. Vol. 1. New York:
        Basic Books, 1959. Pp. 950-963.
0959   *Despert, J. L. Psychosomatic study of fifty stuttering
        children. Round Table. I. Social, physical and psy-
        chiatric findings. *American Journal of Orthopsychia-
        try*, 1946, *16*, 100-113.
0960   Eisenson, J. *Stuttering: A symposium*. New York:
        Harper, 1958.
0961   *Schneer, H. I. & Hewlett, I. W. A family approach to
        stuttering with group therapy techniques. *Interna-
        tional Journal of Group Psychotherapy*, 1958, *8*, 329-
        341.
0962   *Reed, G. F. Elective mutism in children: A re-apprais-
        al. *Journal of Child Psychology and Psychiatry and
        Allied Disciplines*, 1963, *4*, 99-107.
0963   *Browne, E., Wilson, V. & Laybourne, P. C. Diagnosis
        and treatment of elective mutism in children. *Jour-
        nal of the American Academy of Child Psychiatry*, 1963,
        2, 605-617.

0964   Pustrom, E. & Speers, R. W. Elective mutism in chil-
        dren. *Journal of the American Academy of Child Psy-
        chiatry*, 1964, *3*, 287-297.
0965   *Shaw, W. H. Aversive control in the treatment of elec-
        tive mutism. *Journal of the American Academy of Child
        Psychiatry*, 1971, *10*, 572-581.
0966   Schlesinger, H. S. Beyond the range of sound: The
        non-otological aspects of deafness. *California Medi-
        cine*, 1969, *110*, 213-217.
0967   *Schlesinger, H. S. The deaf preschooler and his many
        faces. In *International research seminar on the
        vocational rehabilitation of deaf persons*. Washing-
        ton: Social and Rehabilitation Service, 1968.
        Pp. 345-353.
0968   *Hefferman, A. A psychiatric study of fifty preschool
        children referred to hospital for suspected deafness.
        In G. Caplan (Ed.), *Emotional problems of early child-
        hood*. New York: Basic Books, 1955. Pp. 269-292.
0969   Meadow, K. P. Early manual communication in relation
        to the deaf child's intellectual, social, and communi-
        cative functioning. *American Annals of the Deaf*,
        1968, *113*, 29-41.
0969.1 Schlesinger, H. S. New perspectives on manual communi-
        cation. In H. S. Schlesinger and K. P. Meadow,
        Sound and sign: Childhood deafness and mental health.
        Berkeley: University of California Press, 1972.
        Pp. 31-44.
0970   *Meadow, K. P. Parental response to the medical ambigui-
        ties of congenital deafness. *Journal of Health and
        Social Behavior*, 1968, *9*, 299-309.
0971   *Schlesinger, H. S. & Meadow, K. P. *Sound and sign:
        Childhood deafness and mental health*. Berkeley:
        University of California Press, 1972.
0971.1 Schlesinger, H. S. A developmental model applied to
        problems of deafness. In H. S. Schlesinger and K.
        P. Meadow, *Sound and sign: Childhood deafness and
        mental health*. Berkeley: University of California
        Press, 1972. Pp. 7-30.
0971.2 Meadow, K. P., Schlesinger, H. S. & Holstein, C. B.
        The developmental process in deaf preschool children:
        Communicative competence and socialization. In H. S.
        Schlesinger and K. P. Meadow, *Sound and sign: Child-
        hood deafness and mental health*. Berkeley: Univer-
        sity of California Press, 1972. Pp. 88-110.
0971.3 Schlesinger, H. S. Language acquisition in four deaf
        children. In H. S. Schlesinger and K. P. Meadow,
        *Sound and sign: Childhood deafness and mental
        health*. Berkeley: University of California Press,
        1972. Pp. 45-87.
0971.4 Meadow, K. P. Developmental aspects of deafness in the
        school years. In H. S. Schlesinger and K. P. Meadow,
        Sound and sign: Childhood deafness and mental health.
        Berkeley: University of California Press, 1972.
        Pp. 111-149.

0971.5　　Bolton, B.　A behavior-oriented treatment program for deaf clients in a comprehensive rehabilitation center. *American Journal of Orthopsychiatry*, 1974, *44*, 376-385.

ULCER (PEPTIC)

0972　　*Sultz, H. A. et al.　The epidemiology of peptic ulcer in childhood. *American Journal of Public Health*, 1970, *60*, 492-498.

0973　　*Millar, T. P.　Peptic ulcers in children.　In J. G. Howells (Ed.), *Modern perspectives in international child psychiatry*. Edinburgh: Oliver & Boyd, 1969. Pp. 471-493.　(Modern perspectives in psychiatry, vol. 3)

0974　　*Taboroff, L. H. & Brown, W. H.　A study of the personality patterns of children and adolescents with the peptic ulcer syndrome. *American Journal of Orthopsychiatry*, 1954, *24*, 602-610.

0974.1　　Lidz, T. & Rubenstein, R.　Psychology of gastrointestinal disorders.　In S. Arieti (Ed.), *American Handbook of Psychiatry*. Vol. 1.　New York:　Basic Books, 1959. Pp. 678-689.

0974.2　　Sultz, H. A., Schlesinger, E. R., Mosher, W. E. & Feldman, J. G.　Peptic ulcer.　In *Long-term childhood illness*. Pittsburgh, Pa.:　University of Pittsburgh Press, 1972.　Pp. 381-401.

ULCERATIVE COLITIS

0975　　*Ein, S. H., Lynch, M. J. & Stephens, C. A.　Ulcerative colitis in children under one year:　A twenty-year review. *Journal of Pediatric Surgery*, 1971, *6*, 264-271.

0976　　*McDermott, J. F. & Finch, S. M.　Ulcerative colitis in children:　Reassessment of a dilemma. *Journal of the American Academy of Child Psychiatry*, 1967, *6*, 512-525.

0977　　*Mohr, G. J., Josselyn, I. M., Spurlock, J. & Barron, S. H.　Studies in ulcerative colitis. *American Journal of Psychiatry*, 1958, *114*, 1067-1076.

0978　　*Reinhart, J. B. & Succop, R. A.　Regional enteritis in pediatric patients:　Psychiatric aspects. *Journal of the American Academy of Child Psychiatry*, 1968, *7*, 252-281.

0979　　*Sperling, M.　Ulcerative colitis in children:　Current views and therapies. *Journal of the American Academy of Child Psychiatry*, 1969, *8*, 336-352.

0980　　Sperling, M.　Mucous colitis associated with phobias. *Psychoanalytic Quarterly*, 1950, *19*, 318-326.

0981   McKegney, F. P., Gordon, R. O. & Levine, S. M. A psychosomatic comparison of patients with ulcerative colitis and Crohn's disease. *Psychosomatic Medicine*, 1970, *32*, 153-166.

0982   *Blom, G. E. Ulcerative colitis in a five-year-old boy. In G. Caplan (Ed.), *Emotional problems of early childhood*. New York: Basic Books, 1955. Pp. 169-198.

0983   *Prugh, D. G. & Jordan, K. The management of ulcerative colitis in childhood. In J. G. Howells (Ed.), *Modern perspectives in international child psychiatry*. Edinburgh: Oliver & Boyd, 1969. Pp. 494-530. (Modern perspectives in psychiatry, vol. 3)

0983.1   Finch, S. M. & Hess, J. H. Ulcerative colitis in children. *American Journal of Psychiatry*, 1962, *118*, 819-826.

MISCELLANEOUS CONDITIONS

0984   Richmond, J. B. Discussion of "juvenile paroxysmal supraventricular tachycardia: Psychosomatic and psychodynamic aspects". *Journal of the American Academy of Child Psychiatry*, 1962, *1*, 265-268.

0985   Rahe, R. H. & Christ, A. E. An unusual cardiac (ventricular) arrhythmia in a child: Psychiatric and psychophysiologic aspects. *Psychosomatic Medicine*, 1966, *28*, 181-188.

0986   Falstein, E. I. & Rosenblum, A. H. Juvenile paroxysmal supraventricular tachycardia: Psychosomatic and psychodynamic aspects. *Journal of the American Academy of Child Psychiatry*, 1962, *1*, 246-264.

0987   Boswell, J. I., Lewis, C. P., Freeman, D. F. & Clark, K. M. Hyperthyroid children: Individual and family dynamics. A study of twelve cases. *Journal of the American Academy of Child Psychiatry*, 1967, *6*, 64-85.

0988   Cytryn, L., Cytryn, E. & Rieger, R. E. Psychological implications of cryptorchism. *Journal of the American Academy of Child Psychiatry*, 1967, *6*, 131-165.

0989   Engels, W. D., Pattee, C. J. & Wittkower, E. D. Emotional settings of functional amenorrhea. *Psychosomatic Medicine*, 1964, *26*, 682-700.

0990   Mattsson, A., Gross, S. & Hall, T. Psychoendocrine study of adaptation in young hemophiliacs. *Psychosomatic Medicine*, 1971, *33*, 215-225.

0991   Reinhart, J. B. & Drash, A. L. Psychosocial dwarfism: Environmentally induced recovery. *Psychosomatic Medicine*, 1969, *31*, 165-172.

0992   Thomas, L. A., Milman, D. H. & Rodriguez-Torres, R. Anxiety in children with rheumatic fever: Relation to route of prophylaxis. *Journal of the American Medical Association*, 1970, *212*, 2080-2085.

0993   Schorer, C. E. Muscular dystrophy and the mind. *Psy-chosomatic Medicine*, 1964, *26*, 5-13.
0994   Meares, R. Features which distinguish groups of spas-modic torticollis. *Journal of Psychosomatic Research*, 1971, *15*, 1-11.
0995   Eldridge, R., Riklan, M. & Cooper, I. S. The limited role of psychotherapy in torsion dystonia: Experience with 44 cases. *Journal of the American Medical Asso-ciation*, 1969, *210*, 705-708.
0996   Silberstein, R. M., Blackman, S. & Mandell, W. Auto-erotic head banging: A reflection on the opportunism of infants. *Journal of the American Academy of Child Psychiatry*, 1966, *5*, 235-242.
0997   Greenberg, N. H. Origins of head-rolling (spasmus nu-tans) during early infancy: Clinical observations and theoretical implications. *Psychosomatic Medicine*, 1964, *26*, 162-171.
0998   Meyer, E., Unger, H. T. & Slaughter, R. Investigation of a psychosocial hypothesis in appendectomies. *Psy-chosomatic Medicine*, 1964, *26*, 671-681.
0999   Wolff, S. Illness and going to hospital. In *Children under stress*. London: Allen Lane, Penguin Press, 1969. Pp. 51-74.
1000   Kivowitz, J. & Corcoran, J. Theoretical and practical considerations of Klinefelter's Syndrome in children: A report of three cases of 47 XXY. *Journal of the American Academy of Child Psychiatry*, 1971, *10*, 700-712.
1000.1 Sultz, H. A., Schlesinger, E. R., Mosher, W. E. & Feld-man, J. G. The nephrotic syndrome and related condi-tions. In *Long-term childhood illness*. Pittsburgh, Pa.: University of Pittsburgh Press, 1972. Pp. 345-379.
1000.2 Sultz, H. A., Schlesinger, E. R., Mosher, W. E. & Feld-man, J. G. Blood dyscrasias. In *Long-term childhood illness*. Pittsburgh, Pa.: University of Pittsburgh Press, 1972. Pp. 283-344.
1000.3 Bernstein, D. M. After transplantation: The child's emotional reactions. *American Journal of Psychiatry*, 1971, *127*, 1189-1193.
1000.4 Kaplan De-Nour, A. & Czaczkes, J. W. Emotional prob-lems and reactions of the medical team in a chronic haemodialysis unit. *Lancet*, 1968, *2*, 987-991.
1000.5 Kemph, J. P., Bermann, E. A. & Coppolillo, H. P. Kidney transplants and shifts in family dynamics. *American Journal of Psychiatry*, 1969, *125*, 1485-1490.
1000.6 Korsch, B. M., Fine, R. N., Grushkin, C. M. & Negrete, V. F. Experiences with children and their families during extended hemodialysis and kidney transplanta-tion. *Pediatric Clinics of North America*, 1971, *18*, 625-637.

1000.7   Simmons, R. G. & Klein, S. D. Family noncommunication: the search for kidney donors. *American Journal of Psychiatry*, 1972, *129*, 687-692.
1000.8   Lesser, S. R. & Easser, B. R. Personality differences in the perceptually handicapped. In S. Chess & A. Thomas (Eds.), *Annual progress in child psychiatry and child development: 1973*. New York: Brunner/ Mazel, 1974. Pp. 396-404.
1000.9   Anders, T. F. & Weinstein, P. Sleep and its disorders in infants and children: A review. In S. Chess & A. Thomas (Eds.), *Annual progress in child psychiatry and child development: 1973*. New York: Brunner/ Mazel, 1974. Pp. 377-395.
1000.11 Chess, S. Neurological dysfunction and childhood behavioral pathology. In S. Chess & A. Thomas (Eds.), *Annual progress in child psychiatry and child development: 1973*. New York: Brunner/Mazel, 1974. Pp. 405-418.
1000.12 Sultz, H. A., Schlesinger, E. R., Mosher, W. E. & Feldman, J. G. Encephalitis and encephalomyelitis. In *Long-term childhood illness*. Pittsburgh, Pa.: University of Pittsburgh Press, 1972. Pp. 403-426.

DISABILITY AND WORK WITH THE FAMILY

1001   Offord, D. R. & Aponte, J. F. Distortion of disability and effect on family life. *Journal of the American Academy of Child Psychiatry*, 1967, *6*, 499-511.
1002   Green, M. Care of the child with a long-term, life-threatening illness: Some principles of management. *Pediatrics*, 1967, *39*, 441-445.
1003   Nolfi, M. W. Families in grief: The question of casework intervention. *Social Work*, 1967, *12*(4), 40-46.
1004   Lang, P. & Oppenheimer, J. The influence of social work when parents are faced with the fatal illness of a child. *Social Casework*, 1968, *49*, 161-166.

ADDITIONAL REFERENCES

1005   Caplan, G. *Emotional problems of early childhood.* New York: Basic Books, 1955.
1006   Deutsch, F. *The psychosomatic concept in psychoanalysis.* New York: International Universities Press, 1953.
1007   Engel, G. L. *Psychological development in health and disease.* Philadelphia: Saunders, 1962.
1008   Garner, A. M. & Wenar, C. *The mother-child interaction in psychosomatic disorders.* Urbana: University of Illinois Press, 1959.

1009   Ruesch, J. The infantile personality: The core prob-
        lem of psychosomatic medicine. *Psychosomatic Medi-
        cine*, 1948, *10*, 134-144.
1010   Szasz, T. S. *Pain and pleasure*. New York: Basic
        Books, 1957.

VII. HYPERACTIVITY

OVERVIEW - HISTORICAL - TERMINOLOGY

1011   *Chess, S. Diagnosis and treatment of the hyperactive
        child. *New York State Journal of Medicine*, 1960,
        60, 2379-2385.
1012   *Clements, S. D. & Peters, J. E. Minimal brain dysfunc-
        tions in the schoolage child: Diagnosis and treat-
        ment. *Archives of General Psychiatry*, 1962, *6*, 185-
        197.
1013   *Clements, S. D. Minimal brain dysfunction in children;
        terminology and identification, phase one of three-
        phase project. [Washington] 1966, part 1. (NINDB
        monograph, no. 3)
1014   *O'Malley, J. E. & Eisenberg, L. The hyperkinetic syn-
        drome. *Seminars in Psychiatry*, 1973, *5*, 95-103.
        (Also in S. Walzer & P. H. Wolff (Eds.), *Minimal cere-
        bral dysfunction in children*. New York: Grune &
        Stratton, 1973. Pp. 95-103.
1015   *Stewart, M. A., Pitts, F. N., Craig, A. G. & Dieruf, W.
        The hyperactive child syndrome. *American Journal of
        Orthopsychiatry*, 1966, *36*, 861-867.
1016   *Werry, J. S., Weiss, G. & Douglas, V. Studies on the
        hyperactive child. I: Some preliminary findings.
        Canadian Psychiatric Association Journal, 1964, *9*,
        120-130.
1017   Bakwin, H. Developmental hyperactivity. *Acta Paedia-
        trica Scandinavica*, 1967, *Supplement 172*, 25-29.
1018   Laufer, M. W., Denhoff, E. & Solomons, G. Hyperkinetic
        impulse disorder in children's behavior problems.
        Psychosomatic Medicine, 1957, *19*, 38-49.
1019   Pincus, J. H. & Glaser, G. H. The syndrome of "minimal
        brain damage" in childhood. *New England Journal of
        Medicine*, 1966, *275*, 27-35.
1020   Rutter, M., et al. A tri-axial classification of men-
        tal disorders in childhood: An international study.
        *Journal of Child Psychology and Psychiatry and Allied
        Disciplines*, 1969, *10*, 41-61.
1020.1 Morrison, J. R. & Stewart, M. A. The psychiatric
        status of the legal families of adopted hyperactive
        children. *Archives of General Psychiatry*, 1973, *28*,
        888-891.
1020.2 Gardner, R. W. Evolution and brain injury. In S. G.
        Sapir & A. C. Nitzburg (Eds.), *Children with learning
        problems: Readings in a developmental-interaction*

approach. New York: Brunner/Mazel, 1973. Pp. 241-251.

1020.3   Strother, C. R. Minimal cerebral dysfunction: An historical overview. In S. G. Sapir & A. C. Nitzburg (Eds.), *Children with learning problems: Readings in a developmental-interaction approach.* New York: Brunner/Mazel, 1973. Pp. 173-186.

PREVALENCE

1021   *Huessy, H. R. Study of the prevalence and therapy of the choreatiform syndrome or hyperkinesis in rural Vermont. *Acta Paedopsychiatrica,* 1967, *34,* 130-135.

1022   Minde, K., Weiss, G. & Mendelson, N. A 5-year follow-up study of 91 hyperactive school children. *Journal of the American Academy of Child Psychiatry,* 1972, *11,* 595-610.

1023   Paine, R. S., Werry, J. S. & Quay, H. C. A study of 'minimal cerebral dysfunction'. *Developmental Medicine and Child Neurology,* 1968, *10,* 505.

1024   Prechtl, H. F. R. & Stemmer, C. J. The choreiform syndrome in children. *Developmental Medicine and Child Neurology,* 1962, *4,* 119-127.

1025   Stewart, M. A., Pitts, F. N., Craig, A. G. & Dieruf, W. The hyperactive child syndrome. *American Journal of Orthopsychiatry,* 1966, *36,* 861-867.

1026   Wender, P. H. *Minimal brain dysfunction in children.* New York: Wiley-Interscience, 1971.

1027   Werry, J. S., Weiss, G. & Douglas, V. Studies on the hyperactive child. I: Some preliminary findings. *Canadian Psychiatric Association Journal,* 1964, *9,* 120-130.

1027.1   Birch, H. G. & Lefford, A. Two strategies for studying perception in "brain-damaged" children. In S. G. Sapir & A. C. Nitzburg (Eds.), *Children with learning problems: Readings in a developmental-interaction approach.* New York: Brunner/Mazel, 1973. Pp. 335-349.

1027.2   Kosc, L. Developmental dyscalculia. *Journal of Learning Disabilities,* 1974, *7,* 164-177.

1027.3   Chess, S. Neurological dysfunction and childhood behavioral pathology. *Journal of Autism and Childhood Schizophrenia,* 1972, *2,* 299-311.

NATURAL HISTORY

1028   *Eisenberg, L. The management of the hyperkinetic child. *Developmental Medicine and Child Neurology,* 1966, *8,* 593-598.

1029 *Weiss, G., Minde, K., Werry, J. S., Douglas, V. &
Nemeth, E. Studies on the hyperactive child. VIII.
Five-year follow-up. *Archives of General Psychiatry,*
1971, *24,* 409-414.

1030 Campbell, S. B., Douglas, V. I. & Morgenstern, C. Cognitive styles in hyperactive children and the effect
of methylphenidate. *Journal of Child Psychology and
Psychiatry and Allied Disciplines,* 1971, *12,* 55-67.

1031 Minde, K., Webb, B. & Sykes, D. Studies on the hyperactive child. VI. Prenatal and paranatal factors
associated with hyperactivity. *Developmental Medicine and Child Neurology,* 1968, *10,* 355-363.

1031.1 Carter, S. & Gold, A. P. The nervous system: Diagno-
sis of neurologic disease. In S. G. Sapir & A. C.
Nitzburg (Eds.), *Children with learning problems:
Readings in a developmental-interaction approach.*
New York: Brunner/Mazel, 1973. Pp. 569-585.

1031.2 Myklebust, H. R. Learning disorders--Psychoneurologi-
cal disturbances in childhood. In S. G. Sapir & A. C.
Nitzburg (Eds.), *Children with learning problems:
Readings in a developmental-interaction approach.*
New York: Brunner/Mazel, 1973. Pp. 257-269.

1031.3 Rappaport, S. R. The brain damage syndrome. In S. G.
Sapir & A. C. Nitzburg (Eds.), *Children with learning
problems: Readings in a developmental-interaction
approach.* New York: Brunner/Mazel, 1973. Pp. 252-
256.

1031.4 Satterfield, J. H., Cantwell, D. P., Lesser, L. I. &
Podosin, R. L. Physiological studies of the hyperkinetic child: I. *American Journal of Psychiatry,*
1972, *128,* 1418-1424.

1031.5 de la Cruz, F. F., Fox, B. H. & Roberts, R. H. (Eds.)
Minimal brain dysfunction. New York: New York Academy of Sciences, 1973.

1031.6 Morrison, J. R. & Stewart, M. A. Evidence for poly-
genetic inheritance in the hyperactive child syndrome. *American Journal of Psychiatry,* 1973, *130,*
791-792.

1031.7 Satterfield, J. H., Cantwell, D. P., Saul, R. E. &
Yusin, A. Intelligence, academic achievement, and
EEG abnormalities in hyperactive children. *American
Journal of Psychiatry,* 1974, *131,* 391-395.

TREATMENT

1032 *Conners, C. K. & Eisenberg, L. The effects of methylphenidate on symptomatology and learning in disturbed
children. *American Journal of Psychiatry,* 1963, *120,*
458-464.

1033 *Conners, C. K., Eisenberg, L. & Barcai, A. Effect of
dextroamphetamine on children: Studies on subjects

with learning disabilities and school behavior problems. *Archives of General Psychiatry*, 1967, *17*, 478-485.

1034   *Eisenberg, L. Symposium: Behavior modification by drugs. III. The clinical use of stimulant drugs in children. *Pediatrics*, 1972, *49*, 709-715.

1035   *Millichap, J. G. Drugs in management of hyperkinetic and perceptually handicapped children. *Journal of the American Medical Association*, 1968, *206*, 1527-1530.

1036   Alexandris, A. & Lundell, F. W. Effect of thioridazine, amphetamine and placebo on the hyperkinetic syndrome and cognitive area in mentally deficient children. *Canadian Medical Association Journal*, 1968, *98*, 92-96.

1037   Conners, C. K. A teacher rating scale for use in drug studies with children. *American Journal of Psychiatry*, 1969, *126*, 884-888.

1038   Conners, C. K. & Eisenberg, L. The effects of methylphenidate on symptomatology and learning in disturbed children. *American Journal of Psychiatry*, 1963, *120*, 458-464.

1039   Conners, C. K. & Rothschild, G. H. Drugs and learning in children. In J. Hellmuth (Ed.), *Learning disorders*. Vol. 3. Seattle: Special Child Publications, 1968. Pp. 191-223.

1040   Fish, B. Drug therapy in child psychiatry: Pharmacological aspects. *Comprehensive Psychiatry*, 1960, *1*, 212-227.

1041   Fish, B. Drug use in psychiatric disorders of children. *American Journal of Psychiatry*, 1968, *124*, (no. 8 Supplement), 31-36.

1042   Grant, Q. R. Psychopharmacology in childhood emotional and mental disorders. *Journal of Pediatrics*, 1962, *61*, 626-637.

1043   Greenhill, L. L., Rieder, R. O., Wender, P. H., Buchsbaum, M. & Zahn, T. P. Lithium carbonate in the treatment of hyperactive children. *Archives of General Psychiatry*, 1973, *28*, 636-640.

1044   Lucas, A. R. & Weiss, M. Methylphenidate hallucinosis. *Journal of the American Medical Association*, 1971, *217*, 1079-1081.

1045   Ney, P. G. Psychosis in a child, associated with amphetamine administration. *Canadian Medical Association Journal*, 1967, *97*, 1026-1029.

1046   Sprague, R. L., Barnes, K. R. & Werry, J.S. Methylphenidate and thioridazine: Learning, reaction time, activity, and classroom behavior in disturbed children. *American Journal of Orthopsychiatry*, 1970, *40*, 615-628.

1047   Werry, J. S., Weiss, G., Douglas, V. & Martin, J. Studies on the hyperactive child. III: The effect of chlorpromazine upon behavior and learning ability.

Journal of the American Academy of Child Psychiatry, 1966, *5*, 292-312.

1048   Whitehead, P. L. & Clark, L. D.   Effect of lithium carbonate, placebo, and thioridazine on hyperactive children. *American Journal of Psychiatry*, 1970, *127*, 824-825.

1048.1   Gardner, R. A.   *MBD: The family book about minimal brain dysfunction.*   New York: Jason Aronson, 1973.

1048.2   Weil, A. P.   Children with minimal brain dysfunction: Diagnostic, dynamic and therapeutic considerations. In S. G. Sapir & A. C. Nitzburg (Eds.), *Children with learning problems: Readings in a developmental-interaction approach.*   New York: Brunner/Mazel, 1973. Pp. 551-568.

1048.3   Bateman, B. D.   Educational implications of minimal brain dysfunction.   In S. G. Sapir & A. C. Nitzburg (Eds.), *Children with learning problems: Readings in a developmental-interaction approach.*   New York: Brunner/Mazel, 1973. Pp. 674-681.

1048.4   Furman, S. & Feighner, A.   Video feedback in treating hyperkinetic children: A preliminary report. *American Journal of Psychiatry*, 1973, *130*, 792-796.

1048.5   Schnackenberg, R. C.   Caffeine as a substitute for schedule II stimulants in hyperkinetic children. *American Journal of Psychiatry*, 1973, *130*, 796-798.

1048.6   Grinspoon, L. & Singer, S. B.   Amphetamines in the treatment of hyperkinetic children. *Harvard Educational Review*, 1973, *43*, 515-555.

1048.7   Hoffman, S. P., Engelhardt, D. M., Margolis, R. A., Polizos, P., Waizer, J. & Rosenfeld, R.   Response to methylphenidate in low socioeconomic hyperactive children. *Archives of General Psychiatry*, 1974, *30*, 354-359.

VIII.   CHILDREN IN THE HOSPITAL AND DEATH AND DYING

CHILDREN IN THE HOSPITAL/Developmental Basis of Effects of Hospital Care

1049   *Ainsworth, M. D.   The effects of maternal deprivation: A review of findings and controversy in the context of research strategy.   In *Deprivation of maternal care: A reassessment of its effects.* Public health papers, no. 14. Geneva: World Health Organization, 1962. Pp. 97-165.

1050   *Bakwin, H.   Loneliness in infants. *American Journal of Diseases of Children*, 1942, *63*, 30-40.

1051   *Provence, S. A. & Lipton, R. C.   *Infants in institutions.* New York: International Universities Press, 1963.

1052   Bergmann, T. Observation of children's reactions to
        motor restraint. *Nervous Child*, 1945, *4*, 318-328.
1053   *Spitz, R. A. Hospitalism: An inquiry into the genesis
        of psychiatric conditions in early childhood. *Psycho-
        analytic Study of the Child*, 1946, *1*, 53-74.
1054   Bowlby, J. *Maternal care and mental health.* Geneva:
        World Health Organization, 1951. (Monograph series,
        no. 2)
1055   *Freud, A. The role of bodily illness in the mental
        life of children. *Psychoanalytic Study of the Child*,
        1952, *7*, 69-81. (*Writings*, vol. 4, pp. 260-279)
1056   *Winnicott, D. W. Transitional objects and transitional
        phenomena: A study of the first not-me possession.
        International Journal of Psychoanalysis, 1953, *34*,
        89-97.
1057   *Jessner, L. Some observations on children hospitalized
        during latency. In *Dynamic psychopathology in child-
        hood.* New York: Grune & Stratton, 1959. Pp. 257-
        268.
1058   Freud, A. & Burlingham, D. T. *War and children.* New
        York: Medical War Books, 1943.
1059   *Freud, A. & Burlingham, D. T. *Infants without families.*
        New York: International Universities Press, 1973.
        (*Writings*, vol. 3, pp. 543-664)
1060   Kaufman, R. V. Body-image changes in physically ill
        teen-agers. *Journal of the American Academy of Child
        Psychiatry*, 1972, *11*, 157-170.

CHILDREN IN THE HOSPITAL/Effect of Hospital Care and Procedures
on Children

1061   American Academy of Pediatrics. *Care of children in
        hospitals.* Evanston, Ill.: 1960.
1062   *Stern, R. A hospital is no place for people. *Resident
        and Staff Physician*, August 1971, *17*, 90-92.
1063   Vaughan, G. F. Children in hospital. *Lancet*, 1957,
        272, 1117-1120.
1065   *Great Britain. Play Committee. *The welfare of children
        in hospital.* London: Her Majesty's Stationery
        Office, 1959.
1066   *Bergmann, T. *Children in the hospital.* New York:
        International Universities Press, 1966.
1067   U.S. Department of Health, Education and Welfare. Chil-
        dren's Bureau. *Illness among children.* [Data from
        the U.S. National Health Survey, by C. G. Schiffer
        and E. P. Hunt.] Publication No. 405. Washington,
        D.C.: HEW, 1963.
1068   Vernon, D. T. A. et al. *The psychological responses of
        children to hospitalization and illness.* Springfield,
        Ill.: C. C. Thomas, 1965.

1069   *Prugh, D. G. Children's reactions to illness, hospital-
        ization, and surgery. In A. M. Freedman and H. I.
        Kaplan (Eds.), *Comprehensive textbook of psychiatry*.
        Baltimore: Williams & Wilkins, 1967. Pp. 1369-1376.
1070   Dimock, G. H. *The child in the hospital: A study of
        his emotional and social well-being*. Philadelphia:
        F. A. Davis, 1960.
1071   *Geist, H. *A child goes to the hospital: The psycholo-
        gical aspects of a child going to the hospital*.
        Springfield, Ill.: Thomas, 1965.
1072   Korsch, B. M. Psychologic principles in pediatric
        practice: The pediatrician and the sick child. *Ad-
        vances in Pediatrics*, 1958, *10*, 11-73.
1073   *Richmond, J. B. The pediatric patient in illness. In
        M. H. Hollender (Ed.), *The psychology of medical prac-
        tice*. Philadelphia: Saunders, 1958. Pp. 195-211.
1074   Schaffer, H. R. & Callender, W. M. Psychologic effects
        of hospitalization in infancy. *Pediatrics*, 1959, *24*,
        528-539.
1075   *Shore, M. F. (Ed.) *"Red is the color of hurting"*:
        Planning for children in the hospital. Bethesda:
        National Institute of Mental Health, National Insti-
        tutes of Health, 1967.
1076   Parry, L. A. The urgent need for reforms in hospitals.
        Lancet, 1947, *253*, 881-883.
1077   Loomis, E. A. The child's emotions and surgery. In
        W. B. Kiesewetter (Ed.), *Pre and post operative care
        in the pediatric surgical patient*. Chicago: Year
        Book Publishers, 1956.
1078   Levy, D. M. Psychic trauma of operations in children
        and a note on combat neurosis. *American Journal of
        Diseases of Children*, 1945, *69*, 7-25.
1079   *Pearson, G. H. J. Effect of operative procedures on
        the emotional life of the child. *American Journal of
        Diseases of Children*, 1941, *62*, 716-729.
1080   *Jessner, L., Blom, G. E. & Waldfogel, S. Emotional
        implications of tonsillectomy and adenoidectomy on
        children. *Psychoanalytic Study of the Child*, 1952,
        7, 126-169.
1081   Lipton, S. D. On the psychology of childhood tonsil-
        lectomy. *Psychoanalytic Study of the Child*, 1962,
        17, 363-417.
1083   Garrow, D. H. The tonsil and adenoid problem. *British
        Journal of Clinical Practice*, 1957, *11*, 218-220.
1084   *Werry, J. S. & Davenport, H. T. Effect of surgery and
        anesthesia on post-hospitalization adjustment in
        children. *Scientific Proceedings in Summary Form,
        Annual Meeting of the American Psychiatric Associa-
        tion*, 1969, 208-209.
1085   Toker, E. Psychiatric aspects of cardiac surgery in a
        child. *Journal of the American Academy of Child Psy-
        chiatry*, 1971, *10*, 156-186.

1085.1   Stocking, M., Rothney, W., Grosser, G. & Goodwin, R.
         Psychopathology in the pediatric hospital--Implica-
         tions for community health. In S. Chess & A. Thomas
         (Eds.), *Annual progress in child psychiatry and child
         development: 1973.* New York: Brunner/Mazel, 1974.
         Pp. 654-666.
1085.2   Carey, W. B. & Sibinga, M. S. Avoiding pediatric patho-
         genesis in the management of acute minor illness. In
         S. Chess & A. Thomas (Eds.), *Annual progress in child
         psychiatry and child development: 1973.* New York:
         Brunner/Mazel, 1974. Pp. 639-653.

CHILDREN IN THE HOSPITAL/Effect of Interpersonal Contact or its
   Lack on Child and Mother

1086   *Klaus, M. H. & Kennell, J. H. Mothers separated from
       their newborn infants. *Pediatric Clinics of North
       America,* 1970, *17,* 1015-1037.
1087   Moloney, J. C., Montgomery, J. C. & Trainham, G. The
       newborn, his family and the modern hospital. *Modern
       Hospital,* 1946, *67*(6), 43-46.
1088   *Blake, F. G. *The child, his parents and the nurse.*
       Philadelphia: Lippincott, 1954.
1089   *Riley, I. D., Syme, J., Hall, M. S. & Patrick, M. J.
       Mother and child in hospital -- Two years' experience.
       British Medical Journal, 1965, *2,* no. 5468, 990-992.
1090   Jensen, R. A. & Comly, H. H. Child-parent problems and
       the hospital. *Nervous Child,* 1948, *7,* 200-203.
1091   *MacCarthy, D., Lindsay, M. & Morris, I. Children in
       hospital with mothers. *Lancet,* 1962, *1,* 603-608.
1092   *Prugh, D. G., Staub, E. M., Sands, H. H., Kirschbaum,
       R. M. & Lenihan, E. A. A study of the emotional re-
       actions of children and families to hospitalization
       and illness. *American Journal of Orthopsychiatry,*
       1953, *23,* 70-106.
1094   *Robertson, J. A mother's observations on the tonsillec-
       tomy of her four-year-old daughter. *Psychoanalytic
       Study of the Child,* 1956, *11,* 410-427.
1095   Stevens, M. Visitors are welcome on the pediatric ward:
       Parents and youngsters are happier and there are more
       opportunities for nurses to teach when visiting hours
       are unrestricted. *American Journal of Nursing,* 1949,
       49, 233-235.
1097   *Wessel, M. A. The pediatric nurse and human relations.
       American Journal of Nursing, 1947, *47,* 213-216.

CHILDREN IN THE HOSPITAL/Methods of Helping the Hospitalized
 Child

1098   *Bibring, G. L. The child first. In *Long-term care of
         children*. Washington, D.C.: U.S. Department of
         Health, Education and Welfare, Children's Bureau,
         1949.
1099   *Solnit, A. J. Hospitalization: An aid to physical and
         psychological health in childhood. *American Journal
         of Diseases of Children*, 1960, *99*, 155-163.
1100   *Going to the Hospital*. Oakland, Calif.: Child Develop-
         ment Center, Children's Hospital of the East Bay,
         1951.
1101   Great Britain Ministry of Health. *Hospital building
         note no. 23: Children's ward*. London: Her Majesty's
         Stationery Office, 1964.
1102   *Wallace, M. & Feinauer, V. Understanding a sick child's
         behavior: How to recognize and relieve emotional
         distress and disturbance in the child ill in the hos-
         pital. *American Journal of Nursing*, 1948, *48*, 517-
         522.
1104   *Shore, M. F., Geiser, R. L. & Wolman, H. M. Construc-
         tive uses of a hospital experience. *Children*, 1965,
         12, 3-8.
1105   *Plank, E. N. *Working with children in hospitals*.
         (2nd ed.) Cleveland: Press of Western Reserve Uni-
         versity, 1971.
1106   Powers, G. F. Humanizing hospital experiences. *Ameri-
         can Journal of Diseases of Children*, 1948, *76*, 365-
         379.
1107   *Nuffield Foundation. *Children in hospital: Studies in
         planning*. New York: Oxford University Press, 1963.
1108   *Mason, E. A. The hospitalized child - His emotional
         needs. *New England Journal of Medicine*, 1965, *272*,
         406-414.
1109   *Jackson, E. B. et al. A hospital rooming-in unit for
         four newborn infants and their mothers: Descriptive
         account of background, development, and procedures
         with a few preliminary observations. *Pediatrics*,
         1948, *1*, 28-43.
1110   *Mothers go to babies hospital. *American Journal of
         Nursing*, 1954, *54*, 582-583.
1111   *Jackson, E. B. Treatment of the young child in the
         hospital. *American Journal of Orthopsychiatry*, 1942,
         12, 56-67.
1112   *Klein, D. C. & Lindemann, E. Preventive intervention
         in individual and family crisis situations. In G.
         Caplan (Ed.), *Prevention of mental disorders in chil-
         dren*. New York: Basic Books, 1961. Pp. 283-306.
1113   Chapin, H. D. A plan of dealing with atrophic infants
         and children. *Archives of Pediatrics*, 1908, *25*, 491-
         496.

1114 *Coyle, G. L. & Fisher, R. Helping hospitalized children through social group work. *The Child*, 1952, *16*, 114-117; 126.

1115 Davidson, E. R. Play for the hospitalized child: Play is a serious business, a response to the child's deep emotional urges. *American Journal of Nursing*, 1949, *49*, 138-141.

1116 *Erickson, F. H. Play interviews for four-year-old hospitalized children. *Monographs of the Society for Research in Child Development*, 1958, *23*, Serial no. 69, no. 3.

1117 Richards, S. S. & Wolff, E. The organization and function of play activities in the setup of a pediatric department: A report of a three-year experiment. *Mental Hygiene*, 1940, *24*, 229-237.

1118 *Tisza, V. B. & Angoff, K. A play program and its function in a pediatric hospital. *Pediatrics*, 1957, *19*, 293-302.

1119 *Langdon, G. A study of the uses of toys in a hospital. *Child Development*, 1948, *19*, 197-212.

1121 *Good, L. R., Siegel, S. M. & Bay, A. P. (Eds.) *Therapy by design*. Springfield, Ill.: Thomas, 1965.

1123 *Jackson, K. Psychologic preparation as a method of reducing the emotional trauma of anesthesia in children. *Anesthesiology*, 1951, *12*, 293-300.

1124 *Mellish, R. W. P. Preparation of a child for hospitalization and surgery. *Pediatric Clinics of North America*, 1969, *16*, 543-553.

1124.1 Cline, F. W. & Rothenberg, M. B. Preparation of a child for major surgery: A case report. *Journal of the American Academy of Child Psychiatry*, 1974, *13*, 78-94.

1125 *Howell, D. A. Emotional management of family stressed in care of dying child. *Pediatric Currents*, 1968, *17*, 7.

1126 *Senn, M. J. E. Emotional aspects of convalescence. *The Child*, 1945, *10*, 24-28.

1127 *Harrison, T. R. Abuse of rest as a therapeutic measure for patients with cardiovascular disease. *Journal of the American Medical Association*, 1944, *125*, 1075-1077.

1128 *Lendrum, B. L., Simon, A. J. & Mack, I. Relation of duration of bed rest in acute rheumatic fever to heart disease present 2 to 14 years later. *Pediatrics*, 1959, *24*, 389-394.

1129 *McCrory, W. W., Fleisher, D. S. & Sohn, W. B. Effects of early ambulation on the course of nephritis in children. *Pediatrics*, 1959, *24*, 395-399.

1130 *Bergman, A. B., Shrand, H. & Oppe, T. E. A pediatric home care program in London -- Ten years experience. *Pediatrics*, 1965, *36*, 314-321.

1131   *Shrand, H. Behavior changes in sick children nursed at
        home. *Pediatrics*, 1965, *36*, 604-607.
1132   *Shrand, H. Home care scheme for sick children. *Nursing
        Times*, 1964, *60*, 1113-1116.
1133   Lightwood, R. et al. A London trial of home care for
        sick children. *Lancet*, 1957, *272*, 313-317.
1134   *Lawrie, R. Operating on children as day-cases. *Lancet*,
        1964, *2*, 1289-1291.
1135   *Green, M. Integration of ambulatory services in a chil-
        dren's hospital: A unifying design. *American Journal
        of Diseases of Children*, 1965, *110*, 178-184.
1136   Green, M. & Haggerty, R. J. (Eds.) *Ambulatory pediat-
        rics*. Philadelphia: Saunders, 1968.
1137   *Langford, W. S. Physical illness and convalescence:
        Their meaning to the child. *Journal of Pediatrics*,
        1948, *33*, 242-250.
1138   Schowalter, J. E. The utilization of child psychiatry
        on a pediatric adolescent ward. *Journal of the Ameri-
        can Academy of Child Psychiatry*, 1971, *10*, 684-699.
1139   Mattsson, A. & Agle, D. P. Group therapy with parents
        of hemophiliacs: Therapeutic process and observations
        of parental adaptation to chronic illness in children.
        Journal of the American Academy of Child Psychiatry,
        1972, *11*, 558-571.
1139.1 Nover, R. A. Pain and the burned child. *Journal of the
        American Academy of Child Psychiatry*, 1973, *12*, 499-
        505.
1139.2 Jankowski, J. J. Clinical child psychiatry services on
        a pediatric-adolescent unit. *Journal of the American
        Academy of Child Psychiatry*, 1974, *13*, 95-109.

DEATH AND DYING/Guilt and Mourning and Separation in Children

1140   *Bowlby, J. Grief and mourning in infancy and early
        childhood. *Psychoanalytic Study of the Child*, 1960,
        15, 9-52.
1141   *Freud, A. Discussion of Dr. John Bowlby's paper. *Psy-
        choanalytic Study of the Child*, 1960, *15*, 53-62.
        (Writings, vol. 5, pp. 167-186)
1142   *Harrison, S. I., Davenport, C. W. & McDermott, J. F.
        Children's reactions to bereavement: Adult confu-
        sions and misperceptions. *Archives of General Psy-
        chiatry*, 1967, *17*, 593-597.
1143   *Paul, N. L. The need to mourn. In E. J. Anthony and
        C. Koupernik (Eds.), *The child in his family*. Vol. 2.
        The impact of disease and death. New York: Wiley,
        1973. Pp. 219-225. (International Yearbook for
        Child Psychiatry and Allied Disciplines, vol. 2)
1144   *Furman, R. A. A child's capacity for mourning. In E.
        J. Anthony and C. Koupernik (Eds.), *The child in his*

family. Vol. 2. *The impact of disease and death.* New York: Wiley, 1973. Pp. 225-231. (International Yearbook for Child Psychiatry and Allied Disciplines, vol. 2)

1145   *Winograd, M. Pathological mourning. In E. J. Anthony and C. Koupernik (Eds.), *The child in his family.* Vol. 2. *The impact of disease and death.* New York: Wiley, 1973. Pp. 233-243. (International Yearbook for Child Psychiatry and Allied Disciplines, vol. 2)

1146   *Lindemann, E. Symptomatology and management of acute grief. *American Journal of Psychiatry,* 1944, *101,* 141-148.

1147   *Keinicke, C. M. Some effects of separating two-year-old children from their parents: A comparative study. *Human Relations,* 1956, *9,* 105-176.

1148   Roudinesco, J., David, M. & Nicolas, J. Responses of young children to separation from their mothers. *Courrier du Centre International de L'Enfance,* 1952, *2,* 66-78.

1149   Beverly, B. I. The effect of illness upon emotional development. *Journal of Pediatrics,* 1936, *8,* 533-543.

1150   Siggins, L. D. Mourning: A critical survey of the literature. *International Journal of Psychoanalysis,* 1966, *47,* 14-25.

1151   *Harnik, J. One component of the fear of death in early infancy. *International Journal of Psychoanalysis,* 1930, *11,* 485-491.

1152   *Heuscher, J. E. Death in the fairy-tale. *Diseases of the Nervous System,* 1967, *28,* 462-468.

1153   *Waechter, E. H. Children's awareness of fatal illness. *American Journal of Nursing,* 1971, *71,* 1168-1172.

1154   *Furman, R. A. Death and the young child: Some preliminary considerations. *Psychoanalytic Study of the Child,* 1964, *19,* 321-333.

1155   *Rothenberg, M. B. Too many and too few limitations for children. In R. H. Williams (Ed.), *To live and to die: When, why, and how.* New York: Springer-Verlag, 1973. Pp. 169-179.

1156   Jackson, E. N. *Telling a child about death.* New York: Channel Press, 1965.

1157   *Diggory, J. C. & Rothman, D. Z. Values destroyed by death. *Journal of Abnormal and Social Psychology,* 1961, *63,* 205-210.

1158   *Nagy, M. H. The child's view of death. *Journal of Genetic Psychology,* 1948, *73,* 3-27. (Also in H. Feifel (Ed.), *The meaning of death.* New York: McGraw-Hill, 1959. Pp. 79-98.)

1159   Howell, D. A. A child dies. *Journal of Pediatric Surgery,* 1966, *1,* 2-7.

1159.1   Nagera, H. Children's reactions to the death of important objects: A developmental approach. In

Psychoanalytic Study of the Child, 1970, *25*, 360-400.

DEATH AND DYING/General References

1160   *Anthony, E. J. & Koupernik, C. (Eds.) *The child in his family*. Vol. 2. *The impact of disease and death*. New York: Wiley, 1973. (International Yearbook for Child Psychiatry and Allied Disciplines, vol. 2)

1161   *Anthony, S. *The discovery of death in childhood and after*. New York: Basic Books, 1972.

1162   *Agee, J. *A death in the family*. New York: Avon, 1963.

1163   *Grollman, E. A. *Explaining death to children*. Boston: Beacon Press, 1967.

1164   *Wolf, A. W. M. *Helping your child to understand death*. New York: Child Study Association of America, 1958.

1165   *Mahler, M. S. Helping children to accept death. *Child Study*, 1950, *27*(4), 98-99, 119-120.

1166   *Aldrich, C. K. The dying patient's grief. *Journal of the American Medical Association*, 1963, *184*, 329-331.

1167   *Hicks, W. & Daniels, R. S. The dying patient, his physician and the psychiatric consultant. *Psychosomatics*, 1968, *9*, 47-52.

1168   *Alby, N. & Alby, J. M. The doctor and the dying child. In E. J. Anthony and C. Koupernik (Eds.), *The child in his family*. Vol. 2. *The impact of disease and death*. New York: Wiley, 1973. Pp. 145-157. (International Yearbook for Child Psychiatry and Allied Disciplines, vol. 2)

1169   Pattison, E. M. The experience of dying. *American Journal of Psychotherapy*, 1967, *21*, 32-43.

1170   *Eissler, K. R. *The psychiatrist and the dying patient*. New York: International Universities Press, 1955.

1171   Weisman, A. D. Misgivings and misconceptions in the psychiatric care of terminal patients. *Psychiatry*, 1970, *33*, 67-81.

1172   *Hinton, J. M. Facing death. *Journal of Psychosomatic Research*, 1966, *10*, 22-28.

1173   Weisman, A. D. *On dying and denying*. New York: Behavioral Publications, 1972.

1174   Rothenberg, A. Psychological problems in terminal cancer management. *Cancer*, 1961, *14*, 1063-1073.

1175   Hinton, J. *Dying*. Harmondsworth, Middlesex, Eng.: Penguin, 1967.

1176   Glaser, B. G. & Strauss, A. L. *Awareness of dying*. Chicago: Aldine, 1965.

1177   Pearson, L. (Ed.) *Death and dying*. Cleveland: Press of Case Western Reserve University, 1969.

1178   Gordon, D. C. *Overcoming the fear of death*. New York: Macmillan, 1970.

1179   Feifel, H. (Ed.) *The meaning of death*. New York: McGraw-Hill, 1959.

1180   *Kastenbaum, R. J. & Aisenberg, R. *The psychology of death.* New York: Springer, 1972.
1181   Vernon, G. M. *Sociology of death.* New York: Ronald Press, 1970.
1182   Fulton, R. L. *Death and identity.* New York: Wiley, 1965.
1183   Kutscher, A. H. *Death and bereavement.* Springfield, Ill.: Thomas, 1969.
1184   *Parkes, C. M. *Bereavement.* London: Tavistock, 1972.
1185   Carkhuff, R. R. *Helping and human relations; a primer for lay and professional helpers.* Vol. 1. New York: Holt, Rinehart and Winston, 1969.
1186   Volkan, V. Typical findings in pathological grief. *Psychiatric Quarterly,* 1970, *44,* 231-250.
1186.1 Langford, W. S. Physical illness and convalescence: their meaning to the child. *Journal of Pediatrics,* 1948, *33,* 242-250.
1187   Choron, J. *Death and Western thought.* New York: Collier, 1963.

DEATH AND DYING/Transcultural Approaches to Death and Dying

1188   *Gorer, G. Introduction: Transcultural approaches to the experience of death. In E. J. Anthony and C. Koupernik (Eds.), *The child in his family.* Vol. 2. *The impact of disease and death.* New York: Wiley, 1973. Pp. 419-421. (International Yearbook for Child Psychiatry and Allied Disciplines, vol. 2)
1189   *Khare, R. S. Dying and death: Some Hindu cultural rules and paradigms. In E. J. Anthony and C. Koupernik (Eds.), *The child in his family.* Vol. 2. *The impact of disease and death.* New York: Wiley, 1973. Pp. 465-477. (International Yearbook for Child Psychiatry and Allied Disciplines, vol. 2)
1190   *Asuni, T. Death of a child in Nigeria. In E. J. Anthony and C. Koupernik (Eds.), *The child in his family.* Vol. 2. *The impact of disease and death.* New York: Wiley, 1973. Pp. 491-500. (International Yearbook for Child Psychiatry and Allied Disciplines, vol. 2)
1191   *Gorer, G. Death, grief, and mourning in Britain. In E. J. Anthony and C. Koupernik (Eds.), *The child in his family.* Vol. 2. *The impact of disease and death.* New York: Wiley, 1973. Pp. 423-438. (International Yearbook for Child Psychiatry and Allied Disciplines, vol. 2)

DEATH AND DYING/Therapeutic Efforts with the Dying Child

1192   *Solnit, A. J. & Green, M. The pediatric management of
       the dying child: Part II. The child's reaction to
       the fear of dying. In A. J. Solnit & S. A. Provence
       (Eds.), *Modern perspectives in child development.*
       New York: International Universities Press, 1963.
       Pp. 217-228.

1193   *Wolters, W. H. G. The dying child in hospital. In E.
       J. Anthony and C. Koupernik (Eds.), *The child in his
       family.* Vol. 2. *The impact of disease and death.*
       New York: Wiley, 1973. Pp. 159-168. (International
       Yearbook for Child Psychiatry and Allied Disciplines,
       vol. 2)

1194   *Richmond, J. B. & Waisman, H. A. Psychologic aspects of
       management of children with malignant diseases. *Amer-
       ican Journal of Diseases of Children,* 1955, *89,* 42-47.

1195   *Vernick, J. Meaningful communication with the fatally
       ill child. In E. J. Anthony and C. Koupernik (Eds.),
       The child in his family. Vol. 2. *The impact of
       disease and death.* New York: Wiley, 1973. Pp. 105-
       119. (International Yearbook for Child Psychiatry
       and Allied Disciplines, vol. 2)

1196   *Binger, C. M., Ablin, A. R., Feuerstein, R. C., Kushner,
       J. H., Zoger, S. & Mikkelsen, C. Childhood leukemia:
       Emotional impact on patient and family. *New England
       Journal of Medicine,* 1969, *280,* 414-418.

1197   Waechter, E. The response of children to fatal illness.
       In M. Duffey, et al. (Eds.), *Current concepts in clin-
       ical nursing.* Vol. 3. St. Louis, Mo.: S. V. Mosby,
       1971.

1198   *Binger, C. M. Jimmy--A clinical case presentation of a
       child with a fatal illness. In E. J. Anthony and C.
       Koupernik (Eds.), *The child in his family.* Vol. 2.
       The impact of disease and death. New York: Wiley,
       1973. Pp. 171-188. (International Yearbook for Child
       Psychiatry and Allied Disciplines, vol. 2)

1199   Bergman, A. B. & Schulte, C. J. A. Care of the child
       with cancer. *Pediatrics,* 1967, *40,* 487-546.

1200   *Morse, J. The goal of life enhancement for a fatally
       ill child. *Children,* 1970, *17,* 63-68.

1201   *Morrissey, J. R. Death anxiety in children with fatal
       illness. In H. J. Parad (Ed.), *Crisis intervention:
       Selected readings.* New York: Family Service Associ-
       ation of America, 1965. Pp. 324-328.

1202   *Natterson, J. M. The fear of death in fatally ill chil-
       dren and their parents. In E. J. Anthony and C.
       Koupernik (Eds.), *The child in his family.* Vol. 2.
       The impact of disease and death. New York: Wiley,
       1973. Pp. 121-125. (International Yearbook for Child
       Psychiatry and Allied Disciplines, vol. 2)

1203   Morrissey, J. R. Children's adaptation to fatal ill-
       ness. *Social Work,* 1963, *8*(4), 81-88.

1204   Natterson, J. M. & Knudson, A. G. Observations con-
        cerning fear of death in fatally ill children and
        their mothers. *Psychosomatic Medicine*, 1960, *22*,
        456-465.
1205   Morrissey, J. F. A note of interviews with children
        facing imminent death. *Social Casework*, 1963, *44*,
        343-345.
1206   Karon, M. & Vernick, J. An approach to the emotional
        support of fatally ill children. *Clinical Pediatrics*,
        1968, *7*, 274-280.
1207   *Easson, W. M. Care of the young patient who is dying.
        Journal of the American Medical Association, 1968,
        205, 203-207.
1208   *Green, M. Care of the child with a long-term, life-
        threatening illness: Some principles of management.
        Pediatrics, 1967, *39*, 441-445.
1209   *Schowalter, J. E. The experience of death on an adol-
        escent pediatric ward (as experienced by the nurse in
        dreams and reality). In E. J. Anthony and C. Kouper-
        nik (Eds.), *The child in his family*. Vol. 2. *The
        impact of disease and death*. New York: Wiley, 1973.
        Pp. 211-218. (International Yearbook for Child Psy-
        chiatry and Allied Disciplines, vol. 2)
1210   *Norton, J. Treatment of a dying patient. *Psychoana-
        lytic Study of the Child*, 1963, *18*, 541-560.
1211   *Evans, A. E. If a child must die. *New England Journal
        of Medicine*, 1968, *278*, 138-142.
1212   Bergman, A. B. & Schulte, C. J. A. Care of the child
        with cancer. *Pediatrics*, 1967, *40*, 487-546.
1213   Futterman, E. H. & Hoffman, I. Transient school phobia
        in a leukemic child. *Journal of the American Academy
        of Child Psychiatry*, 1970, *9*, 477-494.
1214   *Ross, E. K. *On death and dying*. New York: Macmillan,
        1969.
1215   *Easson, W. M. *The dying child*. Springfield, Ill.:
        C. C. Thomas, 1970.
1216   Vernick, J. & Lunceford, J. L. Milieu design for ado-
        lescents with leukemia. *American Journal of Nursing*,
        1967, *67*, 559-561.
1217   Clark, M. B. A therapeutic approach to treating a
        grieving 2 1/2-year-old. *Journal of the American
        Academy of Child Psychiatry*, 1972, *11*, 705-711.

DEATH AND DYING/Impact of a Child's Death on Parents

1218   *Kennell, J. H., Slyter, H. & Klaus, M. H. The mourning
        response of parents to the death of a newborn infant.
        New England Journal of Medicine, 1970, *283*, 344-349.
1219   *Ablin, A. R. et al. A conference with the family of a
        leukemic child. *American Journal of Diseases of Chil-
        dren*, 1971, *122*, 362-364.

1220   *Bozeman, M. F., Orbach, C. E. & Sutherland, A. M. Psy-
       chological impact of cancer and its treatment. III.
       The adaptation of mothers to the threatened loss of
       their children through leukemia: Part I. *Cancer*,
       1955, *8*, 1-19.
1221   Orbach, C. E., Sutherland, A. M. & Bozeman, M. F.
       Psychological impact of cancer and its treatment. III.
       The adaptation of mothers to the threatened loss of
       their children through leukemia: Part II. *Cancer*,
       1955, *8*, 20-33.
1222   *Cobb, B. Psychological impact of long illness and death
       of a child on the family circle. *Journal of Pediat-
       rics*, 1956, *49*, 746-751.
1223   *Green, M. & Solnit, A. J. Reactions to the threatened
       loss of a child: A vulnerable child syndrome. Pe-
       diatric management of the dying child, part III.
       Pediatrics, 1964, *34*, 58-66.
1224   Friedman, S. B. Care of the family of the child with
       cancer. *Pediatrics*, 1967, *40*, 498-507.
1226   *Solnit, A. J. & Green, M. Psychologic considerations
       in the management of deaths on pediatric hospital
       services. I. The doctor and the child's family.
       Pediatrics, 1959, *24*, 106-112.
1227   *Knudson, A. G. & Natterson, J. M. Participation of
       parents in the hospital care of fatally ill children.
       Pediatrics, 1960, *26*, 482-490.
1228   *Orbach, C. E. The multiple meanings of the loss of a
       child. *American Journal of Psychotherapy*, 1959, *13*,
       906-915.
1229   Hamovitch, M. B. *The parent and the fatally ill child*.
       Duarte, Calif.: City of Hope Medical Center, 1964.
1230   *Solnit, A. J. Who mourns when a child dies? In E. J.
       Anthony and C. Koupernik (Eds.), *The child in his
       family*. Vol. 2. *The impact of disease and death*.
       New York: Wiley, 1973. Pp. 245-254. (International
       Yearbook for Child Psychiatry and Allied Disciplines,
       vol. 2)
1231   *Friedman, S. B., Chodoff, P., Mason, J. W. & Hamburg,
       D. A. Behavioral observations on parents anticipa-
       ting the death of a child. *Pediatrics*, 1963, *32*,
       610-625.
1232   Friedman, S. B., Mason, J. W. & Hamburg, D. A. Urinary
       17-hydroxycorticosteroid levels in parents of chil-
       dren with neoplastic disease: A study of chronic
       psychological stress. *Psychosomatic Medicine*, 1963,
       25, 364-376.
1233   *Becker, D. & Margolin, F. How surviving parents han-
       dled their young children's adaptation to the crisis
       of loss. *American Journal of Orthopsychiatry*, 1967,
       37, 753-757.
1234   Schoenberg, B., Carr, A. C., Peretz, D. & Kutscher, A.
       H. (Eds.) *Loss and grief: Psychological management
       in medical practice*. New York: Columbia University
       Press, 1970.

1234.1   Burnell, G. M.   Maternal reaction to the loss of multiple births. *Archives of General Psychiatry*, 1974, *30*, 183-184.

DEATH AND DYING/Reactions of Siblings and Other Children to Death in Family

1235   *Weston, D. L. & Irwin, R. C.   Preschool child's response to death of infant sibling. *American Journal of Diseases of Children*, 1963, *106*, 564-567.
1236   *Binger, C. M.   Childhood leukemia--Emotional impact on siblings. In E. J. Anthony and C. Koupernik (Eds.), *The child in his family*. Vol. 2. *The impact of disease and death*. New York: Wiley, 1973. Pp. 195-209. (International Yearbook for Child Psychiatry and Allied Disciplines, vol. 2)
1237   *Rosenblatt, B.   A young boy's reaction to the death of his sister: A report based on brief psychotherapy. *Journal of the American Academy of Child Psychiatry*, 1969, *8*, 321-335.
1238   Rosenzweig, S.   Sibling death as a psychological experience with special reference to schizophrenia. *Psychoanalytic Review*, 1943, *30*, 177-186.
1239   Cain, A. C., Fast, I. & Erickson, M. E.   Children's disturbed reactions to the death of a sibling. *American Journal of Orthopsychiatry*, 1964, *34*, 741-752.
1240   Plank, E. N.   Death on a children's ward. *Medical Times*, 1964, *92*, 638-644.
1241   *Adam, K. S.   Childhood parental loss, suicidal ideation, and suicidal behavior. In E. J. Anthony and C. Koupernik (Eds.), *The child in his family*. Vol. 2. *The impact of disease and death*. New York: Wiley, 1973. Pp. 275-297. (International Yearbook for Child Psychiatry and Allied Disciplines, vol. 2)
1242   *McDonald, M.   A study of the reactions of nursery school children to the death of a child's mother. *Psychoanalytic Study of the Child*, 1964, *19*, 358-376.
1243   *Anthony, E. J.   Mourning and psychic loss of the parent. In E. J. Anthony and C. Koupernik (Eds.), *The child in his family*. Vol. 2. *The impact of disease and death*. New York: Wiley, 1973. Pp. 255-264. (International Yearbook for Child Psychiatry and Allied Disciplines, vol. 2)
1244   Keeler, W. R.   Children's reaction to the death of a parent. *Proceedings of the American Psychopathological Association*, 1954, *42*, 109-120.
1245   *Ilan, E.   The impact of a father's suicide on his latency son. In E. J. Anthony and C. Koupernik (Eds.), *The child in his family*. Vol. 2. *The impact of disease and death*. New York: Wiley, 1973. Pp. 299-306. (International Yearbook for Child Psychiatry and Allied Disciplines, vol. 2)

1246   Gauthier, Y. The mourning reaction of a ten-and-a-half-
        year-old boy. *Psychoanalytic Study of the Child*, 1965,
        20, 481-494.
1247   *Gauthier, Y. The mourning reaction of a ten-year-old boy.
        Canadian Psychiatric Association Journal Special Supple-
        ment, 1966, *11*, 307-308.
1248   Barnes, M. J. Reactions to the death of a mother. *Psycho-*
        analytic Study of the Child, 1964, *19*, 334-357.
1249   *Furman, R. A. Death of a six-year-old's mother during his
        analysis. *Psychoanalytic Study of the Child*, 1964, *19*,
        377-397.
1250   *Sugar, M. Normal adolescent mourning. *American Journal*
        of Psychotherapy, 1968, *22*, 258-269.
1251   Vernick, J. & Karon, M. Who's afraid of death on leukemia
        ward? *American Journal of Diseases of Children*, 1965,
        109, 393-397.
1251.1 Clark, M. B. A therapeutic approach to treating a griev-
        ing 2 1/2-year-old. *Journal of the American Academy of*
        Child Psychiatry, 1972, *11*, 705-711.

DEATH AND DYING/Family Studies

1252   *Anthony, E. J. A working model for family studies. In
        E. J. Anthony & C. Koupernik (Eds.), *The child in his*
        family. Vol. 2. *The impact of disease and death*. New
        York: Wiley, 1973. Pp. 3-20. (International Yearbook
        for Child Psychiatry and Allied Disciplines, vol. 2)
1253   *Gourevitch, M. A survey of family reactions to disease
        and death in a family member. In E. J. Anthony & C.
        Koupernik (Eds.), *The child in his family*. Vol. 2.
        The impact of disease and death. New York: Wiley,
        1973. Pp. 21-28. (International Yearbook for Child
        Psychiatry and Allied Disciplines, vol. 2)
1254   *Futterman, E. H. & Hoffman, I. Crisis and adaptation in
        the families of fatally ill children. In E. J. Anthony
        & C. Koupernik (Eds.), *The child in his family*. Vol. 2.
        The impact of disease and death. New York: Wiley,
        1973. Pp. 127-143. (International Yearbook for Child
        Psychiatry and Allied Disciplines, vol. 2)

DEATH AND DYING/Professional Workers' Role

1255   Quint, J. C. *The nurse and the dying patient*. London:
        Macmillan, 1967.
1256   *Pieroni, A. L. Role of the social worker in a children's
        cancer clinic. *Pediatrics*, 1967, *40*, 534-536.
1257   *Caplan, G. *The theory and practice of mental health con-*
        sultation. New York: Basic Books, 1970.
1257.1 Barton, D., Flexner, J. M., Van Eys, J. et al. Death and
        dying: A course for medical students. *Journal of Med-*
        ical Education, 1972, *47*, 945-951.

1257.2 Barton, D. Teaching psychiatry in the context of dying
and death. *American Journal of Psychiatry*, 1973, *130*,
1290-1291.

1257.3 Barton, D. The need for including instruction on death
and dying in the medical curriculum. *Journal of Medical Education*, 1972, *47*, 169-175.

1257.4 Griffith, J. A., Fabri, P. J., Kies, M. S. & Sinibaldi,
M. R. Three medical students confront death on a pedi-
atric ward: A case report. *Journal of the American
Academy of Child Psychiatry*, 1974, *13*, 72-77.

1257.5 Koocher, G. P. Talking with children about death. *American Journal of Orthopsychiatry*, 1974, *44*, 404-411.

DEATH AND DYING/Holocaust Studies

1258   *Sigal, J. J. Hypotheses and methodology in the study of
families of the holocaust survivors. In E. J. Anthony
& C. Koupernik (Eds.), *The child in his family.* Vol.
2. *The impact of disease and death.* New York: Wiley,
1973. Pp. 411-415. (International Yearbook for Child
Psychiatry and Allied Disciplines, vol. 2)

1259   *Klein, H. Children of the holocaust: Mourning and be-
reavement. In E. J. Anthony & C. Koupernik (Eds.),
The child in his family. Vol. 2. *The impact of disease
and death.* New York: Wiley, 1973. Pp. 393-409.
(International Yearbook for Child Psychiatry and Allied
Disciplines, vol. 2)

1260   *Aleksandrowicz, D. R. Children of concentration camp survivors. In E. J. Anthony & C. Koupernik (Eds.), *The
child in his family.* Vol. 2. *The impact of disease and
death.* New York: Wiley, 1973. Pp. 385-392. (International Yearbook for Child Psychiatry and Allied Disciplines, vol. 2)

1261   *Furman, E. The impact of the Nazi concentration camps on
the children of survivors. In E. J. Anthony & C. Koupernik (Eds.), *The child in his family.* Vol. 2. *The
impact of disease and death.* New York: Wiley, 1973.
Pp. 379-384. (International Yearbook for Child Psychiatry and Allied Disciplines, vol. 2)

1262   *Rosenberger, L. Children of survivors. In E. J. Anthony
& C. Koupernik (Eds.), *The child in his family.* Vol. 2.
The impact of disease and death. New York: Wiley,
1973. Pp. 375-377. (International Yearbook for Child
Psychiatry and Allied Disciplines, vol. 2)

1263   *Laufer, M. The analysis of a child of survivors. In E.
J. Anthony & C. Koupernik (Eds.), *The child in his family.* Vol. 2. *The impact of disease and death.* New
York: Wiley, 1973. Pp. 363-373. (International Yearbook for Child Psychiatry and Allied Disciplines, vol. 2)

DEATH AND DYING/Miscellaneous Studies

1264   *Lebovici, S. Children who torture and kill. In E. J.
Anthony & C. Koupernik (Eds.), *The child in his family.*
Vol. 2. *The impact of disease and death.* New York:
Wiley, 1973. Pp. 307-318. (International Yearbook for
Child Psychiatry and Allied Disciplines, vol. 2)

1265   *Palgi, P. Discontinuity in the female role within the
traditional family in modern society: A case of infanticide. In E. J. Anthony & C. Koupernik (Eds.), *The
child in his family.* Vol. 2. *The impact of disease
and death.* New York: Wiley, 1973. Pp. 453-463. (International Yearbook for Child Psychiatry and Allied
Disciplines, vol. 2)

1266   *Collomb, H. The child who leaves and returns, or the
death of the same child. In E. J. Anthony & C. Koupernik (Eds.), *The child in his family.* Vol. 2. *The impact of disease and death.* New York: Wiley, 1973.
Pp. 439-452. (International Yearbook for Child Psychiatry and Allied Disciplines, vol. 2)

DEATH AND DYING/Texts and Basic Work

1267   Freud, S. (1917) [1915] Mourning and melancholia. In
Standard Edition, 14, 243-260. London: Hogarth Press,
1957.

1268   Spitz, R. A. *No and yes.* New York: International Universities Press, 1957

1268.1 Anthony, E. J. & Koupernik, C. (Eds.) *The child in his
family.* Vol. 2. *The impact of disease and death.* New
York: Wiley, 1973. (International Yearbook for Child
Psychiatry and Allied Disciplines, vol. 2)

DEATH AND DYING/Kidney Studies

1268.2 Kemph. J. P. Renal failure, artificial kidney and kidney
transplant. *American Journal of Psychiatry,* 1966, *122,*
1270-1274.

1268.3 Lewis, M. Kidney donation by a 7-year-old identical twin
child: Psychological, legal, and ethical considerations.
Journal of the American Academy of Child Psychiatry,
1974, *13,* 221-245.

1268.4 Khan, A. N., Herndon, C. H. & Ahmadian, S. Y. Social
and emotional adaptations of children with trans-
planted kidneys and chronic hemodialysis. *American
Journal of Psychiatry,* 1971, *127,* 1194-1198.

1268.5   Muslin, H. L.   On acquiring a kidney. *American Journal of Psychiatry*, 1971, *127*, 1185-1188.
1268.6   Bernstein, D. M.   After transplantation: The child's emotional reactions. *American Journal of Psychiatry*, 1971, *127*, 1189-1193.
1268.7   Korsch, B. M., Fine, R. N., Grushkin, C. M. & Negrete, V. F.   Experiences with children and their families during extended hemodialysis and kidney transplantation. *Pediatric Clinics of North America*, 1971, *18*, 625-637.
1268.8   Kemph, J. P., Bermann, E. A. & Coppolillo, H. P.   Kidney transplants and shifts in family dynamics. *American Journal of Psychiatry*, 1969, *125*, 1485-1490.
1268.9   Simmons, R. G. & Klein, S. D.   Family noncommunication: The search for kidney donors. *American Journal of Psychiatry*, 1972, *129*, 687-692.
1268.11 Reinhart, J. B.   The doctor's dilemma: Whether or not to recommend continuous renal dialysis or renal homotransplantation for the child with end-stage renal disease. *Journal of Pediatrics*, 1970, *77*, 505-506.
1268.12 Kaplan De-Nour, A. & Czaczkes, J. W.   Emotional problems and reactions of the medical team in a chronic haemodialysis unit. *Lancet*, 1968, *2*, 987-991.
1269.13 Curran, W. J.   A problem of consent: Kidney transplant in minors. *New York University Law Review*, 1959, *34*, 891-898.
1268.14 Fellner, C. H. & Marshall, J. R.   Kidney donors: the myth of informed consent. *American Journal of Psychiatry*, 1970, *126*, 1245-1251.
1268.15 Levy, N. B.   *Living or dying: Adaptation to hemodialysis*. Springfield, Ill.:   C. C. Thomas, 1974.

DEATH AND DYING/Bibliographies

1269   Kalish, R. A.   Death and bereavement: A bibliography. *Journal of Human Relations*, 1965, *13*, 118-141.
1270   Vernick, J. J.   *Selected bibliography on death and dying*. Bethesda, Md.:   U.S. National Institutes of Health, 1969.
1270.1   Cook, S. S.   *Children and dying; an exploration and a selective professional bibliography*. New York: Health Sciences, 1973.

IX.   LEARNING AND SCHOOL DISTURBANCES IN CHILDREN

HISTORY OF EDUCATION AND SOCIO-CULTURAL ASPECTS

1271   *Ariès, P.   *Centuries of childhood: A social history of family life*. New York: Knopf, 1962.   Pp. 137-336.

1272   Frost, S. E., Jr. *Essentials of history of education.*
New York: Barron's Educational Series, 1947. Pp.
19-48.
1273   Standing, E. M. *Maria Montessori: Her life and work.*
New York: American Library of World Literature, 1962.
1274   *Levine, M. & Levine, A. *A social history of helping
services: Clinic, court, school and community.* New
York: Appleton/Century/Crofts, 1970.
1275   *Sarason, S. B. *The culture of the school and the problem of change.* Boston: Allyn & Bacon, 1971.
1276   *Harrington, M. *The accidental century.* New York:
Macmillan, 1965.
1277   *Riessman, F., Cohen, J. & Pearl, A. (Eds.) *Mental
health of the poor.* New York: Free Press of Glencoe,
1964.
1278   Mills, C. W. *The power elite.* New York: Oxford University Press, 1956.
1279   Henry, J. *Culture against man.* New York: Random
House, 1963.
1279.1   Friedrich, L. K. & Stein, A. H. *Aggressive and pro-
social television programs and the natural behavior
of preschool children.* Chicago: University of
Chicago Press, 1973. (*Monographs of the Society for
Research in Child Development,* serial no. 151, v. 38,
no. 4)
1279.2   Bernfeld, S. *Sisyphus; or, The limits of education.*
[translated by Frederic Lilge] Berkeley: University
of California Press, 1973.
1279.3   Beit-Hallahmi, B., Catford, J. C., Cooley, R. E., Dull,
C. Y., Guiora, A. Z. & Raluszny, M. Grammatical
gender and gender identity development: Cross-
cultural and cross lingual implications. *American
Journal of Orthopsychiatry,* 1974, *44,* 424-431.

LEARNING THEORIES

1280   *Mowrer, O. H. *Learning theory and personality dynamics:
Selected papers.* New York: Ronald Press, 1950.
1281   *Flavell, J. H. *The developmental psychology of Jean
Piaget.* Princeton, N. J.: Van Nostrand, 1963.
1282   *Elkind, D. *Children and adolescents: Interpretative
essays on Jean Piaget.* New York: Oxford University
Press, 1970.
1283   *Piaget, J. & Inhelder, B. *The psychology of the child.*
New York: Basic Books, 1969.
1284   *Freud, A. Psychoanalysis and education. *Psychoanalytic Study of the Child,* 1954, *9,* 9-15. (*Writings,*
vol. 4, pp. 317-326.)
1285   *Bruner, J. S. *The process of education.* Cambridge:
Harvard University Press, 1960. Pp. 81-91.
1286   Piaget, J. *The child's conception of physical causality.* New York: Harcourt, Brace, 1930.

1287   Piaget, J. *The language and thought of the child.*
         (3rd ed.) New York: Humanities Press, 1959.
1288   Piaget, J. *Play, dreams, and imitation in childhood.*
         New York: Norton, 1951.
1289   Piaget, J. *The construction of reality in the child.*
         New York: Basic Books, 1954.
1290   Piaget, J. *The child's conception of numbers.* New
         York: Humanities Press, 1952.
1291   *Ashton-Warner, S. *Teacher.* New York: Simon & Schu-
         ster, 1961.
1292   Hunt, J. McV. *Intelligence and experience.* New York:
         Ronald Press, 1961.
1293   *Hilgard, E. R. & Bower, G. H. *Theories of learning.*
         (3rd ed.) New York: Appleton-Century-Crofts, 1966.
1294   *Holt, E. B. *Animal drive and the learning process.*
         New York: Octagon, 1973.
1294.1   Freud, A. The concept of developmental lines. In S.
         G. Sapir & A. C. Nitzburg (Eds.), *Children with
         learning problems: Readings in a developmental-
         interaction approach.* New York: Brunner/Mazel, 1973.
         Pp. 19-36.
1294.2   Shapiro, E. & Biber, B. The education of young chil-
         dren: A developmental-interaction approach. In S.
         G. Sapir & A. C. Nitzburg (Eds.), *Children with
         learning problems: Readings in a developmental-
         interaction approach.* New York: Brunner/Mazel, 1973.
         Pp. 682-709.

PSYCHOLOGICAL FACTORS IN LEARNING DISORDERS

1295   *Nagera, H. The concepts of structure and structuraliza-
         tion: Psychoanalytic usage and implications for a
         theory of learning and creativity. *Psychoanalytic
         Study of the Child,* 1967, *22,* 77-102.
1296   *Mahler, M. S. Energy-economic considerations in the
         learning process. *Quarterly Journal of Child Behav-
         ior,* 1950, *2,* 233-236.
1297   White, R. W. *Ego and reality in psychoanalytic theory;
         a proposal regarding independent ego energies.* New
         York: International Universities Press, 1963. (Psy-
         chological issues, v. 3, no. 3. Monograph 11)
1298   *Biber, B. Integration of mental health principles in
         the school setting. In G. Caplan (Ed.), *Prevention
         of mental disorders in children.* New York: Basic
         Books, 1961. Pp. 323-352.
1299   Jacobson, E. The self and the object world. Vicissi-
         tudes of their infantile cathexes and their influence
         on ideational and affective development. *Psychoana-
         lytic Study of the Child,* 1954, *9,* 75-127.
1300   *Peller, L. E. The school's role in promoting sublima-
         tion. *Psychoanalytic Study of the Child,* 1956, *11,*
         437-449.

1301 *Holmes, D. A contribution to a psychoanalytic theory of work. *Psychoanalytic Study of the Child*, 1965, *20*, 384-393.
1302 *Sarnoff, I. Some psychological problems of the incipient artist. *Mental Hygiene*, 1956, *40*, 375-383.
1303 Berlin, I. N. Aspects of creativity and the learning process. *American Imago*, 1960, *17*, 83-99.
1304 *Witmer, H. L. & Kotinsky, R. The school. In H. L. Witmer and R. Kotinsky (Eds.), *Personality in the making*. New York: Harper, 1952. Pp. 230-272.
1306 Liss, E. Motivations in learning. *Psychoanalytic Study of the Child*, 1955, *10*, 100-116.
1307 *Hill, J. C. *Teaching and the unconscious mind*. New York: International Universities Press, 1971.
1308 Fleming, C. M. *Teaching, a psychological analysis*. London: Methuen, 1958.
1309 *Pearson, G. H. A survey of learning difficulties in children. *Psychoanalytic Study of the Child*, 1952, *7*, 322-386.
1310 Klein, E. Psychoanalytic aspects of school problems. *Psychoanalytic Study of the Child*, 1949, *3-4*, 369-390.
1311 *Goldfarb, W. Emotional and intellectual consequences of psychologic deprivation in infancy: A revaluation. *Proceedings of the American Psychopathological Association*, 1955, *44*, 105-119.
1312 *Rubenstein, B. O., Falick, M. L., Levitt, M. & Ekstein, R. Learning problems. 2. Learning impotence: A suggested diagnostic category. *American Journal of Orthopsychiatry*, 1959, *29*, 315-323.
1313 *Sperry, B., Staver, N., Reiner, B. S. & Ulrich, D. Renunciation and denial in learning difficulties. *American Journal of Orthopsychiatry*, 1958, *28*, 98-111.
1314 *Levy, D. M. Oppositional syndromes and oppositional behavior. *Proceedings of the American Psychopathological Association*, 1955, *44*, 204-226.
1315 *Berlin, I. N. & Szurek, S. A. (Eds.) *Learning and its disorders*. Palo Alto: Science and Behavior Books, 1965. (Clinical approaches to problems of childhood; child psychiatry series of the Langley Porter Children's Service, vol. 1)
1316 *Hewett, F. M. *The emotionally disturbed child in the classroom*. Boston: Allyn & Bacon, 1968.
1317 *Szurek, S. A. Emotional factors in the use of authority. In E. L. Ginsburg, *Public health is people*. New York: Commonwealth Fund, 1950. Pp. 206-225.
1318 Strang, R. Students' perception of factors affecting their studying. *Mental Hygiene*, 1957, *41*, 97-102.
1319 *Hellman, I. Some observations on mothers of children with intellectual inhibitions. *Psychoanalytic Study of the Child*, 1954, *9*, 259-273.
1320 Sarason, S. B. et al. *Psychology in community settings*. New York: Wiley, 1966.

1321   Nirk, G. Observations on the relationship of emotional and cognitive development: A psychiatric contribution to compensatory education. *Journal of the American Academy of Child Psychiatry*, 1973, *12*, 93-107.

1321.1 Freeman, R. D. Emotional reactions of handicapped children. In S. G. Sapir & A. C. Nitzburg (Eds.), *Children with learning problems: Readings in a developmental-interaction approach.* New York: Brunner/Mazel, 1973. Pp. 270-286.

1321.2 Sapir, S. G. Sex differences in perceptual motor development. In S. G. Sapir & A. C. Nitzburg (Eds.), *Children with learning problems: Readings in a developmental-interaction approach.* New York: Brunner/Mazel, 1973. Pp. 359-365.

GENERAL LEARNING PROBLEMS

1322   *Wimberger, H. C. Conceptual system for classification of psychogenic school underachievement. *Journal of Pediatrics*, 1966, *69*, 1092-1097.

1323   *Switzer, J. A genetic approach to the understanding of learning problems. *Journal of the American Academy of Child Psychiatry*, 1963, *2*, 653-666.

1324   Long, N. J., Morse, W. C. & Newman, R. G. (Eds.) *Conflict in the classroom: The education of emotionally disturbed children.* Belmont, Calif.: Wentworth, 1965.

1325   *Kounin, J. S. & Obradovic, S. Managing emotionally disturbed children in regular classrooms: A replication and extension. *Journal of Special Education*, 1968, *2*, 129-135.

1326   *Redl, F. The life space interview. 1. Strategy and techniques of the life space interview. *American Journal of Orthopsychiatry*, 1959, *29*, 1-18.

1327   *Blom, G. E., Rudnick, M., & Searless, J. Some principles and practices in the psychoeducational treatment of emotionally disturbed children. *Psychology in the Schools*, 1966, *3*, 30-38.

1328   Cohen, S. Teaching emotionally disturbed children. *Children*, 1966, *13*, 232-236.

1329   *Rubenstein, B. O., Falick, M. L., Levitt, M. & Ekstein, R. Learning problems. 2. Learning impotence: A suggested diagnostic category. *American Journal of Orthopsychiatry*, 1959, *29*, 315-323.

1330   *Mahler, M. S. Pseudoimbecility: A magic cap of invisibility. *Psychoanalytic Quarterly*, 1942, *11*, 149-164.

1331   *Newman, C. J. & Krug, O. Problems in learning arithmetic in emotionally disabled children. *Journal of the American Academy of Child Psychiatry*, 1964, *3*, 413-429.

1332   *Blom, G. E. The concept, "perceptually handicapped": Its assets and limitations. *Seminars in Psychiatry*, 1969, *1*, 253-261.

1333   *Sperry, B., Ulrich, D. N. & Staver, N. The relation
        of motility to boys' learning problems. *American
        Journal of Orthopsychiatry*, 1958, *28*, 640-646.
1334   Freibergs, V. & Douglas, V. I. Concept learning in
        hyperactive and normal children. *Journal of Abnormal
        Psychology*, 1969, *74*, 388-395.
1335   Gyarfas, M. G. *Boys with learning disability: A study
        of ego development, ego functioning, and family
        stress.* Chicago: University of Chicago, 1971.
        (Social service monographs, 2nd ser., no. 7)
1336   Ekanger, C. A. & Westervelt, G. Contributions of ob-
        servation in naturalistic settings to clinical and
        educational practice. *Journal of Special Education*,
        1967, *1*, 207-213.
1337   *Ervin-Tripp, S. Language development. *Review of Child
        Development Research*, 1966, *2*, 55-105.
1337.1 Sapir, S. G. & Nitzburg, A. C. (Eds.) *Children with
        learning problems: Readings in a developmental-inter-
        action approach.* New York: Brunner/Mazel, 1973.
1337.2 Bryan, T. H. Learning disabilities: A new stereotype.
        Journal of Learning Disabilities, 1974, *7*, 304-309.
1337.3 Mattick, I. & Murphy, L. B. Cognitive disturbances in
        young children. In S. G. Sapir & A. C. Nitzburg
        (Eds.), *Children with learning problems: Readings in
        a developmental-interaction approach.* New York:
        Brunner/Mazel, 1973. Pp. 415-460.
1337.4 Werner, H. & Kaplan, B. The organismic-developmental
        framework. In S. G. Sapir & A. C. Nitzburg (Eds.),
        *Children with learning problems: Readings in a
        developmental-interaction approach.* New York:
        Brunner/Mazel, 1973. Pp. 148-155.
1337.5 Frostig, M. & Maslow, P. *Learning problems in the
        classroom.* New York: Grune & Stratton, 1973.
1337.6 Holmes, M., Holmes, D. & Field, J. *The therapeutic
        classroom.* New York: Jason Aronson, 1974.
1337.7 Sapir, S. G. Learning disability and deficit centered
        classroom training. In S. G. Sapir & A. C. Nitzburg
        (Eds.), *Children with learning problems: Readings in
        a developmental-interaction approach.* New York:
        Brunner/Mazel, 1973. Pp. 660-673.

LANGUAGE AND READING DISORDERS

1338   *Eisenberg, L. Reading retardation: I. Psychiatric and
        sociologic aspects. *Pediatrics*, 1966, *37*, 352-365.
1339   Bender, L. Problems in conceptualization and communi-
        cation in children with developmental alexia. *Pro-
        ceedings of the American Psychopathological Associa-
        tion*, 1958, *46*, 155-176.
1339.1 de Hirsch, K. Concepts related to normal reading pro-
        cesses and their application to reading pathology.
        In S. G. Sapir & A. C. Nitzburg (Eds.), *Children with

learning problems: Readings in a developmental-interaction approach. New York: Brunner/Mazel, 1973. Pp. 517-527.

1340   *Rabinovitch, R. D.   Reading and learning disabilities. In S. Arieti (Ed.), *American handbook of psychiatry.* Vol. 1. New York: Basic Books, 1959. Pp. 857-869.

1341   *Blom, G. E., Farley, G. K. & Guthals, C.   The concept of body image and the remediation of body image disorders. *Journal of Learning Disabilities,* 1970, *3*, 440-447.

1342   Natchez, G. (Ed.) *Children with reading problems.* New York: Basic Books, 1968.

1343   *Stewart, R. S.   Personality maladjustment and reading achievement. *American Journal of Orthopsychiatry,* 1950, *20*, 410-417.

1344   *Silverman, J. S., Fite, M. W. & Mosher, M. M.   Learning problems. 1. Clinical findings in reading disability children--Special cases of intellectual inhibition. *American Journal of Orthopsychiatry,* 1959, *29*, 298-314.

1345   Blanchard, P.   Psychoanalytic contributions to the problems of reading disabilities. *Psychoanalytic Study of the Child,* 1946, *2*, 163-187.

1346   Silver, A. A. & Hagin, R. A.   Specific reading disability: Delineation of the syndrome and relationship to cerebral dominance. *Comprehensive Psychiatry,* 1960, *1*, 126-134.

1347   *Silver, A. A. & Hagin, R. A.   Specific reading disability: Follow-up studies. *American Journal of Orthopsychiatry,* 1964, *34*, 95-102.

1348   Critchley, M. *Developmental dyslexia.* London: Heinemann, 1964.

1350   Hellmuth, J. (Ed.) *Learning disorders.* Vols. 1-2. Seattle: Special Child Publications, 1965-1966.

1351   Hellmuth, J. (Ed.) *Disadvantaged child.* Vol. 2. New York: Brunner/Mazel, 1967.

1352   Millman, I. K. & Canter, S. M.   Language disturbances in normal and pathological development: Comparisons and practical considerations. *Journal of the American Academy of Child Psychiatry,* 1972, *11*, 243-254.

1352.1   Johnson, D. J.   The language continuum. In S. G. Sapir & A. C. Nitzburg (Eds.), *Children with learning problems: Readings in a developmental-interaction approach.* New York: Brunner/Mazel, 1973. Pp. 366-377.

1352.2   Brown, R. & Bellugi, U.   Three processes in the child's acquisition of syntax. In S. G. Sapir and A. C. Nitzburg (Eds.), *Children with learning problems: Readings in a developmental-interaction approach.* New York: Brunner/Mazel, 1973. Pp. 388-407.

1352.3   de Hirsch, K.   The concept of plasticity and language disabilities. In S. G. Sapir and A. C. Nitzburg

(Eds.), *Children with learning problems: Readings in a developmental-interaction approach.* New York: Brunner/Mazel, 1973. Pp. 477-484.
1352.4   Frank, J. & Levinson, H.   Dysmetric dyslexia and dyspraxia. *Journal of the American Academy of Child Psychiatry,* 1973, *12,* 690-701.
1352.5   Nelson, K.   Structure and strategy in learning to talk. *Monographs of the Society for Research in Child Development,* 1973, Ser. no. 149, *38,* no. 1-2.
1352.6   Wedell, K.   *Learning and perceptuo-motor disabilities in children.* London: Wiley, 1973.

PARENTS AND SCHOOL PROBLEMS

1353   *Buxbaum, E.   The parents' role in the etiology of learning disabilities. *Psychoanalytic Study of the Child,* 1964, *19,* 421-447.
1354   *Staver, N.   The child's learning difficulty as related to the emotional problem of the mother. *American Journal of Orthopsychiatry,* 1953, *23,* 131-141.
1355   *McCarthy, D.   Language disorders and parent-child relationships. *Journal of Speech and Hearing Disorders,* 1954, *19,* 514-523.
1356   *Hellman, I.   Some observations on mothers of children with intellectual inhibitions. *Psychoanalytic Study of the Child,* 1954, *9,* 259-273.
1357   *Walker, D. R.   Parents as "enablers" in helping the child with a school problem. *Child Welfare,* 1959, *38*(3), 11-16.

X.   PROBLEMS OF ADOLESCENCE

DEVELOPMENTAL ISSUES

1358   *Schonfeld, W. A.   Adolescent development: Biological, psychological, and sociological determinants. In *Annals of the American Society for Adolescent Psychiatry,* 1971, *1,* 296-323.
1359   Young, H. B.   The physiology of adolescence. In J. G. Howells (Ed.), *Modern perspectives in adolescent psychiatry.* Edinburgh: Oliver & Boyd, 1971. Pp. 3-27. (Modern perspectives in psychiatry, vol. 4)
1360   *Rothchild, E.   "Anatomy is destiny": Psychological implications of adolescent physical changes in girls. *Pediatrics,* 1967, *39,* 532-538.
1361   *Tanner, J. M.   Sequence, tempo, and individual variation in the growth and development of boys and girls aged twelve to sixteen. *Daedalus,* 1971, *100,* 907-930.
1362   *Freud, A.   Adolescence as a developmental disturbance. In G. Caplan and S. Lebovici (Eds.), *Adolescence:*

Psychosocial perspectives. New York: Basic Books, 1969. Pp. 5-10.

1363   *Blos, P. The second individuation process of adolescence. *Psychoanalytic Study of the Child,* 1967, *22,* 162-186.

1364   *Erikson, E. H. The problem of ego identity. *Journal of the American Psychoanalytic Association,* 1956, *4,* 56-121.

1365   Geleerd, E. R. Some aspects of ego vicissitudes in adolescence. *Journal of the American Psychoanalytic Association,* 1961, *9,* 394-405.

1366   *Josselyn, I. M. The ego in adolescence. *American Journal of Orthopsychiatry,* 1954, *24,* 223-237.

1367   *Blos, P. Character formation in adolescence. *Psychoanalytic Study of the Child,* 1968, *23,* 245-263.

1368   Offer, D. & Offer, J. Four issues in the developmental psychology of adolescents. In J. G. Howells (Ed.), *Modern perspectives in adolescent psychiatry.* Edinburgh: Oliver & Boyd, 1971. Pp. 28-44. (Modern perspectives in psychiatry, vol. 4)

1369   *Ritvo, S. Late adolescence: Developmental and clinical considerations. *Psychoanalytic Study of the Child,* 1971, *26,* 241-263.

1370   Harley, M. Some observations on the relationship between genitality and structural development at adolescence. *Journal of the American Psychoanalytic Association,* 1961, *9,* 434-460.

1371   *Erikson, E. H. *Identity, youth and crisis.* New York: Norton, 1968.

1372   *Horney, K. Personality changes in female adolescents. *American Journal of Orthopsychiatry,* 1935, *5,* 19-26.

1372.1 Tooley, K. Playing it right. *Journal of the American Academy of Child Psychiatry,* 1973, *12,* 615-631.

1372.2 King, S. H. Coping and growth in adolescence. In S. Chess & A. Thomas (Eds.), *Annual progress in child psychiatry and child development: 1973.* New York: Brunner/Mazel, 1974. Pp. 187-202.

DEVELOPMENTAL ISSUES/Normal Problems of Adolescence

1373   Kiell, N. (Ed.) *The universal experience of adolescence.* New York: International Universities Press, 1964.

1374   *Weiner, I. B. Perspectives on the modern adolescent. *Psychiatry,* 1972, *35,* 20-31.

1375   Adatto, C. P. On the metamorphosis from adolescence into adulthood. *Journal of the American Psychoanalytic Association,* 1966, *14,* 485-509.

1376   Blos, P. *On adolescence: A psychoanalytic interpretation.* New York: Free Press, 1962.

1377   Group for the Advancement of Psychiatry. Committee on
        Adolescence. *Normal adolescence.* GAP report, no.
        68. New York: 1968.
1378   Silber, E., Coelho, G. V., Murphey, E. B., Hamburg, D.
        A., Pearlin, L. I. & Rosenberg, M. Competent adol-
        escents coping with college decisions. *Archives of
        General Psychiatry,* 1961, *5,* 517-527.
1379   *Pumpian-Mindlin, E. Omnipotentiality, youth, and com-
        mitment. *Journal of the American Academy of Child
        Psychiatry,* 1965, *4,* 1-18.
1380   Gustin, J. C. The revolt of youth. *Psychoanalysis and
        the Psychoanalytic Review,* 1961, *48,* 78-90.
1381   *Piaget, J. The intellectual development of the adoles-
        cent. In G. Caplan and S. Lebovici (Eds.), *Adoles-
        cence: Psychosocial perspectives.* New York: Basic
        Books, 1969. Pp. 22-26.
1382   *Schofield, M. Normal sexuality in adolescence. In J.
        G. Howells (Ed.), *Modern perspectives in adolescent
        psychiatry.* Edinburgh: Oliver & Boyd, 1971. Pp.
        45-65. (Modern perspectives in psychiatry, vol. 4)
1383   *Berman, S. Alienation: An essential process of the
        psychology of adolescence. *Journal of the American
        Academy of Child Psychiatry,* 1970, *9,* 233-250.
1384   *Erikson, E. H. The life cycle: Epigenesis of identity.
        In *Identity, youth and crisis.* New York: Norton,
        1968. Pp. 91-141.
1385   Werkman, S. L. Identity and the creative surge in
        adolescence. *Science and Psychoanalysis,* 1966, *9,*
        48-60.
1386   Offer, D. & Sabshin, M. The psychiatrist and the nor-
        mal adolescent. *Archives of General Psychiatry,* 1963,
        9, 427-432.
1387   *Offer, D., Sabshin, M. & Marcus, D. Clinical evalua-
        tion of normal adolescents. *American Journal of Psy-
        chiatry,* 1965, *121,* 864-872.
1388   Masterson, J. F. *The psychiatric dilemma of adoles-
        cence.* Boston: Little, Brown, 1967.
1389   Spiegel, L. A. A review of contributions to a psycho-
        analytic theory of adolescence. *Psychoanalytic Study
        of the Child,* 1951, *6,* 375-393.
1390   *Frued, A. Adolescence. *Psychoanalytic Study of the
        Child,* 1958, *13,* 255-278. (*Writings,* vol. 5, pp. 136-
        166)
1391   Josselyn, I. M. The psychoanalytic psychology of the
        adolescent. In M. Levitt (Ed.), *Readings in psycho-
        analytic psychology.* New York: Appleton-Century-
        Crofts, 1959. Pp. 70-83.
1392   Spiegel, L. A. Disorder and consolidation in adoles-
        cence. *Journal of the American Psychoanalytic As-
        sociation,* 1961, *9,* 406-416.
1393   *Blos, P. The child analyst looks at the young adoles-
        cent. *Daedalus,* 1971, *100,* 961-978.

1394   Tanner, J. M. *Growth at adolescence*. Springfield,
        Ill.: Thomas, 1955.
1395   Sachs, D. M. & Shapiro, S. H. Comments on teaching
        the psychoanalytic psychology of adolescence to resi-
        dents. *Journal of the American Academy of Child Psy-
        chiatry*, 1972, *11*, 201-211.
1395.1 Offer, D. & Offer, J. Normal adolescence in perspec-
        tive. In J. C. Schoolar (Ed.), *Current issues in
        adolescent psychiatry*. New York: Brunner/Mazel,
        1973. Pp. 3-18.
1395.2 Straus, R. Alcohol and youth. *Psychiatric Annals*,
        1973, *3*(10), 95-96.
1395.3 Straus, R. A follow-up study of drinking in college.
        Psychiatric Annals, 1973, *3*(10), 15-23.
1395.4 Straus, R. Some early research on drinking and problem
        drinking. *Psychiatric Annals*, 1973, *3*(10), 13-14.
1395.5 Howell, M. C., Emmons, E. B. & Frank, D. A. Reminis-
        cences of runaway adolescents. *American Journal of
        Orthopsychiatry*, 1973, *43*, 840-853.

DEVELOPMENTAL ISSUES/Familial Determinants

1396   *Shapiro, R. L. Adolescent ego autonomy and the family.
        In G. Caplan and S. Lebovici (Eds.), *Adolescence:
        Psychosocial perspectives*. New York: Basic Books,
        1969. Pp. 113-121.
1397   *McWhinnie, A. M. The adopted child in adolescence. In
        G. Caplan & S. Lebovici (Eds.), *Adolescence: Psycho-
        social perspectives*. New York: Basic Books, 1969.
        Pp. 133-142.
1398   *Lidz, T. F. The adolescent and his family. In G. Cap-
        lan & S. Lebovici (Eds.), *Adolescence: Psychosocial
        perspectives*. New York: Basic Books, 1969. Pp. 105-
        112.
1398.1 Ravenscroft, K. Jr. Normal family regression at adol-
        escence. *American Journal of Psychiatry*, 1974, *131*,
        31-35.
1399   *Biller, H. B. A note on father absence and masculine
        development in lower-class Negro and white boys.
        Child Development, 1968, *39*, 1003-1006.
1399.1 Stierlin, H. A family perspective on adolescent runa-
        ways. *Archives of General Psychiatry*, 1973, *29*, 56-
        62.
1399.2 Paredes, A., Hood, W. R. & Gregory, D. Microecology of
        alcoholism: Implications for the development of the
        adolescent. In J. C. Schoolar (Ed.), *Current issues
        in adolescent psychiatry*. New York: Brunner/Mazel,
        1973. Pp. 158-178.
1399.3 Sobel, R. Adolescence and family stress: A clinician's
        approach. In J. C. Schoolar (Ed.), *Current issues in
        adolescent psychiatry*. New York: Brunner/Mazel,
        1973. Pp. 53-64.

DEVELOPMENTAL ISSUES/Societal Determinants

1400   *Anthony, E. J. The reactions of adults to adolescents
        and their behavior. In G. Caplan & S. Lebovici (Eds.)
        Adolescence: Psychosocial perspectives. New York:
        Basic Books, 1969. Pp. 54-78.
1401   *Gordon, C. Social characteristics of early adolescence.
        Daedalus, 1971, *100*, 931-960.
1402   Marcus, I. M. From school to work: Certain aspects of
        psychosocial interaction. In G. Caplan & S. Lebovici
        (Eds.), *Adolescence: Psychosocial perspectives.* New
        York: Basic Books, 1969. Pp. 157-164.
1403   *Bakan, D. Adolescence in America: From idea to social
        fact. *Daedalus*, 1971, *100*, 979-995.
1404   *Keniston, K. Youth as a stage of life. *Annals of the
        American Society for Adolescent Psychiatry*, 1971, *1*,
        161-175.
1405   *Keniston, K. Student activism, moral development, and
        morality. *American Journal of Orthopsychiatry*, 1970,
        40, 577-592.
1406   *Baittle, B. & Offer, D. On the nature of male adoles-
        cent rebellion. *Annals of the American Society for
        Adolescent Psychiatry*, 1971, *1*, 139-160.
1407   *Noshpitz, J. D. Certain cultural and familial factors
        contributing to adolescent alienation. *Journal of
        the American Academy of Child Psychiatry*, 1970, *9*,
        216-223.
1407.1   Cambor, C. G. Adolescent alienation syndrome. In J. C.
        Schoolar (Ed.), *Current issues in adolescent psychia-
        try*. New York: Brunner/Mazel, 1973. Pp. 101-117.
1408   *Greenacre, P. Youth, growth, and violence. *Psychoana-
        lytic Study of the Child*, 1970, *25*, 340-359.
1409   *Erikson, E. H. Toward contemporary issues: Youth. In
        Identity, youth and crisis. New York: Norton, 1968.
        Pp. 232-260.
1410   Mays, J. B. The adolescent as a social being. In J.
        G. Howells (Ed.), *Modern perspectives in adolescent
        psychiatry*. Edinburgh: Oliver & Boyd, 1971. Pp.
        126-151. (Modern perspectives in psychiatry, vol. 4)
1411   *Mead, M. *From the South Seas: Studies of adolescence
        and sex in primitive societies*. New York: Morrow,
        1939.
1412   *Pierce, C. M. Problems of the Negro adolescent in the
        next decade. In E. B. Brody (Ed.), *Minority group
        adolescents in the United States*. Baltimore: Wil-
        liams & Wilkins, 1968. Pp. 17-47.
1413   *Preble, E. The Puerto Rican-American teen-ager in New
        York City. In E. B. Brody (Ed.), *Minority group adol-
        escents in the United States*. Baltimore: Williams &
        Wilkins, 1968. Pp. 48-72.
1413.1   Yamamoto, J. & Coleman, W. F. Adolescence and poverty--
        From Little Tokyo to black housing projects to the

heartland of America. In J. C. Schoolar (Ed.), *Current issues in adolescent psychiatry*. New York: Brunner/Mazel, 1973. Pp. 65-76.

1414   Mead, M. *Culture and commitment: A study of the generation gap*. Garden City, N.Y.: National History Press, 1970.

1415   Mead, M. Adolescence in primitive and in modern society. In Society for the Psychological Study of Social Issues, *Readings in social psychology*. (3rd ed.) New York: Holt, Rinehart & Winston, 1958. Pp. 341-349.

1416   Fountain, G. Adolescent into adult: An inquiry. *Journal of the American Psychoanalytic Association*, 1961, *9*, 417-433.

1417   *Freeman, D. M. A. Adolescent crises of the Kiowa-Apache Indian male. In E. B. Brody (Ed.), *Minority group adolescents in the United States*. Baltimore: Williams & Wilkins, 1968. Pp. 157-204.

1418   Hollingshead, A. B. *Elmtown's youth*. New York: Science Editions, 1961. Pp. 439-453.

1419   Erikson, E. H. *Identity, youth and crisis*. New York: Norton, 1968.

1419.1   Borus, J. F. Incidence of maladjustment in Vietnam returnees. *Archives of General Psychiatry*, 1974, *30*, 554-557.

1419.2   Shore, M. F. & Massimo, J. L. An innovative approach to the treatment of adolescent delinquent boys within a suburban community. In S. E. Golann and C. Eisdorfer (Eds.), *Handbook of community mental health*. New York: Appleton-Century-Crofts, 1972. Pp. 659-668.

1419.3   Gutmann, D. The vicissitudes of ego identity: Some consequences of the new morality. In J. C. Schoolar (Ed.), *Current issues in adolescent psychiatry*. New York: Brunner/Mazel, 1973. Pp. 34-50.

DEVELOPMENTAL DISORDERS

1420   *Beres, D. & Obers, S. J. The effects of extreme deprivation in infancy on psychic structure in adolescence: A study in ego development. *Psychoanalytic Study of the Child*, 1950, *5*, 212-235.

1421   *Sklarew, B. H. The relationship of early separation from parents to differences in adjustment in adolescent boys and girls. *Psychiatry*, 1959, *22*, 399-405.

1422   *Freud, A. Adolescence. *Psychoanalytic Study of the Child*, 1958, *13*, 255-278. (*Writings*, vol. 5, pp. 136-166)

1423   *Masterson, J. F. The psychiatric significance of adolescent turmoil. *American Journal of Psychiatry*, 1968, *124*, 1549-1554.

1424   *Bruch, H. Obesity in adolescence. In J. G. Howells
(Ed.), *Modern perspectives in adolescent psychiatry.*
Edinburgh: Oliver & Boyd, 1971. Pp. 254-273. (Modern perspectives in psychiatry, vol. 4)

1425   Werkman, S. L. & Greenberg, E. Personality and interest patterns in obese adolescent girls. *Psychosomatic
Medicine*, 1967, *29*, 72-80.

1426   Easson, W. M. *The severely disturbed adolescent.* New
York: International Universities Press, 1969.

1427   *Korkina, M. V. The syndrome of derealisation in adolescence. In J. G. Howells (Ed.), *Modern perspectives
in adolescent psychiatry.* Edinburgh: Oliver & Boyd,
1971. Pp. 329-357. (Modern perspectives in psychiatry, vol. 4)

1428   Laufer, M. Object loss and mourning during adolescence.
Psychoanalytic Study of the Child, 1966, *21*, 269-293.

1429   *Katan, A. The role of "displacement" in agoraphobia.
International Journal of Psychoanalysis, 1951, *32*,
41-50.

1430   *Krevelen, D. A. van Psychoses in adolescence. In J.
G. Howells (Ed.), *Modern perspectives in adolescent
psychiatry.* Edinburgh: Oliver & Boyd, 1971. Pp.
381-403.

1431   *Gardner, G. E. Psychiatric problems of adolescence.
In S. Arieti (Ed.), *American handbook of psychiatry.*
Vol. 1. New York: Basic Books, 1959. Pp. 870-892.

1432   Weiner, I. B. *Psychological disturbance in adolescence.*
New York: Wiley-Interscience, 1970.

1432.1 Holmes, D. J. Superego deficit in incipient sociopathy.
In J. C. Schoolar (Ed.), *Current issues in adolescent
psychiatry.* New York: Brunner/Mazel, 1973. Pp. 118-128.

1432.2 White, R. B. Adolescent identity crisis. In J. C.
Schoolar (Ed.), *Current issues in adolescent psychiatry.* New York: Brunner/Mazel, 1973. Pp. 19-33.

SUICIDE IN ADOLESCENCE

1433   *Mattsson, A., Seese, L. R. & Hawkins, J. W. Suicidal
behavior as a child psychiatric emergency: Clinical
characteristics and follow-up results. *Archives of
General Psychiatry*, 1969, *20*, 100-109.

1434   *Finch, S. M. & Poznanski, E. O. *Adolescent suicide.*
Springfield, Ill.: Thomas, 1971.

1435   *Stanley, E. J. & Barter, J. T. Adolescent suicidal behavior. *American Journal of Orthopsychiatry*, 1970,
40, 87-96.

1436   *Barter, J. T., Swaback, D. O. & Todd, D. Adolescent
suicide attempts: A follow-up study of hospitalized
patients. *Archives of General Psychiatry*, 1968, *19*,
523-527.

1437   Balser, B. H. & Masterson, J. F. Suicide in adolescents. *American Journal of Psychiatry*, 1959, *116*, 400-404.

1438   Wieder, H. & Kaplan, E. H. Drug use in adolescents: Psychodynamic meaning and pharmacogenic effect. *Psychoanalytic Study of the Child*, 1969, *24*, 399-431.

1438.1   Bourne, P. G. Suicide among Chinese in San Francisco. *American Journal of Public Health*, 1973, *63*, 744-750.

1438.2   Tabachnick, N. Creative suicidal crises. *Archives of General Psychiatry*, 1973, *29*, 258-263.

1438.3   Burstein, A. G., Adams, R. L. & Giffen, M. B. Assessment of suicidal risk by psychology and psychiatry trainees. *Archives of General Psychiatry*, 1973, *29*, 792-793.

1438.4   Maltsberger, J. T. & Buie, D. H. Countertransference hate in the treatment of suicidal patients. *Archives of General Psychiatry*, 1974, *30*, 625-633.

1438.5   Teicher, J. D. A solution to the chronic problem of living: Adolescent attempted suicide. In J. C. Schoolar (Ed.), *Current issues in adolescent psychiatry*. New York: Brunner/Mazel, 1973. Pp. 129-147.

1438.6   Dizmang, L. H., Watson, J., May, P. A. & Bopp, J. Adolescent suicide at an Indian reservation. *American Journal of Orthopsychiatry*, 1974, *44*, 43-49.

PSYCHOTHERAPY

1439   *Meeks, J. E. *The fragile alliance: An orientation to the outpatient psychotherapy of the adolescent*. Baltimore: Williams & Wilkins, 1971.

1440   *Gitelson, M. VI. Character synthesis: The psychotherapeutic problem of adolescence. *American Journal of Orthopsychiatry*, 1948, *18*, 422-431.

1441   *Blos, P. Intensive psychotherapy in relation to the various phases of the adolescent period. *American Journal of Orthopsychiatry*, 1962, *32*, 901-910.

1442   *Corday, R. J. Limitations of therapy in adolescence. *Journal of the American Academy of Child Psychiatry*, 1967, *6*, 526-538.

1443   Lorand, S. & Schneer, H. I. (Eds.) *Adolescents: Psychoanalytic approach to problems and therapy*. New York: P. B. Hoeber, 1961.

1444   Holmes, D. J. *The adolescent in psychotherapy*. Boston: Little, Brown, 1964.

1445   *Balser, B. H. (Ed.) *Psychotherapy of the adolescent*. New York: International Universities Press, 1957.

1446   *Mattsson, A. The male therapist and the female adolescent patient. *Journal of the American Academy of Child Psychiatry*, 1970, *9*, 707-721.

1446.1   Pichel, J. I. A long-term follow-up study of 60 adolescent psychiatric outpatients. *American Journal of Psychiatry*, 1974, *131*, 140-144.

1446.2   Marohn, R. C., Dalle-Molle, D., Offer, D. & Ostrov, E.
A hospital riot: Its determinants and implications
for treatment. *American Journal of Psychiatry*, 1973,
130, 631-636.

1446.3   Harley, M. On some problems of technique in the analysis of early adolescents. *Psychoanalytic Study of
the Child*, 1970, *25*, 99-121.

1446.4   Werkman, S. L. Value confrontations between psychotherapists and adolescent patients. *American Journal
of Orthopsychiatry*, 1974, *44*, 337-344.

1466.5   Maltsberger, J. T. & Buie, D. H. Countertransference
hate in the treatment of suicidal patients. *Archives
of General Psychiatry*, 1974, *30*, 625-633.

1446.6   Miller, D. The development of psychiatric treatment
services for adolescents. In J. C. Schoolar (Ed.),
Current issues in adolescent psychiatry. New York:
Brunner/Mazel, 1973. Pp. 189-202.

1446.7   Bauer, R. & Stein, J. Sex counseling on campus: Short-
term treatment techniques. *American Journal of Orthopsychiatry*, 1973, *43*, 824-839.

ADDITIONAL REFERENCES

1447   Blos, P. Prolonged adolescence: The formulation of a
syndrome and its therapeutic implications. *American
Journal of Orthopsychiatry*, 1954, *24*, 733-742.

1448   Douglas, J. D. *Youth in turmoil; America's changing
youth cultures and student protest movements.* Chevy
Chase, Md.: U.S. National Institute of Mental Health,
Center for Studies of Crime and Delinquency, 1970.

1449   Erikson, E. H. *Identity, youth and crisis*. New York:
Norton, 1968.

1450   Deutsch, H. *Selected problems of adolescence; with
special emphasis on group formation*. New York: International Universities Press, 1967.

1450.1   Monsour, K. J. & Stewart, B. Abortion and sexual behavior in college women. *American Journal of Orthopsychiatry*, 1973, *43*, 804-814.

1450.2   Kane, F. J., Jr. & Lachenbruch, P. A. Adolescent pregnancy: A study of aborters and non-aborters. *American Journal of Orthopsychiatry*, 1973, *43*, 796-803.

1450.3   Abernethy, V. & Abernethy, G. L. Risk for unwanted
pregnancy among mentally ill adolescent girls. *American Journal of Orthopsychiatry*, 1974, *44*, 442-449.

1451   Goodman, P. *Growing up absurd*. New York: Random
House, 1960.

1452   Keniston, K. *Young radicals*. New York: Harcourt,
Brace & World, 1968.

1453   *Hartmann, D. A study of drug-taking adolescents. *Psychoanalytic Study of the Child*, 1969, *24*, 384-398.

1454   Keniston, K. *Youth and dissent*. New York: Harcourt,
Brace, Jovanovich, 1971.

1455   Spiegel, L. A. Comments on the psychoanalytic psychol-
        ogy of adolescence. *Psychoanalytic Study of the
        Child*, 1958, *13*, 296-308.
1456   Szurek, S. A. An attitude towards (child) psychiatry.
        Part IV. *Quarterly Journal of Child Behavior*, 1949,
        1, 195-213.
1457   Allen, J. R. & West, L. J. Flight from violence: Hip-
        pies and the green rebellion. *American Journal of
        Psychiatry*, 1968, *125*, 364-370.
1457.1 U.S. National Center for Health Statistics. *Teenagers:
        marriages, divorces, parenthood, and mortality; anal-
        ysis of teenage marriage, divorce, parenthood (includ-
        ing information on illegitimacy rates and ratios),
        and mortality during the 1960's.* Washington: Supt.
        of Docs., 1973. DHEW pub. no. (HRA) 74-1901.
1457.2 U.S. National Center for Health Statistics. *Divorces:
        analysis of changes, United States, 1969; analysis of
        divorce statistics for 1968 and 1969, increases of
        divorces in 1963-69 by characteristics of the divor-
        cing couples, and data on several variables for which
        information was collected for the first time.* Rock-
        ville, Md.: Supt. of Docs., U.S. Govt. Print. Off.,
        1973. (*Vital and health statistics. Ser. 21: Data
        from the National Vital Statistics System, no. 22.*)
1457.3 Sundqvist, U. B. *Academic performance and mental health
        in university students; a two-year follow-up study of
        a sample of first-year students at the University of
        Uppsala 1968.* Copenhagen: Munksgaard, 1973. (*Acta
        psychiatrica Scandinavica.* Supplementum 239.)
1457.4 Glasscote, R. M. & Fishman, M. D. *Mental health on the
        campus; a field study.* Washington: Joint Informa-
        tion Service of the American Psychiatric Association
        and the National Association for Mental Health, 1973.
1457.5 Schoolar, J. C. (Ed.) *Current issues in adolescent
        psychiatry.* New York: Brunner/Mazel, 1973.
1457.6 Gossett, J. T., Lewis, S. B., Lewis, J. M. & Phillips,
        V. A. Follow-up of adolescents in a psychiatric
        hospital: I. A review of studies. *American Journal
        of Orthopsychiatry*, 1973, *43*, 602-610.
1457.7 Ottenberg, P. Delivery of adolescent services: A
        model for the future. In J. C. Schoolar (Ed.),
        Current issues in adolescent psychiatry. New York:
        Brunner/Mazel, 1973. Pp. 181-188.

XI. DELINQUENCY, ANTI-SOCIAL, IMPULSIVE AGGRESSIVE DISORDERS

CLASSICAL STUDIES

1458   *Aichhorn, A. (1925) *Wayward youth.* New York: Viking
        Press, 1935.
1459   *Bowlby, J. Forty-four juvenile thieves: Their charac-
        ters and homelife. *International Journal of Psycho-

analysis, 1944, *25*, 19-53. (Also published separately: London: Bailliere, Tindall & Cox, 1946.)

1460   *Healy, W. & Bronner, A. F. *New light on delinquency and its treatment*. New Haven: Yale University Press, 1936.

1461   Karpman, B., et al. Psychopathic behavior in infants and children: A critical survey of the existing concepts. Round Table, 1950. *American Journal of Orthopsychiatry*, 1951, *21*, 223-272.

1462   Karpman, B., et al. A differential study of psychopathic behavior in infants and children. Round Table, 1951. *American Journal of Orthopsychiatry*, 1952, *22*, 223-267.

1463   Kanner, L. *Delinquency in child psychiatry*. Springfield, Ill.: C. C. Thomas, 1957. Pp. 676-721.

1464   Pearson, G. H. The chronically aggressive child. *Quarterly Journal of Child Behavior*, 1951, *3*, 407-448.

1465   *Redl, F. & Wineman, D. *Children who hate*. Glencoe, Ill.: Free Press, 1951.

1466   *Redl, F. & Wineman, D. *Controls from within*. Glencoe, Ill.: Free Press, 1952.

1467   *Bettelheim, B. *Truants from life*. Glencoe, Ill.: Free Press, 1955.

1468   Glueck, S. *The problem of delinquency*. Boston: Houghton, Mifflin, 1959.

1469   Bovet, L. *Psychiatric aspects of juvenile delinquency*. Geneva: World Health Organization, 1951. (Monograph series, no. 1)

1470   Glueck, S. & Glueck, E. *Toward a typology of juvenile offenders*. New York: Grune & Stratton, 1970.

1471   *Friedlander, K. *The psycho-analytical approach to juvenile delinquency*. London: Kegan Paul, Trench, Trubner, 1947.

DYNAMICS OF ANTISOCIAL AND DELINQUENT BEHAVIOR

1472   *Malmquist, C. P. Conscience development. *Psychoanalytic Study of the Child*, 1968, *23*, 301-331.

1473   *Rexford, E. N. A developmental concept of the problems of acting out. *Journal of the American Academy of Child Psychiatry*, 1963, *2*, 6-21.

1474   *Rexford, E. N. & Van Amerongen, S. T. The influence of unsolved maternal oral conflicts upon impulsive acting out in young children. *American Journal of Orthopsychiatry*, 1957, *27*, 75-87.

1475   *Josselyn, I. M. A type of predelinquent behavior. *American Journal of Orthopsychiatry*, 1958, *28*, 606-612.

1476   Reiser, D. E. Observations of delinquent behavior in very young children. *Journal of the American Academy of Child Psychiatry*, 1963, *2*, 50-71.

1477   Berman, S. Antisocial character disorder: Its etiology
and relationship to delinquency. *American Journal of
Orthopsychiatry*, 1959, *29*, 612-621.
1478   *Bernabeu, E. P. Underlying ego mechanisms in delinquency. *Psychoanalytic Quarterly*, 1958, *27*, 383-396.
1479   *Johnson, A. M. Juvenile delinquency. In S. Arieti
(Ed.), *American handbook of psychiatry*. Vol. 1.
New York: Basic Books, 1959. Pp. 840-856.
1480   *Friedlander, K. Formation of the antisocial character.
Psychoanalytic Study of the Child, 1945, *1*, 189-203.
1481   Van Amerongen, S. T. Permission, promotion, and pro-
vocation of antisocial behavior. *Journal of the
American Academy of Child Psychiatry*, 1963, *2*, 99-
117.
1482   *Noshpitz, J. D. & Spielman, P. Diagnosis: Study of the
differential characteristics of hyperaggressive children. *American Journal of Orthopsychiatry*, 1961, *31*,
111-122.
1483   *Malone, C. A. Some observations on children of disorganized families and problems of acting out. *Journal
of the American Academy of Child Psychiatry*, 1963, *2*,
22-49.
1484   Jenkins, R. L. Motivation and frustration in delinquency. *American Journal of Orthopsychiatry*, 1957,
27, 528-537.
1485   Falstein, E. I. The psychodynamics of male adolescent
delinquency. *American Journal of Orthopsychiatry*,
1958, *28*, 613-626.
1486   *Blos, P. The concept of acting out in relation to the
adolescent process. *Journal of the American Academy
of Child Psychiatry*, 1963, *2*, 118-143.
1487   *Bloch, D. A. The delinquent integration. *Psychiatry*,
1952, *15*, 297-303.
1488   *Johnson, A. M. & Szurek, S. A. The genesis of antisocial acting out in children and adults. *Psychoanalytic Quarterly*, 1952, *21*, 323-343.
1489   Giffin, M. E., Johnson, A. M. & Litin, E. M. Symposium, 1954. Antisocial acting out. 2. Specific factors determining antisocial acting out. *American
Journal of Orthopsychiatry*, 1954, *24*, 668-684.
1490   *Johnson, A. M. Sanctions for superego lacunae of adolescents. In K. R. Eissler (Ed.), *Searchlights on
delinquency*. New York: International Universities
Press, 1949. Pp. 225-245.
1491   Frankenstein, C. The configurational approach to
causation in the study of juvenile delinquents. *Archives of Criminal Psychodynamics*, 1957, *2*, 572-596.
1493   *Levitt, M. & Rubenstein, B. O. Acting out in adolescence: A study in communication. *American Journal
of Orthopsychiatry*, 1959, *29*, 622-632.
1494   Finch, S. M. The psychiatrist and juvenile delinquency. *Journal of the American Academy of Child Psychiatry*, 1962, *1*, 619-635.

1495   *Johnson, A. M. & Robinson, D. B. The sexual deviant
        (Sexual psychopath)--Causes, treatment, and preven-
        tion. *Journal of the American Medical Association*,
        1957, *164*, 1559-1565.
1497   Hirschi, T. *Causes of delinquency*. Berkeley: Univer-
        sity of California Press, 1969.
1498   Bloch, H. A. & Flynn, F. T. *Delinquency*. New York:
        Random House, 1956.

GIRLS AND ANTISOCIAL BEHAVIOR

1499   *Lander, J. Some aspects of female delinquency. *Journal
        of the American Academy of Child Psychiatry*, 1963, *2*,
        549-560.
1500   *Kaufman, I., Makkay, E. S. & Zilbach, J. The impact of
        adolescence on girls with delinquent character forma-
        tion. *American Journal of Orthopsychiatry*, 1959, *29*,
        130-143.

THE FAMILY AND ANTISOCIAL BEHAVIOR

1501   *Rexford, E. N. & Van Amerongen, S. T. The influence of
        unsolved maternal oral conflicts upon impulsive acting
        out in young children. *American Journal of Orthopsy-
        chiatry*, 1957, *27*, 75-87.
1502   *Johnson, A. M. & Szurek, S. A. The genesis of anti-
        social acting out in children and adults. *Psychoana-
        lytic Quarterly*, 1952, *21*, 323-343.
1503   *Rexford, E. N. Antisocial young children and their
        families. In L. Jessner & E. Pavenstedt (Eds.),
        Dynamic psychopathology in childhood. New York:
        Grune & Stratton, 1959. Pp. 186-220.
1504   *Giffin, M. E., Johnson, A. M. & Litin, E. M. Symposium,
        1954. Antisocial acting out. 2. Specific factors
        determining antisocial acting out. *American Journal
        of Orthopsychiatry*, 1954, *24*, 668-684.
1505   *Carek, D. J., Hendrickson, W. J. & Holmes, D. J. Delin-
        quency addiction in parents. *Archives of General Psy-
        chiatry*, 1961, *4*, 357-362.
1506   *Litin, E. M., Giffin, M. E. & Johnson, A. M. Parental
        influence in unusual sexual behavior in children.
        Psychoanalytic Quarterly, 1956, *25*, 37-55.
1507   *Sperling, M. A study of deviate sexual behavior in
        children by the method of simultaneous analysis of
        mother and child. In L. Jessner & E. Pavenstedt
        (Eds.), *Dynamic psychopathology in childhood*. New
        York: Grune & Stratton, 1959. Pp. 221-242.
1508   *Szurek, S. A. & Berlin, I. N. (Eds.) *The antisocial
        child: His family and his community*. Palo Alto,
        Calif.: Science & Behavior Books, 1969.

1509   Andry, R. G. *Delinquency and parental pathology*. London: Methuen, 1960.
1510   Reiner, B. S. & Kaufman, I. *Character disorders in parents of delinquents*. New York: Family Service Association of America, 1959.

TREATMENT

1511   *Rosenberg, R. M. & Mueller, B. C. Preschool antisocial children: Psychodynamic considerations and implications for treatment. *Journal of the American Academy of Child Psychiatry*, 1968, *7*, 421-441.
1512   *Sperling, M. A study of deviate sexual behavior in children by the method of simultaneous analysis of mother and child. In L. Jessner & E. Pavenstedt (Eds.), *Dynamic psychopathology in childhood*. New York: Grune & Stratton, 1959. Pp. 221-242.
1513   *Eissler, K. R. Ego-psychological Implications of the psychoanalytic treatment of delinquents. *Psychoanalytic Study of the Child*, 1950, *5*, 97-121.
1514   *Berman, S. Techniques of treatment of a form of juvenile delinquency, the antisocial character disorder. *Journal of the American Academy of Child Psychiatry*, 1964, *3*, 24-52.
1515   *Minuchin, S., Chamberlain, P. & Graubard, P. A project to teach learning skills to disturbed, delinquent children. *American Journal of Orthopsychiatry*, 1967, *37*, 558-567.
1516   *Gordon, S. A psychotherapeutic approach to adolescents with character disorders. *American Journal of Orthopsychiatry*, 1960, *30*, 757-766.
1517   Schulman, I. Dynamics and treatment of anti-social psychopathology in adolescents. *Nervous Child*, 1955, *11*, 35-41.
1518   Buck, A. E. & Grygier, T. A new attempt in psychotherapy with juvenile delinquents. *American Journal of Psychotherapy*, 1952, *6*, 711-724.
1519   *Shore, M. F., Massimo, J. L., Kisielewski, J. & Moran, J. K. Object relations changes resulting from successful psychotherapy with adolescent delinquents and their relationship to academic performance. *Journal of the American Academy of Child Psychiatry*, 1966, *5*, 93-104.
1520   *Sullivan, C., Grant, M. Q. & Grant, J. D. The development of interpersonal maturity: Applications to delinquency. *Psychiatry*, 1957, *20*, 373-385.
1521   *Szymanski, L. & Fleming, A. Juvenile delinquent and an adult prisoner: A therapeutic encounter? *Journal of the American Academy of Child Psychiatry*, 1971, *10*, 308-320.
1522   Peck, H. B. & Bellsmith, V. *Treatment of the delinquent adolescent: group and individual therapy with parent*

and child. New York: Family Service Association of America, 1954.

1523   Schneer, H., Gottesfeld, H. & Sales, A. Group therapy as an aid with delinquent pubescents in a special public school. *Psychiatric Quarterly*, 1957, *31*(Supplement), 246-260.

1524   *Slavson, S. R. *Reclaiming the delinquent by para-analytic group psychotherapy and the inversion technique*. New York: Free Press, 1965.

1525   *Kaplan, M., Ryan, J. F., Nathan, E. & Bairos, M. The control of acting out the psychotherapy of delinquents. *American Journal of Psychiatry*, 1957, *113*, 1108-1114.

1526   Schmideberg, M. Treating the unwilling patient. *British Journal of Delinquency*, 1958, *9*, 117-122.

1527   *Staats, A. W. & Butterfield, W. H. Treatment of non-reading in a culturally deprived juvenile delinquent: An application of reinforcement principles. *Child Development*, 1965, *36*, 925-942.

1528   *Burchard, J. & Tyler, V. The modification of delinquent behaviour through operant conditioning. *Behaviour Research and Therapy*, 1965, *2*, 245-250.

1529   *Whitaker, C. A. Ormsby Village: An experiment with forced psychotherapy in the rehabilitation of the delinquent adolescent. *Psychiatry*, 1946, *9*, 239-250.

1530   *Willner, M. Treatment of gangs in a delinquent boys' institution. *Child Welfare*, 1957, *36*(6), 1-5.

DRUG ABUSE

1531   *Wieder, H. & Kaplan, E. H. Drug use in adolescents: Psychodynamic meaning and pharmacogenic effect. *Psychoanalytic Study of the Child*, 1969, *24*, 399-431.

1532   *Hartmann, D. A study of drug-taking adolescents. *Psychoanalytic Study of the Child*, 1969, *24*, 384-398.

1533   *Pearlman, S. Drug use and experience in an urban college population. *American Journal of Orthopsychiatry*, 1968, *38*, 503-514.

1534   *Proskauer, S. & Rolland, R. S. Youth who use drugs: Psychodynamic diagnosis and treatment planning. *Journal of the American Academy of Child Psychiatry*, 1973, *12*, 32-47.

1535   *Nichtern, S. The children of drug users. *Journal of the American Academy of Child Psychiatry*, 1973, *12*, 24-31.

1536   *Levitt, L. Rehabilitation of narcotics addicts among lower-class teenagers. *American Journal of Orthopsychiatry*, 1968, *38*, 56-62.

1537   Mason, P. The mother of the addict. *Psychiatric Quarterly*, 1958, *32*(Supplement), 189-199.

1538   Cohen, M. & Klein, D. F. Drug abuse in a young psychiatric population. *American Journal of Orthopsychiatry*, 1970, *40*, 448-455.

1539   *Gershon, S. On the pharmacology of marihuana. *Behavioral Neuropsychiatry*, 1970, *1*(10), 9-18.
1540   Council on Mental Health. Committee on Alcoholism and Drug Dependence. Dependence on cannabis (marihuana). *Journal of the American Medical Association*, 1967, *201*, 368-371.
1541   *Talbott, J. A. & Teague, J. W. Marihuana psychosis: Acute toxic psychosis associated with the use of Cannabis derivatives. *Journal of the American Medical Association*, 1969, *210*, 299-302.
1542   Council on Mental Health. Marihuana and society. *Journal of the American Medical Association*, 1968, *204*, 1181-1182.
1543   Marihuana thing. *Journal of the American Medical Association*, 1968, *204*, 1187-1188.
1544   *Ames, F. A clinical and metabolic study of acute intoxication with Cannabis sativa and its role in the model psychosis. *Journal of Mental Science*, 1958, *104*, 972-999.
1545   Allentuck, S. Medical aspects. In D. Solomon (Ed.), *The marihuana papers*. Indianapolis: Bobbs-Merrill, 1966. Pp. 269-284.
1546   Bromberg, W. Marihuana intoxication: A clinical study of Cannabis sativa intoxication. *American Journal of Psychiatry*, 1934, *91*, 303-330.
1547   Isbell, H., et al. Effects of (-)Δ^9- Trans-Tetrahydrocannabinol in man. *Psychopharmacologia*, 1967, *11*, 184-188.
1548   *Gioscia, V. LSD subcultures: Acidoxy versus orthodoxy. *American Journal of Orthopsychiatry*, 1969, *39*, 428-436.
1549   Smart, R. G. & Bateman, K. Unfavourable reactions to LSD: A review and analysis of the available case reports. *Canadian Medical Association Journal*, 1967, *97*, 1214-1221.
1550   *Wiener, J. M. & Egan, J. H. Heroin addiction in an adolescent population. *Journal of the American Academy of Child Psychiatry*, 1973, *12*, 48-58.
1551   *Corliss, L. M. A review of the evidence on glue-sniffing -- A persistent problem. *Journal of School Health*, 1965, *35*, 442-449.
1552   *Rubin, T. & Babbs, J. The glue sniffer. *Federal Probation*, 1970, *34*(3), 23-28.
1552.1 Shearn, C. R. & Fitzgibbons, D. J. Patterns of drug use in a population of youthful psychiatric patients. *American Journal of Psychiatry*, 1972, *128*, 1381-1387.
1553   Pearson, G. H. J. *Adolescence and the conflict of generations.* (1st ed.) New York: Norton, 1958.
1554   Freud, A. Adolescence. *Psychoanalytic Study of the Child*, 1958, *13*, 255-278. (*Writings*, vol. 5, pp. 136-166)

FOLLOW-UP STUDIES

1555   *Morris, H. H., Escoll, P. J. & Wexler, R. Aggressive
       behavior disorders of childhood: A follow-up study.
       American Journal of Psychiatry, 1956, *112*, 991-997.
1556   *Kaufman, I., Heims, L. W. & Reiser, D. E. A re-evalua-
       tion of the psychodynamics of firesetting. *American
       Journal of Orthopsychiatry*, 1961, *31*, 123-136.

SOCIOLOGICAL STUDIES

1557   *Hollingshead, A. B. *Elmtown's youth*. New York: Sci-
       ence Editions, 1961.
1558   McDonald, L. *Social class and delinquency*. London:
       Faber & Faber, 1969.
1559   *Malmquist, C. P. Dilemmas of the juvenile court. *Jour-
       nal of the American Academy of Child Psychiatry*, 1967,
       6, 723-748.
1560   Matza, D. *Becoming deviant*. Englewood Cliffs, N.J.:
       Prentice Hall, 1969.

ADDITIONAL REFERENCES

1561   Karpman, B., et al. Psychopathic behavior in infants
       and children: A critical survey of the existing
       concepts. Round Table, 1950. *American Journal of
       Orthopsychiatry*, 1951, *21*, 223-272.
1562   Karpman, B., et al. A differential study of psycho-
       pathic behavior in infants and children. Round table,
       1951. *American Journal of Orthopsychiatry*, 1952, *22*,
       223-267.
1563   Karpman, B., et al. Psychodynamics of child delinquen-
       cy. Round table, 1952. *American Journal of Orthopsy-
       chiatry*, 1953, *23*, 1-69.
1564   Karpman, B., et al. Psychodynamics of child delinquen-
       cy: Further contributions. Round table, 1953. *Amer-
       ican Journal of Orthopsychiatry*, 1955, *25*, 238-282.
1565   Maenchen, A. A case of superego disintegration. *Psy-
       choanalytic Study of the Child*, 1946, *2*, 257-262.
1566   *Redl, F. & Wineman, D. *The aggressive child*. Glencoe,
       Ill.: Free Press, 1957.
1567   Eissler, K. R. (Ed.) *Searchlights on delinquency*. New
       York: International Universities Press, 1949.
1568   Healy, W. & Bronner, A. F. *New light on delinquency and
       its treatment*. New Haven: Yale University Press,
       1936.

XII. FAILURE TO THRIVE, CHILD NEGLECT AND ABUSE

BIBLIOGRAPHIES

1569   Jones, D. M. *Children who need protection: An annotated bibliography.* Washington: U.S. Dept. of Health, Education, and Welfare, Welfare Administration. Children's Bureau, 1966.
1570   U.S. Children's Bureau. Clearinghouse for Research in Child Life. *Bibliography on the battered child, July 1969 (revised).* Washington: U.S. Dept. of Health, Education, and Welfare, Social and Rehabilitation Service, Children's Bureau Clearinghouse for Research on Child Life, 1969.

HISTORICAL ASPECTS

1573   *Aries, P. *Centuries of childhood: A social history of family life.* New York: Knopf, 1962.
1574   Radbill, S. X. A history of child abuse and infanticide. In R. E. Helfer & C. H. Kempe (Eds.), *The battered child.* Chicago: University of Chicago Press, 1968. Pp. 3-17.
1575   *Kempe, C. H., Silverman, F. N., Steele, B. F., Droegemueller, W. & Silver, H. K. The battered-child syndrome. *Journal of the American Medical Association,* 1962, *181,* 17-24.
1576   Allen, A. & Morton, A. *This is your child: The story of the National Society for the Prevention of Cruelty to Children.* London: Routledge & Kegan Paul, 1961.
1577   *Isaacs, S. Physical ill-treatment of children. *Lancet,* 1968, *1,* 37-39.
1578   Earl, H. G. 10,000 children battered and starved. *Today's Health,* 1965, *43*(9), 24-31.
1579   Coles, R. Terror-struck children. *New Republic,* 1964, *150*(22), 11-13.
1580   *Adelson, L. Slaughter of the innocents: A study of 46 homicides in which the victims were children. *New England Journal of Medicine,* 1961, *264,* 1345-1349.
1581   Barta, R. A. & Smith, N. J. Willful trauma to young children: A challenge to the physician. *Clinical Pediatrics,* 1963, *2,* 545-554.
1582   *Helfer, R. E. & Kempe, C. H. (Eds.) *The battered child.* Chicago: University of Chicago Press, 1968.

DYNAMICS OF CHILD ABUSE

1583   *Bellak, L. & Hurvich, M. A systematic study of ego functions. *Journal of Nervous and Mental Disease,* 1969, *148,* 569-585.

1584   *Ainsworth, M. D. The effects of maternal deprivation:
       A review of findings and controversy in the context of
       research strategy. In World Health Organization,
       *Deprivation of maternal care; a reassessment of its
       effects.* (Public health papers, no. 14) Geneva:
       World Health Organization, 1962. Pp. 97-165.
1585   *Pavenstedt, E. A study of immature mothers and their
       children. In G. Caplan (Ed.), *Prevention of mental
       disorders in children.* New York: Basic Books, 1961.
       Pp. 192-217.
1586   *Malone, C. A. Safety first: Comments on the influence
       of external danger in the lives of children of disor-
       ganized families. *American Journal of Orthopsychia-
       try,* 1966, *36,* 3-12.
1587   *Spitz, R. A. & Wolf, K. M. Anaclitic depression. An
       inquiry into the genesis of psychiatric conditions in
       early childhood, II. *Psychoanalytic Study of the
       Child,* 1946, *2,* 313-342.
1588   Provence, S. A. & Lipton, R. C. *Infants in institu-
       tions.* New York: International Universities Press,
       1963.
1589   Bowlby, J. *Maternal care and mental health.* Geneva:
       World Health Organization, 1951. (Monograph series,
       no. 2)
1590   Winnicott, D. W. *The maturational processes and the
       facilitating environment.* London: Hogarth, 1965.
1591   Thomas, A. et al. *Behavioral individuality in early
       childhood.* New York: New York University Press,
       1963.
1592   Schilder, P. *The image and appearance of the human
       body.* New York: International Universities Press,
       1950.
1593   Whiting, B. B. (Ed.) *Six cultures: Studies of child
       rearing.* New York: Wiley, 1963.
1594   Hurley, R. L. *Poverty and mental retardation.* New
       York: Random House, 1969.
1595   *Reinhart, J. B. & Elmer, E. Love of children -- A
       myth? *Clinical Pediatrics,* 1968, *7,* 703-705.
1596   *Brazelton, T. B. Psychophysiologic reactions in the
       neonate. I: The values of observation of the neo-
       nate. *Journal of Pediatrics,* 1961, *58,* 508-512.
1597   Marans, A. E. & Lourie, R. Hypotheses regarding the
       effects of childrearing patterns on the disadvantaged
       child. In J. Hellmuth (Ed.), *Disadvantaged child.*
       Vol. 1. New York: Brunner/Mazel, 1967. Pp. 17-41.
1598   *Martin, H. The child and his development. In C. H.
       Kempe & R. E. Helfer (Eds.), *Helping the battered
       child and his family.* Philadelphia: J. B. Lippin-
       cott, 1972. Pp. 93-114.
1599   Elmer, E. & Gregg, G. S. Developmental characteristics
       of abused children. *Pediatrics,* 1967, *40,* 596-602.
1600   *Silver, L. B. The psychological aspects of the battered
       child and his parents. *Clinical Proceedings of the
       Children's Hospital,* 1968, *24,* 355-364.

1601   *Milowe, I. D. & Lourie, R. S.   9.   The child's role in
       the battered child syndrome. *Journal of Pediatrics,*
       1964, *65,* 1079-1081.
1602   *Cohen, M. I., Raphling, D. L. & Green, P. E.   Psycho-
       logic aspects of the maltreatment syndrome of child-
       hood. *Journal of Pediatrics,* 1966, *69,* 279-284.
1603   *Morris, M. G. & Gould, R. W.   Neglected children.   Role
       reversal: A necessary concept in dealing with the
       "battered child syndrome". *American Journal of Ortho-*
       psychiatry, 1963, *33,* 298-299.   (Also in *The neglected*
       battered child syndrome.   New York: Child Welfare
       League of America, 1963.)
1604   Morris, M. G.   Psychological miscarriage: An end to
       mother love. *Trans-action,* 1966, *3*(2), 8-13.
1605   *Curtis, G. C.   Violence breeds violence--perhaps?
       American Journal of Psychiatry, 1963, *120,* 386-387.
1606   Green, A. H.   Self-destructive behavior in physically
       abused schizophrenic children. *Archives of General*
       Psychiatry, 1968, *19,* 171-179.
1607   *Benedek, T.   Parenthood as a developmental phase: A
       contribution to the libido theory. *Journal of the*
       American Psychoanalytic Association, 1959, *7,* 389-
       417.
1608   Nurse, S.   Familial patterns of parents who abuse their
       children. *Smith College Studies in Social Work,* 1964,
       35, 11-25.
1609   *Melnick, B. & Hurley, J. R.   Distinctive personality
       attributes of child-abusing mothers. *Journal of Con-*
       sulting and Clinical Psychology, 1969, *33,* 746-749.
1610   *Galdston, R.   Dysfunctions of parenting: The battered
       child, the neglected child, the exploited child.   In
       J. G. Howells (Ed.), *Modern perspectives in inter-*
       national child psychiatry.   Edinburgh: Oliver & Boyd,
       1969.   Pp. 571-588.   (Modern perspectives in psychia-
       try, vol. 3)
1611   *Steele, B. F.   Parental abuse of infants and small chil-
       dren.   In E. J. Anthony & T. Benedek (Eds.), *Parent-*
       hood: Its psychology and psychopathology.   Boston:
       Little, Brown, 1970.   Pp. 449-477.
1612   *Wasserman, S.   The abused parent of the abused child.
       Children, 1967, *14,* 175-179.
1613   Williams, A. E.   *Barnardo of Stepney: The father of*
       nobody's children.   London: George Allen & Unwin,
       1966.
1613.1 Gelles, R. J.   Child abuse as psychopathology: A socio-
       logical critique and reformulation. *American Journal*
       of Orthopsychiatry, 1973, *43,* 611-621.

DIAGNOSIS OF CHILD ABUSE

1614   *Baron, M. A., Bejar, R. L. & Sheaff, P. J. Neurologic
        manifestations of the battered child syndrome. *Pedi-
        atrics*, 1970, *45*, 1003-1007.
1615   Hawkes, C. D. Craniocerebral trauma in infancy and
        childhood. *Clinical Neurosurgery*, 1963, *11*, 66-75.
1616   Russell, P. A. Subdural haematoma in infancy. *British
        Medical Journal*, 1965, *2*, no. 5459, 446-448.
1617   *McHenry, T., Girdany, B. R. & Elmer, E. Unsuspected
        trauma with multiple skeletal injuries during infancy
        and childhood. *Pediatrics*, 1963, *31*, 903-908.
1618   Lis, E. F. & Frauenberger, G. S. Multiple fractures
        associated with subdural hematoma in infancy. *Pedi-
        atrics*, 1950, *6*, 890-892.
1619   *Griffiths, D. L. & Moynihan, F. J. Multiple epiphysial
        injuries in babies ("battered baby" syndrome). *Brit-
        ish Medical Journal*, 1963, *2*, no. 5372, 1558-1561.
1620   Nelson, G. D. & Paletta, F. X. Burns in children.
        Surgery, Gynecology and Obstetrics, 1969, *128*, 518-
        522.
1621   McCort, J. & Vaudagna, J. Visceral injuries in battered
        children. *Radiology*, 1964, *82*, 424-428.
1622   Polomeque, F. E. et al. "Battered child" syndrome:
        Unusual dermatological manifestation. *Archives of
        Dermatology*, 1964, *90*, 326-327.
1623   Gillespie, R. W. The battered child syndrome: Thermal
        and caustic manifestations. *Journal of Trauma*, 1965,
        5, 523-534.
1624   *Dine, M. S. Tranquilizer poisoning: An example of
        child abuse. *Pediatrics*, 1965, *36*, 782-785.
1625   *Murdock, C. G. The abused child and the school system.
        American Journal of Public Health, 1970, *60*, 105-109.
1626   *Holter, J. C. & Friedman, S. B. Child abuse: Early
        case finding in the emergency department. *Pediatrics*,
        1968, *42*, 128-138.
1627   *Rowe, D. S. et al. A hospital program for the detection
        and registration of abused and neglected children.
        New England Journal of Medicine, 1970, *282*, 950-952.
1628   Berlow, L. Recognition and rescue of the "battered
        child". *Hospitals*, 1967, *41*(2), 58-61.
1629   *Werry, J. S. Studies on the hyperactive child. IV. An
        empirical analysis of the minimal brain dysfunction
        syndrome. *Archives of General Psychiatry*, 1968, *19*,
        9-16.
1630   Paine, R. S., Werry, J. S. & Quay, H. C. A study of
        'minimal cerebral dysfunction'. *Developmental Medi-
        cine and Child Neurology*, 1968, *10*, 505-520.
1631   Prechtl, H. F. R. & Stemmer, C. J. The choreiform syn-
        drome in children. *Developmental Medicine and Child
        Neurology*, 1962, *4*, 119-127.
1632   *Berant, M. & Jacobs, J. A "pseudo" battered child.
        Clinical Pediatrics, 1966, *5*, 230-237.

1633   *Caffey, J. Significance of the history in the diagnosis
        of traumatic injury to children. *Journal of Pediat-
        rics*, 1965, *67*, 1008-1014.
1634   Elmer, E. Hazards in determining child abuse. *Child
        Welfare*, 1966, *45*, 28-33.
1635   Elmer, E. Abused young children seen in hospitals.
        Social Work, 1960, *5*, 98-102.
1636   *Silver, L. B., Dublin, C. C. & Lourie, R. S. Child
        abuse syndrome: The "gray areas" in establishing a
        diagnosis. *Pediatrics*, 1969, *44*, 594-600.
1637   *Fontana, V. J. Recognition of maltreatment and pre-
        vention of the battered child syndrome. *Pediatrics*,
        1966, *38*, 1078.
1638   Helfer, R. E. & Pollock, C. B. The battered child syn-
        drome. *Advances in Pediatrics*, 1968, *15*, 9-27.
1639   *Galdston, R. Violence begins at home: The Parents'
        Center Project for the Study and Prevention of Child
        Abuse. *Journal of the American Academy of Child Psy-
        chiatry*, 1971, *10*, 336-350.
1640   *Helfer, R. E. The responsibility and role of the phy-
        sician. In R. E. Helfer & C. H. Kempe (Eds.), *The
        battered child*. Chicago: University of Chicago
        Press, 1968. Pp. 43-57.
1641   Holder, A. R. Child abuse and the physician. *Journal
        of the American Medical Association*, 1972, *222*, 517-
        518.
1642   *Golub, S. The battered child: What the nurse can do.
        Registered Nurse, 1968, *31*, 42-45; 66-68.

CHILD NEGLECT

1643   *Polansky, N. A., De Saix, C. & Sharlin, S. A. *Child
        neglect: Understanding and reaching the parent*. New
        York: Child Welfare League of America, 1972.
1644   Sandusky, A. L. Services to neglected children. *Chil-
        dren*, 1960, *7*, 23-28.
1645   *Adelson, L. Homicide by starvation: The nutritional
        variant of the "battered child". *Journal of the Amer-
        ican Medical Association*, 1963, *186*, 458-460.
1646   *Pickel, S., Anderson, C. & Holliday, M. A. Thirsting
        and hypernatremic dehydration -- A form of child
        abuse. *Pediatrics*, 1970, *45*, 54-59.

FAILURE TO THRIVE

1647   *Bullard, D. M., Glasser, H. H., Heagarty, M. C. &
        Pivchik, E. Failure to thrive in the "neglected"
        child. *American Journal of Orthopsychiatry*, 1967,
        37, 680-690.
1648   Leonard, M. F., Rhymes, J. P. & Solnit, A. J. Failure
        to thrive in infants: A family problem. *American
        Journal of Diseases of Children*, 1966, *111*, 600-612.

1649   Coleman, R. W. & Provence, S. Environmental retarda-
        tion (hospitalism) in infants living in families.
        Pediatrics, 1957, *19*, 285-292.
1650   *Koel, B. S. Failure to thrive and fatal injury as a
        continuum. *American Journal of Diseases of Children*,
        1969, *118*, 565-567.
1651   *Prugh, D. G. & Harlow, R. G. "Masked deprivation" in
        infants and young children. In World Health Organi-
        zation, *Deprivation of maternal care; a reassessment
        of its effects*. (Public health papers, no. 14)
        Geneva: World Health Organization, 1962. Pp. 9-29.
1652   *Blodgett, F. M. Growth retardation related to maternal
        deprivation. In A. J. Solnit & S. A. Provence (Eds.),
        Modern perspectives in child development. New York:
        International Universities Press, 1963. Pp. 83-93.
1653   *Barbero, G. J., Morris, M. G. & Reford, M. T. Maliden-
        tification of mother-baby-father relationships ex-
        pressed in infant failure to thrive. In *The neglect-
        ed battered child syndrome: Role reversal in parents*.
        New York: Child Welfare League of America, 1963.
        Pp. 13-28.
1654   *Whitten, C. F., Pettit, M. G. & Fischhoff, J. Evidence
        that growth failure from maternal deprivation is
        secondary to undereating. *Journal of the American
        Medical Association*, 1969, *209*, 1675-1682.
1655   Silver, H. K. & Finkelstein, M. Deprivation **dwarfism**.
        Journal of Pediatrics, 1967, *70*, 317-324.
1656   *Elmer, E. Failure to thrive: Role of the mother.
        Pediatrics, 1960, *25*, 717-725.
1657   *Whitten, C. F. T.L.C. and the hungry child. *Nutrition
        Today*, 1972, *7*, 10-14.
1658   *Elmer, E., Gregg, G. S. & Ellison, P. Late results of
        the "failure to thrive" syndrome. *Clinical Pediatrics*,
        1969, *8*, 584-589.
1659   Patton, R. G. & Gardner, L. I. *Growth failure in mater-
        nal deprivation*. Springfield, Ill.: Thomas, 1963.

CHILD ABUSE STUDIES

1660   *Simons, B., Downs, E. F., Hurster, M. M. & Archer, M.
        Child abuse: Epidemiologic study of medically re-
        ported cases. *New York State Journal of Medicine*,
        1966, *66*, 2783-2788.
1661   *Silver, L. B. Child abuse syndrome: A review. *Medi-
        cal Times*, 1968, *96*, 803-820.
1662   *Morse, C. W., Sahler, O. J. Z. & Friedman, S. B. A
        three-year follow-up study of abused and neglected
        children. *American Journal of Diseases of Children*,
        1970, *120*, 439-446.
1663   *Gil, D. G. Physical abuse of children: Findings and
        implications of a nationwide survey. *Pediatrics*, 1969,
        44, 857-864.

1664   Resnick, P. J. Child murder by parents: A psychiatric review of filicide. *American Journal of Psychiatry,* 1969, *126,* 325-334.

1665   Kempe, C. H. & Silver, H. K. The problem of parental criminal neglect and severe physical abuse of children. *American Journal of Diseases of Children,* 1959, *98,* 528.

1666   Lonsdale, D. & Evarts, C. M. Guide to the battered child syndrome. *Hospital Medicine,* 1972, *8*(3), 8.

1667   *Galdston, R. Observations on children who have been physically abused and their parents. *American Journal of Psychiatry,* 1965, *122,* 440-443.

1668   Gil, D. G. *Violence against children; physical child abuse in the United States.* Cambridge, Mass.: Harvard University Press, 1970.

1670   Elmer, E. et al. *Children in jeopardy: A study of abused minors and their families.* Pittsburgh: University of Pittsburgh Press, 1967.

1671   Gil, D. G. *Violence against children; physical child abuse in the United States.* Cambridge, Mass.: Harvard University Press, 1970.

1672   Young, L. R. *Wednesday's children: A study of child neglect and abuse.* New York: McGraw-Hill, 1964.

PREVENTION AND TREATMENT

1673   *Morris, M. G., Gould, R. W. & Matthews, P. J. Toward prevention of child abuse. *Children,* 1964, *11,* 55-60.

1674   Birch, H. G. & Gussow, J. D. *Disadvantaged children: Health, nutrition and school failure.* New York: Grune & Stratton, 1970.

1675   *Taylor, A. Deprived infants: Potential for affective adjustment. *American Journal of Orthopsychiatry,* 1968, *38,* 835-845.

1676   Leaverton, D. R. The pediatrician's role in maternal deprivation: Illustrative cases and an approach to early recognition. *Clinical Pediatrics,* 1968, *7,* 340-343.

1677   *Pollock, C. B. Early case finding as a means of prevention of child abuse. In R. E. Helfer & C. H. Kempe (Eds.), *The battered child.* Chicago: University of Chicago Press, 1968. Pp. 149-152.

1678   Jacobziner, H. Rescuing the battered child. *American Journal of Nursing,* 1964, *64*(6), 92-97.

1679   *Holter, J. C. et al. Principles of management in child abuse cases. *American Journal of Orthopsychiatry,* 1968, *38,* 127-136.

1680   *Delsordo, J. D. Protective casework for abused children. *Children,* 1963, *10,* 213-218.

1681   *Rappaport, M. F. & Finberg, L. The neglected child: Collaborative approaches to recognition and management. *Clinical Pediatrics*, 1963, *2*, 521-524.

1682   Silver, L., Dublin, C. C. & Lourie, R. S. Agency action
and interaction in cases of child abuse. *Social Casework*, 1971, *52*, 164-171.

1683   *Schwartz, L. H., Snider, J. & Schwartz, J. E. Psychiatric case report of nutritional battering with implications for community agencies. *Community Mental
Health Journal*, 1967, *3*, 163-169.

1684   *Foresman, L. Homemaker service in neglect and abuse.
I. Strengthening family life. *Children*, 1965, *12*,
23-26.

1685   Stringer, E. A. Homemaker service in neglect and abuse.
II. A tool for case evaluation. *Children*, 1965, *12*,
26-29.

1686   Gil, D. G. What schools can do about child abuse.
American Education, 1969, *5*(4), 2-4.

1687   *Loomis, W. G. Management of children's emotional reactions to severe body damage (burns). *Clinical Pediatrics*, 1970, *9*, 362-367.

1688   *Schulman, J. L. The management of the irate parent.
Journal of Pediatrics, 1970, *77*, 338-340.

1689   *Feinstein, H. M., et al. Group therapy for mothers with
infanticidal impulses. *American Journal of Psychiatry*, 1964, *120*, 882-886.

1690   Kempe, C. H. & Helfer, R. E. *Helping the battered child
and his family*. Philadelphia: Lippincott, 1972.

1690.1   Light, R. J. Abused and neglected children in America:
A study of alternative policies. *Harvard Educational
Review*, 1973, *43*, 556-598.

THE LAW AND RESPONSIBILITY AND CHILD ABUSE

1691   *Curran, W. J. The revolution in American criminal law:
Its significance for psychiatric diagnosis and treatment. *American Journal of Public Health*, 1968, *58*,
2209-2216.

1692   *Paulsen, M. G. The law and abused children. In R. E.
Helfer & C. H. Kempe (Eds.), *The battered child*.
Chicago: University of Chicago Press, 1968. Pp. 175-
200.

1693   Cameron, J. M., Johnson, H. R. M. & Camps, F. E. The
battered child syndrome. *Medicine, Science and the
Law*, 1966, *6*, 2-21.

1694   *Terr, L. C. & Watson, A. The battered child rebrutal-
ized: Ten cases of medical-legal confusion. *American Journal of Psychiatry*, 1968, *124*, 1432-1439.

1695   *Gil, T. D. The legal nature of neglect. *Crime and
Delinquency*, 1960, *6*, 1-16.

1696   *Silver, L. B., Barton, W. & Dublin, C. C. Child abuse
laws--Are they enough? *Journal of the American Medical Association*, 1967, *199*, 65-68.

1697   *Reinhart, J. B. & Elmer, E. The abused child: Manda-
       tory reporting legislation. *Journal of the American
       Medical Association,* 1964, *188,* 358-362.
1698   *Ireland, W. H. A registry on child abuse. *Children,*
       1966, *13,* 113-115.
1700   *Cheney, K. B. Safeguarding legal rights in providing
       protective services. *Children,* 1966, *13,* 87-92.
1701   *Kempe, C. H. Some problems encountered by welfare de-
       partments in the management of the battered child syn-
       drome. In R. E. Helfer & C. H. Kempe (Eds.), *The
       battered child.* Chicago: University of Chicago
       Press, 1968. Pp. 169-171.
1702   Tracy, J. E. *The doctor as a witness.* Philadelphia:
       Saunders, 1957.
1703   Paull, D., Lawrence, R. J. & Schimel, B. A new approach
       to reporting child abuse. *Hospitals,* 1967, *41*(2),
       62-64.
1704   Harper, F. V. The physician, the battered child, and
       the law. *Pediatrics,* 1963, *31,* 899-902.
1705   Hopkins, J. The nurse and the abused child. *Nursing
       Clinics of North America,* 1970, *5*(4), 589-598.
1706   Miller, M. B. Community action and child abuse. *Nurs-
       ing Outlook,* 1969, *17*(3), 44-46.
1707   *Kempe, C. H. The battered child and the hospital.
       Hospital Practice, 1969, *4*(10), 44-57.
1708   Paulsen, M. G. Legal protections against child abuse.
       Children, 1966, *13,* 42-48.
1709   De Francis, V. The battered child--A role for the ju-
       venile court, the legislature and the child welfare
       agency. *Juvenile Court Judges Journal,* 1963, *14*(2),
       27-29;33.
1710   Driscoll, P. & Hickey, J. P. Child abuse legal aspects
       of the physician's duty. In M. Belli (Ed.), *Trial
       and Tort Trends of 1967.* Vienna, Va.: Coiner Publi-
       cations, 1968. Pp. 394-419.

                    XIII. PSYCHOSES IN CHILDHOOD

ANNOTATED BIBLIOGRAPHIES

1711   Bryson, C. Q. & Hingtgen, J. N. *Early childhood psy-
       chosis: Infantile autism, childhood schizophrenia
       and related disorders. An annotated bibliography,
       1964-1969.* Rockville, Md.: U.S. National Institute
       of Mental Health, 1971.
1712   Tilton, J. R., DeMyer, M. K. & Loew, L. H. *Annotated
       bibliography on childhood schizophrenia, 1955-1964.*
       New York: Grune & Stratton, 1966.
1713   Ekstein, R., Bryant, K. & Friedman, S. W. Childhood
       schizophrenia and allied conditions. In L. Bellak
       (Ed.), *Schizophrenia: A review of the syndrome.* New

York: Logos Press, 1958. Pp. 555-693.
1714   Goldfarb, W. & Dorsen, M. M. *Annotated bibliography of childhood schizophrenia and related disorders.* New York: Basic Books, 1956.
1715   Laufer, M. W. & Gair, D. S. Childhood schizophrenia. In L. Bellak & L. Loeb (Eds.), *The schizophrenic syndrome.* New York: Grune & Stratton, 1969. Pp. 378-461.

HISTORICAL PERSPECTIVES

1716   *Witmer, L. What I did with Don. In S. A. Szurek & I. N. Berlin (Eds.), *Clinical studies in childhood psychoses.* New York: Brunner/Mazel, 1973. Pp. 48-64.
1717   Potter, H. W. Schizophrenia in children. *American Journal of Psychiatry,* 1933, *89*[Old Series, vol. 12], 1253-1270.
1718   *Vaillant, G. E. John Haslam on early infantile autism. *American Journal of Psychiatry,* 1962, *119,* 376.
1719   Bradley, C. *Schizophrenia in childhood.* New York: Macmillan, 1941.
1720   *Bender, L. Childhood schizophrenia. *Nervous Child,* 1942, *1,* 138-140.
1721   *Despert, J. L. Schizophrenia in children. *Psychiatric Quarterly,* 1938, *12,* 366-371.
1722   *Kanner, L. Early infantile autism. *Journal of Pediatrics,* 1944, *25,* 211-217.
1723   *Putnam, M. C. Case study of an atypical two-and-a-half-year-old. *American Journal of Orthopsychiatry,* 1948, *18,* 1-30.
1724   *Mahler, M. S. On childhood psychosis and schizophrenia: Autistic and symbiotic infantile psychoses. *Psychoanalytic Study of the Child,* 1952, *7,* 286-305.
1725   *Rank, B. & Kaplan, S. A case of pseudoschizophrenia in a child. Workshop, 1950. *American Journal of Orthopsychiatry,* 1951, *21,* 155-181.
1726   *Darr, G. C. & Worden, F. G. Case report twenty-eight years after an infantile autistic disorder. *American Journal of Orthopsychiatry,* 1951, *21,* 559-570.
1727   Hingtgen, J. N. & Bryson, C. Q. Recent developments in the study of early childhood psychoses: Infantile autism, childhood schizophrenia, and related disorders. *Schizophrenia Bulletin,* 1972, *5,* 8-54.
1727.1 Despert, J. L. Reflections on early infantile autism. *Journal of Autism and Childhood Schizophrenia,* 1971, *1,* 363-367.
1728   Bradley, C. Psychoses in children. In N. D. C. Lewis & B. L. Pacella (Eds.), *Modern trends in child psychiatry.* New York: International Universities Press, 1945. Pp. 135-154.
1729   Bradley, C. & Bowen, M. Behavior characteristics of

schizophrenic children. *Psychiatric Quarterly*, 1941, *15*, 296-315.

1730   Bradley, C. Biography of a schizophrenic child. *Nervous Child*, 1942, *1*, 141-171.

1731   Kanner, L. Autistic disturbances of affective contact. *Nervous Child*, 1943, *2*, 217-250.

1732   *Kanner, L. Irrelevant and metaphorical language in early infantile autism. *American Journal of Psychiatry*, 1946, *103*, 242-246.

1733   *Kanner, L. Problems of nosology and psychodynamics of early infantile autism. *American Journal of Orthopsychiatry*, 1949, *19*, 416-426.

1734   *Mahler, M. S. Autism and symbiosis, two extreme disturbances of identity. *International Journal of Psychoanalysis*, 1958, *39*, 77-83.

1735   Mahler, M. S. & Gosliner, B. J. On symbiotic child psychosis: Genetic, dynamic and restitutive aspects. *Psychoanalytic Study of the Child*, 1955, *10*, 195-212.

1736   Klein, M. Personification in the play of children. *International Journal of Psychoanalysis*, 1929, *10*, 193-204.

1737   *De Sanctis, S. On some varieties of dementia praecox. In S. A. Szurek & I. N. Berlin (Eds.), *Clinical studies in childhood psychoses*. New York: Brunner/Mazel, 1973. Pp. 31-47.

1737.1   Harlow, H. F. & McKinney, W. T. Nonhuman primates and psychoses. *Journal of Autism and Childhood Schizophrenia*, 1971, *1*, 368-375.

DIAGNOSIS, CLASSIFICATION AND EVALUATION/Diagnostic and Descriptive Factors

1738   *Kanner, L. Early infantile autism. *Journal of Pediatrics*, 1944, *25*, 211-217.

1739   *Mahler, M. S., Furer, M. & Settlage, C. F. Severe emotional disturbances in childhood: Psychosis. In S. Arieti (Ed.), *American handbook of psychiatry*. Vol. 1. New York: Basic Books, 1959. Pp. 816-839.

1740   *Fish, B. Longitudinal observations of biological deviations in a schizophrenic infant. *American Journal of Psychiatry*, 1959, *116*, 25-31.

1741   *Creak, M., et al. Schizophrenic syndrome in childhood: Further progress report of a working party (April, 1964). *Developmental Medicine and Child Neurology*, 1964, *6*, 530-535.

1742   *DesLauriers, A. M. The schizophrenic child. *Archives of General Psychiatry*, 1967, *16*, 194-201.

1743   *Despert, J. L. & Sherwin, A. C. Further examination of diagnostic criteria in schizophrenic illness and psychoses of infancy and early childhood. *American Journal of Psychiatry*, 1958, *114*, 784-790.

1744 *Wing, J. K. Diagnosis, epidemiology, etiology. In J. K. Wing (Ed.), *Early childhood autism: Clinical, educational and social aspects.* Oxford: Pergamon Press, 1966. Pp. 3-49.

1745 *Ward, A. J. Early infantile autism: Diagnosis, etiology, and treatment. *Psychological Bulletin,* 1970, *73,* 350-362.

1746 *Menolascino, F. J. Autistic reactions in early childhood: Differential diagnostic considerations. *Journal of Child Psychology and Psychiatry and Allied Disciplines,* 1965, *6,* 203-218.

1747 *Boatman, M. J. & Szurek, S. A. A clinical study of childhood schizophrenia. In D. D. Jackson (Ed.), *The etiology of schizophrenia.* New York: Basic Books, 1960. Pp. 389-440.

1748 Wysocki, B. A. & Wysocki, A. C. Behavior symptoms as a basis for a new diagnostic classification of problem children. *Journal of Clinical Psychology,* 1970, *26,* 41-45.

1749 Kolvin, I., Ounsted, C., Humphrey, M. & McNay, A. Studies in the childhood psychoses. II. The phenomenology of childhood psychoses. *British Journal of Psychiatry,* 1971, *118,* 385-395.

1750 *Kolvin, I. Studies in the childhood psychoses. I. Diagnostic criteria and classification. *British Journal of Psychiatry,* 1971, *118,* 381-384.

1751 *Rutter, M. Childhood schizophrenia reconsidered. *Journal of Autism and Childhood Schizophrenia,* 1972, *2,* 315-337.

1752 *Eisenberg, L. The classification of childhood psychosis reconsidered. *Journal of Autism and Childhood Schizophrenia,* 1972, *2,* 338-342.

1752.1 Stutte, H. & Dauner, I. Systematized delusions in early life schizophrenia. *Journal of Autism and Childhood Schizophrenia,* 1971, *1,* 411-420.

1752.2 Hingtgen, J. N. & Bryson, C. Q. Recent developments in the study of early childhood psychoses: Infantile autism, childhood schizophrenia, and related disorders. In S. Chess & A. Thomas (Eds.), *Annual progress in child psychiatry and child development.* New York: Brunner/Mazel, 1974. Pp. 503-575.

1752.3 Polizos, P., Engelhardt, D. M., Hoffman, S. P. & Waizer, J. Schizophrenic children. *Journal of Autism and Childhood Schizophrenia,* 1973, *3,* 247-253.

1752.4 Rutter, M. Childhood schizophrenia reconsidered. *Journal of Autism and Childhood Schizophrenia,* 1972, *2,* 315-337.

1752.5 Simons, J. M. Observations on compulsive behavior in autism. *Journal of Autism and Childhood Schizophrenia,* 1974, *4,* 1-10.

DIAGNOSIS, DESCRIPTION AND EVALUATION/Issues in Evaluation/*PRE-
PERI-, AND POST NATAL FACTORS*

1753   *Wing, J. K., O'Connor, N. & Lotter, V. Autistic condi-
       tions in early childhood: A survey in Middlesex.
       British Medical Journal, 1967, *3,* no. 5562, 389-392.
1754   *Gittelman, M. & Birch, H. G. Childhood schizophrenia:
       Intellect, neurologic status, perinatal risk, progno-
       sis, and family pathology. *Archives of General Psy-
       chiatry,* 1967, *17,* 16-25.
1755   *Pollack, M. & Woerner, M. G. Pre- and perinatal com-
       plications and "childhood schizophrenia": A compari-
       son of five controlled studies. *Journal of Child Psy-
       chology and Psychiatry and Allied Disciplines,* 1966,
       7, 235-242.
1756   *Terris, M., Lapouse, R. & Monk, M. A. The relation of
       prematurity and previous fetal loss to childhood schiz-
       ophrenia. *American Journal of Psychiatry,* 1964, *121,*
       476-481.
1757   Taft, L. T. & Goldfarb, W. Prenatal and perinatal fac-
       tors in childhood schizophrenia. *Developmental Medi-
       cine and Child Neurology,* 1964, *6,* 32-43.

DIAGNOSIS, DESCRIPTION AND EVALUATION/Issues in Evaluation/
CLASSIFICATION

1758   *Fish, B., Shapiro, T., Campbell, M. & Wile, R. A clas-
       sification of schizophrenic children under five years.
       American Journal of Psychiatry, 1968, *124,* 1415-1423.
1759   *Eisenberg, L. The classification of the psychotic dis-
       orders in childhood. In L. D. Eron (Ed.), *The clas-
       sification of behavior disorders.* Chicago: Aldine,
       1966. Pp. 87-114.
1760   *Rutter, M. et al. A tri-axial classification of mental
       disorders in childhood: An international study.
       *Journal of Child Psychology and Psychiatry and Allied
       Disciplines,* 1969, *10,* 41-61.
1761   *Rutter, M. Classification and categorization in child
       psychiatry. *Journal of Child Psychology and Psychia-
       try and Allied Disciplines,* 1965, *6,* 71-83.
1762   *Rutter, M. Concepts of autism: A review of research.
       *Journal of Child Psychology and Psychiatry and Allied
       Disciplines,* 1968, *9,* 1-25.

DIAGNOSIS, DESCRIPTION AND EVALUATION/Issues in Evaluation/*SIGNS
AND SYMPTOMS NONVERBAL*

1763   *Wing, L. The handicaps of autistic children--A compara-
       tive study. *Journal of Child Psychology and Psychia-
       try and Allied Disciplines,* 1969, *10,* 1-40.

1764   Fish, B. & Shapiro, T. A descriptive typology of child-
        ren's psychiatric disorders: II. A behavioral clas-
        sification. *Psychiatric Research Reports of the Amer-*
        ican Psychiatric Association, 1964, *18,* 75-86.
1765   *Hutt, S. J. & Hutt, C. Stereotypy, arousal and autism.
        Human Development, 1968, *11,* 277-286.
1766   Ritvo, E. R., Ornitz, E. M. & LaFranchi, S. Frequency
        of repetitive behaviors in early infantile autism and
        its variants. *Archives of General Psychiatry,* 1968,
        19, 341-347.
1767   *Ruttenberg, B. A., Dratman, M. L., Fraknoi, J. & Wenar,
        C. An instrument for evaluating autistic children.
        Journal of the American Academy of Child Psychiatry,
        1966, *5,* 453-478.
1768   Sorosky, A. D., Ornitz, E. M., Brown, M. B. & Ritvo, E.
        R. Systematic observations of autistic behavior. *Ar-*
        chives of General Psychiatry, 1968, *18,* 439-449.
1769   Douglas, V. I. & Sanders, F. A. A pilot study of Rim-
        land's diagnostic check list with autistic and men-
        tally retarded children. *Journal of Child Psychology*
        and Psychiatry and Allied Disciplines, 1968, *9,* 105-
        109.
1770   *Smolen, E. M. Some thoughts on schizophrenia in child-
        hood. *Journal of the American Academy of Child Psy-*
        chiatry, 1965, *4,* 443-472.
1771   *Weiland, I. H. Development of object relationships and
        childhood psychosis. *Journal of the American Academy*
        of Child Psychiatry, 1964, *3,* 317-329.
1772   Sussman, S. & Sklar, J. L. The social awareness of au-
        tistic children. *American Journal of Orthopsychiatry,*
        1969, *39,* 798-806.
1773   *Weiner, B. J., Ottinger, D. R. & Tilton, J. R. Compari-
        son of the toy-play behavior of autistic, retarded and
        normal children: A reanalysis. *Psychological Reports,*
        1969, *25,* 223-227.
1774   DeMyer, M. K., Mann, N. A., Tilton, J. R. & Loew, L. H.
        Toy-play behavior and the use of body by autistic and
        normal children as reported by mothers. *Psychological*
        Reports, 1967, *21,* 973-981.

DIAGNOSIS, DESCRIPTION AND EVALUATION/Issues in Evaluation/
MEASUREMENT OF INTELLIGENCE

1775   *Alpern, G. D. Measurement of "untestable" autistic
        children. *Journal of Abnormal Psychology,* 1967, *72,*
        478-486.
1776   *Allen, C. E. & Toomey, L. C. Use of the Vineland Social
        Maturity Scale for evaluating progress of psychotic
        children in a therapeutic nursery school. *American*
        Journal of Orthopsychiatry, 1965, *35,* 152-159.
1777   Goldfarb, W., Goldfarb, N. & Pollack, R. C. Changes in

IQ of schizophrenic children during residential treatment. *Archives of General Psychiatry*, 1969, *21*, 673-
690.

1778   *Spurgeon, R. K. Some problems in measuring nonverbal
behavior of autistic children. *Nursing Research*, 1967
16, 212-218.

DIAGNOSIS, DESCRIPTION AND EVALUATION/Issues in Evaluation/*SELF-
DESTRUCTIVE BEHAVIOR*

1779   Shodell, M. J. & Reiter, H. H. Self-mutilative behavior
in verbal and nonverbal schizophrenic children. *Archives of General Psychiatry*, 1968, *19*, 453-455.
1780   *Green, A. H. Self-mutilation in schizophrenic children.
Archives of General Psychiatry, 1967, *17*, 234-244.
1781   Green, A. H. Self-destructive behavior in physically
abused schizophrenic children. *Archives of General
Psychiatry*, 1968, *19*, 171-179.
1782   Haworth, M. R. & Menolascino, F. J. Video-tape observations of disturbed young children. *Journal of Clinical Psychology*, 1967, *23*, 135-140.

DIAGNOSIS, DESCRIPTION AND EVALUATION/Issues in Evaluation/
COGNITIVE-LINGUISTIC ASPECTS

1783   *Hagen, J. W., Winsberg, B. G. & Wolff, P. Cognitive and
linguistic deficits in psychotic children. *Child Development*, 1968, *39*, 1103-1117.
1784   Fay, W. H. On the basis of autistic echolalia. *Journal
of Communication Disorders*, 1969, *2*, 38-47.
1785   Griffith, R. J. & Ritvo, E. R. Echolalia: Concerning
the dynamics of the syndrome. *Journal of the American
Academy of Child Psychiatry*, 1967, *6*, 184-193.
1786   *Weiland, I. H. & Legg, D. R. Formal speech characteristics as a diagnostic aid in childhood psychosis.
American Journal of Orthopsychiatry, 1964, *34*, 91-94.
1787   *Pronovost, W., Wakstein, M. P. & Wakstein, D. J. A
longitudinal study of the speech behavior and language
comprehension of fourteen children diagnosed atypical
or autistic. *Exceptional Children*, 1966, *33*, 19-26.
1788   *Shapiro, T. & Fish, B. A method to study language deviation as an aspect of ego organization in young
schizophrenic children. *Journal of the American A-
cademy of Child Psychiatry*, 1969, *8*, 36-56.
1789   Ruttenberg, B. A. & Wolf, E. G. Evaluating the communication of the autistic child. *Journal of Speech and
Hearing Disorders*, 1967, *32*, 314-324.
1790   de Hirsch, K. Differential diagnosis between aphasic
and schizophrenic language in children. *Journal of
Speech and Hearing Disorders*, 1967, *32*, 3-10.

DIAGNOSIS, DESCRIPTION AND EVALUATION/Issues in Evaluation/
NEUROPHYSIOLOGICAL ASPECTS

1791   Birch, H. G. & Walker, H. A. Perceptual and perceptual-
        motor dissociation: Studies in schizophrenic and
        brain-damaged psychotic children. *Archives of General
        Psychiatry*, 1966, *14*, 113-118.
1792   *Bryson, C. Q. Systematic identification of perceptual
        disabilities in autistic children. *Perceptual and
        Motor Skills*, 1970, *31*, 239-246.
1793   *Ornitz, E. M. & Ritvo, E. R. Neurophysiologic mecha-
        nisms underlying perceptual inconstancy in autistic
        and schizophrenic children. *Archives of General Psy-
        chiatry*, 1968, *19*, 22-27.
1794   White, P. T., DeMyer, W. & DeMyer, M. EEG abnormalities
        in early childhood schizophrenia: A double-blind
        study of psychiatrically disturbed and normal children
        during promazine sedation. *American Journal of Psy-
        chiatry*, 1964, *120*, 950-958.

DIAGNOSIS, DESCRIPTION AND EVALUATION/Additional Readings

1795   *Despert, J. L. *Schizophrenia in children; collected
        papers*. New York: Brunner, 1968.
1796   *O'Gorman, G. The psychoses of childhood. In J. G.
        Howells (Ed.), *Modern perspectives in child psychia-
        try*. London: Oliver & Boyd, 1965. Pp. 473-495.
        (*Modern perspectives in psychiatry*. Vol. 1)
1797   Haworth, M. R. & Menolascino, F. J. Some aspects of
        psychotic behavior in young children: Thoughts on the
        etiology. *Archives of General Psychiatry*, 1968, *18*,
        355-359.
1798   Mahler, M. S. Diagnostic considerations. In *On human
        symbiosis and the vicissitudes of individuation*. Vol.
        1. New York: International Universities Press, 1968.
        Pp. 66-81.
1799   Hermelin, B. Recent psychological research. In J. K.
        Wing (Ed.), *Early childhood autism: Clinical, educa-
        tional and social aspects*. Oxford: Pergamon Press,
        1966. Pp. 159-173.
1800   *Yates, A. J. The psychoses: Children. In *Behavior
        therapy*. New York: Wiley, 1970. Pp. 246-272.
1800.1 Shapiro, T., Fish, B. & Ginsberg, G. L. The speech of
        a schizophrenic child from two to six. *American Jour-
        nal of Psychiatry*, 1972, *128*, 1408-1413.

THEORIES OF ETIOLOGY

1801   *Chambers, C. H. Leo Kanner's concept of early infantile
        autism. *British Journal of Medical Psychology*, 1969,
        42, 51-54.

1802   Kanner, L. Problems of nosology and psychodynamics of early infantile autism. *American Journal of Orthopsychiatry*, 1949, *19*, 416-426.
1803   *Lotter, V. Epidemiology of autistic conditions in young children. I. Prevalence. *Social Psychiatry*, 1966, *1*, 124-137.
1804   Rutter, M. (Ed.) *Infantile autism: Concepts, characteristics and treatment.* Edinburgh: Churchill Livingstone, 1971.

THEORIES OF ETIOLOGY/Psychoanalytic

1805   *Despert, J. L. *The emotionally disturbed child--then and now.* New York: Vantage Press, 1965.
1806   *Bettelheim, B. *The empty fortress: Infantile autism and the birth of the self.* New York: Free Press, 1967.
1807   *Ekstein, R. & Wallerstein J. Observations on the psychology of borderline and psychotic children. *Psychoanalytic Study of the Child*, 1954, *9*, 344-369.
1808   *Beres, D. Ego deviation and the concept of schizophrenia. *Psychoanalytic Study of the Child*, 1956, *11*, 164-235.
1809   *Johnson, A. M., Giffin, M. E., Watson, E. J. & Beckett, P. G. S. Studies in schizophrenia at the Mayo Clinic. II. Observations on ego functions in schizophrenia. *Psychiatry*, 1956, *19*, 143-148.
1810   *Klein, M. Notes on some schizoid mechanisms. *International Journal of Psychoanalysis*, 1946, *27*, 99-110.
1811   *Mahler, M. S., Furer, M. & Settlage, C. F. Severe emotional disturbance in childhood: Psychosis. In S. Arieti (Ed.), *American handbook of psychiatry*. Vol. 1. New York: Basic Books, 1959. Pp. 816-839.
1812   *Ruttenberg, B. A. A psychoanalytic understanding of infantile autism and its treatment. In D. W. Churchill, G. D. Alpern, & M. K. DeMyer (Eds.), *Infantile autism: Proceedings of the Indiana University colloquium.* Springfield, Ill.: Thomas, 1971. Pp. 145-184.
1813   Mahler, M. S. & Furer, M. Child psychosis: A theoretical statement and its implications. *Journal of Autism and Childhood Schizophrenia*, 1972, *2*, 213-218.
1814   *Mahler, M. S. On childhood psychosis and schizophrenia: Autistic and symbiotic infantile psychoses. *Psychoanalytic Study of the Child*, 1952, *7*, 286-305.
1815   *Weiland, I. H. Development of object relationships and childhood psychosis. *Journal of the American Academy of Child Psychiatry*, 1964, *3*, 317-329.
1816   *Mahler, M. S. Thoughts about development and individuation. *Psychoanalytic Study of the Child*, 1963, *18*, 307-324.
1817   Bettelheim, B. Feral children and autistic children.

American Journal of Sociology, 1959, *64*, 455-467.

1818   *Ekstein, R. *Children of time and space, of action and impulse.* New York: Appleton-Century-Crofts, 1966.

1819   Bettelheim, B. Joey: A "mechanical boy". *Scientific American*, 1959, *200*(3), 116-127.

1820   *Elkisch, P. Initiating separation-individuation in the simultaneous treatment of a child and his mother. In J. B. McDevitt & C. F. Settlage (Eds.), *Separation-individuation: Essays in honor of Margaret S. Mahler.* New York: International Universities Press, 1971. Pp. 356-376.

1821   Hendrick, I. Early development of the ego: Identification in infancy. *Psychoanalytic Quarterly*, 1951, *20*, 44-61.

1822   Mahler, M. S. On the significance of the normal separation-individuation phase with reference to research in symbiotic child psychosis. In M. Schur (Ed.), *Drives, affects, behavior.* Vol. 2. New York: International Universities Press, 1965. Pp. 161-169.

1823   Thomas, R. Comments on some aspects of self and object representation in a group of psychotic children. An application of Anna Freud's diagnostic profile. *Psychoanalytic Study of the Child*, 1966, *21*, 527-580.

1824   Mahler, M. S. On early infantile psychosis: The symbiotic and autistic syndromes. *Journal of the American Academy of Child Psychiatry*, 1965, *4*, 554-568.

1825   Furer, M. The development of a preschool symbiotic psychotic boy. *Psychoanalytic Study of the Child*, 1964, *19*, 448-469.

1826   Klein, M. Personification in the play of children. *International Journal of Psychoanalysis*, 1929, *10*, 193-204.

1827   Elkisch, P. & Mahler, M. S. On infantile precursors of the "influencing machine" (Tausk). *Psychoanalytic Study of the Child*, 1959, *14*, 219-235.

1828   Rodrigue, E. The analysis of a three-year-old mute schizophrenic. In M. Klein, P. Heimann, & R. E. Money-Kyrle (Eds.), *New directions in psycho-analysis: The significance of infant conflict in the pattern of adult behaviour.* New York: Basic Books, 1955. Pp. 140-179.

1829   Morrow, T. & Loomis, E. A. Symbiotic aspects of a seven-year-old psychotic. In G. Caplan (Ed.), *Emotional problems of early childhood.* New York: Basic Books, 1955. Pp. 337-361.

1830   Modell, A. Some recent psychoanalytic theories of schizophrenia. *Psychoanalytic Review*, 1956, *43*, 181-194.

1831   Ekstein, R., Bryant, K. & Friedman, S. W. Childhood schizophrenia and allied conditions. In L. Bellak (Ed.), *Schizophrenia: A review of the syndrome.* New York: Logos Press, 1958. Pp. 555-693.

1831.1   Mahler, M. S. & Furer, M. Child psychosis: A theoretical statement and its implications. *Journal of Autism
and Childhood Schizophrenia,* 1972, *2,* 213-218.

THEORIES OF ETIOLOGY/Interpersonal and Developmental/*DEVELOP-
MENTAL*

1832   *Bowlby, J. *Attachment and loss.* Vol. 1. *Attachment.*
New York: Basic Books, 1969.
1833   Szurek, S. A. Attachment and psychotic detachment. In
S. A. Szurek & I. N. Berlin (Eds.), *Clinical studies
in childhood psychoses.* New York: Brunner/Mazel,
1973. Pp. 191-277.
1834   *Weil,·A. P. Some evidences of deviational development
in infancy and early childhood. *Psychoanalytic Study
of the Child,* 1956, *11,* 293-299.
1835   Hendrick, I. Early development of the ego: Identification in infancy. *Psychoanalytic Quarterly,* 1951, *20,*
44-61.
1836   Elkisch, P. The struggle for ego boundaries in a psychotic child. *American Journal of Psychotherapy,*
1956, *10,* 578-602.
1837   *Erikson, E. H. Early ego failure: Jean. In *Childhood
and society.* New York: Norton, 1963. Pp. 195-208.
1838   *Bergman, P. & Escalona, S. K. Unusual sensitivities in
very young children. *Psychoanalytic Study of the
Child,* 1949, *3-4,* 333-352.
1839   *Johnson, A. M., Giffin, M. E., Watson, E. J. & Beckett,
P. G. S. Studies in schizophrenia at the Mayo Clinic.
II. Observations on ego functions in schizophrenia.
Psychiatry, 1956, *19,* 143-148.
1840   Weil, A. P. Certain severe disturbances of ego development in childhood. *Psychoanalytic Study of the Child,*
1953, *8,* 271-287.
1841   *Szurek, S. A. Childhood schizophrenia. Symposium, 1955.
4. Psychotic episodes and psychotic maldevelopment.
American Journal of Orthopsychiatry, 1956, *26,* 519-543.
1842   *Shapiro, T. & Fish, B. A method to study language deviation as an aspect of ego organization in young schizophrenic children. *Journal of the American Academy of
Child Psychiatry,* 1969, *8,* 36-56.
1843   *Loomis, E. A., Hilgeman, L. M. & Meyer, L. R. Childhood
psychosis. 2. Play patterns as nonverbal indices of
ego functions: A preliminary report. *American Journal of Orthopsychiatry,* 1957, *27,* 691-700.
1844   *Bettelheim, B. Childhood schizophrenia. Symposium,
1955. 3. Schizophrenia as a reaction to extreme situations. *American Journal of Orthopsychiatry,* 1956,
26, 507-518.
1845   Beckett, P. G. S., et al. Studies in schizophrenia at
the Mayo Clinic. I. The significance of exogenous

traumata in the genesis of schizophrenia. *Psychiatry,* 1956, *19,* 137-142.

1846   Cain, A. C. Special "isolated" abilities in severely psychotic young children. *Psychiatry,* 1969, *32,* 137-149.

1847   *Kramer, S. The adolescent recapitulation of a childhood psychosis. In J. B. McDevitt & C. F. Settlage (Eds.), *Separation-individuation: Essays in honor of Margaret S. Mahler.* New York: International Universities Press, 1971. Pp. 416-440.

THEORIES OF ETIOLOGY/Interpersonal and Developmental/*INTER-PERSONAL*

1848   *Boatman. M. J. & Szurek, S. A. A clinical study of childhood schizophrenia. In D. D. Jackson (Ed.), *The etiology of schizophrenia.* New York: Basic Books, 1960. Pp. 389-440.

1849   *Block, J. Parents of schizophrenic, neurotic, asthmatic, and congenitally ill children: A comparative study. *Archives of General Psychiatry,* 1969, *20,* 659-674.

1850   Kaufman, I., Frank, T., Heims, L., Herrick, J. & Willer, L. Parents of schizophrenic children. Workshop, 1958. 3. Four types of defense in mothers and fathers of schizophrenic children. *American Journal of Orthopsychiatry,* 1959, *29,* 460-472.

1851   *Pitfield, M. & Oppenheim, A. N. Child rearing attitudes of mothers of psychotic children. *Journal of Child Psychology and Psychiatry and Allied Disciplines,* 1964, *5,* 51-57.

1852   *Rice, G., Kepecs, J. G. & Yahalom, I. Differences in communicative impact between mothers of psychotic and nonpsychotic children. *American Journal of Orthopsychiatry,* 1966, *36,* 529-543.

1853   Schopler, E. & Loftin, J. Thought disorders in parents of psychotic children: A function of test anxiety. *Archives of General Psychiatry,* 1969, *20,* 174-181.

1854   *Bowen, M. A family concept of schizophrenia. In D. D. Jackson (Ed.), *The etiology of schizophrenia.* New York: Basic Books, 1960. Pp. 346-372.

1855   *McDermott, J. F., Jr., Harrison, S. I., Schrager, J., Lindy, J. & Killins, E. Social class and mental illness in children: The question of childhood psychosis. In S. Chess & A. Thomas (Eds.), *Annual progress in child psychiatry and child development.* New York: Brunner/Mazel, 1968. Pp. 437-448.

1855.1 Fish, B. & Hagin, R. Visual-motor disorders in infants at risk for schizophrenia. *Archives of General Psychiatry,* 1973, *28,* 900-904.

1855.2 Goldfarb, W., Yudkovitz, E. & Goldfarb, N. Verbal symbols to designate objects: An experimental study of communication in mothers of schizophrenic children. *Journal of Autism and Childhood Schizophrenia,* 1973, *3,* 281-298.

1855.3   Spitz, R. A.   The adaptive viewpoint: Its role in autism and child psychiatry. *Journal of Autism and Childhood Schizophrenia,* 1971, *1,* 239-245.

THEORIES OF ETIOLOGY/Genetic

1856   Stabenau, J. R. & Pollin, W.   Early characteristics of monozygotic twins discordant for schizophrenia. In S. Chess & A. Thomas (Eds.), *Annual progress in child psychiatry and child development.*   New York: Brunner/Mazel, 1968.   Pp. 497-515.

1857   *Chapman, A. H.   Early infantile autism in identical twins: Report of a case. *Archives of Neurology and Psychiatry,* 1957, *78,* 621-623.

1858   *Gregory, I.   Genetic factors in schizophrenia. *American Journal of Psychiatry,* 1960, *116,* 961-972.

1859   *Jackson, D. D.   A critique of the literature on the genetics of schizophrenia.   In *The etiology of schizophrenia.*   New York: Basic Books, 1960.   Pp. 37-87.

1860   *Nielson, J., et al.   Childhood of males with the XYY syndrome. *Journal of Autism and Childhood Schizophrenia,* 1973, *3,* 5-26.

1860.1   Jarvik, L. F., Yen, F-S. & Goldstein, F.   Chromosomes and mental status. *Archives of General Psychiatry,* 1974, *30,* 186-190.

1860.2   Belmaker, R., Pollin, W., Wyatt, R. J. & Cohen, S.   A follow-up of monozygotic twins discordant for schizophrenia. *Archives of General Psychiatry,* 1974, *30,* 219-222.

1860.3   Campbell, M., Wolman, S. R., Breuer, H., Miller, F. T. & Perlman, B. B.   Klinefelter's syndrome in a three-year-old severely disturbed child. *Journal of Autism and Childhood Schizophrenia,* 1972, *2,* 34-48.

THEORIES OF ETIOLOGY/Learning Theory and Others

1861   *Phillips, E. L.   Contributions to a learning theory account of childhood autism. *Journal of Psychology,* 1957, *43,* 117-124.

1862   *Ferster, C. B.   Positive reinforcement and behavioral deficits of autistic children. *Child Development,* 1961, *32,* 437-456.

1863   Ferster, C. B.   The repertoire of the autistic child in relation to principles of reinforcement.   In L. A. Gottschalk & A. H. Auerbach (Eds.), *Methods of research in psychotherapy.*   New York: Appleton-Century-Crofts, 1966.   Pp. 312-333.

1864   Kolvin, I., Humphrey, M. & McNay, A.   Studies in the
            childhood psychoses. VI. Cognitive factors in child-
            hood psychoses. *British Journal of Psychiatry*, 1971,
            118, 415-419.
1864.1   Creak, M.   Reflections on communication and autistic
            children. *Journal of Autism and Childhood Schizophre-
            nia*, 1972, *2*, 1-8.
1864.2   Wax, D. E.   Psychotic recognizing and the process of
            primary elaboration. *Journal of the American Academy
            of Child Psychiatry*, 1973, *12*, 632-640.

THEORIES OF ETIOLOGY/Other Concepts

1865   *Moloney, J. C.   The precognitive cultural ingredients of
            schizophrenia. *International Journal of Psychoanal-
            sis*, 1957, *38*, 325-340.
1866   *Bateson, G., Jackson, D. D., Haley, J. & Weakland, J.
            Toward a theory of schizophrenia. *Behavioral Science*,
            1956, *1*, 251-264.
1867   *Anthony, E. J.   Clinical evaluation of children with psy-
            chotic parents. *American Journal of Psychiatry*, 1969,
            126, 177-184.
1868   DesLauriers, A. M. & Carlson, C. F.   *Your child is a-
            sleep; early infantile autism: Etiology; treatment,
            parental influences*. Homewood, Ill.:   Dorsey Press,
            1969.
1869   Goldfarb, W.   *Childhood schizophrenia*.   Cambridge, Mass.:
            Harvard University Press, 1961.
1870   Bosch, G.   *Infantile autism*.   New York: Springer-Verlag,
            1970.
1870.1   Campbell, M. & Hersh, S. P.   Observations on the vicis-
            situdes of aggression in two siblings. *Journal of
            Autism and Childhood Schizophrenia*, 1971, *1*, 398-410.

NEUROPHYSIOLOGICAL AND BIOLOGICAL RESEARCH/Introduction

1871   *Taft, L. T. & Goldfarb, W.   Prenatal and perinatal fac-
            tors in childhood schizophrenia. *Developmental Medi-
            cine and Child Neurology*, 1964, *6*, 32-43.
1872   *Berkowitz, P. H.   Some psychophysical aspects of mental
            illness in children. *Genetic Psychology Monographs*,
            1961, *63*, 103-148.
1873   *Fish, B.   Longitudinal observations of biological de-
            viations in a schizophrenic infant. *American Journal
            of Psychiatry*, 1959, *116*, 25-31.
1874   Fish, B.   The detection of schizophrenia in infancy: A
            preliminary report. *Journal of Nervous and Mental
            Disease*, 1957, *125*, 1-24.
1875   Goldfarb, W.   Receptor preferences in schizophrenic
            children. *Archives of Neurology and Psychiatry*, 1956,
            76, 643-652.

1876   *O'Connor, N. & Hermelin, B. Sensory dominance in autis-
       tic children and subnormal controls. *Perceptual and
       Motor Skills*, 1963, *16*, 920.
1877   *Ornitz, E. M. & Ritvo, E. R. Perceptual inconstancy in
       early infantile autism: The syndrome of early infant
       autism and its variants including certain cases of
       childhood schizophrenia. *Archives of General Psychi-
       atry*, 1968, *18*, 76-98.
1878   Ritvo, E. R. et al. Decreased postrotatory nystagmus
       in early infantile autism. *Neurology*, 1969, *19*, 653-
       658.
1879   *Silver, A. & Gabriel, H. P. The association of schizo-
       phrenia in childhood with primitive postural responses
       and decreased muscle tone. *Developmental Medicine and
       Child Neurology*, 1964, *6*, 495-497.
1880   *Hutt, S. J., Hutt, C., Lee, D. & Ounsted, C. A behav-
       ioural and electroencephalographic study of autistic
       children. *Journal of Psychiatric Research*, 1965, *3*,
       181-197.
1881   Ornitz, E. M., et al. The EEG and rapid eye movements
       during REM sleep in normal and autistic children.
       Electroencephalography and Clinical Neurophysiology,
       1969, *26*, 167-175.
1882   White, P. T., DeMyer, W. & DeMyer, M. EEG abnormalities
       in early childhood schizophrenia: A double-blind study
       of psychiatrically disturbed and normal children during
       promazine sedation. *American Journal of Psychiatry*,
       1964, *120*, 950-958.
1883   *Satterfield, J. H., et al. Response to stimulant drug
       treatment in hyperactive children: Prediction from
       EEG and neurological findings. *Journal of Autism and
       Childhood Schizophrenia*, 1973, *3*, 36-48.
1883.1 Wing, L. & Wing, J. K. Multiple impairments in early
       childhood autism. *Journal of Autism and Childhood
       Schizophrenia*, 1971, *1*, 256-266.

NEUROPHYSIOLOGICAL AND BIOLOGICAL RESEARCH/Neurophysiological

1884   *Pasamanick, B. & Knobloch, H. Early feeding and birth
       difficulties in childhood schizophrenia: An explana-
       tory note. *Journal of Psychology*, 1963, *56*, 73-77.
1885   Goldstein, K. Abnormal mental conditions in infancy.
       Journal of Nervous and Mental Disease, 1959, *128*,
       538-557.
1886   *Fish, B. Longitudinal observations of biological de-
       viations in a schizophrenic infant. *American Journal
       of Psychiatry*, 1959, *116*, 25-31.
1887   *Bender, L. The concept of plasticity in childhoood
       schizophrenia. *Proceedings of the American Psycho-
       pathological Association*, 1966, *54*, 354-365.
1888   Fish, B. & Alpert, M. Abnormal states of consciousness

and muscle tone in infants born to schizophrenic mothers. *American Journal of Psychiatry*, 1962, *119*, 439-445.

1889   Fish, B. Involvement of the central nervous system in infants with schizophrenia. *Archives of Neurology*, 1960, *2*, 115-121.

1890   *Rabinovitch, R. D. Observations on the differential study of severely disturbed children. *American Journal of Orthopsychiatry*, 1952, *22*, 230-236.

1891   Vorster, D. An investigation into the part played by organic factors in childhood schizophrenia. *Journal of Mental Science*, 1960, *106*, 494-522.

1892   *Goldfarb, W. An investigation of childhood schizophrenia: A retrospective view. *Archives of General Psychiatry*, 1964, *11*, 620-634.

1893   *Bender, L. Childhood schizophrenia: Clinical study of one hundred schizophrenic children. *American Journal of Orthopsychiatry*, 1947, *17*, 40-56.

1894   Haworth, M. R. & Menolascino, F. J. Some aspects of psychotic behavior in young children: Thoughts on the etiology. *Archives of General Psychiatry*, 1968, *18*, 355-359.

1895   Bender, L. Childhood schizophrenia. Symposium, 1955. 2. Schizophrenia in childhood--Its recognition, description and treatment. *American Journal of Orthopsychiatry*, 1956, *26*, 499-506.

1896   *Kolvin, I., Ounsted, C. & Roth, M. Studies in the childhood psychoses. V. Cerebral dysfunction and childhood psychoses. *British Journal of Psychiatry*, 1971, *118*, 407-414.

1897   *DeMyer, M. K. Perceptual limitations in autistic children and their relation to social and intellectual deficits. In M. Rutter (Ed.), *Infantile autism: Concepts, characteristics and treatment*. Edinburgh: Churchill Livingstone, 1971. Pp. 81-96.

1897.1   Taft, L. T. & Cohen, H. J. Hypsarrhythmia and infantile autism: A clinical report. *Journal of Autism and Childhood Schizophrenia*, 1971, *1*, 327-336.

1897.2   DeMyer, M. K., Barton, S., Alpern, G. D., Kimberlin, C., Allen, J., Yang, E. & Steele, R. The measured intelligence of autistic children. *Journal of Autism and Childhood Schizophrenia*, 1974, *4*, 42-60.

NEUROPHYSIOLOGICAL AND BIOLOGICAL RESEARCH/Genetic

1898   *Judd, L. L. & Mandell, A. J. Chromosome studies in early infantile autism. *Archives of General Psychiatry*, 1968, *18*, 450-457.

1899   Book, J. A., Nichtern, S. & Gruenberg, E. Cytogenetical investigations in childhood schizophrenia. *Acta Psychiatrica Scandinavica*, 1963, *39*, 309-323.

1899.1   Sperber, M. A., Salomon, L., Collins, M. H. & Stambler,
M. Childhood schizophrenia and 47,XXY Klinefelter's
Syndrome. *American Journal of Psychiatry*, 1972, *128*,
1400-1407.

NEUROPHYSIOLOGICAL AND BIOLOGICAL RESEARCH/Biochemical

1900   *Sankar, S. D., Cates, N., Broer, H. H. & Sankar, D. B.
Biochemical parameters of childhood schizophrenia
(autism) and growth. *Recent Advances in Biological
Psychiatry*, 1961, *5*, 76-83.
1901   *Schain, R. J. & Freedman, D. X. Studies on 5-hydroxy-
indole metabolism in autistic and other mentally retarded children. *Journal of Pediatrics*, 1961, *58*,
315-320.
1902   *Heeley, A. F. & Roberts, G. E. Tryptophan metabolism
in psychotic children. *Developmental Medicine and
Child Neurology*, 1965, *7*, 46-49.
1903   Shaw, C. R., Lucas, J. & Rabinovitch, R. D. Metabolic
studies in childhood schizophrenia: Effects of tryptophan loading on indole excretion. *Archives of General Psychiatry*, 1959, *1*, 366-371.
1904   Shaw, C. R. & Sutton, H. E. Metabolic studies in childhood schizophrenia. II. Amino acid excretion patterns. *Archives of General Psychiatry*, 1960, *3*, 519-
522.
1906   DeMyer, M. K., Ward, S. D. & Lintzenich, J. Comparison
of macronutrients in the diets of psychotic and normal children. *Archives of General Psychiatry*, 1968,
18, 584-590.
1907   Rimland, B. *Infantile autism: The syndrome and its
implications for a neural theory of behavior*. New
York: Appleton-Century-Crofts, 1964.
1908   *Coleman, M. Serotonin and central nervous system syndromes of childhood: A review. *Journal of Autism
and Childhood Schizophrenia*, 1973, *3*, 27-35.
1908.1   Campbell, M., Friedman, E., DeVito, E., Greenspan, L.
& Collins, P. J. Blood serotonin in psychotic and
brain damaged children. *Journal of Autism and Childhood Schizophrenia*, 1974, *4*, 33-41.

DATA ON FAMILY BACKGROUND AND INTERACTION

1909   *Creak, M. & Ini, S. Families of psychotic children.
*Journal of Child Psychology and Psychiatry and Allied
Disciplines*, 1960, *1*, 156-175.
1910   *Szurek, S. A. Childhood schizophrenia. Symposium, 1955.
4. Psychotic episodes and psychotic maldevelopment.
American Journal of Orthopsychiatry, 1956, *26*, 519-
543.

1911   Behrens, M. L. & Goldfarb, W. A study of patterns of
        interaction of families of schizophrenic children in
        residential treatment. *American Journal of Orthopsy-
        chiatry*, 1958, *28*, 300-312.
1912   *Lordi, W. M. & Silverberg, J. Infantile autism: A
        family approach. *International Journal of Group Psy-
        chotherapy*, 1964, *14*, 360-365.
1913   *Goldfarb, W. The mutual impact of mother and child in
        childhood schizophrenia. *American Journal of Ortho-
        psychiatry*, 1961, *31*, 738-747.
1914   Meyers, D. I. & Goldfarb, W. Studies of perplexity in
        mothers of schizophrenic children. *American Journal
        of Orthopsychiatry*, 1961, *31*, 551-564.
1915   Bene, E. A Rorschach investigation into the mothers of
        autistic children. *British Journal of Medical Psy-
        chology*, 1958, *31*, 226-227.
1916   *Call, J. D. Interlocking affective freeze between an
        autistic child and his "as-if" mother. *Journal of the
        American Academy of Child Psychiatry*, 1963, *2*, 319-
        344.
1917   *Eisenberg, L. The fathers of autistic children. *Amer-
        ican Journal of Orthopsychiatry*, 1957, *27*, 715-724.
1918   Bowen, M., Dysinger, R. H. & Basamania, B. The role of
        the father in families with a schizophrenic patient.
        American Journal of Psychiatry, 1959, *115*, 1017-1020.
1919   Lidz, T. F., Parker, B. & Cornelison, A. The role of
        the father in the family environment of the schizo-
        phrenic patient. *American Journal of Psychiatry*,
        1956, *113*, 126-132.
1920   Brodey, W. M. Some family operations and schizophrenia:
        A study of five hospitalized families each with a
        schizophrenic member. *Archives of General Psychiatry*,
        1959, *1*, 379-402.
1921   Clausen, J. A. & Kohn, M. L. Social relations and
        schizophrenia: A research report and a perspective.
        In D. D. Jackson (Ed.), *The etiology of schizophrenia*.
        New York: Basic Books, 1960. Pp. 295-320.
1922   *Lidz, T. F., Cornelison, A. R., Fleck, S. & Terry, D.
        The intrafamilial environment of the schizophrenic
        patient. I. The father. *Psychiatry*, 1957, *20*,
        329-342.
1923   Lidz, T. F. Schizophrenia and the family. *Psychiatry*,
        1958, *21*, 21-27.
1924   *McDermott, J. F., Harrison, S. I., Schrager, J., Lindy,
        J. & Killins, E. Social class and mental illness in
        children: The question of childhood psychosis. *Amer-
        ican Journal of Orthopsychiatry*, 1967, *37*, 548-557.
1925   Chapman, L. F., Hinkle, L. E. & Wolff, H. G. Human
        ecology, disease, and schizophrenia. *American Jour-
        nal of Psychiatry*, 1960, *117*, 193-204.
1926   Kolvin, I., Ounsted, C., Richardson, L. M. & Garside,
        R. F. Studies in the childhood psychoses. III. The

family and social background in childhood psychoses. *British Journal of Psychiatry*, 1971, *118*, 396-402.

1927   Kolvin, I., Garside, R. F. & Kidd, J. S. H. Studies in the childhood psychoses. IV. Parental personality and attitude and childhood psychoses. *British Journal of Psychiatry*, 1971, *118*, 403-406.

1927.1   Stabenau, J. R. Schizophrenia: A family's projective identification. *American Journal of Psychiatry*, 1973 *130*, 19-23.

1927.2   Wright, D. M. Thought disorder in the parents of poor-premorbid male schizophrenics. *Archives of General Psychiatry*, 1973, *29*, 472-475.

1927.3   Schopler, E. & Reichler, R. J. How well do parents understand their own psychotic child? *Journal of Autism and Childhood Schizophrenia*, 1972, *2*, 387-400.

1927.4   Reed, S. C., et al. *The psychoses; family studies.* Philadelphia: W. B. Saunders, 1973.

1927.5   Lotter, V. Social adjustment and placement of autistic children in Middlesex: A follow-up study. *Journal of Autism and Childhood Schizophrenia*, 1974, *4*, 11-32

1927.6   Florsheim, J. & Peterfreund, O. The intelligence of parents of psychotic children. *Journal of Autism and Childhood Schizophrenia*, 1974, *4*, 61-70.

TREATMENT AND MANAGEMENT/Individual Psychotherapy

1928   *Tessman, L. H. & Kaufman, I. Treatment techniques, the primary process, and ego development in schizophrenic children. *Journal of the American Academy of Child Psychiatry*, 1967, *6*, 98-115.

1929   Speers, R. W. & Lansing, C. Group psychotherapy with preschool psychotic children and collateral group therapy of their parents: A preliminary report of the first two years. *American Journal of Orthopsychiatry*, 1964, *34*, 659-666.

1930   *Weiland, I. H. & Rudnick, R. Considerations of the development and treatment of autistic childhood psychosis. *Psychoanalytic Study of the Child*, 1961, *16*, 549-563.

1931   *Ekstein, R. & Friedman, S. W. On the meaning of play in childhood psychosis. In L. Jessner & E. Pavenstedt (Eds.), *Dynamic psychopathology in childhood.* New York: Grune & Stratton, 1959. Pp. 269-292.

1932   Cain, A. C. On the meaning of "playing crazy" in borderline children. *Psychiatry*, 1964, *27*, 278-289.

1933   *Harrison, S. I. Symbiotic infantile psychosis: Observation of an acute episode. In J. B. McDevitt & C. F. Settlage (Eds.), *Separation-individuation: Essays in honor of Margaret S. Mahler.* New York: International Universities Press, 1971. Pp. 404-415.

1934   *Rank, B. Adaptation of the psychoanalytic technique for the treatment of young children with atypical development. *American Journal of Orthopsychiatry*, 1949, *19*, 130-139.

1935   Pavenstedt, E. History of a child with an atypical development and some vicissitudes of his treatment. In G. Caplan (Ed.), *Emotional problems of early childhood*. New York: Basic Books, 1955. Pp. 379-406.

1936   *Rank, B. Intensive study and treatment of preschool children who show marked personality deviations, or "atypical development," and their parents. In G. Caplan (Ed.), *Emotional problems of early childhood*. New York: Basic Books, 1955. Pp. 491-501.

1937   *Rice, G. & Klein, A. Getting the message from a schizophrenic child. *Psychiatry*, 1964, *27*, 163-169.

1938   *Miller, B. M. Communication with a non-verbal child. *American Journal of Psychoanalysis*, 1960, *20*, 79-82.

1939   *Alpert, A. & Pfeiffer, E. Treatment of an autistic child: Introduction and theoretical discussion, treatment diaries--first two years. *Journal of the American Academy of Child Psychiatry*, 1964, *3*, 591-616.

1940   Ekstein, R. & Caruth, E. Distancing and distance devices in childhood schizophrenia and borderline states: Revised concepts and new directions in research. *Psychological Reports*, 1967, *20*, 109-110.

1941   *Ekstein, R. & Wallerstein, J. Choice of interpretation in the treatment of borderline and psychotic children. *Bulletin of the Menninger Clinic*, 1957, *21*, 199-207.

1942   *Hirsch, E. A. Interpretive flexibility as a condition set by schizophrenic children in psychotherapy. *American Journal of Orthopsychiatry*, 1960, *30*, 397-404.

1943   *Kemph, J. P. Communicating with the psychotic child. *International Psychiatry Clinics*, 1964, *1*(1), 53-72.

1944   Geleerd, E. R. The psychoanalysis of a psychotic child. *Psychoanalytic Study of the Child*, 1949, *3-4*, 311-332.

1945   Gurevitz, S. Direct analytic therapy and symbolical fulfilment reviewed as to their applicability in childhood schizophrenia. *Quarterly Journal of Child Behavior*, 1951, *3*, 276-288.

1946   Fabian, A. A. & Holden, M. A. Treatment of childhood schizophrenia in a child guidance clinic. *American Journal of Orthopsychiatry*, 1951, *21*, 571-583.

1947   Kemph, J. P., Harrison, S. I. & Finch, S. M. Promoting the development of ego functions in the middle phase of treatment of psychotic children. *Journal of the American Academy of Child Psychiatry*, 1965, *4*, 401-412.

1948   *Maslow, A. R. A concentrated therapeutic relationship with a psychotic child. *Journal of the American Academy of Child Psychiatry*, 1964, *3*, 140-150.

1949   Ekstein, R. & Caruth, E. The working alliance with the monster. *Bulletin of the Menninger Clinic*, 1965, *29*, 189-197.

1950   Bender, L. & Gurevitz, S. Results of psychotherapy with
         young schizophrenic children. *American Journal of
         Orthopsychiatry*, 1955, *25*, 162-170.
1951   Kaufman, I., et al. Success and failure in the treat-
         ment of childhood schizophrenia. *American Journal of
         Psychiatry*, 1962, *118*, 909-915.
1952   Seidman, F. Outpatient treatment of a seriously dis-
         turbed child in a child guidance center. *Journal of
         Clinical Psychology*, 1961, *17*, 220-225.
1953   *Wilkins, A. The meaning of external control to a schiz-
         ophrenic adolescent girl. *Bulletin of the Menninger
         Clinic*, 1957, *21*, 140-152.
1954   *Betz, B. A study of tactics for resolving the autistic
         barrier in the psychotherapy of the schizophrenic per-
         sonality. *American Journal of Psychiatry*, 1947, *104*,
         267-273.
1955   Sechehaye, M. A. The transference in symbolic realiza-
         tion. *International Journal of Psychoanalysis*, 1956,
         37, 270-277.
1956   *Ekstein, R. Special training problems in psychothera-
         peutic work with psychotic and borderline children.
         American Journal of Orthopsychiatry, 1962, *32*, 569-
         583.
1957   Durham, M. S. Pandora's box: The fantasies of an au-
         tisticlike child. *Journal of the American Academy of
         Child Psychiatry*, 1972, *11*, 255-269.
1958   *Berlin, I. N. Intrapersonal, interpersonal, and im-
         personal factors in the genesis of childhood schizo-
         phrenia. In S. A. Szurek & I. N. Berlin (Eds.),
         Clinical studies in childhood psychoses. New York:
         Brunner/Mazel, 1973. Pp. 551-593.
1959   *Gianascol, A. J. Experiences in the psychotherapy of
         a non-verbal, self-destructive, psychotic child. In
         S. A. Szurek & I. N. Berlin (Eds.), *Clinical studies
         in childhood psychoses*. New York: Brunner/Mazel,
         1973. Pp. 540-550.
1960   *Susselman, S. Work with a psychotic boy: An illustra-
         tion of concepts of authority and physical interven-
         tion. In S. A. Szurek & I. N. Berlin (Eds.), *Clini-
         cal studies in childhood psychoses*. New York: Brun-
         ner/Mazel, 1973. Pp. 594-625.
1961   *Berlin, I. N. Lessons from failure in ten years of
         psychotherapeutic work with a schizophrenic boy and
         his parents. In S. A. Szurek & I. N. Berlin (Eds.),
         Clinical studies in childhood psychoses. New York:
         Brunner/Mazel, 1973. Pp. 697-767.

TREATMENT AND MANAGEMENT/Group Therapy

1962   *Speers, R. W. & Lansing, C. Group psychotherapy with
         preschool psychotic children and collateral group

therapy of their parents: A preliminary report of the first two years. *American Journal of Orthopsychiatry*, 1964, *34*, 659-666.

1963   *Coffey, H. S. & Wiener, L. L.   *Group treatment of autistic children*. Englewood Cliffs, N.J.: Prentice-Hall, 1967.

1964   *King, C. H.   Activity group therapy with a schizophrenic boy--Follow-up two years later. *International Journal of Group Psychotherapy*, 1959, *9*, 184-194.

1965   Speers, R. W. & Lansing, C.   *Group therapy in childhood psychosis*. Chapel Hill: University of North Carolina Press, 1965.

1966   Bauer, I. L. & Gurevitz, S.   Group therapy with parents of schizophrenic children. *International Journal of Group Psychotherapy*, 1952, *2*, 344-357.

TREATMENT AND MANAGEMENT/Residential Care

1967   Silberstein, R. M., Mandell, W., Dalack, J. D. & Cooper, A.   Avoiding institutionalization of psychotic children. *Archives of General Psychiatry*, 1968, *19*, 17-21.

1968   *Davids, A., Ryan, R. & Salvatore, P. D.   Effectiveness of residential treatment for psychotic and other disturbed children. *American Journal of Orthopsychiatry*, 1968, *38*, 469-475.

1969   *Krug, O.   The application of principles of child psychotherapy in residential treatment. *American Journal of Psychiatry*, 1952, *108*, 695-700.

1970   *Kemph, J. P., Cain, A. C. & Finch, S. M.   New directions in the inpatient treatment of psychotic children in a training center. *American Journal of Psychiatry*, 1963, *119*, 934-939.

1971   *Goldfarb, W. & Goldfarb, N.   Evaluation of behavioral changes of schizophrenic children in residential treatment. *American Journal of Psychotherapy*, 1965, *19*, 185-204.

1972   Gerard, M. W. & Overstreet, H. M.   Technical modification in the treatment of a schizoid boy within a treatment institution. *American Journal of Orthopsychiatry*, 1953, *23*, 171-185.

1973   *Freedman, A. M.   Day hospitals for severely disturbed schizophrenic children. *American Journal of Psychiatry*, 1959, *115*, 893-898.

1974   *Ekstein, R., Wallerstein, J. & Mandelbaum, A.   Countertransference in the residential treatment of children: Treatment failure in a child with symbiotic psychosis. *Psychoanalytic Study of the Child*, 1959, *14*, 186-218.

TREATMENT AND MANAGEMENT/Collaborative Therapy

1975   *Langdell, J. I. Family treatment of childhood schizo-
        phrenia. *Mental Hygiene*, 1967, *51*, 387-392.
1976   Pavenstedt, E. & Andersen, I. N. Complementary treat-
        ment of mother and child with atypical development.
        American Journal of Orthopsychiatry, 1952, *22*, 607-
        641.
1977   *Szurek, S. A. & Berlin, I. N. Elements of psychothera-
        peutics with the schizophrenic child and his parents.
        Psychiatry, 1956, *19*, 1-9.
1978   *Tec, L. Vicissitudes in guidance of parents of schizo-
        phrenic children. *Journal of Nervous and Mental Dis-
        ease*, 1956, *124*, 233-238.
1979   *Elkisch, P. Initiating separation-individuation in the
        simultaneous treatment of a child and his mother. In
        J. B. McDevitt & C. F. Settlage (Eds.), *Separation-
        individuation: Essays in honor of Margaret S. Mahler*.
        New York: International Universities Press, 1971.
        Pp. 356-376.
1980   Bergman, A. "I and you." The separation-individuation
        process in the treatment of a symbiotic-psychotic
        child. In J. B. McDevitt & C. F. Settlage (Eds.),
        *Separation-individuation: Essays in honor of Margaret
        S. Mahler*. New York: International Universities
        Press, 1971. Pp. 325-355.
1981   Furer, M. Observations on the treatment of the symbiot-
        ic syndrome of infantile psychosis:--Reality, recon-
        struction, and drive maturation. In J. B. McDevitt
        & C. F. Settlage (Eds.), *Separation-individuation:
        Essays in honor of Margaret S. Mahler*. New York:
        International Universities Press, 1971. Pp. 473-485.
1982   *Kysar, J. E. Reactions of professionals to disturbed
        children and their parents. *Archives of General Psy-
        chiatry*, 1968, *19*, 562-570.
1983   *Kysar, J. E. The two camps in child psychiatry: A re-
        port from a psychiatrist-father of an autistic and
        retarded child. *American Journal of Psychiatry*, 1968,
        125, 103-109.
1984   *Berlin, I. N. & Szurek, S. A. Parental blame: An ob-
        stacle in psychotherapeutic work with schizophrenic
        children and their families. In S. A. Szurek & I. N.
        Berlin (Eds.), *Clinical studies in childhood psycho-
        ses*. New York: Brunner/Mazel, 1973. Pp. 115-126.
1984.1 Howlin, P., Marchant, R., Rutter, M., Berger, M., Hersov,
        L. & Yule, W. A home-based approach to the treatment
        of autistic children. *Journal of Autism and Childhood
        Schizophrenia*, 1973, *3*, 308-336.

TREATMENT AND MANAGEMENT/Psychoeducational Therapies/*TUTORING*

1985   *Cohen, R. S. Some childhood identity disturbances: Ed-
       ucational implementation of a psychiatric treatment
       plan. *Journal of the American Academy of Child Psychi-
       atry*, 1964, *3*, 488-499.
1986   *Dubnoff, B. Education of autistic children. The habil-
       itation and education of the autistic child in a ther-
       apeutic day school. *American Journal of Orthopsychi-
       atry*, 1965, *35*, 385-386.
1987   *Elgar, S. Teaching autistic children. In J. K. Wing
       (Ed.), *Early childhood autism: Clinical, educational
       and social aspects*. Oxford: Pergamon Press, 1966.
       Pp. 205-237.
1988   *Wing, J. K. & Wing, L. A clinical interpretation of
       remedial teaching. In J. K. Wing (Ed.), *Early child-
       hood autism: Clinical, educational and social aspects*.
       Oxford: Pergamon Press, 1966. Pp. 185-203.
1989   *Hirschberg, J. C. Symposium, 1953. The education of
       emotionally disturbed children. 4. The role of edu-
       cation in the treatment of emotionally disturbed chil-
       dren through planned ego development. *American Journal
       of Orthopsychiatry*, 1953, *23*, 684-690.
1990   Goldfarb, W. & Pollack, R. C. The childhood schizo-
       phrenic's response to schooling in a residential treat-
       ment center. *Proceedings of the American Psychopatho-
       logical Association*, 1964, *52*, 221-246.
1991   *Rutter, M. Schooling and the autistic child. *Special
       Education*, 1967, *56*, 19-24.
1992   *Smolen, E. M. & Lifton, N. A special treatment program
       for schizophrenic children in a child guidance clinic.
       American Journal of Orthopsychiatry, 1966, *36*, 736-
       742.
1993   Goldberg, I. Use of remedial reading tutoring as a
       method of psychotherapy for schizophrenic children
       with reading disabilities. *Quarterly Journal of Child
       Behavior*, 1952, *4*, 273-280.
1994   Weston, P. T. B. (Ed.) *Some approaches to teaching
       autistic children*. Oxford: Pergamon Press, 1965.

TREATMENT AND MANAGEMENT/Psychoeducational Therapies/*SPEECH*

1995   *Wolf, E. G. & Ruttenberg, B. A. Communication therapy
       for the autistic child. *Journal of Speech and Hearing
       Disorders*, 1967, *32*, 331-335.
1996   *Rubin, H., Bar, A. & Dwyer, J. H. An experimental
       speech and language program for psychotic children.
       Journal of Speech and Hearing Disorders, 1967, *32*,
       242-248.
1997   *Ekstein, R. On the acquisition of speech in the autistic
       child. *Reiss-Davis Clinic Bulletin*, 1964, *1*, 63-79.

1998   *Shapiro, T., Roberts, A. & Fish, B. Imitation and echo-
       ing in young schizophrenic children. *Journal of the
       American Academy of Child Psychiatry*, 1970, *9*, 548-
       567.
1999   *Goldfarb, W., Braunstein, P. & Scholl, H. An approach
       to the investigation of childhood schizophrenia: The
       speech of schizophrenic children and their mothers.
       American Journal of Orthopsychiatry, 1959, *29*, 481-486.
1999.1 Ratusnik, C. M. & Ratusnik, D. L. A comprehensive com-
       munication approach for a ten-year-old nonverbal au-
       tistic child. *American Journal of Orthopsychiatry*,
       1974, *44*, 396-403.
1999.2 Goldfarb, W., Goldfarb, N., Braunstein, P. & Scholl, H.
       Speech and language faults of schizophrenic children.
       Journal of Autism and Childhood Schizophrenia, 1972,
       2, 219-233.
1999.3 Shapiro, T., Huebner, H. F. & Campbell, M. Language be-
       havior and hierarchic integration in a psychotic child.
       Journal of Autism and Childhood Schizophrenia, 1974,
       4, 71-90.

TREATMENT AND MANAGEMENT/Psychoeducational Therapies/*BODY
   CONTACT, DANCE, AND MUSIC*

2000   *Schopler, E. The development of body image and symbol
       formation through bodily contact with an autistic
       child. *Journal of Child Psychology and Psychiatry and
       Allied Disciplines*, 1962, *3*, 191-202.
2001   Schopler, E. Treatment of the schizophrenic child. The
       relationship between early tactile experience and the
       treatment of an autistic and a schizophrenic child.
       American Journal of Orthopsychiatry, 1964, *34*, 339-340.
2002   *Dreikurs, R. Music therapy with psychotic children.
       Psychiatric Quarterly, 1960, *34*, 722-734.
2002.1 Webster, C. D., McPherson, H., Sloman, L., Evans, M. A.
       & Kuchar, E. Communicating with an autistic boy by
       gestures. *Journal of Autism and Childhood Schizo-
       phrenia*, 1973, *3*, 337-346.
2002.2 Schoop, T. & Mitchell, P. *Won't you join the dance?
       A dancer's essay into the treatment of psychosis*.
       Palo Alto, Calif.: National Press, 1974.

TREATMENT AND MANAGEMENT/Behavior Modification

2003   *Werry, J. S. & Wollersheim, J. P. Behavior therapy with
       children: A broad overview. *Journal of the American
       Academy of Child Psychiatry*, 1967, *6*, 346-370.
2004   Hingtgen, J. N., Coulter, S. K. & Churchill, D. W. In-
       tensive reinforcement of imitative behavior in mute
       autistic children. *Archives of General Psychiatry*,
       1967, *17*, 36-43.

2005   *Jensen, G. D. & Womack, M. Operant conditioning tech-
        niques applied in the treatment of an autistic child.
        American Journal of Orthopsychiatry, 1967, *37*, 30-34.
2006   *Hewett, F. M. Teaching speech to an autistic child
        through operant conditioning. *American Journal of
        Orthopsychiatry*, 1965, *35*, 927-936.
2007   *Ferster, C. B. Positive reinforcement and behavioral
        deficits of autistic children. *Child Development*,
        1961, *32*, 437-456.
2008   *DeMyer, M. K. & Ferster, C. B. Teaching new social be-
        havior to schizophrenic children. *Journal of the A-
        merican Academy of Child Psychiatry*, 1962, *1*, 443-461.
2009   *Churchill, D. W. Psychotic children and behavior modi-
        fication. *American Journal of Psychiatry*, 1969, *125*,
        1585-1590.
2010   *Carlin, A. S. & Armstrong, H. E. Rewarding social re-
        sponsibility in disturbed children: A group play
        technique. *Psychotherapy: Theory, Reseach and Prac-
        tice*, 1968, *5*, 169-174.
2011   Hewett, F. M., Mayhew, D. & Rabb, E. An experimental
        reading program for neurologically impaired, mentally
        retarded, and severely emotionally disturbed children.
        American Journal of Orthopsychiatry, 1967, *37*, 35-48.
2012   *Colligan, R. C. & Bellamy, C. M. Effects of a two year
        treatment program for a young autistic child. *Psy-
        chotherapy: Theory, Research and Practice*, 1968, *5*,
        214-219.
2013   Ferster, C. B. Operant reinforcement of infantile au-
        tism. In S. Lesse (Ed.), *An evaluation of the results
        of the psychotherapies*. Springfield, Ill.: Thomas,
        1968. Pp. 221-236.
2014   *Baroff, G. S. & Tate, B. G. The use of aversive stimu-
        lation in the treatment of chronic self-injurious be-
        havior. *Journal of the American Academy of Child Psy-
        chiatry*, 1968, *7*, 454-470.
2015   *Lovaas, O. I., Schaeffer, B. & Simmons, J. Q. Building
        social behavior in autistic children by use of elec-
        tric shock. *Journal of Experimental Research in Per-
        sonality*, 1965, *1*, 99-109.
2016   *Simmons, J. Q. & Lovaas, O. I. Use of pain and punish-
        ment as treatment techniques with childhood schizo-
        phrenics. *American Journal of Psychotherapy*, 1969,
        23, 23-36.
2017   *Schell, R. E. & Adams, W. P. Training parents of a
        young child with profound behavior deficits to be
        teacher-therapists. *Journal of Special Education*,
        1968, *2*, 439-454.

TREATMENT AND MANAGEMENT/Somatic Therapies

2018   *Bender, L. One hundred cases of childhood schizophrenia
        treated with electric shock. *Transactions of the
        American Neurological Association*, 1947, *72*, 165-169.
2019   *Fish, B., Shapiro, T. & Campbell, M. Long-term prog-
        nosis and the response of schizophrenic children to
        drug therapy: A controlled study of trifluoperazine.
        American Journal of Psychiatry, 1966, *123*, 32-39.
2020   Connell, P. H. Medical treatment. In J. K. Wing (Ed.),
        *Early childhood autism: Clinical, educational and
        social aspects*. Oxford: Pergamon Press, 1966.
        Pp. 101-111.
2021   Schulman, J. L. Management of the child with early in-
        fantile autism. *American Journal of Psychiatry*, 1963,
        120, 250-254.
2022   *Schopler, E. & Reichler, R. J. Psychobiological re-
        ferents for the treatment of autism. In D. W. Church-
        ill, G. D. Alpern & M. K. DeMyer (Eds.), *Infantile
        autism: Proceedings of the Indiana University Col-
        loquium*. Springfield, Ill.: C. C. Thomas, 1971.
        Pp. 243-264.
2023   Freedman, A. M. Treatment of autistic schizophrenic
        children with marsilid. *Journal of Clinical and Ex-
        perimental Psychopathology and Quarterly Review of
        Psychiatry and Neurology Special Supplement*, 1958, *19*,
        138-145.
2024   *Freedman, A. M., Ebin, E. V. & Wilson, E. A. Autistic
        schizophrenic children: An experiment in the use of
        d-lysergic acid diethylamide (LSD-25). *Archives of
        General Psychiatry*, 1962, *6*, 203-213.
2025   Bender, L., Goldschmidt, L. & Sankar, S. D. V. Treat-
        ment of autistic schizophrenic children with LSD-25
        and UML-491. *Recent Advances in Biological Psychiatry*,
        1961, *4*, 170-179.
2026   Ferster, C. B. & DeMyer, M. K. Increased performances
        of an autistic child with prochlorperazine administra-
        tion. *Journal of the Experimental Analysis of Behav-
        ior*, 1961, *4*, 84.
2027   Rimland, B. High-dosage levels of certain vitamins in
        the treatment of children with severe mental disorders.
        In D. Hawkins & L. C. Pauling (Eds.), *Orthomolecular
        psychiatry: Treatment of schizophrenia*. San Francis-
        co: Freeman, 1973. Pp. 513-539.
2027.1 Campbell, M., Fish, B., David, R., Shapiro, T., Collins,
        P. & Koh, C. Response to triiodothyronine and dextro-
        amphetamine: A study of preschool schizophrenic
        children. *Journal of Autism and Childhood Schizo-
        phrenia*, 1972, *2*, 343-358.
2027.2 McAndrew, J. B., Case, Q. & Treffert, D. A. Effects of
        prolonged phenothiazine intake on psychotic and other
        hospitalized children. *Journal of Autism and Child-
        hood Schizophrenia*, 1972, *2*, 75-91.

TREATMENT AND MANAGEMENT/Other Modalities

2028   *Garcia, B. & Sarvis, M. A. Evaluation and treatment
        planning for autistic children. *Archives of General
        Psychiatry*, 1964, *10*, 530-541.
2029   *Wing, L. Counselling and the principles of management.
        In J. K. Wing (Ed.), *Early childhood autism: Clinical,
        educational and social aspects*. Oxford: Pergamon
        Press, 1966. Pp. 257-277.
2030   *Schechter, M. D., Shurley, J. T., Sexauer, J. D. & Tous-
        sieng, P. W. Perceptual isolation therapy: A new
        experimental approach in the treatment of children
        using infantile autistic defenses, a preliminary re-
        port. *Journal of the American Academy of Child Psy-
        chiatry*, 1969, *8*, 97-139.
2031   *Schechter, M. D., Shurley, J. T., Toussieng, P. W. &
        Maier, W. J. Sensory isolation therapy of autistic
        children: A preliminary report. *Journal of Pediat-
        rics*, 1969, *74*, 564-569.
2032   Ferster, C. B. & DeMyer, M. K. The development of per-
        formances in autistic children in an automatically
        controlled environment. *Journal of Chronic Diseases*,
        1961, *13*, 312-345.
2033   *Colby, K. M. Computer-aided language development in
        nonspeaking children. *Archives of General Psychiatry*,
        1968, *19*, 641-651.
2034   Ferster, C. B. Psychotherapy by machine communication.
        *Research Publications of the Association for Research
        in Nervous and Mental Disease*, 1964, *42*, 317-333.
2035   *Bakwin, H. The home management of children with schizo-
        phrenia. *Journal of Pediatrics*, 1955, *47*, 514-519.

TREATMENT AND MANAGEMENT/Additional Readings

2036   DesLauriers, A. M. *The experience of reality in child-
        hood schizophrenia*. New York: International Univer-
        sities Press, 1962.
2037   King, P. D. Theoretical considerations of psychotherapy
        with a schizophrenic child. *Journal of the American
        Academy of Child Psychiatry*, 1964, *3*, 638-649.
2038   Azima, H. & Wittkower, E. D. Gratification of basic
        needs in treatment of schizophrenics. *Psychiatry*,
        1956, *19*, 121-129.
2039   Tessman, L. H. & Kaufman, I. Treatment techniques, the
        primary process, and ego development in schizophrenic
        children. *Journal of the American Academy of Child
        Psychiatry*, 1967, *6*, 98-115.
2040   *Wing, L. *Autistic children*. London: Constable, 1971.
2041   *Weiland, I. H. Discussion of treatment approaches. In
        D. W. Churchill, G. D. Alpern & M. K. DeMyer (Eds.),
        Infantile autism: Proceedings of the Indiana Univer-

sity colloquium. Springfield, Ill.: C. C. Thomas, 1971. Pp. 200-211.

2042 Alpert, A. & Krown, S. Treatment of a child with severe ego restrictions in a therapeutic nursery. *Psychoanalytic Study of the Child*, 1953, *8*, 333-354.

2043 Ekstein, R. & Caruth, E. Levels of verbal communication in the schizophrenic child's struggle against, for, and with the world of objects. *Psychoanalytic Study of the Child*, 1969, *24*, 115-137.

2044 King, P. D. & Ekstein, R. The search for ego controls: Progression of play activity in psychotherapy with a schizophrenic child. *Psychoanalytic Review*, 1967, *54*, 639-648.

2045 Sechehaye, M. A. *Symbolic realization.* New York: International Universities Press, 1951.

2046 Ekstein, R. *Children of time and space, of action and impulse.* New York: Appleton-Century-Crofts, 1966.

2047 Park, C. C. *The siege.* New York: Harcourt, Brace & World, 1967.

2048 Renee, pseud. *Autobiography of a schizophrenic girl.* New York: Grune & Stratton, 1951.

2048.1 Kanner, L., Rodriguez, A. & Ashenden, B. How far can autistic children go in matters of social adaptation? *Journal of Autism and Childhood Schizophrenia*, 1972, *2*, 9-33.

BORDERLINE CONDITIONS

2049 *Knight, R. P. Management and psychotherapy of the borderline schizophrenic patient. In *Psychoanalytic psychiatry and psychology.* New York: International Universities Press, 1954. Pp. 110-122. (Also in *Bulletin of the Menninger Clinic*, 1953, *17*, 139-150.)

2050 *Ekstein, R. & Wallerstein, J. Observations on the psychotherapy of borderline and psychotic children. *Psychoanalytic Study of the Child*, 1956, *11*, 303-311.

2051 *Cain, A. C. On the meaning of "playing crazy" in borderline children. *Psychiatry*, 1964, *27*, 278-289.

2052 *Ekstein, R. & Friedman, S. W. A technical problem in the beginning phase of psychotherapy with a borderline psychotic child. In G. E. Gardner (Ed.), *Case studies in childhood emotional disabilities.* Vol. 2. New York: American Orthopsychiatric Association, 1956. Pp. 353-367.

2053 Geleerd, E. R. Borderline states in childhood and adolescence. *Psychoanalytic Study of the Child*, 1958, *13*, 279-295.

2054 Ekstein, R. & Wallerstein, J. Choice of interpretation in the treatment of borderline and psychotic children. *Bulletin of the Menninger Clinic*, 1957, *21*, 199-207.

2055 Frijling-Schreuder, E. C. M. Borderline states in

children. *Psychoanalytic Study of the Child,* 1969, *24,* 307-327.

2056   Ekstein, R. & Wallerstein, J. Observations on the psychology of borderline and psychotic children. *Psychoanalytic Study of the Child,* 1954, *9,* 344-369.

DEPRESSIONS AND MANIC-DEPRESSIVE DISORDERS

2057   *Anthony, E. J. & Scott, P. Manic-depressive psychosis in childhood. *Journal of Child Psychology and Psychiatry and Allied Disciplines,* 1960, *1,* 53-72.

2058   *Hall, M. B. Our present knowledge about manic-depressive states in childhood. *Nervous Child,* 1951-52, *9,* 319-325.

2059   *Spitz, R. A. & Wolf, K. M. Anaclitic depression. An inquiry into the genesis of psychiatric conditions in early childhood, II. *Psychoanalytic Study of the Child,* 1946, *2,* 313-342.

2060   *Mahler, M. S. On sadness and grief in infancy and childhood: Loss and restoration of the symbiotic love object. *Psychoanalytic Study of the Child,* 1961, *16,* 332-351.

2061   *Zetzel, E. R. "The depressive position." In P. Greenacre (Ed.), *Affective disorders.* New York: International Universities Press, 1953. Pp. 84-116.

2062   *Bowlby, J. Grief and mourning in infancy and early childhood. *Psychoanalytic Study of the Child,* 1960, *15,* 9-52.

2063   *Freud, A. Discussion of Dr. John Bowlby's paper. *Psychoanalytic Study of the Child,* 1960, *15,* 53-62. (Writings, vol. 5. Pp. 167-186.)

2064   *Spitz, R. A. Discussion of Dr. Bowlby's paper. *Psychoanalytic Study of the Child,* 1960, *15,* 85-94.

2065   *Schur, M. Discussion of Dr. John Bowlby's paper. *Psychoanalytic Study of the Child,* 1960, *15,* 63-84.

2066   Rochlin, G. The disorder of depression and elation: A clinical study of the changes from one state to the other. *Journal of the American Psychoanalytic Association,* 1953, *1,* 438-457.

2067   Campbell, J. Manic depressive psychosis in children: Report of 18 cases. *Quarterly Journal of Child Behavior,* 1952, *4,* 389-406.

2068   Greenacre, P. (Ed.) *Affective disorders.* New York: International Universities Press, 1953.

2069   Bibring, E. The mechanism of depression. In P. Greenacre (Ed.), *Affective disorders.* New York: International Universities Press, 1953. Pp. 13-48.

2070   Jacobson, E. Normal and pathological moods: Their nature and functions. *Psychoanalytic Study of the Child,* 1957, *12,* 73-113.

2071   Kasanin, J. The affective psychoses in children.

American Journal of Psychiatry, 1931, *87*, 897-926.
2072 *Putnam, M. C., Rank, B. & Kaplan, S. Notes on John I. A case of primal depression in an infant. *Psycho-analytic Study of the Child*, 1951, *6*, 38-58.
2073 Spitz, R. A. Hospitalism. An inquiry into the genesis of psychiatric conditions in early childhood. *Psychoanalytic Study of the Child*, 1945, *1*, 53-74.
2074 Gero, G. An equivalent of depression: Anorexia. In P. Greenacre (Ed.), *Affective disorders*. New York: International Universities Press, 1953. Pp. 117-139.
2075 *Beres, D. & Alpert, A. Analysis of a prolonged hypomanic episode in a five year old child. *American Journal of Orthopsychiatry*, 1940, *10*, 794-800.
2076 Katan, M. Mania and the pleasure principle. In P. Greenacre (Ed.), *Affective disorders*. New York: International Universities Press, 1953. Pp. 140-209.
2077 Barrett, A. M. Manic depressive psychosis in childhood. *International Clinics*, 1931, *3*, 205-217.
2078 McHarg, J. F. Mania in childhood: Report of a case. *Archives of Neurology and Psychiatry*, 1954, *72*, 531-539.

DEPRESSIONS AND MANIC-DEPRESSIVE DISORDERS IN CHILDHOOD/Use of Drugs in Affective Disorders

2079 *Annell, A. L. Lithium in the treatment of children and adolescents. *Acta Psychiatrica Scandinavica*, 1969, *207*(Suppl.), 19-33.
2080 Schou, M. Lithium in psychiatric therapy: Stock-taking after ten years. *Psychopharmacologia*, 1959, *1*, 65-78.
2081 Baastrup, P. C. & Schou, M. Lithium as a prophylactic agent: Its effect against recurrent depressions and manic-depressive psychosis. *Archives of General Psychiatry*, 1967, *16*, 162-172.
2082 Wolpert, E. A. & Mueller, P. Lithium carbonate in the treatment of manic-depressive disorders. *Archives of General Psychiatry*, 1969, *21*, 155-159.

COUNTERTRANSFERENCE PROBLEMS

2083 *Ekstein, R. Special training problems in psychotherapeutic work with psychotic and borderline children. *American Journal of Orthopsychiatry*, 1962, *32*, 569-583.
2084 *Prall, R. C. & Dealy, M. N. Countertransference in therapy of childhood psychosis. *Journal of the Hillside Hospital*, 1965, *14*, 69-82.
2085 *Searles, H. F. The schizophrenic's vulnerability to the therapist's unconscious processes. *Journal of Nervous and Mental Disease*, 1958, *127*, 247-262.
2086 Mann, J., Menzer, D. & Standish, C. Psychotherapy of

psychoses: Some attitudes in the therapist influencing
the course of treatment. *Psychiatry*, 1950, *13*, 17-23.

2087   Caruth, E. & Ekstein, R. Certain phenomenological aspects of the counter-transference in the treatment of
schizophrenic children. *Reiss-Davis Clinic Bulletin*,
1964, *1*, 80-88.

2088   *Christ, A. E. Sexual countertransference problems with
a psychotic child. *Journal of the American Academy of
Child Psychiatry*, 1964, *3*, 298-316.

2089   Frijling-Schreuder, E. C. M. Borderline states in children. *Psychoanalytic Study of the Child*, 1969, *24*,
307-327.

2090   Ekstein, R. & Wallerstein, J. Observations on the psychology of borderline and psychotic children. *Psychoanalytic Study of the Child*, 1954, *9*, 344-369.

PROGNOSIS AND FOLLOW-UP

2091   *Kanner, L. & Eisenberg, L. Notes on the follow-up
studies of autistic children. *Proceedings of the
American Psychopathological Association*, 1955, *44*,
227-239.

2092   Freedman, A. M. & Bender, L. When the childhood schizophrenic grows up. *American Journal of Orthopsychiatry*, 1957, *27*, 553-565.

2093   *Fish, B., et al. The prediction of schizophrenia in
infancy: II. A ten-year follow-up report of pre-
dictions made at one month of age. *Proceedings of
the American Psychopathological Association*, 1966,
54, 335-353.

2094   *Eisenberg, L. The autistic child in adolescence.
American Journal of Psychiatry, 1956, *112*, 607-612.

2095   *Rutter, M. Prognosis: Psychotic children in adolescence and early adult life. In J. K. Wing (Ed.),
*Early childhood autism: Clinical, educational and
social aspects*. Oxford: Pergamon Press, 1966.
Pp. 83-99.

2096   *Rutter, M., Greenfield, D. & Lockyer, L. A five to
fifteen year follow-up study of infantile psychosis.
II. Social and behavioural outcome. *British Journal
of Psychiatry*, 1967, *113*, 1183-1199.

2097   *Rutter, M. & Lockyer, L. A five to fifteen year follow-
up study of infantile psychosis. I. Description of
sample. *British Journal of Psychiatry*, 1967, *113*,
1169-1182.

2098   *Bennett, S. & Klein, H. R. Childhood schizophrenia:
30 years later. *American Journal of Psychiatry*,
1966, *122*, 1121-1124.

2099   Mittler, P., Gillies, S. & Jukes, E. Prognosis in psychotic children: Report of a follow-up study. *Journal of Mental Deficiency Research*, 1966, *10*, 73-83.

2100   *Menolascino, F. J. & Eaton, L. Psychoses of childhood:

A five year follow-up study of experiences in a mental retardation clinic. *American Journal of Mental Deficiency*, 1967, *72*, 370-380.

2101   *Levy, E. Z. Long-term follow-up of former inpatients at the Children's Hospital of the Menninger Clinic. *American Journal of Psychiatry*, 1969, *125*, 1633-1639.

2102   *Jackson, L. Non-speaking children: Seven years later. *British Journal of Medical Psychology*, 1958, *31*, 92-103.

2103   Reiser, D. E. & Brown, J. L. Patterns of later development in children with infantile psychosis. *Journal of the American Academy of Child Psychiatry*, 1964, *3*, 650-667.

2104   Eisenberg, L. The course of childhood schizophrenia. *Archives of Neurology and Psychiatry*, 1957, *78*, 69-83.

2105   *Brown, J. L. Follow-up of children with atypical development (infantile psychosis). *American Journal of Orthopsychiatry*, 1963, *33*, 855-861.

2106   Clardy, E. R. A study of the development and course of schizophrenia in children. *Psychiatric Quarterly*, 1951, *25*, 81-90.

2107   Fish, B., Shapiro, T., Halpern, F. & Wile, R. The prediction of schizophrenia in infancy: III. A ten-year follow-up report of neurological and psychological development. *American Journal of Psychiatry*, 1965, *121*, 768-775.

2108   *Brown, J. L. Prognosis from presenting symptoms of preschool children with atypical development. *American Journal of Orthopsychiatry*, 1960, *30*, 382-390.

2109   *Bomberg, D., Szurek, S. A. & Etemad, J. G. A statistical study of a group of psychotic children. In S. A. Szurek & I. N. Berlin (Eds.), *Clinical studies in childhood psychoses*. New York: Brunner/Mazel, 1973. Pp. 303-347.

2110   *Etemad, J. G. & Szurek, S. A. A modified follow-up study of a group of psychotic children. In S. A. Szurek & I. N. Berlin (Eds.), *Clinical studies in childhood psychoses*. New York: Brunner/Mazel, 1973. Pp. 348-371.

2110.1 Bender, L. The life course of children with schizophrenia. *American Journal of Psychiatry*, 1973, *130*, 783-786.

ADDITIONAL READINGS

2111   Hoedemaker, E. D. The therapeutic process in the treatment of schizophrenia. *Journal of the American Psychoanalytic Association*, 1955, *3*, 89-109.

2112   Kanner, L., Hirschberg, J., Bryant, K. & Bender, L. Symposium on juvenile schizophrenia. *Research Publications of the Association for Research in Nervous and Mental Disease*, 1954, *34*, 451-477.

2113   Bender, L. *Child psychiatric techniques.* Springfield, Ill.: C. C. Thomas, 1952.

2114   Pollack, M. & Krieger, H. P. Oculomotor and postural patterns in schizophrenic children. *Archives of Neurology and Psychiatry,* 1958, *79,* 720-726.

2115   Sackler, M. D., et al. A psychobiologic viewpoint on schizophrenias of childhood. *Nervous Child,* 1952, *10,* 43-59.

2116   *Singer, R. D. Organization as a unifying concept in schizophrenia. *Archives of General Psychiatry,* 1960, *2,* 61-74.

2117   Arieti, S. *Interpretation of schizophrenia.* New York: Brunner, 1955.

2118   Federn, P. *Ego psychology and the psychoses.* New York: Basic Books, 1952.

2119   Hartmann, H. Contribution to the metapsychology of schizophrenia. *Psychoanalytic Study of the Child,* 1953, *8,* 177-198.

2120   Hoch, P. H. & Zubin, J. (Eds.) *Psychopathology of communication.* New York: Grune & Stratton, 1958. (*Proceedings of the American Psychopathological Association,* 1958, *46*)

2121   Hill, L. B. *Psychotherapeutic intervention in schizophrenia.* Chicago: University of Chicago Press, 1955.

2122   Rosen, J. N. The treatment of schizophrenic psychosis by direct analytic therapy. *Psychiatric Quarterly,* 1947, *21,* 3-37.

2123   Brody, E. B. & Redlich, F. C. (Eds.) *Psychotherapy with schizophrenics.* New York: International Universities Press, 1952.

2123.1 Kanner, L. *Childhood psychosis: Initial studies and new insights.* New York: Wiley, 1973.

2123.2 Wing, L. *Autistic children: A guide for parents and professionals.* New York: Brunner/Mazel, 1972.

XIV. MENTAL RETARDATION

GENERAL REFERENCES

2124   U.S. President's Panel on Mental Retardation. *Report to the president: A proposed program for national action to combat mental retardation.* Washington: U.S. President's Panel on Mental Retardation, 1962.

2125   Perry, S. E. Some theoretic problems of mental deficiency and their action implications. *Psychiatry,* 1954, *17,* 45-73.

2126   Zigler, E. Familial mental retardation: A continuing dilemma. *Science,* 1967, *155,* 292-298.

2127   Group for the Advancement of Psychiatry. Committee on Mental Retardation. *Basic considerations in mental retardation.* GAP report, no. 43. New York: Group

for the Advancement of Psychiatry, 1959.
2128   Knobloch, H. & Pasamanick, B. Mental subnormality.
New England Journal of Medicine, 1962, *266*, 1045-1051;
1155-1161.
2129   *Cytryn, L. & Lourie, R. S. Mental retardation. In A.
M. Freedman & H. I. Kaplan (Eds.), *Comprehensive textbook of psychiatry*. Baltimore: Williams & Wilkins,
1967. Pp. 817-856.
2130   *Pasamanick, B. & Knobloch, H. Brain behavior: Session
II. Symposium, 1959. 2. Brain damage and reproductive casualty. *American Journal of Orthopsychiatry*,
1960, *30*, 298-305.
2130.1 Tarjan, G. & Keeran, C. V., Jr. An overview of mental
retardation. *Psychiatric Annals*, 1974, *4*(2), 6-21.
2130.2 Mental Health Law Project. *Basic rights of the mentally
handicapped*. Washington, D.C.: Mental Health Law
Project, 1973.

ETIOLOGY

2131   *Chase, H. P., Dabiere, C. S., Welch, N. N. & O'Brien, D.
Intrauterine undernutrition and brain development.
Pediatrics, 1971, *47*, 491-500.
2132   *Cravioto, J., DeLicardie, E. R. & Birch, H. G. Nutrition,
growth and neurointegrative development: An experimental and ecologic study. *Pediatrics*, 1966, *38*,
319-372.
2133   Barnes, R. H. Nutrition and man's intellect and behavior. *Federation Proceedings*, 1971, *30*, 1429-1433.
2134   Scrimshaw, N. S. Malnutrition, learning and behavior.
American Journal of Clinical Nutrition, 1967, *20*,
493-502.
2135   *Tompkins, W. T., et al. Maternal and newborn nutrition
studies at Philadelphia Lying-in Hospital. Maternal
studies. II. Prematurity and maternal nutrition. In
Milbank Memorial Fund, *The promotion of maternal and
newborn health: Papers presented at the 1954 annual
conference of the Milbank Memorial Fund*. New York,
1955. Pp. 25-50.
2136   *O'Connell, E. J., Feldt, R. H. & Stickler, G. B. Head
circumference, mental retardation, and growth failure.
Pediatrics, 1965, *36*, 62-66.
2137   *Winick, M. Cellular growth during early malnutrition.
Pediatrics, 1971, *47*, 969-978.
2138   Winick, M. & Coombs, J. Nutrition, environment, and behavioral development. *Annual Review of Medicine*,
1972, *23*, 149-160.
2139   Krech, D. The chemistry of learning. *Saturday Review*,
1968, *51*(3), 48-50;68.
2140   *Pasamanick, B. & Knobloch, H. Retrospective studies on
the epidemiology of reproductive casualty: Old and

new. *Merrill-Palmer Quarterly,* 1966, *12,* 7-26.

2141   Knobloch, H. & Pasamanick, B. Environmental factors affecting human development, before and after birth.
Pediatrics, 1960, *26,* 210-218.

2142   *Knobloch, H. & Pasamanick, B. Distribution of intellectual potential in an infant population. In B. Pasamanick (Ed.), *Epidemiology of mental disorder.* Washington: American Association for the Advancement of
Science, 1959. Pp. 249-272.

2143   *Frisch, R. E. Present status of the supposition that
malnutrition causes permanent mental retardation.
American Journal of Clinical Nutrition, 1970, *23,*
189-195.

2144   Harrell, R. F., Woodyard, E. R. & Gates, A. I. The influence of vitamin supplementation of diets of pregnant and lactating women on the intelligence of their
offspring. *Metabolism: Clinical and Experimental,*
1956, *5,* 555-562.

2145   Dobbing, J. Effects of experimental undernutrition on
development of the nervous system. In N. S. Scrimshaw & J. E. Gordon (Eds.), *Malnutrition, learning,
and behavior.* Cambridge: M.I.T. Press, 1968. Pp.
181-202.

2146   *Drillien, C. M. The incidence of mental and physical
handicaps in school age children of very low birth
weight. *Pediatrics,* 1967, *39,* 238-247.

2147   *Earle, K. M., Baldwin, M. & Penfield, W. Incisural
sclerosis and temporal lobe seizures produced by hippo-
campal herniation at birth. *Archives of Neurology
and Psychiatry,* 1953, *69,* 27-42.

2148   *Gerver, J. M. & Day, R. Intelligence quotient of children who have recovered from erythroblastosis fetalis.
Journal of Pediatrics, 1950, *36,* 342-348.

2149   Knobloch, H. & Pasamanick, B. An evaluation of the con-
sistency and predictive value of the 40 week Gesell
developmental schedule. In C. Shagass & B. Pasamanick
(Eds.), *Child development and child psychiatry.* Washington: American Psychiatric Association, 1960. Pp.
10-31. (*Psychiatric Research Reports,* No. 13)

2150   Keith, H. M. & Gage, R. P. Neurologic lesions in relation to asphyxia of the newborn and factors of pregnancy: Long-term follow-up. *Pediatrics,* 1960, *26,*
616-622.

2151   Windle, W. F. Effects of asphyxiation of the fetus and
the newborn infant. *Pediatrics,* 1960, *26,* 565-569.

2152   *Zuelzer, W. W. & Brown, A. K. Neonatal jaundice: A
review. *American Journal of Diseases of Children,*
1961, *101,* 87-127.

2153   *Thurston, D., Graham, F. K., Ernhart, C. B., Eichman, P.
L. & Craft, M. Neurologic status of 3-year-old children originally studied at birth. *Neurology,* 1960, *10,*
680-690.

2154   *Knobloch, H. & Pasamanick, B.   Syndrome of minimal cere-
        bral damage in infancy. *Journal of the American Medi-
        cal Association,* 1959, *170,* 1384-1387.
2155   *Goldfarb, W.   Effects of psychological deprivation in
        infancy and subsequent stimulation. *American Journal
        of Psychiatry,* 1945, *102,* 18-33.
2156   *Bowlby, J., Ainsworth, M., Boston, M. & Rosenbluth, D.
        The effects of mother-child separation: A follow-up
        study. *British Journal of Medical Psychology,* 1956,
        29, 211-247.
2157   *Pinneau, S. R.   Infantile disorders of hospitalism and
        anaclitic depression. *Psychological Bulletin,* 1955,
        52, 429-452.
2158   *Stott, D. H.   Infantile illness and subsequent mental
        and emotional development. *Journal of Genetic Psy-
        chology,* 1959, *94,* 233-251.
2158.1 Mercer, J. R. *Labeling the mentally retarded; clinical
        and social system perspectives on mental retardation.*
        Berkeley: University of California Press, 1973.
2158.2 Douglas, C. P. & Holt, K. S. (Eds.) *Mental retardation;
        prenatal diagnosis and infant assessment.* London:
        Butterworths, 1972. (Institute for Research into
        Mental Retardation. Symposia nos. 6 and 8)
2158.3 Valente, M. & Tarjan, G.   Etiologic factors in mental
        retardation. *Psychiatric Annals,* 1974, *4*(2), 22-37.
2158.4 Murphy, A. & Pounds, L.   Repeat evaluations of retarded
        children. In S. Chess & A. Thomas (Eds.), *Annual
        progress in child psychiatry and child development:
        1973.* New York: Brunner/Mazel, 1974. Pp. 479-488.
2158.5 DeMyer, M. K., Alpern, G. D., Barton, S., DeMyer, W. E.,
        Churchill, D. W., Hingtgen, J. N., Bryson, C. Q.,
        Pontius, W. & Kimberlin, C.   Subnormal children.
        Journal of Autism and Childhood Schizophrenia, 1972,
        2, 264-287.
2158.6 Begab, M. J. & LaVeck, G. D.   Mental retardation: De-
        velopment of an international classification scheme.
        American Journal of Psychiatry, 1972, *128,* 1437-1438.

HISTORY

2159   *Silberstein, R. M. & Irwin, H.   Jean-Marc-Gaspard Itard
        and the savage of Aveyron: An unsolved diagnostic
        problem in child psychiatry. *Journal of the American
        Academy of Child Psychiatry,* 1962, *1,* 314-322.
2160   *Kanner, L. *A history of the care and study of the men-
        tally retarded.* Springfield, Ill.: Thomas, 1964.
2161   Haskell, R. H.   Mental deficiency over a hundred years:
        A brief historical sketch of trends in this field.
        American Journal of Psychiatry, 1944, *100,* 107-118.
2162   *Potter, H. W.   The needs of mentally retarded children
        for child psychiatry services. *Journal of the American*

Academy of Child Psychiatry, 1964, 3, 352-374.
2163   *Menolascino, F. J. Psychiatry's past, current and
        future role in mental retardation. In Psychiatric
        approaches to mental retardation. New York: Basic
        Books, 1970. Pp. 709-744.
2164   Davies, S. P. Social control of the mentally deficient.
        New York: Crowell, 1930.

THE FAMILY

2165   *Begab, M. J. The mentally retarded and the family. In
        I. Philips (Ed.), Prevention and treatment of mental
        retardation. New York: Basic Books, 1966. Pp. 71-84.
2166   *Group for the Advancement of Psychiatry. Committee on
        Mental Retardation. Mental retardation: A family
        crisis--the therapeutic role of the physician. GAP
        report, no. 56. New York: Group for the Advancement
        of Psychiatry, 1963.
2167   Matheny, A. P. & Vernick, J. Parents of the mentally
        retarded child: Emotionally overwhelmed or informa-
        tionally deprived? Journal of Pediatrics, 1969, 74,
        953-959.
2168   *Solnit, A. J. & Stark, M. H. Mourning and the birth of
        a defective child. Psychoanalytic Study of the Child,
        1961, 16, 523-537.
2169   *Mandelbaum, A. & Wheeler, M. E. The meaning of a de-
        fective child to parents. Social Casework, 1960, 41,
        360-367.
2170   Wolfensberger, W. & Menolascino, F. J. A theoretical
        framework for the management of parents of the men-
        tally retarded. In F. J. Menolascino (Ed.), Psychiat-
        ric approaches to mental retardation. New York:
        Basic Books, 1970. Pp. 475-493.
2171   Caldwell, B. M. & Guze, S. B. A study of the adjust-
        ment of parents and siblings of institutionalized and
        non-institutionalized retarded children. American
        Journal of Mental Deficiency, 1960, 64, 845-861.
2171.1 Crandall, B. F. Genetic counseling and mental retarda-
        tion. Psychiatric Annals, 1974, 4(2), 70-95.
2171.2 Golden, D. A. & Davis, J. G. Counseling parents after
        the birth of an infant with Down's Syndrome. Chil-
        dren Today, 1974, 3(2), 7-11, 36-37.
2171.3 Carver, J. N. & Carver, N. E. The family of the retard-
        ed child. Syracuse: Syracuse University Division of
        Special Education and Rehabilitation, 1972.
2171.4 Mannoni, M. The retarded child and the mother; a psy-
        choanalytic study. London: Tavistock, 1973.
2171.5 Weinrott, M. R. A training program in behavior modifi-
        cation for siblings of the retarded. American Journal
        of Orthopsychiatry, 1974, 44, 362-375.

PSYCHOPATHOLOGY

2172   *Duhl, L. J. Mental retardation: A review of mental
        health implications. *American Journal of Mental De-
        ficiency,* 1957, *62,* 5-13.
2173   *Philips, I. Psychopathology and mental retardation.
        American Journal of Psychiatry, 1967, *124,* 29-35.
2174   Provence, S. A. & Lipton, R. C. *Infants in institutions.*
        New York: International Universities Press, 1963.
2175   Webster, T. Problems of emotional development in young
        retarded children. *American Journal of Psychiatry,*
        1963, *120,* 37-43.
2176   Eisenberg, L. Emotional determinants of mental defi-
        ciency. *Archives of Neurology and Psychiatry,* 1958,
        80, 114-121.
2177   *Bender, L. The life course of children with autism and
        mental retardation. In F. J. Menolascino (Ed.), *Psy-
        chiatric approaches to mental retardation.* New York:
        Basic Books, 1970. Pp. 149-191.
2178   Bender, L. Autism in children with mental deficiency.
        American Journal of Mental Deficiency, 1959, *64,* 81-
        86.

THERAPEUTIC INTERVENTION/Psychotherapy-Individual and Group

2179   *Philips, I., Jeffress, M., Koch, E. & Boatman, M. J.
        The application of psychiatric clinic services for
        the retarded child and his family. *Journal of the
        American Academy of Child Psychiatry,* 1962, *1,* 297-
        313.
2180   *Lott, G. M. Psychotherapy of the mentally retarded:
        Values and cautions. *Journal of the American Medical
        Association,* 1966, *196,* 229-232.
2181   *Szurek, S. A. & Philips, I. Mental retardation and psy-
        chotherapy. In I. Philips (Ed.), *Prevention and treat-
        ment of mental retardation.* New York: Basic Books,
        1966. Pp. 221-246.
2182   Sheimo, S. L. Problems encountered in dealing with
        handicapped and emotionally disturbed children. *Amer-
        ican Journal of Occupational Therapy,* 1949, *3,* 303-307.
2183   *Slivkin, S. E. & Bernstein, N. R. Goal-directed group
        psychotherapy for retarded adolescents. *American
        Journal of Psychotherapy,* 1968, *22,* 35-45.
2184   Woodward, K. F., Jaffe, N. & Brown, D. Psychiatric pro-
        gram for very young retarded children. *American Jour-
        nal of Diseases of Children,* 1964, *108,* 221-229.
2185   Chess, S. Psychiatric treatment of the mentally retarded
        child with behavior problems. *American Journal of
        Orthopsychiatry,* 1962, *32,* 863-869.
2186   Gunzburg, H. C. Psychotherapy with the feeble-minded.
        In A. M. Clarke & A. D. B. Clarke (Eds.), *Mental De-*

ficiency: The changing outlook. New York: Free
Press, 1965. Pp. 417-446.

2187 Jakab, I. Psychotherapy of the mentally retarded child.
In N. R. Bernstein (Ed.), *Diminished people.* Boston:
Little, Brown, 1970. Pp. 223-261.

2188 *Gardner, W. I. Use of behavior therapy with the mentally retarded. In F. J. Menolascino (Ed.), *Psychiatric approaches to mental retardation.* New York:
Basic Books, 1970. Pp. 250-275.

2190 *Blatt, A. Group therapy with parents of severely retarded children: A preliminary report. *Group Psychotherapy,* 1957, *10,* 133-140.

2191 *Colodny, D. & Kurlander, L. F. Psychopharmacology as a
treatment adjunct for the mentally retarded: Problems
and issues. In F. J. Menolascino (Ed.), *Psychiatric
approaches to mental retardation.* New York: Basic
Books, 1970. Pp. 368-386.

2192 Freeman, R. D. Psychopharmacology and the retarded
child. In F. J. Menolascino (Ed.), *Psychiatric approaches to mental retardation.* New York: Basic
Books, 1970. Pp. 294-368.

2192.1 Simmons, J. Q., Tymchuk, A. J. & Valente, M. Treatment
and care of the mentally retarded. *Psychiatric Annals,* 1974, *4*(2), 38-69.

RESIDENTIAL INSTITUTIONS

2193 *Wolfensberger, W. The origin and nature of our institutional models. In R. B. Kugel & W. Wolfensberger
(Eds.), *Changing patterns in residential services for
the mentally retarded.* Washington, D.C.: President's
Committee on Mental Retardation, 1969. Pp. 59-171.

2194 *Kugel, R. B. & Wolfensberger, W. (Eds.) *Changing patterns in residential services for the mentally retarded.* Washington: President's Committee on Mental
Retardation, 1969.

2195 Nirje, B. The normalization principle and its human
management implications. In R. B. Kugel & W. Wolfensberger (Eds.), *Changing patterns in residential
services for the mentally retarded.* Washington, D.C.:
President's Committee on Mental Retardation, 1969.
Pp. 179-195.

2196 Dybwad, G. Action implications, U.S.A. today. In R.
B. Kugel & W. Wolfensberger (Eds.), *Changing patterns
in residential services for the mentally retarded.*
Washington, D.C.: President's Committee on Mental
Retardation, 1969. Pp. 383-428.

2196.1 Clayton, B. E. (Ed.) *Mental retardation: environmental hazards.* London: Butterworth's, 1973. (Institute for Research into Mental Retardation. Sym-
posia nos. 9, 10, & 11)

2196.2   Joint Commission on Accreditation of Hospitals. Accreditation Council for Facilities for the Mentally Retarded. *Standards for community agencies serving persons with mental retardation and other developmental disabilities, adopted July 25, 1973.* Chicago, 1973.

RESIDENT TRAINING AND TEACHING

2197   *Philips, I.   Problems of training the professional in the field of mental retardation: A review of a training program. *Journal of the American Academy of Child Psychiatry,* 1966, *5,* 693-705.

2198   *Bernstein, N. R.   Psychiatric training in a state school for the retarded: Establishing an environment for teaching, evaluation and treatment. *Journal of the American Academy of Child Psychiatry,* 1969, *8,* 68-83.

2199   Gardner, G. E.   Mental retardation as part of the training program in child psychiatry.   In P. W. Bowman & H. V. Mautner (Eds.), *Mental retardation: Proceedings of the 1st International Medical Conference.* New York: Grune & Stratton, 1960.   Pp. 505-515.

2200   Cytryn, L. & Milowe, I. D.   Development of a training program in mental retardation for psychiatric and pediatric residents. *Mental Retardation,* 1966, *4*(5), 2-5.

CONSULTATION AND COMMUNITY PSYCHIATRY

2201   *Tarjan, G.   Prevention, a program goal in mental deficiency. *American Journal of Mental Deficiency,* 1959, *64,* 4-11.

2202   Barton, W. E.   The psychiatrist's responsibility for mental retardation. *American Journal of Psychiatry,* 1961, *118,* 362-363.

2203   Potter, H. W.   The needs of mentally retarded children for child psychiatry services. *Journal of the American Academy of Child Psychiatry,* 1964, *3,* 352-374.

2204   *Philips, I.   Children, mental retardation and planning. *American Journal of Orthopsychiatry,* 1965, *35,* 899-902.

2205   *Chope, H. D.   The organization of community services for the mentally retarded.   In I. Philips (Ed.), *Prevention and treatment of mental retardation.* New York: Basic Books, 1966.   Pp. 398-406.

2206   Gardner, W. I. & Nisonger, H. W.   A manual on program development in mental retardation: Guidelines for planning, development, and coordination of programs for the mentally retarded at state and local levels. Section VIII. Community planning. *American Journal of Mental Deficiency,* 1962, *66*(Monogr. Suppl.), 137-148.

2207   *Boggs, E. M.   Legal aspects of mental retardation.   In
        I. Philips (Ed.), *Prevention and treatment of mental
        retardation.* New York: Basic Books, 1966. Pp. 407-
        428.
2208   *Berlin, I. N.   Consultation and special education.   In
        I. Philips (Ed.), *Prevention and treatment of mental
        retardation.* New York: Basic Books, 1966. Pp. 279-
        293.

CARE AND MANAGEMENT

2209   *Boggs, E. M. & Jervis, G. A.   Care and management of the
        retarded.   In S. Arieti (Ed.), *American handbook of
        psychiatry.* Vol. 3. New York: Basic Books, 1966.
        Pp. 31-46.
2210   *Hurley, R. L.   Public education and mental retardation.
        In *Poverty and mental retardation.* New York: Random
        House, 1969. Pp. 91-127.
2211   *Blatt, B.   A concept of educability and the correlates
        of mental illness, mental retardation, and cultural
        deprivation.   In N. R. Bernstein (Ed.), *Diminished
        people.* Boston: Little, Brown, 1970. Pp. 7-27.
2212   *Tarjan, G.   Rehabilitation of the mentally retarded.
        Journal of the American Medical Association, 1964,
        187, 867-870.
2213   U.S. President's Panel on Mental Retardation. *Report
        to the president: A proposed program for national
        action to combat mental retardation.* Washington:
        U.S. President's Panel on Mental Retardation, 1962.
        Pp. 73-130.
2213.1 Griffiths, M. I. (Ed.) *The young retarded child; medi-
        cal aspects of care.* Edinburgh: Churchill Living-
        stone, 1973.
2213.2 de la Cruz, F. F. & LaVeck, G. D. (Eds.) *Human sex-
        uality and the mentally retarded.* New York: Brunner/
        Mazel, 1973.

DEVELOPMENT OF INTELLIGENCE

2214   *McClearn, G. E.   Genetic influences on behavior and
        development.   In L. Carmichael, *Manual of child psy-
        chology.* (3rd ed.) Vol. 1. New York: Wiley, 1970.
        Pp. 39-76.
2215   Clarke, A. D. B.   Genetic and environmental studies of
        intelligence.   In A. M. Clarke & A. D. B. Clarke
        (Eds.), *Mental deficiency: The changing outlook.*
        (Rev. ed.) New York: Free Press, 1965. Pp. 92-137.
2216   Jensen, A. A.   A theory of primary and secondary famil-
        ial mental retardation.   *International Review of Re-
        search in Mental Retardation,* 1970, *4,* 33-106.

2217   *Hurley, R. L. Poverty and organic impairment, and the
        effects of cultural deprivation on intellectual per-
        formance. In *Poverty and mental retardation*. New
        York: Random House, 1969. Pp. 53-90.
2218   *Robinson, H. B. & Robinson, N. M. The physical environ-
        ment as a factor in mental retardation. In *The men-
        tally retarded child: A psychological approach*. New
        York: McGraw-Hill, 1965. Pp. 124-157.
2219   *Stein, Z. & Susser, M. Families of dull children. Part
        IV.--Increments in intelligence. *Journal of Mental
        Science*, 1960, *106*, 1311-1319.
2220   *Bayley, N. Development of mental abilities. In L. Car-
        michael, *Manual of child psychology*. (3rd ed.) Vol. 1.
        New York: Wiley, 1970. Pp. 1163-1209.
2221   *Bayley, N. Value and limitations of infant testing.
        Children, 1958, *5*, 129-133.
2222   *Bayley, N. Comparisons of mental and motor test scores
        for ages 1-15 months by sex, birth order, race, geo-
        graphical location and education of parents. *Child
        Development*, 1965, *36*, 379-411.
2223   *Bernstein, N. R. Intellectual defect and personality
        development. In *Diminished people*. Boston: Little,
        Brown, 1970. Pp. 165-200.
2224   Heber, R. Personality. In H. A. Stevens & R. Heber
        (Eds.), *Mental retardation: A review of research*.
        Chicago: University of Chicago Press, 1964. Pp.
        143-174.
2225   Weiner, G. Scholastic achievement at age 12-13 of pre-
        maturely born infants. *Journal of Special Education*,
        1968, *2*(3), 237-250.

SELECTED BOOKS AND PAMPHLETS

2226   American Medical Association. *Mental retardation: A
        handbook for the primary physician*. Chicago, 1965.
2227   Baumeister, A. A. *Mental retardation: Appraisal, edu-
        cation and rehabilitation*. Chicago: Aldine, 1967.
2228   Bender, L. *Psychopathology of children with organic
        brain disorders*. Springfield, Ill.: Thomas, 1956.
2229   Bernstein, N. R. *Diminished people*. Boston: Little,
        Brown, 1970.
2230   Carter, C. H. *Medical aspects of mental retardation*.
        Springfield, Ill.: Thomas, 1965.
2231   Clarke, A. M. *Mental deficiency: The changing outlook*.
        (Rev. ed.) New York: Free Press, 1965.
2232   Ford, F. R. *Diseases of the nervous system in infancy,
        childhood, and adolescence*. (6th ed.) Springfield,
        Ill.: Thomas, 1973.
2233   Gardner, W. I. & Nisonger, H. W. A manual on program
        development in mental retardation: Guidelines for
        planning, development, and coordination of programs

for the mentally retarded at state and local levels. *American Journal of Mental Deficiency*, 1962, *66*(Monogr. Suppl.), 1-192.

2234 Group for the Advancement of Psychiatry. Committee on Mental Retardation. *Mild mental retardation: A growing challenge to the physician.* GAP report, no. 66. New York: Group for the Advancement of Psychiatry, 1967.

2235 Haywood, H. C. (Ed.) *Social-cultural aspects of mental retardation.* New York: Appleton-Century-Crofts, 1970.

2236 Hunt, J. McV. *Intelligence and experience.* New York: Roland Press, 1961.

2237 Hurley, R. L. *Poverty and mental retardation.* New York: Random House, 1969.

2238 Masland, R. L., Sarason, S. B. & Gladwin, T. *Mental subnormality.* New York: Basic Books, 1958.

2239 Menolascino, F. J. (Ed.) *Psychiatric approaches to mental retardation.* New York: Basic Books, 1970.

2240 Penrose, L. S. *The biology of mental defect.* (3rd rev. and reset ed.) London: Sidgwick & Jackson, 1963.

2241 Philips, I. (Ed.) *Prevention and treatment of mental retardation.* New York: Basic Books, 1966.

2242 Robinson, H. B. & Robinson, N. M. *The mentally retarded child: A psychological approach.* New York: McGraw-Hill, 1965.

2243 Sarason, S. B. & Doris, J. L. *Psychological problems in mental deficiency.* (4th ed.) New York: Harper & Row, 1969.

2244 Stevens, H. A. & Heber, R. (Eds.) *Mental retardation: A review of research.* Chicago: University of Chicago Press, 1964.

2245 Tredgold, A. F. *Tredgold's mental retardation.* (11th ed.) London: Bailliere, Tindall and Cassell, 1970.

2246 Wortis, J. (Ed.) *Mental retardation and developmental disabilities.* New York: Brunner/Mazel, 1973.

2247 Zubin, J. & Jervis, G. A. (Eds.) *Psychopathology of mental development.* New York: Grune & Stratton, 1967.

2247.1 Clarke, A. D. B. & Clarke, A. M. *Mental retardation and behavioural research.* Edinburgh: Churchill Livingstone, 1973.

XV. SOCIO-CULTURAL ISSUES IN CHILD PSYCHIATRY

RESEARCH IN SOCIO-CULTURAL FACTORS IN HEALTH AND MENTAL HEALTH

2248 *Bertalanffy, L. Von. System, symbol and the image of man (Man's immediate socio-ecological world). In I. Galdston (Ed.), *The interface between psychiatry and anthropology.* New York: Brunner/Mazel, 1971. Pp. 88-119.

2249 *Schon, D. A. Technology and social change. In M.

Levitt & B. Rubenstein (Eds.), *The mental health field: A critical appraisal.* Detroit: Wayne State University Press, 1971. Pp. 353-375.

2250   *Leighton, A. H. & Murphy, J. M. Cross-cultural psychiatry. In J. M. Murphy & A. H. Leighton (Eds.), *Approaches to cross-cultural psychiatry.* Ithaca, N.Y.: Cornell University Press, 1965. Pp. 3-20.

2251   *Chance, N. A. Conceptual and methodological problems in cross-cultural health research. *American Journal of Public Health,* 1962, *52,* 410-417.

2252   Butts, R. F. & Cremin, L. A. *A history of education in American culture.* New York: Holt, Rinehart, and Winston, 1953.

2253   *Cassel, J. The use of medical records: Opportunity for epidemiological studies. *Journal of Occupational Medicine,* 1963, *5,* 185-190.

2254   Driver, E. D. *The sociology and anthropology of mental illness; a reference guide.* Amherst: University of Massachusetts Press, 1972.

2255   *Becker, E. *The revolution in psychiatry: The new understanding of man.* New York: Free Press of Glencoe, 1964.

2256   Hendin, H. M., Gaylin, W. & Carr, A. C. *Psychoanalysis and social research.* Garden City, N.Y.: Doubleday, 1965.

2257   *Reid, D. D. *Epidemiological methods in the study of mental disorders.* Geneva: World Health Organization, 1960. (Public health papers, no. 2)

2258   *Brown, A. C. & Fry, J. The Cornell Medical Index Health Questionnaire in the identification of neurotic patients in general practice. *Journal of Psychosomatic Research,* 1962, *6,* 185-190.

2259   *Langner, T. S. A twenty-two item screening score of psychiatric symptoms indicating impairment. *Journal of Health and Human Behavior,* 1962, *3,* 269-276.

2259.1   Hong, K-E. M. & Holmes, T. H. Transient diabetes mellitus associated with culture change. *Archives of General Psychiatry,* 1973, *29,* 683-687.

2259.2   Ward, S. H. & Braun, J. Self-esteem and racial preference in black children. In S. Chess & A. Thomas (Eds.), *Annual progress in child psychiatry and child development: 1973.* New York: Brunner/Mazel, 1974. Pp. 358-362.

2259.3   Johnson, L. B. & Proskauer, S. Hysterical psychosis in a prepubescent Navajo girl. *Journal of the American Academy of Child Psychiatry,* 1974, *13,* 17-19.

2259.4   Joint Commission on Mental Health of Children. *Social change and the mental health of children; report of Task Force VI and excerpts from the report of the Committee on Children of Minority Groups.* New York: Harper & Row, 1973.

SOCIO-CULTURAL INFLUENCES ON THE FAMILY AND CHILD'S DEVELOPMENT

2261   Whiting, B. B. (Ed.) *Six cultures: Studies of child rearing.* New York: Wiley, 1963.

2262   Brazelton, T. B. Sucking in infancy. *Pediatrics,* 1956, *17,* 400-404.

2263   Kluckhohn, F. R. Variations in the basic values of family systems. In N. W. Bell & E. F. Vogel (Eds.), *A modern introduction to the family.* New York: Free Press, 1968. Pp. 319-330.

2264   Bronfenbrenner, U. Socialization and social class through time and space. In Society for the Psychological Study of Social Issues, *Readings in social psychology.* (3rd ed.) New York: Holt, Rinehart & Winston, 1958. Pp. 400-425.

2265   *Chen, E. & Cobb, S. Family structure in relation to health and disease: A review of the literature. *Journal of Chronic Diseases,* 1960, *12,* 544-567.

2266   Bronfenbrenner, U. Toward a theoretical model for the analysis of parent-child relationships in a social context. In J. C. Glidewell (Ed.), *Parental attitudes and child behavior.* Springfield, Ill.: Thomas, 1961. Pp. 90-109.

2267   Hoffman, L. W. & Lippitt, R. The measurement of family life variables. In P. H. Mussen (Ed.), *Handbook of research methods in child development.* New York: Wiley, 1960. Pp. 945-1013.

2268   *Rosen, B. C. Family structure and value transmission. *Merrill-Palmer Quarterly,* 1964, *10,* 59-76.

2269   Yarrow, M. R., Scott, P., DeLeeuw, L. & Heinig, C. Child-rearing in families of working and nonworking mothers. *Sociometry,* 1962, *25,* 122-140.

2270   *Harris, D. B., Gough, H. G. & Martin, W. E. Children's ethnic attitudes: II. Relationship to parental beliefs concerning child training. *Child Development,* 1950, *21,* 169-181.

2271   *Hoffman, M. L. Personality, family structure, and social class as antecedents of parental power assertion. *Child Development,* 1963, *34,* 869-884.

2272   Littman, R. A., Moore, R. C. A. & Pierce-Jones, J. Social class differences in child rearing: A third community for comparison with Chicago and Newton. *American Sociological Review,* 1957, *22,* 694-704.

2273   *Hess, R. D. & Shipman, V. C. Early experience and the socialization of cognitive modes in children. *Child Development,* 1965, *36,* 869-886.

2273.1 Goldstein, H. S. & Peck, R. Maternal differentiation, father absence and cognitive differentiation in children. *Archives of General Psychiatry,* 1973, *29,* 370-373.

2274   Price-Williams, D., Gordon, W. & Ramirez, M. Skill and conservation: A study of pottery-making children.

Developmental Psychology, 1969, *1*, 769.

2275 Riesman, D. *The oral tradition, the written word, and the screen image.* Yellow Springs, Ohio: Antioch Press, 1956.

2276 *Cazden, C. B. Subcultural differences in child language: An interdisciplinary review. *Merrill-Palmer Quarterly*, 1966, *12*, 185-219.

2277 Koch, H. L. The relation of "primary mental abilities" in five- and six-year-olds to sex of child and characteristics of his sibling. *Child Development*, 1954, *25*, 209-223.

2278 *John, V. P. & Goldstein, L. S. The social context of language acquisition. *Merrill-Palmer Quarterly*, 1964, *10*, 265-275.

2279 *McCandless, B. R. & Hoyt, J. M. Sex, ethnicity, and play preferences of preschool children. *Journal of Abnormal and Social Psychology*, 1961, *62*, 683-685.

2280 Sears, P. S. Doll play aggression in normal young children: Influence of sex, age, sibling status, father's absence. *Psychological Monographs*, 1951, *65*(6, Whole No. 323).

2281 *Stotland, E. & Dunn, R. E. Identification, "opposite-ness," authoritarianism, self-esteem and birth order. *Psychological Monographs*, 1962, *76*(9, Whole No. 528), 1-21.

2282 *Stevenson, H. W. & Stewart, E. C. A developmental study of racial awareness in young children. *Child Development*, 1958, *29*, 399-409.

2283 Koch, H. L. The relation of certain formal attributes of siblings to attitudes held toward each other and toward their parents. *Monographs of the Society for Research in Child Development*, 1960, *25*(4, Serial No. 78).

2284 *Stone, C. L. Three-generation influences on teen-agers' conceptions of family culture patterns and parent-child relationships. *Marriage and Family Living*, 1962, *24*, 287-288.

2285 *Hoffman, L. W. Effects of maternal employment on the child. *Child Development*, 1961, *32*, 187-197.

2286 *Nash, J. The father in contemporary culture and current psychological literature. *Child Development*, 1965, *36*, 261-297.

2287 Hoffman, L. W. The father's role in the family and the child's peergroup adjustment. *Merrill-Palmer Quarterly*, 1961, *7*, 97-105.

2288 *LaBarre, M. B., Jessner, L. & Ussery, L. The significance of grandmothers in the psychopathology of children. *American Journal of Orthopsychiatry*, 1960, *30*, 175-185.

2289 Barron, F. What is psychological health? *California Monthly*, 1957, *68*, 22-25.

2289.1 Pinderhughes, C. A. Ego development and cultural

differences. *American Journal of Psychiatry,* 1974,
131, 171-176.
2289.2   Golden, M., Bridger, W. H. & Montare, A.   Social class
differences in the ability of young children to use
verbal information to facilitate learning. *American
Journal of Orthopsychiatry,* 1974, *44,* 86-91.
2289.3   Scheflen, A. E. & Scheflen, A.   *Body language and social
order.*   Englewood Cliffs, N.J.:   Prentice-Hall, 1972.
2289.4   Hertzig, M. E., Birch, H. G., Richardson, S. A. & Tizard,
J.   Intellectual levels of school children severely
malnourished during the first two years of life.   In S.
Chess & A. Thomas (Eds.), *Annual progress in child psychiatry and child development: 1973.*   New York:
Brunner/Mazel, 1974.   Pp. 156-171.

THE BLACK, SPANISH-SPEAKING AMERICAN, AND AMERICAN INDIAN
EXPERIENCE IN THE UNITED STATES

2290   U.S. President's Commission on Law Enforcement and Administration of Justice. *The challenge of crime in
a free society.*   Washington: U.S. Govt. Print. Off.,
1967.
2291   *U.S. President's National Advisory Commission on Civil
Disorders. *Report.*   New York: Bantam Books, 1968.
2292   *U.S. National Commission on the Causes and Prevention of
Violence.   *To establish justice, to insure domestic
tranquility.*   New York: Bantam Books, 1970.
2293   *Berreman, G. D.   Caste in India and the United States.
American Journal of Sociology, 1960, *66,* 120-127.
2294   *Frazier, E. F.   *The Negro family in the United States.*
Chicago: University of Chicago Press, 1939.
2296   *Brink, W. & Harris, L.   *The Negro revolution in America.*
New York: Simon & Schuster, 1964.
2297   *Baldwin, J.   *Nobody knows my name.*   New York: Dial,
1961.
2298   *Bruce, L. (J. Cohen, Ed.)   *The essential Lenny Bruce.*
New York: Ballantine, 1968.
2299   *Grier, W. H. & Cobbs, P. M.   *Black rage.*   New York:
Basic Books, 1968.
2300   *Hanke, L.   *The Spanish struggle for justice in the conquest of America.*   Philadelphia: University of Pennsylvania Press, 1949.
2300.1   Serrano, A. C. & Gibson, G.   Mental health services to
the Mexican-American community in San Antonio, Texas.
American Journal of Public Health, 1973, *63,* 1055-
1057.
2301   *Lewis, O.   *Five families.*   New York: Basic Books, 1959.
2302   *Sexton, P.   *Spanish Harlem: An anatomy of poverty.*
New York: Harper & Row, 1965.
2303   *McNickle, D.   The sociocultural setting of Indian life.
American Journal of Psychiatry, 1968, *125,* 219-223.

2304   *Washburn, W. E. (Ed.) *The Indian and the white man.*
        New York: New York University Press, 1964.
2305   *Havighurst, R. J. & Neugarten, B. L. *American Indian
        and white children.* Chicago: University of Chicago
        Press, 1955.
2306   *Deloria, V. *Custer died for your sins.* New York:
        Macmillan, 1969.
2307   *Deloria, V. *We talk, you listen; New tribes, new turf.*
        New York: Macmillan, 1970.
2308   *Farb, P. The American Indian: A portrait in limbo.
        Saturday Review, 1968, *51*(41), 26-29.
2309   Kluckhohn, C. *Navaho witchcraft.* Boston: Beacon
        Press, 1944.
2310   Sturtevant, W. C. *Bibliography on American Indian med-
        icine and health.* Washington: U.S. Bureau of Ameri-
        can Ethnology, 1962.
2310.1 Allen, J. R. The Indian adolescent: Psychosocial tasks
        of the Plains Indian of western Oklahoma. *American
        Journal of Orthopsychiatry,* 1973, *43*, 368-375.
2310.2 Hammerschlag, C. A., Alderfer, C. P. & Berg, D. Indian
        education: A human systems analysis. *American Jour-
        nal of Psychiatry,* 1973, *130*, 1098-1102.
2310.3 Shore, J. H. & Von Fumetti, B. Three alcohol programs
        for American Indians. *American Journal of Psychiatry,*
        1972, *128*, 1450-1454.

POVERTY IN THE UNITED STATES

2311   *Harrington, M. *The other America: Poverty in the
        United States.* Harmondsworth, Middlesex, Eng.:
        Penguin, 1963.
2312   Myrdal, G. *Challenge to affluence.* New York: Pan-
        theon Books, 1963.
2313   Conference on Economic Progress. *Poverty and depriva-
        tion in the United States--The plight of two-fifths
        of a nation.* Washington, D.C.: The Conference on
        Economic Progress, 1962.
2314   *Cohen, W. J. & Sullivan, E. Poverty in the United
        States. *Health, Education, and Welfare Indicators,*
        February. 1964, vi-xxii.
2315   *U.S. President's Task Force on Manpower Conservation.
        *One-third of a nation, report on young men found un-
        qualified for military service.* Washington, D.C.:
        U.S. Govt. Print. Off., 1964.
2316   *Rainwater, L. & Weinstein, K. K. *And the poor get
        children.* Chicago: Quadrangle Books, 1960.
2317   Bendiner, R. Poverty is a tougher problem than ever.
        New York Times Magazine, February 4, 1968, 22-23;
        59-62;69-72.
2318   *Alinsky, S. D. The poor and the powerful. *Psychiatric
        Research Reports of the American Psychiatric Associa-
        tion,* 1967, *21*, 22-28.

2319   Klein, P. *From philanthropy to social welfare.* San
          Francisco: Jossey-Bass, 1968.
2319.1   Ohlin, L. E., Coates, R. B. & Miller, A. D.   Radical
          correctional reform: A case study of the Massachu-
          setts youth correctional system. *Harvard Educational
          Review,* 1974, *44,* 74-111.

SOCIAL CLASS, POVERTY, AND MENTAL HEALTH

2320   *Hollingshead, A. B. & Redlich, F. C. *Social class and
          mental illness.* New York: Wiley, 1958.
2321   *Hunt, R. Social class and mental illness: Some impli-
          cations for clinical theory and practice. *American
          Journal of Psychiatry,* 1960, *116,* 1065-1069.
2322   Srole, L., Langner, T. S., Michael, S. T., Opler, M. K.
          & Rennie, T. A. C. *The Midtown Manhattan Study.*
          Vol. 1. *Mental health in the metropolis.* New York:
          McGraw-Hill, 1962.
2323   *Leighton, A. H. *My name is legion: Foundations for a
          theory of man in relation to culture.* New York:
          Basic Books, 1959. (Stirling County study of psychi-
          atric disorder and sociocultural environment, vol. 1)
2324   Leighton, D. C., Harding, J. S., Macklin, D. B., Mac-
          millan, A. M. & Leighton, A. H. *The character of dan-
          ger.* New York: Basic Books, 1963. (Stirling County
          study of psychiatric disorder and sociocultural en-
          vironment, vol. 3)
2325   *Linton, R. *Culture and mental disorders.* Springfield,
          Ill.: Thomas, 1956.
2326   *Levitt, M. & Rubenstein, B. Some observations on the
          relationship between cultural variants and emotional
          disorders. *American Journal of Orthopsychiatry,* 1964,
          34, 423-435.
2327   Parker, S. & Kleiner, R. J. Social status and mental
          disorder. In *Mental illness in the urban Negro com-
          munity.* New York: Free Press, 1966. Pp. 237-266.
2328   *Pasamanick, B., Knobloch, H. & Lilienfeld, A. M. Socio-
          economic status and some precursors of neuropsychiat-
          ric disorder. *American Journal of Orthopsychiatry,*
          1956, *26,* 594-601.
2329   Scheff, T. J. (Ed.) *Mental illness and social processes.*
          New York: Harper & Row, 1967.
2330   Srole, L. & Langner, T. Socioeconomic status groups:
          Their mental health composition. In S. K. Weinberg
          (Ed.), *The sociology of mental disorders.* Chicago:
          Aldine, 1967. Pp. 33-47.
2331   Opler, M. K. *Culture & social psychiatry.* New York:
          Atherton Press, 1967.
2332   *Robins, L. N. Social correlates of psychiatric dis-
          orders: Can we tell causes from consequences? *Jour-
          nal of Health and Social Behavior,* 1969, *10,* 95-104.

2333   Freeman, H. E. & Giovannoni, J. M. Social psychology of
         mental health. In G. Lindzey & E. Aronson (Eds.),
         Handbook of social psychology. (2nd ed.) Vol. 5.
         Reading, Mass.: Addison-Wesley, 1969. Pp. 660-719.
2334   Kleiner, R. J. & Parker, S. Goal-striving, social sta-
         tus, and mental disorder: A research review. In S.
         K. Weinberg (Ed.), *The sociology of mental disorders.*
         Chicago: Aldine, 1967. Pp. 55-66.
2335   *Murphy, H. B. M. Migration and the major mental dis-
         orders: A reappraisal. In M. B. Kantor (Ed.), *Mobil-
         ity and mental health.* Springfield, Ill.: Thomas,
         1965. Pp. 5-29.
2336   Malzberg, B. & Lee, E. S. *Migration and mental disease:
         A study of first admissions to hospitals for mental
         disease, New York, 1939-1941.* New York: Social
         Science Research Council, 1956.
2337   *Goffman, E. *Asylums: Essays on the social situation of
         mental patients and other inmates.* Garden City, N.Y.:
         Anchor Books, 1961.
2338   *Roman, P. M. & Trice, H. M. *Schizophrenia and the poor.*
         Ithaca, N.Y.: New York State School of Industrial
         and Labor Relations, Cornell University, 1967.
2339   *Scott, R. D. & Ashworth, P. L. 'Closure' at the first
         schizophrenic break-down: A family study. *British
         Journal of Medical Psychology,* 1967, *40,* 109-145.
2340   *Freeman, H. E. & Simmons, O. G. *The mental patient
         comes home.* New York: Wiley, 1963.
2341   *Ohlin, L. E. Conflicting interests in correctional
         objectives. In R. A. Cloward et al. (Eds.), *Theoret-
         ical studies in social organization of the prison.*
         New York: Social Science Research Council, 1960.
         Pp. 111-129.
2343   Kogelschatz, J. L., Adams, P. L. & Tucker, D. McK.
         Family styles of fatherless households. *Journal of
         the American Academy of Child Psychiatry,* 1972, *11,*
         365-383.

EFFECT OF POVERTY ON CHILDREN AND FAMILIES

2344   *Clarke, A. D. B. & Clarke, A. M. Some recent advances
         in the study of early deprivation. *Journal of Child
         Psychology and Psychiatry and Allied Disciplines,*
         1960, *1,* 26-36.
2345   *Pavenstedt, E. A comparison of the child-rearing en-
         vironment of upper-lower and very low-lower class
         families. *American Journal of Orthopsychiatry,* 1965,
         35, 89-98.
2346   Pavenstedt, E. (Ed.) *The drifters: Children of dis-
         organized lower-class families.* Boston: Little,
         Brown, 1967.
2347   Looff, D. H. *Appalachia's children.* Lexington: Uni-
         versity Press of Kentucky, 1971.

2348   *Deutsch, M. P. The disadvantaged child and the learn-
        ing process. In F. Riessman, J. Cohen & A. Pearl
        (Eds.), *Mental health of the poor*. New York: Free
        Press, 1964. Pp. 172-187.
2349   Kohn, M. L. Social class and parent-child relation-
        ships: An interpretation. *American Journal of So-
        ciology*, 1963, *68*, 471-480. (Also in F. Riessman,
        J. Cohen & A. Pearl (Eds.), *Mental health of the
        poor*. New York: Free Press, 1964. Pp. 159-171.)
2350   *Duvall, E. M. Conceptions of parenthood. *American
        Journal of Sociology*, 1946, *52*, 193-203.
2351   Deutsch, M. *Minority group and class status as related
        to social and personality factors in scholastic a-
        chievement*. Ithaca, N.Y.: Society for Applied An-
        thropology, 1960. (Society for Applied Anthropology.
        Monograph no. 2)
2352   Sears, R. R., Maccoby, E. E. & Levin, H. *Patterns of
        child rearing*. Evanston, Ill.: Row, Peterson, 1957.
2353   *Burchinal, L. G., Gardner, B. & Hawkes, G. R. Child-
        ren's personality adjustment and the socio-economic
        status of their families. *Journal of Genetic Psy-
        chology*, 1958, *92*, 149-159.
2354   *Middleton, R. Alienation, race, and education. *Ameri-
        can Sociological Review*, 1963, *28*, 973-977.
2355   Riessman, F. *The culturally deprived child*. New York:
        Harper, 1962.
2356   *Toby, J. Orientation to education as a factor in the
        school maladjustment of lower-class children. *Social
        Forces*, 1957, *35*, 259-266.
2357   *Meier, D. L. & Bell, W. Anomia and differential access
        to the achievement of life goals. *American Socio-
        logical Review*, 1959, *24*, 189-202.
2358   *Malone, C. A. Safety first: Comments on the influence
        of external danger in the lives of children of dis-
        organized families. *American Journal of Orthopsychi-
        atry*, 1966, *36*, 3-12.
2359   Conant, J. B. *Slums and suburbs; A commentary on
        schools in metropolitan areas*. New York: McGraw-
        Hill, 1961.
2360   Clark, J. P. Measuring alienation within a social
        system. *American Sociological Review*, 1959, *24*,
        849-852.
2361   *Minuchin, S., et al. *Families of the slums: An ex-
        ploration of their structure and treatment*. New York:
        Basic Books, 1967.
2362   Bowlby, J. *Forty-four juvenile thieves: Their charac-
        ters and home life*. London: Bailliere, Tindall &
        Cox, 1946. (Also in *International Journal of Psycho-
        analysis*, 1944, *25*, 19-53;107-128.)
2363   *Waring, M. & Ricks, D. Family patterns of children who
        became adult schizophrenics. *Journal of Nervous and
        Mental Disease*, 1965, *140*, 351-364.

2363.1 Polier, J. W. Myths and realities in the search for juvenile justice. *Harvard Educational Review,* 1974, *44,* 112-124.

POVERTY AND PSYCHIATRIC TREATMENT OF CHILDREN

2364 Baratz, S. S. & Baratz, J. C. Early childhood intervention: The social science base of institutional racism. *Harvard Educational Review,* 1970, *40,* 29-50.

2365 *Pasamanick, B. & Knobloch, H. Epidemiologic studies on the complications of pregnancy and the birth process. In G. Caplan (Ed.), *Prevention of mental disorders in children.* New York: Basic Books, 1961. Pp. 74-94.

2366 *Harrison, S. I., McDermott, J. F., Schrager, J. & Showerman, E. R. Social status and child psychiatric practice: The influence of the clinician's socioeconomic origin. *American Journal of Psychiatry,* 1970, *127,* 652-658.

2367 *Cole, N., Branch, C. H. H. & Allison, R. Some relationships between social class and the practice of dynamic psychotherapy. *American Journal of Psychiatry,* 1962, *118,* 1004-1012.

2368 *McDermott, J. F., Harrison, S. I., Schrager, J., Wilson, P., Killins, E., Lindy, J. & Waggoner, R. W. Social class and mental illness in children: The diagnosis of organicity and mental retardation. *Journal of the American Academy of Child Psychiatry,* 1967, *6,* 309-320. (Also in S. Chess & A. Thomas (Eds.), *Annual progress in child psychiatry and child development.* New York: Brunner/Mazel, 1968. Pp. 300-310.)

2369 Kahn, R. L., Pink, M. & Siegel, N. Sociopsychological aspects of psychiatric treatment: A report of treatment in three voluntary hospitals. *Archives of General Psychiatry,* 1966, *14,* 20-25.

2370 *McDermott, J. F., Harrison, S. I., Schrager, J. & Wilson, P. Social class and mental illness in children: Observations on the children of blue-collar families. *American Journal of Orthopsychiatry,* 1965, *35,* 500-508. (Also in E. Thomas (Ed.), *Behavioral science for social workers.* New York: Free Press, 1967. Pp. 332-340.)

2371 *Maas, H. Socio-cultural factors in psychiatric clinic services for children. *Smith College Studies in Social Work,* 1955, *25,* 1-90.

2372 *Malmquist, C. P. Psychiatric perspectives on the socially-disadvantaged child. *Comprehensive Psychiatry,* 1965, *6,* 176-183.

2373 *Heine, R. W. & Trosman, H. Initial expectations of the doctor-patient interaction as a factor in continuance in psychotherapy. *Psychiatry,* 1960, *23,* 275-278.

2374   *Rosengren, W. R. The hospital careers of lower- and
        middle-class child psychiatric patients. *Psychiatry*,
        1962, *25*, 16-22.
2375   Myers, J. K. & Auld, F. Some variables related to out-
        come of psychotherapy. *Journal of Clinical Psychology*,
        1955, *11*, 51-54.
2376   Wood, A. C., Jr., Friedman, C. J. & Steisel, I. M. Psy-
        chosocial factors in phenylketonuria. *American Jour-
        nal of Orthopsychiatry*, 1967, *37*, 671-679.
2377   Hetznecker, W. & Forman, M. A. Community child psychia-
        try: Evolution and direction. *American Journal of
        Orthopsychiatry*, 1971, *41*, 350-370.
2377.1 Garber, N. Pediatric-child psychiatry collaboration in
        a health maintenance organization. *American Journal
        of Psychiatry*, 1973, *130*, 1227-1231.
2377.2 Jackson, A. M., Berkowitz, H. & Farley, G. K. Race as a
        variable affecting the treatment involvement of chil-
        dren. *Journal of the American Academy of Child Psychi-
        atry*, 1974, *13*, 20-31.
2377.3 Capron, A. M. Legal considerations affecting clinical
        pharmacological studies in children. *Clinical Re-
        search*, 1973, *21*, 141-150.
2377.4 Leonard, C. O., Chase, G. A. & Childs, B. Genetic coun-
        seling: A consumer's view. *New England Journal of
        Medicine*, 1972, *287*, 433-439.

DIVORCE AND CUSTODY: EFFECT ON CHILDREN

2377.5 *Westman, J. C. & Cline, D. W. Divorce is a family
        affair. *Family Law Quarterly*, 1971, *5*, 1-10.
2377.6 *Goldstein, J., Freud, A. & Solnit, A. J. *Beyond the
        best interests of the child*. New York: Free Press,
        1970.
2377.7 *Westman, J. C., Cline, D. W., Swift, W. J. & Kramer, D.
        A. Role of child psychiatry in divorce. *Archives of
        General Psychiatry*, 1970, *23*, 416-420.
2377.8 *Benedek, E. P. & Benedek, R. S. New child custody laws:
        Making them do what they say. *American Journal of
        Orthopsychiatry*, 1972, *42*, 825-834.
2377.9 *Comment: Psychological parenthood as the controlling
        factor in determining the best interests of the child.
        Rutgers Law Review, 1973, *26*, 693-713.
2377.11 Hansen, R. W. The role and rights of children in di-
        vorce actions. *Journal of Family Law*, 1966, *6*, 1-14.
2377.12 *Bradbrook, A. The relevance of psychological and psy-
        chiatric studies to the future development of the
        laws governing the settlement of inter-parental child
        custody disputes. *Journal of Family Law*, 1971, *11*,
        557-587.
2377.13 Shepherd, R. E., Jr. Solomon's sword: Adjudication of
        child custody questions. *University of Richmond Law
        Review*, 1974, *8*, 151-200.

2377.14   Clark, H. H., Jr.   The law of domestic relations in the
          United States.   In *Custody of children*.   St. Paul,
          Minn.:   West, 1968.   Pp. 572-601.
2377.15 *Kren, G. M. & Rappoport, L.   Clio and psyche.   *History
          of Childhood Quarterly*, 1973, *1*, 151-163.
2377.16   Zuckman, H. L. & Fox, W. F.   The ferment in divorce
          legislation.   *Journal of Family Law*, 1973, *12*, 515-605.
2377.17 *Kleinfield, A. J.   The balance of power among infants,
          their parents and the State.   *Family Law Quarterly*,
          1971, *5*, 63-107.
2377.18 *Proposed Revised Uniform Marriage and Divorce Act.
          Family Law Quarterly, 1973, *7*, 135-167.
2377.19   Foster, H. H.   Adoption and child custody: Best in-
          terests of the child?   *Buffalo Law Review*, 1973, *22*,
          1-16.

PART III

THERAPEUTICS

XVI. PSYCHOTHERAPY OF CHILDREN AND ADOLESCENTS

PLAY THERAPY/General Theory

2378   *Murphy, L. B. Infant's play and cognitive development.
        In M. W. Piers (Ed.), *Play and development*. New York:
        Norton, 1972. Pp. 119-126.
2379   Spitz, R. A. Fundamental education. In M. W. Piers
        (Ed.), *Play and development*. New York: Norton, 1972.
        Pp. 43-63.
2380   Brody, S. & Axelrad, S. Anxiety, socialization, and ego
        formation in infancy. *International Journal of Psycho-
        analysis*, 1966, *47*, 218-229.
2381   *Emmerich, W. Continuity and stability in early social
        development: II. Teacher ratings. *Child Development*,
        1966, *37*, 17-27.
2382   Escalona, S. K. Patterns of infantile experience and
        the developmental process. *Psychoanalytic Study of the
        Child*, 1963, *18*, 197-244.
2383   Freud, A. The role of regression in mental development.
        In A. J. Solnit & S. A. Provence (Eds.), *Modern per-
        spectives in child development*. New York: Interna-
        tional Universities Press, 1963. Pp. 97-106.
        (*Writings*, vol. 5. Pp. 407-418)
2384   *Loewenstein, R. M. On the theory of superego: A dis-
        cussion. In R. M. Loewenstein, et al. (Eds.), *Psycho-
        analysis: A general psychology*. New York: Interna-
        tional Universities Press, 1966. Pp. 298-314.
2385   *Khan, M. M. R. The concept of cumulative trauma. *Psycho-
        analytic Study of the Child*, 1963, *18*, 286-306.
2386   *Lustman, S. L. Impulse control, structure, and the syn-
        thetic function. In R. M. Loewenstein, et al. (Eds.),
        Psychoanalysis: A general psychology. New York: In-
        ternational Universities Press, 1966. Pp. 190-221.
2387   Ostfeld, B. & Katz, P. A. The effect of threat severity
        in children of varying socioeconomic levels. *Develop-
        mental Psychology*, 1969, *1*, 205-210.
2388   *Spock, B. Innate inhibition of aggressiveness in in-
        fancy. *Psychoanalytic Study of the Child*, 1965, *20*,
        340-343.
2389   *Sandler, J. & Hagera, H. Aspects of the metapsychology
        of fantasy. *Psychoanalytic Study of the Child*, 1963,
        18, 159-194.

2390   *Wolff, P. H. Operational thought and social adaptation.
        In M. W. Piers (Ed.), *Play and development*. New York:
        Norton, 1972. Pp. 28-42.
2391   *Piaget, J. Some aspects of operations. In M. W. Piers
        (Ed.), *Play and development*. New York: Norton, 1972.
        Pp. 15-27.
2392   *Kardos, E. & Peto, A. Contributions to the theory of
        play. *British Journal of Medical Psychology*, 1956, *29*,
        100-112.
2393   *Erikson, E. H. Play and actuality. In M. W. Piers (Ed.),
        Play and development. New York: Norton, 1972.
        Pp. 127-167.
2394   *Woltmann, A. G. Concepts of play therapy techniques. In
        M. R. Haworth, *Child psychotherapy*. New York: Basic
        Books, 1964. Pp. 20-32.
2395   Dorfman, E. Play therapy. In C. R. Rogers, *Client-
        centered therapy*. Boston: Houghton Mifflin, 1951.
        Pp. 235-277.
2395.1 Klein, M. The psychoanalytic play technique. *American
        Journal of Orthopsychiatry*, 1955, *25*, 223-237.
2396   *Erikson, E. H. Toys and reasons. In M. R. Haworth,
        Child psychotherapy. New York: Basic Books, 1964,
        Pp. 3-11.
2397   *Amster, F. Differential uses of play in treatment of
        young children. In M. R. Haworth, *Child psychotherapy*.
        New York: Basic Books, 1964. Pp. 11-19.
2397.1 Haworth, M. R. & Keller, M. J. The use of food in the
        diagnosis and therapy of emotionally disturbed children.
        Journal of the American Academy of Child Psychiatry,
        1962, *1*, 548-563.
2397.2 Levin, S. & Wermer, H. The significance of giving gifts
        to children in therapy. *Journal of the American Acad-
        emy of Child Psychiatry*, 1966, *5*, 630-652.
2397.3 Kay, P. A boy's wish to give his analyst a gift. *Jour-
        nal of the American Academy of Child Psychiatry*, 1967,
        6, 38-50.
2397.4 Moustakas, C. E. *Children in play therapy*. New York:
        J. Aronson, 1973.
2398   Lovell, K., Hoyle, H. W. & Siddall, M. Q. A study of
        some aspects of the play and language of young children
        with delayed speech. *Journal of Child Psychology and
        Psychiatry and Allied Disciplines*, 1968, *9*, 41-50.
2399   *Beiser, H. R. Therapeutic play techniques. Symposium,
        1954. 8. Play equipment for diagnosis and therapy.
        American Journal of Orthopsychiatry, 1955, *25*, 761-770.
2400   Moore, T. & Ucko, L. E. Four to six: Constructiveness
        and conflict in meeting doll play problems. *Journal of
        Child Psychology and Psychiatry and Allied Disciplines*,
        1961, *2*, 21-47.
2400.1 Meeks, J. E. Children who cheat at games. *Journal of
        the American Academy of Child Psychiatry*, 1970, *9*,
        157-170.

Psychotherapy of Children and Adolescents   207

2401   *Moore, T.   Realism and fantasy in children's play. *Journal of Child Psychology and Psychiatry and Allied Disciplines*, 1964, *5*, 15-36.
2402   Singer, J. L. *Daydreaming*. New York: Random House, 1966.
2403   Lebo, D. The expressive value of toys recommended for nondirective play therapy. *Journal of Clinical Psychology*, 1955, *11*, 144-148.
2404   Scott, W. C. M. Differences between the playroom used in child psychiatric treatment and in child analysis. *Canadian Psychiatric Association Journal*, 1961, *6*, 281-285.
2405   *Lebo, D. A theoretical framework for nondirective play therapy: Concepts from psychoanalysis and learning theory. *Journal of Consulting Psychology*, 1958, *22*, 275-279.
2406   Witmer, H. L. (Ed.), *Psychiatric interviews with children*. Cambridge, Mass.: Harvard University Press, 1946.
2406.1 Group for the Advancement of Psychiatry. Committee on Child Psychiatry. *From diagnosis to treatment: an approach to treatment planning for the emotionally disturbed child*. GAP report, no. 87. New York: Group for the Advancement of Psychiatry, 1973.
2407   Herron, W. G. The child therapy scene. *Psychology in the Schools*, 1968, *5*, 351-355.
2408   *Taft, J. J. *The dynamics of therapy in a controlled relationship*. New York: Dover, 1962.
2408.1 Haley, J. Strategic therapy when a child is presented as the problem. *Journal of the American Academy of Child Psychiatry*, 1973, *12*, 641-659.
2409   Axline, V. M. The eight basic principles. In M. R. Haworth, *Child psychotherapy*. New York: Basic Books, 1964. Pp. 93-94.
2410   Lederer, W. *Dragons, delinquents, and destiny: An essay on positive superego functions*. New York: International Universities Press, 1964. (*Psychological Issues*, 1964, *4*(3, mono. no. 15)
2411   Piers, M. W. (Ed.) *Play and development*. New York: Norton, 1972.
2411.1 Gardner, R. A. *Understanding children*. New York: J. Aronson, 1973.
2412   Axline, V. M. *Dibs*. New York: Ballantine Books, 1964.
2412.1 Geleerd, E. R. *The child analyst at work*. New York: International Universities Press, 1967.
2412.2 Freud, A. *The psycho-analytical treatment of children*. London: Imago, 1946.
2412.3 Anthony, E. J. Communicating therapeutically with the child. *Journal of the American Academy of Child Psychiatry*, 1964, *3*, 106-125.
2412.4 Korner, A. F. & Opsvig, P. Developmental considerations in diagnosis and treatment: A case illustration. *Journal of the American Academy of Child Psychiatry*, 1966, *5*, 594-616.

2412.5 Kramer, S. & Settlage, C. F. On the concepts and technique of child analysis. *Journal of the American Academy of Child Psychiatry*, 1962, *1*, 509-535.
2412.6 Frankl, L. & Hellman, I. Symposium on child analysis. II. The ego's participation in the therapeutic alliance. *International Journal of Psychoanalysis*, 1962, *43*, 333-337.
2412.7 Hamm, M. Some aspects of a difficult therapeutic (working) alliance. In E. R. Geleerd, *The child analyst at work*. New York: International Universities Press, 1967. Pp. 185-205.
2412.8 Fraiberg, S. Clinical notes on the nature of transference in child analysis. *Psychoanalytic Study of the Child*, 1951, *6*, 286-306.

PLAY THERAPY/Early Sessions

2413 Swanson, F. L. The initial therapy interview. In *Psychotherapists and children*. New York: Pitman, 1970. Pp. 43-55.
2414 *Axline, V. M. Establishing rapport. In M. R. Haworth, *Child psychotherapy*. New York: Basic Books, 1964. Pp. 95-101.
2415 *Allen, F. H. The beginning phase of therapy. In M. R. Haworth, *Child psychotherapy*. New York: Basic Books, 1964. Pp. 101-105.
2416 *Erikson, E. H. Play and cure. In *Childhood and society*. New York: Norton, 1963. Pp. 222-234.
2417 Lorenz, K. The enmity between generations and its probable ethological causes. In M. W. Piers (Ed.), *Play and development*. New York: Norton, 1972. Pp. 64-118.
2417.1 Loomis, E. A. The use of checkers in handling certain resistances in child therapy and child analysis. *Journal of the American Psychoanalytic Association*, 1957, *5*, 130-135.

PLAY THERAPY/Limits and Structure

2418 *Ross, A. O. Techniques of therapy. In M. R. Haworth, *Child psychotherapy*. New York: Basic Books, 1964. Pp. 121-125.
2419 *Ginott, H. G. Problems in the playroom. In M. R. Haworth, *Child psychotherapy*. New York: Basic Books, 1964. Pp. 125-130.
2420 *Despert, J. L. Technical approaches used in the study and treatment of emotional problems in children. *Psychiatric Quarterly*, 1937, *11*, 677-693.
2420.1 Fraiberg, S. Technical aspects of the analysis of a child with a severe behavior disorder. *Journal of the American Psychoanalytic Association*, 1962, *10*, 338-367.

2421   Ginott, H. G. & Lebo, D. Play therapy limits and theoretical orientation. *Journal of Consulting Psychology*, 1961, *25*, 337-340.

2421.1 Wenar, C. The therapeutic value of setting limits with inhibited children. *Journal of Nervous and Mental Disease*, 1957, *125*, 390-395.

2422   *Bixler, R. H. Limits are therapy. In M. R. Haworth, *Child psychotherapy*. New York: Basic Books, 1964. Pp. 134-147.

2422.1 Finzer, W. F. & Waite, R. R. The relationship between accumulated knowledge and therapeutic techniques. *Journal of the American Academy of Child Psychiatry*, 1964, *3*, 709-720.

2422.2 Furman, R. A. A technical problem: The child who has difficulty in controlling his behavior in analytic sessions. In E. R. Geleerd, *The child analyst at work*. New York: International Universities Press, 1967. Pp. 59-84.

2423   *Ginott, H. G. The theory and practice of "therapeutic intervention" in child treatment. In M. R. Haworth, *Child psychotherapy*. New York: Basic Books, 1964. Pp. 148-158.

2423.1 Heinicke, C. M. Frequency of psychotherapeutic session as a factor affecting the child's developmental status. *Psychoanalytic Study of the Child*, 1965, *20*, 42-98.

PLAY THERAPY/Special Play Therapy Methods

2424   *Hambidge, G., Jr. Therapeutic play techniques. Symposium, 1954. 4. Structured play therapy. *American Journal of Orthopsychiatry*, 1955, *25*, 601-617.

2425   *Solomon, J. C. Active play therapy. *American Journal of Orthopsychiatry*, 1938, *8*, 479-498.

2426   *Axline, V. M. Nondirective therapy. In M. R. Haworth, *Child psychotherapy*. New York: Basic Books, 1964. Pp. 34-39.

2427   Goldings, C. R. & Goldings, H. J. Books in the playroom: A dimension of child psychiatric technique. *Journal of the American Academy of Child Psychiatry*, 1972, *11*, 52-65.

2427.1 Loomis, E. A. The use of checkers in handling certain resistances in child therapy and child analysis. *Journal of the American Psychoanalytic Association*, 1957, *5*, 130-135.

2427.2 Gardner, R. A. The mutual storytelling technique in the treatment of psychogenic problems secondary to minimal brain dysfunction. *Journal of Learning Disabilities*, 1974, *7*, 135-143.

PLAY THERAPY/Special Situations: Group Therapy

2428 *Ginott, H. G. Play group therapy: A theoretical frame-
       work. *International Journal of Group Psychotherapy*,
       1958, *8*, 410-418.
2429 *Schiffer, M. *The therapeutic play group*. New York:
       Grune & Stratton, 1969.

PLAY THERAPY/Research in Play Therapy

2430 *Lebo, D. Age and suitability for nondirective play
       therapy. *Journal of Genetic Psychology*, 1956, *89*,
       231-238.
2430.1 Freud, A. Indications for child analysis. *Psychoana-
       lytic Study of the Child*, 1945, *1*, 127-149. (*Writings*,
       vol. 4, Pp. 3-38)
2430.2 Korner, A. F. & Opsvig, P. Developmental considerations
       in diagnosis and treatment: A case illustration.
       Journal of the American Academy of Child Psychiatry,
       1966, *5*, 594-616.
2430.3 Bernstein, I. Indications and goals of child analysis as
       compared with child psychotherapy. *Journal of the Amer-
       ican Psychoanalytic Association*, 1957, *5*, 158-163.
2431 *Moustakas, C. E. Emotional adjustment and the play
       therapy process. *Journal of Genetic Psychology*, 1955,
       86, 79-99.
2432 *Lebo, D. The relationship of response categories in play
       therapy to chronological age. *Journal of Child Psy-
       chiatry*, 1952, *2*, 330-336.
2432.1 Erikson, E. H. Studies in the interpretation of play:
       I. Clinical observation of play disruption in young
       children. *Genetic Psychology Monographs*, 1940, *22*,
       557-671.
2433 *Pumfrey, P. D. & Elliott, C. D. Play therapy, social ad-
       justment and reading attainment. *Educational Research*,
       1970, *12*, 183-193.
2434 Moustakas, C. E. & Schalock, H. D. An analysis of thera-
       pist-child interaction in play therapy. *Child Develop-
       ment*, 1955, *26*, 143-157.
2435 *Lebo, D. & Lebo, E. Aggression and age in relation to
       verbal expression in nondirective play therapy. *Psy-
       chological Monographs*, 1957, *71*, (20, Whole No. 449).
2435.1 Furman, E. The latency child as an active participant
       in the analytic work. In E. R. Geleerd, *The child ana-
       lyst at work*. New York: International Universities
       Press, 1967. Pp. 142-184.
2435.2 Maenchen, A. On the technique of child analysis in rela-
       tion to stages of development. *Psychoanalytic Study of
       the Child*, 1970, *25*, 175-208.
2435.3 Ables, B. S. The loss of a therapist through suicide.
       Journal of the American Academy of Child Psychiatry,
       1974, *13*, 143-152.

VARIOUS MODALITIES OF THERAPEUTIC INTERVENTION/Evaluating the
Child for Therapy

2436   *Rabinovitch, R. D. An evaluation of present trends in
psychotherapy with children. In M. R. Haworth, *Child
psychotherapy*. New York: Basic Books, 1964.
Pp. 39-45.

2437   *Werkman, S. L. The psychiatric diagnostic interview with
children. *American Journal of Orthopsychiatry*, 1965,
35, 764-771.

2438   *McDonald, M. The psychiatric evaluation of children.
Journal of the American Academy of Child Psychiatry,
1965, *4*, 569-612.

2439   *Beiser, H. R. Psychiatric diagnostic interviews with
children. *Journal of the American Academy of Child
Psychiatry*, 1962, *1*, 656-670.

2440   *Koppitz, E. M. Psychotherapy and children's drawings.
In *Psychological evaluation of children's figure drawings*. New York: Grune & Stratton, 1968. Pp. 245-157.

2441   *Shearn, C. R. & Russell, K. R. Use of the family drawing
as a technique for studying parent-child interaction.
*Journal of Projective Techniques and Personality Assess-
ment*, 1969, *33*, 35-44.

2442   Bersoff, D. N. & Grieger, R. M. An interview model for
the psycho-situational assessment of children's behavior. *American Journal of Orthopsychiatry*, 1971, *41*,
483-493.

2443   Hundleby, J. D. The trait of anxiety, as defined by objective performance measures, and indices of emotional
disturbance in middle childhood. *Multivariate Behavioral Research*, 1968, *3*, 7-14.

2444   *Hafner, A. J., Quast, W., Speer, D. C. & Grams, A. Children's anxiety scales in relation to self, parental,
and psychiatric ratings of anxiety. *Journal of Consulting Psychology*, 1964 *28*, 555-558.

2445   *Goodman, J. D. & Sours, J. A. A mental status examination for children. In *The child mental status examination*. New York: Basic Books, 1967. Pp. 41-86.

2446   *Group for the Advancement of Psychiatry. Committee on
Child Psychiatry. *The diagnostic process in child
psychiatry*. GAP report, no. 38. New York: Group for
the Advancement of Psychiatry, 1957.

2447   *Coppolillo, H. P. A technical consideration in child
analysis and child therapy. *Journal of the American
Academy of Child Psychiatry*, 1969, *8*, 411-435.

2447.1 Di Leo, J. H. *Children's drawings as diagnostic aids*.
New York: Brunner/Mazel, 1973.

VARIOUS MODALITIES OF THERAPEUTIC INTERVENTION/Treatment of
Some Specific Presenting Problems

2448   *Mattsson, A., Hawkins, J. W. & Seese, L. R.   Child psychiatric emergencies: Clinical characteristics and
follow-up results. *Archives of General Psychiatry*,
1967, *17*, 584-592.

2449   *Mattsson, A., Seese, L. R. & Hawkins, J. W.   Suicidal behavior as a child psychiatric emergency: Clinical
characteristics and follow-up results. *Archives of
General Psychiatry*, 1969, *20*, 100-109.

2449.1 Wieder, H.   Intellectuality: Aspects of its development
from the analysis of a precocious four-and-a-half-
year-old boy. *Psychoanalytic Study of the Child*, 1966,
21, 294-323.

2450   *Farragher, M. E.   Therapeutic tutoring as an approach to
psychogenic learning disturbances. *Journal of Special
Education*, 1968, *2*, 117-127.

2451   *Defries, Z., Natchez, G. & Verdiani, F.   Treatment of
secondary reading disability in young boys: A pilot
study. *Science and Psychoanalysis*, 1969, *14*, 89-107.

2452   *Malone, A. J. & Massler, M.   Index of nailbiting in
children. *Journal of Abnormal and Social Psychology*,
1952, *47*, 193-202.

2453   Billig, A. L.   Finger nail-biting: Its incipience, incidence, and amelioration. *Genetic Psychology Monographs*, 1941, *24*, 123-218.

2454   *Mowrer, O. H. & Mowrer, W. M.   Enuresis--A method for its
study and treatment. *American Journal of Orthopsychiatry*, 1938, *8*, 436-459.

2455   Stehbens, J. A.   Enuresis in school children. *Journal
of School Psychology*, 1970, *8*, 145-151.

2456   Lovibond, S. H. *Conditioning and enuresis.* New York:
Macmillan, 1964.

2457   Werry, J. S.   Enuresis--A psychosomatic entity? *Canadian Medical Association Journal*, 1967, *97*, 319-327.

2458   Wolters, W. H. G.   Encopresis. *Psychotherapy and Psychosomatics*, 1971, *19*, 266-287.

2458.1 Shane, M.   Encopresis in a latency boy: An arrest along
a developmental line. *Psychoanalytic Study of the
Child*, 1967, *22*, 296-314.

2459   Frick, W. B.   School phobia: A critical review of the
literature. *Merrill-Palmer Quarterly*, 1964, *10*, 361-
373.

2460   Hersov, L. A.   Persistent non-attendance at school.
*Journal of Child Psychology and Psychiatry and Allied
Disciplines*, 1960, *1*, 130-136.

2461   *Hersov, L. A.   Refusal to go to school. *Journal of
Child Psychology and Psychiatry and Allied Disciplines*,
1960, *1*, 137-145.

2462   Rae-Grant, Q. & Levine, S. V.   School phobia. *Modern
Medicine of Canada*, 1969, *24*, 21-24.

2463   *Smith, S. L.   School refusal with anxiety: A review of
       sixty-three cases. *Canadian Psychiatric Association
       Journal*, 1970, *15*, 257-264.
2464   *Eisenberg, L.   The pediatric management of school
       phobia. *Journal of Pediatrics*, 1959, *55*, 758-766.
2465   *Eisenberg, L.   School phobia: A study in the communica-
       tion of anxiety. *American Journal of Psychiatry*, 1958,
       114, 712-718.
2466   *Kennedy, W. A.   School phobia: Rapid treatment of fifty
       cases. *Journal of Abnormal Psychology*, 1965, *70*,
       285-289.
2467   *Berecz, J. M.   Phobias of childhood: Etiology and treat-
       ment. *Psychological Bulletin*, 1968, *70*, 694-720.
2468   *Rachman, S. & Costello, C. G.   The aetiology and treat-
       ment of children's phobias: A review. *American Jour-
       nal of Psychiatry*, 1961, *118*, 97-105.
2468.1 Sperling, M.   Animal phobias in a two-year-old child.
       Psychoanalytic Study of the Child, 1952, *7*, 115-125.
2468.2 Kolansky, H.   Treatment of a three-year-old girl's se-
       vere infantile neurosis: Stammering and insect phobia.
       Psychoanalytic Study of the Child, 1960, *15*, 261-285.
2469   Schmitt, B. D.   School phobia--The great imitator: A
       pediatrician's viewpoint. *Pediatrics*, 1971, *48*,
       433-441.
2470   *Corbett, J. A., Matthews, A. M., Connell, P. H. &
       Shapiro, D. A.   Tics and Gilles de la Tourette's syn-
       drome: A follow-up study and critical review. *British
       Journal of Psychiatry*, 1969, *115*, 1229-1241.
2471   *Zausmer, D. M.   The treatment of tics in childhood: A
       review and a follow-up study. *Archives of Diseases in
       Childhood*, 1954, *29*, 537-542.
2471.1 Sylvester, E.   Analysis of psychogenic anorexia in a
       four-year-old-child. *Psychoanalytic Study of the Child*,
       1945, *1*, 167-187.
2472   *Rollins, N. & Blackwell, A.   The treatment of anorexia
       nervosa in children and adolescents: Stage 1. *Jour-
       nal of Child Psychology and Psychiatry and Allied
       Disciplines*, 1968, *9*, 81-91.
2473   Berlin, I. N., Boatman, M. J., Sheimo, S. L. & Szurek, S.
       A.   Adolescent alternation of anorexia and obesity.
       Workshop, 1950. *American Journal of Orthopsychiatry*,
       1951, *21*, 387-419. (Also in G. E. Gardner (Ed.),
       Case studies in childhood emotional disabilities.
       New York: American Orthopsychiatric Association, 1953.)
2474   *Caplan, M. G. & Douglas, V. I.   Incidence of parental
       loss in children with depressed mood. *Journal of Child
       Psychology and Psychiatry and Allied Disciplines*, 1969,
       10, 225-232.
2475   *Feinstein, S. C. & Wolpert, E. A.   Juvenile manic-
       depressive illness: Clinical and therapeutic con-
       siderations. *Journal of the American Academy of Child
       Psychiatry*, 1973, *12*, 123-136.

2476   Brown, F. Depression and childhood bereavement. *Journal of Mental Science,* 1961, *107,* 754-777.
2477   *Brown, F. Bereavement and lack of a parent in childhood. In E. Miller (Ed.), *Foundations of child psychiatry.* Oxford: Pergamon, 1968. Pp. 435-455.
2478   *Poznanski, E. & Zrull, J. P. Childhood depression: Clinical characteristics of overtly depressed children. *Archives of General Psychiatry,* 1970, *23,* 8-15.
2479   *Waal, N. A special technique of psychotherapy with an autistic child. In G. Caplan (Ed.), *Emotional problems of early childhood.* New York: Basic Books, 1955. Pp. 431-449.
2480   *Ekstein, R. & Wallerstein, J. Choice of interpretation in the treatment of borderline and psychotic children. In *Children of time and space, of action and impulse.* New York: Appleton/Century/Crofts, 1966. Pp. 148-157.
2481   *Szurek, S. A. & Berlin, I. N. Elements of psychotherapeutics with the schizophrenic child and his parents. *Psychiatry,* 1956, *19,* 1-9.
2482   *Marcus, J. Borderline states in childhood. *Journal of Child Psychology and Psychiatry and Allied Disciplines,* 1963, *4,* 207-218.
2483   *Szurek, S. A. Playfulness, creativity and schisis. *American Journal of Orthopsychiatry,* 1959, *29,* 667-683.
2484   *Laufer, M. W., Denhoff, E. & Solomons, G. Hyperkinetic impulse disorder in children's behavior problems. *Psychosomatic Medicine,* 1957, *19,* 38-49.
2485   *Eisenberg, L. The management of the hyperkinetic child. *Developmental Medicine and Child Neurology,* 1966, *8,* 593-598.
2486   Werry, J. S. Studies on the hyperactive child. IV. An empirical analysis of the minimal brain dysfunction syndrome. *Archives of General Psychiatry,* 1968, *19,* 9-16.
2487   *Elonen, A. S. & Cain, A. C. Diagnostic evaluation and treatment of deviant blind children. *American Journal of Orthopsychiatry,* 1964, *34,* 625-633.
2488   Blom, G. E., et al. A psychoeducational approach to day care treatment. *Journal of the American Academy of Child Psychiatry,* 1972, *11,* 492-510.
2488.1 Razani, J. Treatment of phobias by systematic desensitization. *Archives of General Psychiatry,* 1974, *30,* 291-293.
2488.2 Chethik, M. Amy: The intensive treatment of an elective mute. *Journal of the American Academy of Child Psychiatry,* 1973, *12,* 482-498.
2488.3 Geist, R. A. Some observations on adolescent drug use: Therapeutic implications. *Journal of the American Academy of Child Psychiatry,* 1974, *13.* 54-71.

VARIOUS MODALITIES OF THERAPEUTIC INTERVENTION/A Variety of
Therapeutic Techniques

2489   Gardner, R. A. The mutual storytelling technique: Use
         in alleviating childhood oedipal problems. *Contempo-*
         rary Psychoanalysis, 1968, *4*, 161-177.
2490   *Redl, F. & Wineman, D. Programming for ego support. In
         Controls from within. New York: Free Press, 1952.
         Pp. 76-152.
2491   *Furman, R. A. & Katan, A. (Eds.) *The therapeutic nurs-*
         ery school. New York: International Universities
         Press, 1969.
2492   Kohn, M. & Rosman, B. L. Therapeutic intervention with
         disturbed children in day care: Implications of the
         deprivation hypothesis. *Child Care Quarterly*, 1971, *1*,
         21-46.
2493   *Tolor, A. & Lane, P. A. Some characteristics of children
         treated by subprofessionals at a novel therapeutic
         setting. *Journal of School Psychology*, 1968-1969, *7*,
         57-62.
2494   *Josselyn, I. M. Psychotherapy of adolescents at the level
         of private practice. In B. H. Balser (Ed.), *Psychother-*
         apy of the adolescent. New York: International Uni-
         versities Press, 1957. Pp. 13-38.
2495   *Berman, S. Psychotherapeutic techniques with adolescents.
         American Journal of Orthopsychiatry, 1954, *24*, 238-245.
2496   *Kaplan, S. L. & Escoll, P. Treatment of two silent ado-
         lescent girls. *Journal of the American Academy of*
         Child Psychiatry, 1973, *12*, 59-72.
2497   *Fraiberg, S. Some considerations in the introduction to
         therapy in puberty. *Psychoanalytic Study of the Child*,
         1955, *10*, 264-286.
2498   *Eissler, K. R. Notes on the problems of technique in the
         psychoanalytic treatment of adolescents, with some re-
         marks on perversions. *Psychoanalytic Study of the*
         Child, 1958, *13*, 223-254.
2498.1   Geleerd, E. R. Some aspects of psychoanalytic technique
         in adolescence. *Psychoanalytic Study of the Child*,
         1957, *12*, 263-283.
2498.2   Blos, P. The contribution of psychoanalysis to the
         treatment of adolescents. In M. Heiman (Ed.), *Psycho-*
         analysis and social work. New York: International
         Universities Press, 1953. Pp. 210-241.
2499   *Weinreb, J. & Counts, R. M. Impulsivity in adolescents
         and its therapeutic management. *Archives of General*
         Psychiatry, 1960, *2*, 548-558.
2500   Patton, J. D. Joint treatment of adolescent and mother.
         Diseases of the Nervous System, 1957, *18*, 220-222.
2501   *Greaves, D. C. Practical and theoretical aspects of the
         treatment in psychotherapy of the adolescent patient.
         Psychotherapy and Psychosomatics, 1967, *15*, 25.

2502   Sachs, D. M. & Shapiro, S. H. Comments on teaching the psychoanalytic psychology of adolescence to residents. *Journal of the American Academy of Child Psychiatry*, 1972, *11*, 201-211.
2503   Subotnik, L. Transference toward the child therapist and other parent surrogates. *Journal of Genetic Psychology*, 1971, *119*, 215-231.
2504   *Minuchin, S., Chamberlain, P. & Graubard, P. A project to teach learning skills to disturbed, delinquent children. *American Journal of Orthopsychiatry*, 1967, *37*, 558-567.
2505   *Newman, M. B. & San Martino, M. The child and the seriously disturbed parent: Treatment issues. *Journal of the American Academy of Child Psychiatry*, 1973, *12*, 162-181.
2506   Proskauer, S. Focused time-limited psychotherapy with children. *Journal of the American Academy of Child Psychiatry*, 1971, *10*, 619-639.
2506.1 Wolpe, J., Brady, J. P., Serber, M., Agras, W. S. & Liberman, R. P. The current status of systematic desensitization. *American Journal of Psychiatry*, 1973, *130*, 961-965.
2506.2 Havens, L. L. The existential use of the self. *American Journal of Psychiatry*, 1974, *131*, 1-10.
2506.3 Goldstein, A. P. *Structured learning therapy: Toward a psychotherapy for the poor.* New York: Academic Press, 1973.
2506.4 Naumburg, M. *An introduction to art therapy; studies of the "free" art expression of behavior problem children and adolescents as a means of diagnosis and therapy.* New York: Teachers College Press, 1973.
2506.5 Betensky, M. *Self-discovery through self-expression: Use of art in psychotherapy with children and adolescents.* Springfield: Thomas, 1973.
2506.6 Lewis, M. Interpretation in child analysis: Developmental considerations. *Journal of the American Academy of Child Psychiatry*, 1974, *13*, 32-53.

VARIOUS MODALITIES OF THERAPEUTIC INTERVENTION/Behavior Modification

2507   *Ross, A. O. Learning theory and therapy with children. *Psychotherapy: Theory, Research and Practice*, 1963, *1*, 102-108.
2508   *Eysenck, H. J. & Rachman, S. J. The application of learning theory to child psychiatry. In J. G. Howells (Ed.), *Modern perspectives in child psychiatry*. London: Oliver & Boyd, 1965. Pp. 104-169. (*Modern perspectives in psychiatry*, vol. 1)

2509   *Bijou, S. W. Child behavior and development: A behavioral analysis. *International Journal of Psychology*, 1968, *3*, 221-238.

2510   *Werry, J. S. & Wollersheim, J. P. Behavior therapy with children: A broad overview. *Journal of the American Academy of Child Psychiatry*, 1967, *6*, 346-370.

2511   Gelfand, D. M. & Hartmann, D. P. Behavior therapy with children: A review and evaluation of research methodology. *Psychological Bulletin*, 1968, *69*, 204-215.

2512   *Churchill, D. W. Psychotic children and behavior modification. *American Journal of Psychiatry*, 1969, *125*, 1585-1590.

2513   Leff, R. Behavior modification and the psychoses of childhood: A review. *Psychological Bulletin*, 1968, *69*, 396-409.

2514   Wahler, R. G. Oppositional children: A quest for parental reinforcement control. *Journal of Applied Behavior Analysis*, 1969, *2*, 159-170.

2515   Gardner, J. E. A blending of behavior therapy techniques in an approach to an asthmatic child. *Psychotherapy: Theory, Research and Practice*, 1968, *5*, 46-49.

2516   *Garvey, W. P. & Hegrenes, J. R. Desensitization techniques in the treatment of school phobia. *American Journal of Orthopsychiatry*, 1966, *36*, 147-152.

2517   Lazarus, A. A., Davison, G. C. & Polefka, D. A. Classical and operant factors in the treatment of a school phobia. *Journal of Abnormal Psychology*, 1965, *70*, 225-229.

2518   Ayllon, T., Smith, D. & Rogers, M. Behavioral management of school phobia. *Journal of Behavior Therapy and Experimental Psychiatry*, 1970, *1*, 125-138.

2519   *Clement, P. W. Please, Mother, I'd rather you did it yourself: Training parents to treat their own children. *Journal of School Health*, 1971, *41*, 65-69.

2520   *Clement, P. W., Fazzone, R. A. & Goldstein, B. Tangible reinforcers and child group therapy. *Journal of the American Academy of Child Psychiatry*, 1970, *9*, 409-427.

2521   Wahler, R. G. & Erickson, M. Child behavior therapy: A community program in Appalachia. *Behaviour Research and Therapy*, 1969, *7*, 71-78.

2522   Liberman, R. Behavioral approaches to family and couple therapy. *American Journal of Orthopsychiatry*, 1970, *40*, 106-118.

2523   Engeln, R., Knutson, J., Laughy, L. & Garlington, W. Behaviour modification techniques applied to a family unit--A case study. *Journal of Child Psychology and Psychiatry and Allied Disciplines*, 1968, *9*, 245-252.

2523.1   Rhoads, J. M. & Feather, B. W. The application of psychodynamics to behavior therapy. *American Journal of Psychiatry*, 1974, *131*, 17-20.

2523.2   Birk, L. Intensive group therapy: An effective behav-

ioral-psychoanalytic method. *American Journal of Psychiatry*, 1974, *131*, 11-16.
2523.3   Klein, H. A. Behavior modification as therapeutic paradox. *American Journal of Orthopsychiatry*, 1974, *44*, 353-361.

VARIOUS MODALITIES OF THERAPEUTIC INTERVENTION/Group, Family and Filial Therapy

2524   *Ginott, H. G. *Group psychotherapy with children: The theory and practice of play-therapy.* New York: McGraw-Hill, 1961.
2525   *Ganter, G., Yeakel, M. & Polansky, N. A. *Retrieval from limbo: The intermediary group treatment of inaccessible children.* New York: Child Welfare League of America, 1967.
2526   *Scheidlinger, S. Three group approaches with socially deprived latency-age children. *International Journal of Group Psychotherapy*, 1965, *15*, 434-445.
2527   Dana, R. H. & Dana, J. M. Systematic observation of children's behavior in group therapy. *Psychological Reports*, 1969, *24*, 134.
2528   *Berkovitz, I. H. *Adolescents grow in groups: Experiences in adolescent group psychotherapy.* New York: Brunner/Mazel, 1972.
2529   Slivkin, S. E. & Bernstein, N. R. Goal-directed group psychotherapy for retarded adolescents. *American Journal of Psychotherapy*, 1968, *22*, 35-45.
2530   *Williams, F. S. Family therapy: A critical assessment. *American Journal of Orthopsychiatry*, 1967, *37*, 912-919.
2531   *Minuchin, S. Conflict-resolution family therapy. *Psychiatry*, 1965, *28*, 278-286.
2532   *Minuchin, S. & Montalvo, B. Techniques for working with disorganized low socioeconomic families. *American Journal of Orthopsychiatry*, 1967, *37*, 880-887.
2533   *Markowitz, I. Family therapy in a child guidance clinic. *Psychiatric Quarterly*, 1966, *40*, 308-318.
2533.1   Kolansky, H. & Moore, W. T. Some comments on the simultaneous analysis of a father and his adolescent son. *Psychoanalytic Study of the Child*, 1966, *21*, 237-268.
2533.2   Rosenthal, P. A., Mosteller, S., Wells, J. L. & Rolland, R. S. Family therapy with multiproblem multichildren families in a court clinic setting. *Journal of the American Academy of Child Psychiatry*, 1974, *13*, 126-142.
2534   Morrison, G. C. & Collier, J. G. Family treatment approaches to suicidal children and adolescents. *Journal of the American Academy of Child Psychiatry*, 1969, *8*, 140-153.
2535   Safer, D. J. Family therapy for children with behavior disorders. *Family Process*, 1966, *5*, 243-255.

2536   Minuchin, S. & Barcai, A. Therapeutically induced family
        crisis. *Science and Psychoanalysis*, 1969, *14*, 199-205.
2537   *Andronico, M. P., Fidler, J., Guerney, B. Jr. & Guerney,
        L. F. The combination of didactic and dynamic elements
        in filial therapy. *International Journal of Group Psy-
        chotherapy*, 1967, *17*, 10-17.
2537.1 Burlingham, D. T. Present trends in handling the mother-
        child relationship during the therapeutic process.
        Psychoanalytic Study of the Child, 1951, *6*, 31-37.
2537.2 Bonnard, A. The mother as therapist, in a case of ob-
        sessional neurosis. *Psychoanalytic Study of the Child*,
        1950, *5*, 391-408.
2537.3 Furman, E. Treatment of under-fives by way of their
        parents. *Psychoanalytic Study of the Child*, 1957, *12*,
        250-262.
2538   Guerney, B. G. Filial therapy: Description and rationale.
        Journal of Consulting Psychology, 1964, *28*, 304-310.
2538.1 White, J. H., Hornsby, L. G. & Gordon, R. Treating in-
        fantile autism with parent therapists. *International
        Journal of Child Psychotherapy*, 1972, *1(3)*, 83-95.
2539   Cooper, M. M. Evaluation of the mothers' advisory serv-
        ice. *Monographs of the Society for Research in Child
        Development*, 1948, *12*(1, Serial No. 44).
2540   *Wahler, R. G., Winkel, G. H., Peterson, R. F. & Morrison,
        D. C. Mothers as behavior therapists for their own
        children. *Behaviour Research and Therapy*, 1965, *3*,
        113-124.
2540.1 Minuchin, S. *Families and family therapy: A structural
        approach.* Cambridge: Harvard Press, 1974.
2540.2 Hawkins, D. M., Norton, C. B., Eisdorfer, C. & Gianturco,
        D. Group process research: A factor analytical study.
        American Journal of Psychiatry, 1973, *130*, 916-919.

VARIOUS MODALITIES OF THERAPEUTIC INTERVENTION/Brief Therapy

2541   *Rosenthal, A. J. & Levine, S. V. Brief psychotherapy
        with children: Process of therapy. *American Journal
        of Psychiatry*, 1971, *128*, 141-146.
2542   *Berlin, I. N. Crisis intervention and short-term ther-
        apy: An approach in a child-psychiatric clinic. In
        H. H. Barten & S. S. Barten (Eds.), *Children and their
        parents in brief therapy.* New York: Behavioral Pub-
        lications, 1973. Pp. 49-62. (Also in *Journal of the
        American Academy of Child Psychiatry*, 1970, *9*, 595-606)
2543   *Proskauer, S. Focused time-limited psychotherapy with
        children. *Journal of the American Academy of Child
        Psychiatry*, 1971, *10*, 619-639.
2544   *Augenbraun, B., Reid, H. L. & Friedman, D. B. Brief in-
        tervention as a preventive force in disorders of early
        childhood. *American Journal of Orthopsychiatry*, 1967,
        37, 697-702.

2545   Lester, E. P. Brief psychotherapies in child psychiatry.
        Canadian Psychiatric Association Journal, 1968, *13*,
        301-309.
2546   Mackay, J. The use of brief psychotherapy with children.
        Canadian Psychiatric Association Journal, 1967, *12*,
        269-279.
2547   *Morrison, G. C. Therapeutic intervention in a child psy-
        chiatry emergency service. *Journal of the American
        Academy of Child Psychiatry*, 1969, *8*, 542-558.
2548   Baldwin, K. A. Crisis-focused casework in a child guid-
        ance clinic. *Social Casework*, 1968, *49*, 28-34.
2549   *Hare, M. K. Shortened treatment in a child guidance
        clinic: The results in 119 cases. *British Journal of
        Psychiatry*, 1966, *112*, 613-616.
2550   Proskauer, S. Some technical issues in time-limited psy-
        chotherapy with children. *Journal of the American
        Academy of Child Psychiatry*, 1969, *8*, 154-169.
2551   *Rosenthal, A. J. & Levine, S. V. Brief psychotherapy with
        children: A preliminary report. *American Journal of
        Psychiatry*, 1970, *127*, 646-651.
2552   Schulman, J. L. One-visit psychotherapy with children.
        In *Progress in Psychotherapy*, 1960, *5*, 86-93.
2553   Shaw, R., Blumenfeld, H. & Senf, R. A short-term treat-
        ment program in a child guidance clinic. *Social Work*,
        1968, *13(3)*, 81-90.
2554   *Parad, H. J. & Parad, L. G. A study of crisis-oriented
        planned short-term treatment: Part I. *Social Case-
        work*, 1968, *49*, 346-355.
2555   Phillips, E. L. & Johnston, M. S. H. Theoretical and
        clinical aspects of short-term parent-child psycho-
        therapy. *Psychiatry*, 1954, *17*, 267-275.
2555.1 Mann, J. *Time-limited psychotherapy*. Cambridge: Har-
        vard University Press, 1973.

FOLLOW-UP AND EVALUATION RESEARCH

2556   Bennett, C. C. & Rogers, C. R. Predicting the outcomes
        of treatment. *American Journal of Orthopsychiatry*,
        1941, *11*, 210-221.
2557   Wimberger, H. C. & Millar, G. The psychotherapeutic
        effects of initial clinical contact on child psychiatry
        patients. In S. Lesse (Ed.), *An evaluation of the re-
        sults of the psychotherapies*. Springfield, Ill.:
        Thomas, 1968. Pp. 179-189.
2558   *Axline, V. M. Therapeutic play techniques. Symposium,
        1954. 5. Play therapy procedures and results.
        American Journal of Orthopsychiatry, 1955, *25*, 618-
        626.
2559   *Maclay, I. Prognostic factors in child guidance practice.
        *Journal of Child Psychology and Psychiatry and Allied
        Disciplines*, 1967, *8*, 207-215.

2560   *Rutter, M.   Discussion.   In E. H. Hare & J. K. Wing
        (Eds.), *Psychiatric Epidemiology*. London: Oxford
        University Press, 1970. Pp. 69-86.
2561   *Heinicke, C. M. Frequency of psychotherapeutic session
        as a factor affecting the child's developmental status.
        Psychoanalytic Study of the Child, 1965, *20*, 42-98.
2562   *Heinicke, C. M. Frequency of psychotherapeutic session
        as a factor affecting outcome: Analysis of clinical
        ratings and test results. *Journal of Abnormal Psy-
        chology*, 1969, *74*, 553-560.
2563   *Morris, D. P., Soroker, E. & Burruss, G. Follow-up
        studies of shy, withdrawn children--I. Evaluation of
        later adjustment. *American Journal of Orthopsychiatry*,
        1954, *24*, 743-754.
2564   *Michael, C. M., Morris, D. P. & Soroker, E. Follow-up
        studies of shy withdrawn children. II: Relative in-
        cidence of schizophrenia. *American Journal of Ortho-
        psychiatry*, 1957, *27*, 331-337.
2565   *Rodriguez, A., Rodriguez, M. & Eisenberg, L. The outcome
        of school phobia: A follow-up study based on 41 cases.
        American Journal of Psychiatry, 1959, *116*, 540-544.
2566   *Coolidge, J. C., Brodie, R. D. & Feeney, B. A ten-year
        follow-up study of sixty-six school-phobic children.
        American Journal of Orthopsychiatry, 1964, *34*, 675-684.
2567   *Rexford, E. N., Schleifer, M. & Van Amerongen, S. T.
        A follow-up of a psychiatric study of 57 antisocial
        young children. *Mental Hygiene*, 1956, *40*, 196-214.
2568   *Rexford, E. N. Antisocial young children and their fam-
        ilies. In L. Jessner & E. Pavenstedt (Eds.), *Dynamic
        psychopathology in childhood*. New York: Grune &
        Stratton, 1959. Pp. 186-220.
2569   Morris, H. H., Escoll, P. J. & Wexler, R. Aggressive be-
        havior disorders of childhood: A follow-up study.
        American Journal of Psychiatry, 1956, *112*, 991-997.
2570   *Wattenberg, W. W. & Quiroz, F. Follow-up study of ten-
        year-old boys with police records. *Journal of Con-
        sulting Psychology*, 1953, *17*, 309-313.
2571   Wattenberg, W. W. & Saunders, F. Recidivism among girls.
        Journal of Abnormal and Social Psychology, 1955, *50*,
        405-406.
2572   Stott, D. H. Prediction of success or failure on proba-
        tion: A follow-up study. *International Journal of
        Social Psychiatry*, 1964, *10*, 27-29.
2573   *Phillips, E. L. Parent-child psychotherapy: A follow-
        up study comparing two techniques. *Journal of Psy-
        chology*, 1960, *49*, 195-202.
2574   Robins, L. N. *Deviant children grown up: A sociological
        and psychiatric study of sociopathic personality*.
        Baltimore: Williams & Wilkins, 1966.
2575   Robins, L. N. Antecedents of character disorder. In M.
        Roff & D. F. Ricks (Eds.), *Life history research in
        psychopathology*. Minneapolis: University of Minnesota
        Press, 1970. Pp. 226-239.

2576   Bronner, A. F. Treatment and what happened afterward
       (A second report). *American Journal of Orthopsychia-*
       try, 1944, *14,* 28-35.
2577   Levitt, E. E. Psychotherapy with children: A further
       evaluation. *Behaviour Research and Therapy,* 1963, *1,*
       45-51.
2578   Lewis, W. W. Continuity and intervention in emotional
       disturbance: A review. *Exceptional Children,* 1965,
       31, 465-475.
2579   Kellner, R. The evidence in favour of psychotherapy.
       British Journal of Medical Psychology, 1967, *40,*
       341-358.

OTHER RESEARCH IN TREATMENT OF CHILDREN/Paraprofessionals and
Other Helping Persons

2580   *Tuckman, J. & Regan, R. A. A note on secondary preven-
       tion. *Mental Hygiene,* 1965, *49,* 334-336.
2581   Tolor, A. Teachers' evaluations of children in short-
       term treatment with subprofessionals. *Journal of*
       Clinical Psychology, 1968, *24,* 377-378.
2582   *Tolor, A. The effectiveness of various therapeutic
       approaches: A study of subprofessional therapists.
       International Journal of Group Psychotherapy, 1970,
       20, 48-62.
2583   Guerney, B. G. & Flumen, A. B. Teachers as psychothera-
       peutic agents for withdrawn children. *Journal of*
       School Psychology, 1970, *8,* 107-113.
2584   *Minde, K. K. & Werry, J. S. Intensive psychiatric teach-
       er counseling in a low socioeconomic area: A con-
       trolled evaluation. *American Journal of Orthopsy-*
       chiatry, 1969, *39,* 595-608.
2585   *Tolor, A. & Lane, P. A. An experimental approach to the
       treatment of disturbed school-age children. *Journal*
       of School Psychology, 1968, *6,* 97-103.
2586   *Linden, J. I. & Stollak, G. E. The training of under-
       graduates in play techniques. *Journal of Clinical*
       Psychology, 1969, *25,* 213-218.
2587   *Cowen, E. L., Leibowitz, E. & Leibowitz, G. Utilization
       of retired people as mental health aides with children.
       American Journal of Orthopsychiatry, 1968, *38,* 900-909.
2588   *Kauffman, J. M. School and family as potential change
       agents in the mental health of children. *Journal of*
       School Health, 1970, *40,* 443-446.
2589   Mira, M. Case histories and shorter communications:
       Results of a behavior modification training program
       for parents and teachers. *Behaviour Research and*
       Therapy, 1970, *8,* 309-311.
2590   *Fidler, J. W., et al. Filial therapy as a logical ex-
       tension of current trends in psychotherapy. In B. G.
       Guerney (Ed.), *Psychotherapeutic agents: New roles*

for nonprofessionals, parents, and teachers. New York: Holt, Rinehart & Winston, 1969. Pp. 47-55.

2591 *Guerney, B. G., Stover, L. & Andronico, M. P. On educating disadvantaged parents to motivate children for learning: A filial approach. *Community Mental Health Journal,* 1967, *3,* 66-72.

2592 *Andronico, M. P. & Guerney, B. The potential application of filial therapy to the school situation. *Journal of School Psychology,* 1967, *6,* 2-7.

2593 Stover, L. & Guerney, B. G. The efficacy of training procedures for mothers in filial therapy. *Psychotherapy: Theory, Research and Practice,* 1967, *4,* 110-115.

2594 Zeilberger, J., Sampen, S. E. & Sloane, H. N. Modification of a child's problem behaviors in the home with the mother as therapist. *Journal of Applied Behavior Analysis,* 1968, *1,* 47-53.

2595 Guerney, B. G., Guerney, L. F. & Andronico, M. P. Filial therapy: A case illustration. In B. G. Guerney (Ed.), *Psychotherapeutic agents: New roles for nonprofessionals, parents, and teachers.* New York: Holt, Rinehart & Winston, 1969. Pp. 461-465.

OTHER RESEARCH IN TREATMENT OF CHILDREN/The Community Context

2596 *Gath, D. Child guidance and the general practitioner: A study of factors influencing referrals made by general practitioners to a child psychiatric department. *Journal of Child Psychology and Psychiatry and Allied Disciplines,* 1968, *9,* 213-227.

2597 *Engel, M. Public education and the "emotionally disturbed" child. *Journal of the American Academy of Child Psychiatry,* 1964, *3,* 617-637.

2598 *Morse, W. C., Finger, C. & Gilmore, G. C. Innovations in school mental health programs. *Review of Educational Research,* 1968, *38,* 460-477.

2599 *Hobbs, N. Helping disturbed children: Psychological and ecological strategies. *American Psychologist,* 1966, *21,* 1105-1115.

2600 *Chess, S. & Lyman, M. S. A psychiatric unit in a general hospital pediatric clinic. *American Journal of Orthopsychiatry,* 1969, *39,* 77-85.

2601 *Eisenberg, L., Marlowe, B. & Hastings, M. Diagnostic services for maladjusted foster children: An orientation toward an acute need. *American Journal of Orthopsychiatry,* 1958, *28,* 750-763.

2602 Rosenthal, A. J. & Langee, H. The development of a service-oriented psychiatric program in a disadvantaged area. *American Journal of Psychiatry,* 1970, *126,* 1436-1443

2603 *Berkowitz, P. H. A preliminary assessment of the extent of interaction between child psychiatric clinics and public schools. *Psychology in the Schools*, 1968, *5*, 291-295.

2604   Joint Commission on Mental Health of Children. *Crisis in child mental health: Challenge for the 1970's.* New York: Harper & Row, 1970.

OTHER RESEARCH IN TREATMENT OF CHILDREN/Prevention and Early Intervention/*PREVENTION*

2605   *Bolman, W. M. & Westman, J. C. Prevention of mental disorder: An overview of current programs. *American Journal of Psychiatry*, 1967, *123*, 1058-1068.

2606   *Stringer, L. A. Research interviews with mothers as entry into primary prevention. *American Journal of Public Health*, 1969, *59*, 485-489.

2607   *Cary, A. C. & Reveal, M. T. Prevention and detection of emotional disturbances in preschool children. *American Journal of Orthopsychiatry*, 1967, *37*, 719-724.

2608   *Zax, M. & Cowen, E. L. Research on early detection and prevention of emotional dysfunction in young school children. *Current Topics in Clinical and Community Psychology*, 1969, *1*, 67-108.

2609   *Bower, E. M. *Early identification of emotionally handicapped children in school.* (2nd ed.) Springfield, Ill.: Thomas, 1969.

2609.1 Meier, J. *Screening and assessment of young children at developmental risk.* Washington, D.C.: U.S. President's Committee on Mental Retardation, 1973. (DHEW publication no. (OS) 73-90)

OTHER RESEARCH IN TREATMENT OF CHILDREN/Prevention and Early Intervention/*EARLY INTERVENTION*

2609.2 Powell, L. F. The effect of extra stimulation and maternal involvement on the development of low-birthweight infants and on maternal behavior. *Child Development*, 1974, *45*, 106-113.

2609.3 Korner, A. F. & Thoman, E. B. The relative efficacy of contact and vestibular-proprioceptive stimulation in soothing neonates. *Child Development*, 1972, *43*, 443-453.

2609.4 Jones, S. J. & Moss, H. A. Age, state, and maternal behavior associated with infant vocalizations. *Child Behavior*, 1971, *42*, 1039-1052.

2609.5 Radin, N. Three degrees of maternal involvement in a preschool program: Impact on mothers and children. *Child Development*, 1972, *43*, 1355-1364.

2609.6   Saltz, R.   Effects of part-time "mothering" on IQ and
         SQ of young institutionalized children. *Child Devel-
         opment,* 1973, *44,* 166-170.
2609.7   Tizard, B. & Rees, J.   A comparison of the effects of
         adoption, restoration to the natural mother, and con-
         tinued institutionalization on the cognitive develop-
         ment of four-year-old children. *Child Development,*
         1974, *45,* 92-99.
2609.8   Alford, G. S. & Rosenthal, T. L.   Process and products
         of modeling in observational concept attainment.
         Child Development, 1973, *44,* 714-720.
2609.9   Nelson, K. E. & Earl, N.   Information search by pre-
         school children: Induced use of categories and
         category hierarchies. *Child Development,* 1973, *44,*
         682-685.
2609.11 Wimberger, H. C. & Kogan, K. L.   A direct approach to
         altering mother-child interaction in disturbed chil-
         dren. *Archives of General Psychiatry,* 1974, *30,*
         636-639.
2609.12 Bryant, B. K.   Locus of control related to teacher-
         child interperceptual experiences. *Child Develop-
         ment,* 1974, *45,* 157-164.
2609.13 Egeland, B.   Training impulsive children in the use of
         more efficient scanning techniques. *Child Develop-
         ment,* 1974, *45,* 165-171.
2609.14 Zelniker, T. & Oppenheimer, L.   Modification of infor-
         mation processing of impulsive children. *Child Devel-
         opment,* 1973, *44,* 445-450.

XVII.   FAMILY INTERACTION AND FAMILY THERAPY

GENERAL REFERENCES

2610   *Glick, I. D. & Haley, J. *Family therapy and research:
       An annotated bibliography of articles and books pub-
       lished 1950-1970.* New York: Grune & Stratton, 1971.
2611   Sander, F. M. & Beels, C. C.   A didactic course for
       family therapy trainees. *Family Process,* 1970, *9,*
       411-423.
2612   Aldous, J. & Hill, R.   *International bibliography of
       research in marriage and the family, 1900-1964.*
       Minneapolis: University of Minnesota Press, 1967.

FAMILY: HISTORY AND FUNCTION

2613   *Aries, P. *Centuries of childhood: A social history of
       family life.* New York: Knopf, 1962.
2614   *Bell, N. W. & Vogel, E. F.   (Eds.) *A modern introduction*

to the family. (Rev. ed.) New York: Free Press, 1968.

2615   *Lidz, T. F. *The family and human adaptation.* New York: International Universities Press, 1963.

2616   *Parsons, T. & Bales, R. F. *Family socialization and interaction process.* Glencoe, Ill.: Free Press, 1954.

2617   Handel, G. (Comp.) *The psychosocial interior of the family: A sourcebook for the study of whole families.* Chicago: Aldine, 1967.

2618   Group for the Advancement of Psychiatry. *Integration and conflict in family behavior.* New York: Group for the Advancement of Psychiatry, 1968.

2620   *Toman, W. *Family constellation.* (2nd ed.) New York: Springer, 1969.

2621   Ryle, A. *Neuroses in the ordinary family.* London: Tavistock, 1967.

2623   Burgess, E. W. & Locke, H. J. *The family: From institution to companionship.* New York: American Books, 1953.

2624   Bott, E. *Family and social network.* (2nd ed.) London: Tavistock, 1971.

2625   Foote, N. N. & Cottrell, L. S. *Identity and interpersonal competence: A new direction in family research.* Chicago: University of Chicago Press, 1955.

2626   Galdston, I. (Ed.) *The family in contemporary society.* New York: International Universities Press, 1958.

2627   Hess, R. D. & Handel, G. *Family worlds.* Chicago: University of Chicago Press, 1959.

2628   Liebman, S. (Ed.) *Emotional forces in the family.* Philadelphia: Lippincott, 1959.

2630   Myers, J. K. & Roberts, B. H. *Family and class dynamics in mental illness.* New York: Wiley, 1959.

2630.1 Willie, C. V. The black family and social class. *American Journal of Orthopsychiatry,* 1974, *44,* 50-60.

2630.2 Lurie, O. R. Parents' attitudes toward children's problems and toward use of mental health services: Socioeconomic differences. *American Journal of Orthopsychiatry,* 1974, *44,* 109-120.

THEORY OF FAMILY DYNAMICS AND THERAPY

2631   *Ackerman, N. W. *Treating the troubled family.* New York: Basic Books, 1966.

2632   *Bowen, M. The use of family theory in clinical practice. *Comprehensive Psychiatry,* 1966, *7,* 345-374.

2633   *Jackson, D. D. Family interaction, family homeostasis and some implications for conjoint family psychotherapy. *Science and Psychoanalysis,* 1959, *2,* 122-141.

2634   *Boszormenyi-Nagy, I. & Framo, J. L. *Intensive family therapy: Theoretical and practical aspects.* New York: Harper & Row, 1965.

2635   *MacGregor, R., et al. *Multiple impact therapy with families.* New York: McGraw-Hill, 1964.

2636   *Haley, J. Whither family therapy. *Family Process,*
       1962, *1,* 69-100.

2637   *Beels, C. C. & Ferber, A. Family therapy: A view.
       Family Process, 1969, *8,* 280-318.

2638   *Spiegel, J. P. Cultural strain, family role patterns,
       and intrapsychic conflict. In J. G. Howells, *Theory
       and practice of family psychiatry.* Edinburgh:
       Oliver & Boyd, 1968. Pp. 367-389.

2639   *Ackerman, N. W. *The psychodynamics of family life.*
       New York: Basic Books, 1958.

2640   *Howells, J. G. *Family psychiatry.* London: Oliver &
       Boyd, 1963.

2641   *Williams, F. S. Family therapy: A critical assessment.
       American Journal of Orthopsychiatry, 1967, *37,* 912-919.

2642   *Zuk, G. H. Family therapy. *Archives of General Psy-
       chiatry,* 1967, *16,* 71-79.

2643   *Zuk, G. H. & Boszormenyi-Nagy, I. (Eds.) *Family ther-
       apy and disturbed families.* Palo Alto, Calif.:
       Science and Behavior Books, 1967.

2644   *Ferber, A., Mendelsohn, M. & Napier, A. *The book of
       family therapy.* New York: Science House, 1972.

2645   Ackerman, N. W. (Ed.) *Family process.* New York:
       Basic Books, 1970.

2646   Ackerman, N. W. Family therapy. In S. Arieti (Ed.),
       American handbook of psychiatry. Vol. 3. New York:
       Basic Books, 1966. Pp. 201-212.

2647   Ackerman, N. W. Family psychotherapy today: Some areas
       of controversy. *Comprehensive Psychiatry,* 1966, *7,*
       375-388.

2648   Bell, J. E. *Family group therapy: A method for the psy-
       chological treatment of older children, adolescents,
       and their parents.* Washington, D.C.: U.S. Dept. of
       Health, Education, and Welfare, Public Health Service,
       1971. (Public health monograph no. 64)

2649   Fleck, S. An approach to family pathology. *Comprehen-
       sive Psychiatry,* 1966, *7,* 307-320.

2650   Bowen, M. The family as the unit of study and treatment.
       Workshop, 1959. 1. Family psychotherapy. *American
       Journal of Orthopsychiatry,* 1961, *31,* 40-60.

2651   Ackerman, N. W., Beatman, F. L. & Sherman, S. N. (Eds.)
       Exploring the base for family therapy. New York:
       Family Service Association of America, 1961.

2652   Bell, N. W. & Vogel, E. F. The emotionally disturbed
       child as the family scapegoat. In N. W. Bell and E. F.
       Vogel (Eds.), *A modern introduction to the family.*
       New York: Free Press, 1968. Pp. 412-427.

2653   Koos, E. L. *Families in trouble.* New York: King's
       Crown Press, 1946.

2654   Cohen, I. M. (Ed.) *Family structure, dynamics, and
       therapy.* Washington: American Psychiatric Associa-
       tion, 1966.

2655   Masserman, J. H. (Ed.) Individual and familial dynamics.
       Science and Psychoanalysis, 1958, *2.*

2656   Richardson, H. B. *Patients have families*. New York:
        Commonwealth Fund, 1945.
2657   Friedman, A. S., et al. *Psychotherapy for the whole
        family*. New York: Springer, 1965.
2658   Chance, E. *Families in treatment*. New York: Basic
        Books, 1959.
2661   Midelfort, C. F. *The family in psychotherapy*. New York:
        McGraw-Hill, 1957.
2661.1 Mishler, E. G. & Waxler, N. E. Family interaction pro-
        cesses and schizophrenia: A review of current theories.
        International Journal of Psychiatry, 1966, *2*, 375-428.
2661.2 DeMyer, M. K., Pontius, W., Norton, J. A., Barton, S.,
        Allen, J. & Steele, R. Parental practices and innate
        activity in normal, autistic, and brain-damaged in-
        fants. *Journal of Autism and Childhood Schizophrenia*,
        1972, *2*, 49-66.
2661.3 Williams, T. M. Childrearing practices of young mothers:
        What we know, how it matters, why it's so little.
        American Journal of Orthopsychiatry, 1974, *44*, 70-75.
2661.4 Mannino, F. V. & Shore, M. F. Family structure, after-
        care, and post-hospital adjustment. *American Journal
        of Orthopsychiatry*, 1974, *44*, 76-85.
2661.5 Ford, F. R. & Herrick, J. Family rules: Family life
        styles. *American Journal of Orthopsychiatry*, 1974, *44*,
        61-69.
2661.6 Rollins, N., Lord, J. P., Walsh, E. & Weil, G. Some roles
        children play in their families: Scapegoat, baby, pet,
        and peacemaker. *Journal of the American Academy of
        Child Psychiatry*, 1973, *12*, 511-530.

FAMILY THERAPY: TECHNIQUE

2662   *Haley, J. & Hoffman, L. *Techniques of family therapy*.
        New York: Basic Books, 1967.
2663   *Satir, V. M. *Conjoint family therapy*. Palo Alto, Calif.:
        Science & Behavior Books, 1967.
2664   *Minuchin, S. Conflict-resolution family therapy. *Psy-
        chiatry*, 1965, *28*, 278-286.
2665   *Haley, J. *Strategies of psychotherapy*. New York:
        Grune & Stratton, 1963.
2666   Zuk, G. H. The side-taking function in family therapy.
        American Journal of Orthopsychiatry, 1968, *38*, 553-559.
2667   Zuk, G. H. The go-between process in family therapy.
        Family Process, 1966, *5*, 162-178.
2668   Minuchin, S. & Montalvo, B. Techniques for working with
        disorganized low socioeconomic families. *American
        Journal of Orthopsychiatry*, 1967, *37*, 880-887.
2669   Lessing, E. E. & Phillips, R. L. Reduction of children's
        symptomatology through reduction of parental, child-
        focused anxiety: An exploratory study. *Psychotherapy:
        Theory, Research and Practice*, 1971, *8*, 158-164.

2670   Speck, R. B. Family therapy in the home. *Journal of Marriage and the Family*, 1964, *26*, 72-76.
2671   Weiner, L, Becker, A. & Friedmann, T. T. *Home treatment.* Pittsburgh: University of Pittsburgh Press, 1967.
2672   Chappel, J. N. & Daniels, R. S. Home visiting in a black urban ghetto. *American Journal of Psychiatry*, 1970, *126*, 1455-1460.
2673   Coughlin, F. & Wimberger, H. C. Group family therapy. *Family Process*, 1968, *7*, 37-50.
2674   Myrick, R. D. & Kelly, F. D. Group counseling with primary school-age children. *Journal of School Psychology*, 1971, *9*, 137-143.
2675   Pasnau, R. O., Williams, L. & Tallman, F. F. Small activity groups in the school: Report of a twelve year research project in community psychiatry. *Community Mental Health Journal*, 1971, *7*, 303-311.
2676   Stedman, J. M., Peterson, T. L. & Cardarelle, J. Application of a token system in a pre-adolescent boys' group. *Journal of Behavior Therapy and Experimental Psychiatry*, 1971, *2*, 23-29.
2677   Boll, T. J. Systematic observation of behavior change with older children in group therapy. *Psychological Reports*, 1971, *28*, 26.
2677.1 Boszormenyi-Nagy, I. & Spark, G. M. *Invisible loyalties; reciprocity in intergenerational family therapy.* Hagerstown, Md.: Medical Dept., Harper & Row, 1973.
2677.2 Liebman, R., Minuchin, S. & Baker, L. The role of the family in the treatment of anorexia nervosa. *Journal of the American Academy of Child Psychiatry*, 1974, *13*, 264-274.
2677.3 Liebman, R., Minuchin, S. & Baker, L. The use of structural family therapy in the treatment of intractable asthma. *American Journal of Psychiatry*, 1974, *131*, 535-540.
2677.4 Wellisch, D. & Hays, J. R. Development of family therapy as a new treatment modality in a drug abuse program for adolescents. In J. C. Schoolar (Ed.), *Current issues in adolescent psychiatry*. New York: Brunner/Mazel, 1973. Pp. 221-232.

GENERAL THEORETICAL/CLINICAL STUDIES

2678   *Winter W. D. & Ferreira, A. J. (Eds.) *Research in family interaction: Readings and commentary*. Palo Alto, Calif.: Science and Behavior Books, 1969.
2679   *Minuchin, S., et al. *Families of the slums: An exploration of their structure and treatment*. New York: Basic Books, 1967.
2680   Philp, A. F. *Family failure: A study of 129 families with multiple problems*. London: Faber & Faber, 1963.
2681   Ehrenwald, J. *Neuroses in the family and patterns of psychosocial defense*. New York: Hoeber, 1963.

2682   Fisher, S. & Mendell, D. The communication of neurotic patterns over two and three generations. *Psychiatry*, 1956, *19*, 41-46.

2683   Becker, J. & Iwakami, E. Conflict and dominance within families of disturbed children. *Journal of Abnormal Psychology*, 1969, *74*, 330-335.

2684   Stachowiak, J. G. Psychological disturbances in children as related to disturbances in family interaction. *Journal of Marriage and the Family*, 1968, *30*, 123-127.

2685   Spiegel, J. P. Some cultural aspects of transference and countertransference. *Science and Psychoanalysis*, 1959, *2*, 160-182.

2686   Speer, D. C., Fossum, M., Lippman, H. S., Schwartz, R. & Slocum, B. A comparison of middle-and lower-class families in treatment at a child guidance clinic. *American Journal of Orthopsychiatry*, 1968, *38*, 814-822.

2687   Serrano, A. C., et al. Adolescent maladjustment and family dynamics. *American Journal of Psychiatry*, 1962, *118*, 897-901.

2688   Counts, R. M. Family crises and the impulsive adolescent. *Archives of General Psychiatry*, 1967, *17*, 64-71.

2689   Miller, D. R. & Swanson, G. E. *The changing American parent: A study in the Detroit area.* New York: Wiley, 1958.

2690   Young, M. D. & Willmott, P. *Family and kinship in East London.* Harmondsworth, Middlesex, Eng.: Penguin Books, 1957.

2691   Hill, R. *Families under stress: Adjustment to the crises of war separation and reunion.* Westport, Conn.: Greenwood Press, 1971.

2692   Langsley, D. G., et al. Followup evaluation of family crisis therapy. *American Journal of Orthopsychiatry*, 1969, *39*, 753-759.

2693   Greenblatt, M., et al. *The prevention of hospitalization: Treatment without admission for psychiatric patients.* New York: Grune & Stratton, 1963.

2694   Newman, M. B. & San Martino, M. The child and the seriously disturbed parent: Treatment issues. *Journal of the American Academy of Child Psychiatry*, 1973, *12*, 162-181.

2695   Taylor, D. A. & Starr, P. The use of clinical services by adoptive parents: A review of some practice assumptions. *Journal of the American Academy of Child Psychiatry*, 1972, *11*, 384-399.

INTERACTIONAL AND TRANSACTIONAL THEORY

2696   *Watzlawick, P., Beavin, J. H. & Jackson, D. D. *Pragmatics of human communication.* New York: Norton, 1967.

2697   *Ruesch, J. & Bateson, G. *Communication, the social matrix of psychiatry.* New York: Norton, 1951.

2698   *Spiegel, J. P. *Transactions: The interplay between individual, family, and society.* New York: Science House, 1971.

2699   *Berne, E. *Transactional analysis in psychotherapy: A systematic approach to individual and social psychiatry.* New York: Grove Press, 1961.

2700   *Riskin, J. & Faunce, E. E. An evaluative review of family interaction research. *Family Process,* 1972, *11,* 365-455.

2701   Berne, E. *Games people play.* New York: Grove Press, 1964.

2702   Raybin, J. B. The curse: A study in family communication. *American Journal of Psychiatry,* 1970, *127,* 617-625.

2703   Dicks, H. V. *Marital tensions; clinical studies towards a psychological theory of interaction.* London: Routledge and Kegan Paul, 1967.

2704   Garner, A. M. & Wenar, C. *The mother-child interaction in psychosomatic disorders.* Urbana: University of Illinois Press, 1959.

2705   Wimberger, H. C. & Kogan, K. L. Interpersonal behavior ratings. *Journal of Nervous and Mental Diseases,* 1968, *147,* 260-271.

2706   Curry, A. E. The family therapy situation as a system. *Family Process,* 1966, *5,* 131-141.

2706.1 Wimberger, H. C. & Kogan, K. L. A direct approach to altering mother-child interaction in disturbed children. *Archives of General Psychiatry,* 1974, *30,* 636-639.

STUDIES OF SCHIZOPHRENIC FAMILIES

2707   *Mishler, E. G. & Waxler, N. E. Family interaction processes and schizophrenia: A review of current theories. *International Journal of Psychiatry,* 1966, *2,* 375-428.

2708   *Lidz, T. F., Fleck, S. & Cornelison, A. R. *Schizophrenia and the family.* New York: International Universities Press, 1965.

2709   *Zuk, G. H. & Rubinstein, D. A review of concepts in the study and treatment of families of schizophrenics. In I. Boszormenyi-Nagy & J. L. Framo (Eds.), *Intensive family therapy.* New York: Harper & Row, 1965. Pp. 1-37.

2710   *Laing, R. D. & Esterson, A. *Sanity, madness and the family.* (2nd ed.) London: Tavistock, 1970.

2711   Mosher, L. R., Wild, C., Valcov, A. & Feinstein, A. E. Cognitive style, schizophrenia, and the family: Methodological implications of contextual effects. *Family Process,* 1972, *11,* 125-146.

2712   Crabtree, L. H., Brecht, J. A. & Sonne, J. C. Monadic orientation: A contribution to the structure of families with autistic children. *Family Process,* 1972, *11,* 255-274.

2713   Sampson, H., Messinger, S. L. & Towne, R. D. *Schizophrenic women: Studies in marital crisis.* New York:
Atherton, 1964.

PSYCHOANALYTIC STUDIES OF FAMILIES

2714   *Winnicott, D. W. *The family and individual development.*
London: Tavistock, 1965.
2715   *Erikson, E. H. The life cycle: Epigenesis of identity.
In *Identity, youth and crisis.* New York: Norton,
1968. Pp. 91-141.
2716   Lomas, P. (Ed.) *The predicament of the family.* London:
Hogarth Press, 1967.
2717   Grotjahn, M. *Psychoanalysis and the family neurosis.*
New York: Norton, 1960.
2718   Ehrenwald, J. *Neurosis in the family and patterns of
psychosocial defense.* New York: Harper & Row, 1963.
2719   Flugel, J. C. *Man, morals and society: A psycho-
analytical study.* New York: International Universities
Press, 1945.
2720   Flugel, J. C. *The psycho-analytic study of the family.*
(6th ed.) London: Hogarth Press, 1939.

SPECIFIC SOCIAL WORK APPROACHES

2721   *The family is the patient: The group approach to treatment of family health problems.* New York: National
Association of Social Workers, 1965.
2722   Howarth, E., et al. *The Canford families; a study in
social casework and group work.* Keele, England:
University of Keele, 1962. (The Sociological Review. Monograph no. 6)
2723   Voiland, A. L., et al. *Family casework diagnosis.* New
York: Columbia University Press, 1962.

NETWORK THERAPY

2724   *Speck, R. V. & Attneave, C. L. *Family networks.* New
York: Pantheon Books, 1973.
2725   *Speck, R. V. & Rueveni, U. Network therapy--A developing
concept. *Family Process,* 1969, *8,* 182-191.
2726   Leichter, H. J. & Mitchell, W. E. *Kinship and casework.*
New York: Russell Sage Foundation, 1967.
2726.1 Johnson, D. L., Leler, H., Rios, L., Brandt, L., Kahn, A.
J., Mazeika, E., Frede, M. & Bisett, B. The Houston
parent-child development center: A parent education
program for Mexican-American families. *American Journal of Orthopsychiatry,* 1974, *44,* 121-128.

MARRIAGE THERAPY

2727   *Olsen, E. H. The marriage--A basic unit for psychother-
        apy. *American Journal of Psychiatry*, 1971, *127*,
        945-948.
2728   *O'Neill, N. & O'Neill, G. *Open marriage: A new life
        style for couples.* New York: M. Evans, 1972.
2729   *Haley, J. Marriage therapy. *Archives of General Psy-
        chiatry*, 1963, *8*, 213-234.
2730   *Jackson, D. D. Family rules: Marital quid pro quo.
        Archives of General Psychiatry, 1965, *12*, 589-594.
2731   Bach, G. R. & Wyden, P. *The intimate enemy.* New York:
        Morrow, 1969.
2732   Ryder, R. G., Kafka, J. S. & Olson, D. H. Separating and
        joining influences in courtship and early marriage.
        American Journal of Orthopsychiatry, 1971, *41*, 450-464.
2733   Greene, B. L. (Ed.) *The psychotherapies of marital dis-
        harmony.* New York: Free Press, 1965.
2734   Eisenstein, V. W. (Ed.) *Neurotic interaction in mar-
        riage.* New York: Basic Books, 1956.
2735   Bannister, K. & Pincus, L. *Shared phantasy in marital
        problems: Therapy in a four-person relationship.*
        London: Tavistock, 1965.

XVIII.   GROUP THERAPY

GENERAL THEORY OF GROUP THERAPY AND OF ADOLESCENTS IN GROUPS

2736   *Kestenberg, J. S. Phases of adolescence, with sugges-
        tions for a correlation of psychic and hormonal organ-
        izations: Part III. Puberty growth, differentiation,
        and consolidation. *Journal of the American Academy of
        Child Psychiatry*, 1968, *7*, 108-151.
2737   *Keniston, K. Social change and youth in America. In E.
        H. Erikson (Ed.), *The challenge of youth.* Garden
        City, N.Y.: Doubleday, 1965. Pp. 191-222.
2738   Fleck, S. An approach to family pathology. *Comprehen-
        sive Psychiatry*, 1966, *7*, 307-320.
2739   *Counts, R. M. Family crises and the impulsive adoles-
        cent. *Archives of General Psychiatry*, 1967, *17*, 64-71.
2740   *Freud, A. Adolescence as a developmental disturbance.
        In G. Caplan & S. Lebovici (Eds.), *Adolescence: Psy-
        chosocial perspectives.* New York: Basic Books, 1969.
        Pp. 5-10.
2741   *Anthony, E. J. The reactions of adults to adolescents
        and their behavior. In G. Caplan & S. Lebovici (Eds.),
        Adolescence: Psychosocial perspectives. New York:
        Basic Books, 1969. Pp. 54-78.
2742   *Foulkes, S. H. & Anthony, E. J. *Group psychotherapy:
        The psychoanalytic approach.* (2nd ed.) Harmondsworth,
        Middlesex, Eng.: Penguin, 1964.

2743   *Foulkes, S. H. Some basic concepts in group psychother-
       apy. In J. L. Moreno, et al. (Eds.), *The international
       handbook of group psychotherapy*. New York: Philosoph-
       ical Library, 1966. Pp. 166-172.
2744   *Sherwood, M. Bion's experiences in groups: A critical
       evaluation. *Human Relations*, 1964, *17*, 113-130.
2745   *Stoller, F. H. Accelerated interaction: A time-limited
       approach based on the brief, intensive group. *Inter-
       national Journal of Group Psychotherapy*, 1968, *18*,
       220-235.
2746   Sugar, M. Network psychotherapy of an adolescent. *Amer-
       ican Society for Adolescent Psychiatry*, 1971, *1*, 464-478.
2747   Speck, R. V. Psychotherapy of the social network of a
       schizophrenic family. *Family Process*, 1967, *6*, 208-214.
2748   Scheidlinger, S. The relationship of group therapy to
       other group influence attempts. *Mental Hygiene*, 1955,
       39, 376-390.
2749   *Parloff, M. B. Analytic group psychotherapy. In J.
       Marmor (Ed.). *Modern psychoanalysis*. New York: Basic
       Books, 1968. Pp. 492-531.
2750   *Bion, W. R. *Experiences in groups*. New York: Basic
       Books, 1961.
2751   *Yalom, I. D. *The theory and practice of group psycho-
       therapy*. New York: Basic Books, 1970.
2752   *Parad, H. J. *Crisis intervention: Selected readings*.
       New York: Family Service Association of America, 1965.
2753   Langsley, D. G., Kaplan, D. M., et al. *The treatment of
       families in crisis*. New York: Grune & Stratton, 1968.
2754   Berne, E. *Principles of group treatment*. New York:
       Oxford University Press, 1966.
2755   Perls, F. S., Hefferline, R. F. & Goodman, P. *Gestalt
       therapy*. New York: Julian Press, 1951.
2756   Slavson, S. R. *A textbook in analytic group psycho-
       therapy*. New York: International Universities Press,
       1964. Pp. 398-399.
2757   Malamud, D. I. & Machover, S. *Toward self-understanding:
       Group techniques in self-confrontation*. Springfield,
       Ill.: Thomas, 1965.
2758   *Jones, M. S., et al. *The therapeutic community*. New
       York: Basic Books, 1953.
2759   *Durkin, H. E. *The group in depth*. New York: Inter-
       national Universities Press, 1964.
2760   MacGregor, R., et al. *Multiple impact therapy with
       families*. New York: McGraw-Hill, 1964.
2761   Berne, E. *Games people play*. New York: Grove Press,
       1964.
2761.1 Sager, C. J. & Kaplan, H. S. (Eds.) *Progress in group
       and family therapy*. New York: Brunner/Mazel, 1972.
2761.2 Rose, S. D. *Treating children in groups*. San Francisco:
       Jossey-Bass, 1973.

YOUNG CHILDREN IN GROUP THERAPY/General Theory of Group Therapy
with Children

2762   *Ginott, H. G. Group therapy with children. In G. M.
        Gazda (Ed.), *Basic approaches to group psychotherapy
        and group counseling*. Springfield, Ill.: Thomas,
        1968. Pp. 176-194.
2763   *Coolidge, J. C. & Grunebaum, M. G. Individual and group
        therapy of a latency age child. *International Journal
        of Group Psychotherapy*, 1964, *14*, 84-96.
2764   *Kraft, I. A. Child and adolescent group psychotherapy.
        In H. I. Kaplan & B. J. Sadock (Eds.), *Comprehensive
        group psychotherapy*. Baltimore: Williams & Wilkins,
        1971. Pp. 534-565.
2765   *Geller, J. J. Group psychotherapy in child guidance
        clinics. *Current Psychiatric Therapies*, 1963, *3*,
        219-228.
2766   Rosenbaum, M. & Kraft, I. A. Group psychotherapy for
        children. In B. B. Wolman (Ed.), *Manual of child psy-
        chopathology*. New York: McGraw-Hill, 1972. Pp. 935-
        950.
2767   Epstein, N. Recent observations on group psychotherapy
        with adolescent delinquent boys in residential treat-
        ment. Round table. III. Activity group therapy.
        International Journal of Group Psychotherapy, 1960, *10*,
        180-194.
2768   *Field, L. W. An ego-programmed group treatment approach
        with emotionally disturbed boys. *Psychological Reports*,
        1966, *18*, 47-50.
2769   Boulanger, J. B. Group psychoanalytic therapy in child
        psychiatry. *Canadian Psychiatric Association Journal*,
        1961, *6*, 272-275.
2770   *Berkovitz, I. H., Chikahisa, P., Lee, M. L. & Murasaki,
        E. M. Psychosexual development of latency-age children
        and adolescents in group therapy in a residential set-
        ting. *International Journal of Group Psychotherapy*,
        1966, *16*, 344-356.
2771   Quinn, D. C., Robison, O. L. & Egan, M. H. Preadoles-
        cent girls in "transitional" group therapy. *American
        Journal of Orthopsychiatry*, 1969, *39*, 263-264.
2772   *Peck, M. L. & Stewart, R. H. Current practices in selec-
        tion criteria for goup play-therapy. *Journal of Clini-
        cal Psychology*, 1964, *20*, 146.
2773   Rickers-Ovsiankina, M. Social accessibility in three age
        groups. *Psychological Reports*, 1956, *2*, 283-294.
2774   Hart, J. T., et al. Interview group psychotherapy of
        boys and girls of latency age: A preliminary study.
        Journal of Psychoanalysis in Groups, 1968, *2(2)*, 9-14.
2775   Novick, J. I. Comparison between short-term group and
        individual psychotherapy in effecting change in non-
        desirable behavior in children. *International Journal
        of Group Psychotherapy*, 1965, *15*, 366-373.

2776   *Heinicke, C. M. & Goldman, A. Research on psychotherapy
        with children: A review and suggestions for further
        study. *American Journal of Orthopsychiatry*, 1960, *30*,
        483-494.
2777   *Watson, K. W. & Boverman, H. Preadolescent foster chil-
        dren in group discussions. *Children*, 1968, *15*, 65-70.
2778   Speroff, B. J. & Simon, D. Problems and approaches in
        child group psychotherapy in a public school milieu.
        Group Psychotherapy, 1963, *16*, 39-45.
2779   *Davidson, P. W. Comment on the small activity group
        (SAG) project of the Montebello Unified School District.
        Journal of School Health, 1965, *35*, 423-429.
2780   Ginott, H. G. *Group psychotherapy with children: The
        theory and practice of play-therapy.* New York: McGraw-
        Hill, 1961.
2781   *Schiffer, M. *The therapeutic play group.* New York:
        Grune & Stratton, 1969.
2781.1 Semonsky, C. & Zicht, G. Activity group parameters.
        Journal of the American Academy of Child Psychiatry,
        1974, *13*, 166-179.
2781.2 Abramowitz, S. I. & Abramowitz, C. V. Psychological-
        mindedness and benefit from insight-oriented group
        therapy. *Archives of General Psychiatry*, 1974, *30*,
        610-615.

YOUNG CHILDREN IN GROUP THERAPY/Behavior Modification in Groups

2782   *Hinds, W. C. A learning theory approach to group coun-
        seling with elementary school children. *Dissertation
        Abstracts*, 1969, *29*, 2524-2525.
2783   *Clement, P. W. & Milne, D. C. Group play therapy and
        tangible reinforcers used to modify the behavior of
        8-year-old boys. *Behaviour Research and Therapy*, 1967,
        5, 301-312.
2784   *Patterson, G. R. & Anderson, D. Peers as social rein-
        forcers. *Child Development*, 1964, *35*, 951-960.
2785   *Lazarus, A. A. Group therapy of phobic disorders by
        systematic desensitization. *Journal of Abnormal and
        Social Psychology*, 1961, *63*, 504-510.
2786   Paul, G. L. & Shannon, D. T. Treatment of anxiety
        through systematic desensitization in therapy groups.
        Journal of Abnormal Psychology, 1966, *71*, 124-135.
2787   Laws, D. R., Brown, R. A., Epstein, J. & Hocking, N.
        Reduction of inappropriate social behavior in dis-
        turbed children by an untrained paraprofessional ther-
        apist. *Behavior Therapy*, 1971, *2*, 519-533.
2788   *Gittelman, M. Behavior rehearsal as a technique in child
        treatment. *Journal of Child Psychology and Psychiatry
        and Allied Disciplines*, 1965, *6*, 251-255.

YOUNG CHILDREN IN GROUP THERAPY/Deprived Children

2789   *Ganter, G., Yeakel, M. & Polansky, N. A.   Intermediate
        group treatment of inaccessible children. *American
        Journal of Orthopsychiatry*, 1965, *35*, 739-746.
2790   *Frey, L. A. & Kolodny, R. L.   Group treatment for the
        alienated child in the school. *International Journal
        of Group Psychotherapy*, 1966, *16*, 321-337.
2791   *Scheidlinger, S.   Experiential group treatment of severely
        deprived latency-age children. *American Journal of
        Orthopsychiatry*, 1960, *30*, 356-368.
2792   *Christmas, J. J.   Group therapy with the disadvantaged.
        Current Psychiatric Therapies, 1966, *6*, 163-171.
2793   Westman, J. C., et al.   Parallel group psychotherapy with
        the parents of emotionally disturbed children. *Inter-
        national Journal of Group Psychotherapy*, 1963, *13*,
        52-60.

YOUNG CHILDREN IN GROUP THERAPY/Psychotic Children

2794   *Speers, R. W. & Lansing, C.   Group psychotherapy with
        preschool psychotic children and collateral group ther-
        apy of their parents: A preliminary report of the
        first two years. *American Journal of Orthopsychiatry*,
        1964, *34*, 659-666.
2795   Soble, D. & Geller, J. J.   A type of group psychotherapy
        in the children's unit of a mental hospital. *Psychiat-
        ric Quarterly*, 1964, *38*, 262-270.
2796   *Smolen, E. M. & Lifton, N.   A special treatment program
        for schizophrenic children in a child guidance clinic.
        American Journal of Orthopsychiatry, 1966, *36*, 736-742.
2797   *Anker, J. M. & Walsh, R. P.   Group psychotherapy, a spe-
        cial activity program, and group structure in the treat-
        ment of chronic schizophrenics. *Journal of Consulting
        Psychology*, 1961, *25*, 476-481.
2798   Gratton, L. & Rizzo, A. E.   Group therapy with young psy-
        chotic children. *International Journal of Group Psy-
        chotherapy*, 1969, *19*, 63-71.
2799   *Speers, R. W. & Lansing, C. *Group therapy in childhood
        psychosis.* Chapel Hill: University of North Carolina
        Press, 1965.
2800   Coffey, H. S. & Wiener, L. L. *Group treatment of autistic
        children.* Englewood Cliffs, N.J.: Prentice-Hall, 1967.

YOUNG CHILDREN IN GROUP THERAPY/Special Problems

2801   *Crutcher, R.   The usefulness of group therapy with char-
        acter disorders. *International Journal of Group Psy-
        chotherapy*, 1961, *11*, 431-439.
2802   Anderson, J. E   Group therapy with brain-damaged children.
        Hospital and Community Psychiatry, 1968, *19*, 175-176.

2803   *Cowen, E. L.   Psychotherapy and play techniques with the
       exceptional child and youth.   In W. M. Cruickshank (Ed.)
       Psychology of exceptional children and youth.   Engle-
       wood Cliffs, N.J.:   Prentice-Hall, 1962.   Pp. 520-575.
2804   *Burdon, A. P. & Neely, J. H.   Chronic school failure in
       boys: A short-term group therapy and educational ap-
       proach.   *American Journal of Psychiatry,* 1966, *122,*
       1211-1219.
2805   *Wohl, T. H.   The group approach to the asthmatic child
       and family.   *Journal of Asthma Research,* 1967, *4,*
       237-239.
2806   *Perl, W. R.   Use of fantasy for a breakthrough in psycho-
       therapy groups of hard-to-reach delinquent boys.   *In-
       ternational Journal of Group Psychotherapy,* 1963, *13,*
       27-33.
2807   *Morrison, G. C. & Collier, J. G.   Family treatment ap-
       proaches to suicidal children and adolescents.   *Journal
       of the American Academy of Child Psychiatry,* 1969, *8,*
       140-153.
2808   Heacock, D. R.   Modifications of the standard techniques
       for out-patient group psychotherapy with delinquent
       boys.   *Journal of the National Medical Association,*
       1966, *58,* 41-47.
2809   Taylor, A. J. W.   An evaluation of group psychotherapy in
       a girls' borstal.   *International Journal of Group Psy-
       chotherapy,* 1967, *17,* 168-177.
2810   Feder, B.   Limited goals in short-term group psychotherapy
       with institutionalized delinquent adolescent boys.   *In-
       ternational Journal of Group Psychotherapy,* 1962, *12,*
       503-507.
2811   Straight, B. & Werkman, S. L.   Control problems in group
       therapy with aggressive adolescent boys in a mental
       hospital.   *American Journal of Psychiatry,* 1958, *114,*
       998-1001.
2812   *Epstein, N. & Slavson, S. R.   Further observations on
       group psychotherapy with adolescent delinquent boys in
       residential treatment.   I.   "Breakthrough" in group
       treatment of hardened delinquent adolescent boys.   *In-
       ternational Journal of Group Psychotherapy,* 1962, *12,*
       199-210.
2813   *McNeil, E. B. & Morse, W. C.   The institutional manage-
       ment of sex in emotionally disturbed children.   *Ameri-
       can Journal of Orthopsychiatry,* 1964, *34,* 115-124.
2814   *Sadock, B. & Gould, R. E.   A preliminary report on short-
       term group psychotherapy on an acute adolescent male
       service.   *International Journal of Group Psychotherapy,*
       1964, *14,* 465-473.
2815   Rinsley, D. B.   The adolescent inpatient: Patterns of
       depersonification.   *Psychiatric Quarterly,* 1971, *45,*
       3-22.
2816   *Miezio, S.   Group therapy with mentally retarded adoles-
       cents in institutional settings.   *International Journal
       of Group Psychotherapy,* 1967, *17,* 321-327.

2816.1 Brandt, D. E. A descriptive analysis of selected aspects of group therapy with severely delinquent boys. *Journal of the American Academy of Child Psychiatry*, 1973, *12*, 473-481.

ADOLESCENTS IN GROUP THERAPY

2817 *Kraft, I. A. An overview of group therapy with adolescents. *International Journal of Group Psychotherapy*, 1968, *18*, 461-480.

2818 MacLennan, B. W., et al. *Group counseling and group psychotherapy with adolescents*. Washington: Institute for Youth Studies, Howard University, 1966.

2819 *Berkovitz, I. H. (Ed.) *Adolescents grow in groups*. New York: Brunner/Mazel, 1972.

2820 Richmond, A. H. & Schecter, S. A spontaneous request for treatment by a group of adolescents. *International Journal of Group Psychotherapy*, 1964, *14*, 97-106.

2821 *Kraft, I. A. The nature of sociodynamics and psychodynamics in a therapy group of adolescents. *International Journal of Group Psychotherapy*, 1960, *10*, 313-320.

2822 *Lebovici, S. Psychodrama as applied to adolescents. *Journal of Child Psychology and Psychiatry and Allied Disciplines*, 1961, *1*, 298-305.

2823 *Pumpian-Mindlin, E. Omnipotentiality, youth, and commitment. *Journal of the American Academy of Child Psychiatry*, 1965, *4*, 1-18.

2824 *Fried, E. Ego emancipation of adolescents through group psychotherapy. *International Journal of Group Psychotherapy*, 1956, *6*, 358-373.

2825 Rosenbaum, M. Group therapy with adolescents. In B. B. Wolman (Ed.), *Manual of child psychopathology*. New York: McGraw-Hill, 1972. Pp. 951-968.

2826 Duffy, J. H. & Kraft, I. A. Beginning and middle phase characteristics of group psychotherapy of early adolescent boys and girls. *Journal of Psychoanalysis in Groups*, 1966-67, *2(1)*, 23-29.

2827 *Godenne, G. D. Outpatient adolescent group psychotherapy. I. Review of the literature on use of co-therapists, psychodrama, and parent group therapy. *American Journal of Psychotherapy*, 1964, *18*, 584-593.

2828 Godenne, G. D. Outpatient adolescent group psychotherapy. II. Use of co-therapists, psychodrama, and parent group therapy. *American Journal of Psychotherapy*, 1965, *19*, 40-53.

2829 Kaufmann, P. N. & Deutsch, A. L. Group therapy for pregnant unwed adolescents in the prenatal clinic of a general hospital. *International Journal of Group Psychotherapy*, 1967, *17*, 309-320.

2830 Knorr, N. J., Clower, C. G. & Schmidt, C. W. Mixed adult and adolescent group therapy. *American Journal of Psychotherapy*, 1966, *20*, 323-331.

2831   Slavson, S. R. Further observations on group psychotherapy with adolescent delinquent boys in residential treatment. II. Patterns of acting out of a transference neurosis by an adolescent boy. *International Journal of Group Psychotherapy*, 1962, *12*, 211-224.

2832   *Schulman, I. The dynamics of certain reactions of delinquents to group psychotherapy. *International Journal of Group Psychotherapy*, 1952, *2*, 334-343.

2833   *Westman, J. C. Group psychotherapy with hospitalized delinquent adolescents. *International Journal of Group Psychotherapy*, 1961, *11*, 410-418.

2834   *Sarason, I. G. & Ganzer, V. J. Developing appropriate social behaviors of juvenile delinquents. In J. D. Krumboltz & C. E. Thoresen (Eds.), *Behavioral counseling: Cases and techniques*. New York: Holt, Rinehart & Winston, 1969. Pp. 178-193.

2834.1   Herrick, R. H. & Binger, C. M. Group psychotherapy for early adolescents: An adjunct to a comprehensive treatment program. *Journal of the American Academy of Child Psychiatry*, 1974, *13*, 110-125.

TRAINING IN GROUP THERAPY

2835   *Stein, A. The training of the group psychotherapist. In M. Rosenbaum & M. Berger (Eds.), *Group psychotherapy and group function*. New York: Basic Books, 1963. Pp. 558-576.

2836   Ebersole, G. O., Leiderman, P. H. & Yalom, I. D. Training the nonprofessional group therapist. *Journal of Nervous and Mental Disease*, 1969, *149*, 294-302.

2837   *Berger, M. M. Problems of anxiety in group psychotherapy trainees. In M. Rosenbaum & M. M. Berger (Eds.), *Group psychotherapy and group function*. New York: Basic Books, 1963. Pp. 555-557.

2838   *Yalom, I. D. Problems of neophyte group therapists. *International Journal of Social Psychiatry*, 1966, *12*, 52-59.

2839   Harrow, M., et al. Influence of the psychotherapist on the emotional climate in group therapy. *Human Relations*, 1967, *20*, 49-64.

2840   *Horwitz, L. Transference in training groups and therapy groups. *International Journal of Group Psychotherapy*, 1964, *14*, 202-213.

2841   Schulman, I. Transference, resistance and communication problems in adolescent psychotherapy groups. *International Journal of Group Psychotherapy*, 1959, *9*, 496-503.

2842   *Spruiell, V. Countertransference and an adolescent group crisis. *International Journal of Group Psychotherapy*, 1967, *17*, 298-308.

2843 *Goodman, M., Marks, M. & Rockberger, H. Resistance in group psychotherapy enhanced by the countertransference reactions of the therapist: A peer group experience. *International Journal of Group Psychotherapy*, 1964, *14*, 332-343.

2844 *Grotjahn, M. Special aspects of countertransference in analytic group psychotherapy. *International Journal of Group Psychotherapy*, 1953, *3*, 407-416.

2845 Slavson, S. R. Sources of countertransference and group-induced anxiety. *International Journal of Group Psychotherapy*, 1953, *3*, 373-388.

2846 *Truax, C. B., Carkhuff, R. R. & Kodman, F. Relationships between therapist-offered conditions and patient change in group psychotherapy. *Journal of Clinical Psychology*, 1965, *21*, 327-329.

2847 Morton, R. B. The uses of the laboratory method in a psychiatric hospital. In E. H. Schein & W. G. Bennis, *Personal and organizational change through group methods: The laboratory approach.* New York: Wiley, 1965. Pp. 114-151.

2848 *Frank, J. D. Training and therapy. In L. P. Bradford, J. R. Gibb & K. D. Benne (Eds.), *T-Group theory and laboratory method: Innovation in re-education.* New York: Wiley, 1964. Pp. 442-451.

2849 Kaplan, S. R. Therapy groups and training groups: Similarities and differences. *International Journal of Group Psychotherapy*, 1967, *17*, 473-504.

2850 *Warkentin, J. An experience in teaching psychotherapy by means of group therapy. In M. Rosenbaum & M. Berger (Eds.), *Group psychotherapy and group function.* New York: Basic Books, 1963. Pp. 577-584.

2851 Grotjahn, M. Analytic group therapy with psychotherapists. *International Journal of Group Psychotherapy*, 1969, *19*, 326-333.

2852 *Yalom, I. D. & Handlon, J. H. The use of multiple therapists in the teaching of psychiatric residents. *Journal of Nervous and Mental Disease*, 1965, *141*, 684-692.

2853 *Kraft, I. A. Multiple impact therapy as a teaching device. *Psychiatric Research Reports of the American Psychiatric Association*, 1966, *20*, 218-223.

ISSUES AND RESEARCH IN GROUP THERAPY

2854 *Maslow, A. H. The need to know and the fear of knowing. *Journal of General Psychology*, 1963, *68*, 111-125.

2855 Culbert, S. A. *The interpersonal process of self-disclosure: It takes two to see one.* (Explorations in Applied Behavioral Science, No. 3) New York: Renaissance Editions, 1968.

2856 *Masterson, J. F. The symptomatic adolescent five years later: He didn't grow out of it. *American Journal of Psychiatry*, 1967, *123*, 1338-1345.

2857   *Rinsley, D. B. Theory and practice of intensive residential treatment of adolescents. The fifth annual Edward A. Strecker Memorial Lecture. *Psychiatric Quarterly*, 1968, *42*, 611-638.

2858   Cartwright, D. & Zander, A. (Eds.) *Group dynamics: Research and theory.* (3rd ed.) New York: Harper & Row, 1968.

2859   *Yalom, I. D., Houts, P. S., Newell, G. & Rand, K. H. Preparation of patients for group therapy: A controlled study. *Archives of General Psychiatry*, 1967, *17*, 416-427.

2860   Tuckman, B. Developmental sequence in small groups. *Psychological Bulletin*, 1965, *63*, 384-399.

2861   *Kline, F. M. Dynamics of a leaderless group. *International Journal of Group Psychotherapy*, 1972, *22*, 234-242.

2862   Slavson, S. R. Criteria for selection and rejection of patients for various types of group therapy. *International Journal of Group Psychotherapy*, 1955, *5*, 3-30.

2863   *Yalom, I. D. & Rand, K. Compatibility and cohesiveness in therapy groups. *Archives of General Psychiatry*, 1966, *15*, 267-275.

2864   Cartwright, D. The nature of group cohesiveness. In D. Cartwright & A. Zander (Eds.), *Group dynamics: Research and theory.* (3rd ed.) New York: Harper & Row, 1968. Pp. 91-109.

2865   *Anthony, E. J. Age and syndrome in group psychotherapy. In A. L. Kadis & C. Winick, (Eds.), *Topical problems of psychotherapy.* Vol. 5. *Group psychotherapy today.* New York: Karger, 1965. Pp. 80-89.

2866   Lieberman, M. A. The implications of a total group phenomena: Analysis for patients and therapists. *International Journal of Group Psychotherapy*, 1967, *17*, 71-81.

2867   *Bandura, A. Modelling approaches to the modification of phobic disorders. In *The role of learning in psychotherapy.* London: J. & A. Churchill, 1968. Pp. 201-217. (CIBA Foundation Symposium)

2868   *Brown, S. L. Diagnosis, clinical management and family interviewing. *Science and Psychoanalysis*, 1969, *14*, 188-198.

2869   *Anthony, E. J. Reflections on twenty-five years of group psychotherapy. *International Journal of Group Psychotherapy*, 1968, *18*, 277-301.

2870   *Pattison, E. M. Evaluation studies of group psychotherapy. *International Journal of Group Psychotherapy*, 1965, *15*, 382-397.

2871   *Feifel, H. & Eells, J. Patients and therapists assess the same psychotherapy. *Journal of Consulting Psychology*, 1963, *27*, 310-318.

2872 *Shapiro, D. & Birk, L. Group therapy in experimental per-
      spective. *International Journal of Group Psychotherapy*,
      1967, *17*, 211-224.
2873 Polansky, N. A., Miller, S. C. & White, R. B. Some res-
      ervations regarding group psychotherapy in inpatient
      psychiatric treatment. *Group Psychotherapy*, 1955, *8*,
      254-262.
2874 *Yalom, I. D., Houts, P. S., Zimerberg, S. M. & Rand, K. H.
      Prediction of improvement in group therapy: An explor-
      atory study. *Archives of General Psychiatry*, 1967, *17*,
      159-168.
2875 *Pattison, E. M., Brissenden, A. & Wohl, T. Assessing
      specific effects of inpatient group psychotherapy. *In-
      ternational Journal of Group Psychotherapy*, 1967, *17*,
      283-297.
2876 Bavelas, A., et al. Experiments on the alteration of
      group structure. In D. Cartwright & A. Zander (Eds.),
      Group dynamics: Research and theory. (3rd ed.) New
      York: Harper & Row, 1968. Pp. 527-537.
2877 Burnstein, E. & Zajonc, R. B. The effect of group success
      on the reduction of status incongruence in task-oriented
      groups. *Sociometry*, 1965, *28*, 349-362.
2878 Berger, M. M. & Rosenbaum, M. Notes on help-rejecting
      complainers. *International Journal of Group Psychother-
      apy*, 1967, *17*, 357-370.
2879 *Kanter, S. S., et al. A comparison of oral and genital
      aspects in group psychotherapy. *International Journal
      of Group Psychotherapy*, 1964, *14*, 158-165.
2880 *Yalom, I. D. A study of group therapy dropouts. *Archives
      of General Psychiatry*, 1966, *14*, 393-414.
2881 Berzon, B., Pious, C. & Farson, R. E. The therapeutic
      event in group psychotherapy: A study of subjective
      reports by group members. *Journal of Individual Psy-
      chology*, 1963, *19*, 204-212.
2882 Kassoff, A. I. Advantages of multiple therapists in a
      group of severely acting-out adolescent boys. *Inter-
      national Journal of Group Psychotherapy*, 1958, *8*, 70-75.
2883 *Churchill, S. R. Social group work: A diagnostic tool
      in child guidance. *American Journal of Orthopsychiatry*,
      1965, *35*, 581-588.
2884 Abrahams, D. & Enright, J. Psychiatric intake in groups:
      A pilot study of procedures, problems and prospects.
      American Journal of Psychiatry, 1965, *122*, 170-174.
2884.1 Kronick, D. Some thoughts on group identification: So-
      cial needs. *Journal of Learning Disabilities*, 1974, *7*,
      144-147.

XIX. BEHAVIOR MODIFICATION IN LEARNING
AND BEHAVIOR PROBLEMS

2885 *Baer, D. M. & Wolf, M. M. The reinforcement contingency in pre-school and remedial education. In R. D. Hess & R. M. Bear (Eds.), *Early education*. Chicago: Aldine, 1968. Pp. 119-129.

2886 *Allen, K. E., Turner, K. D. & Everett, P. M. A behavior modification classroom for Head Start children with behavior problems. *Exceptional Children*, 1970, *37*, 119-127.

2887 *Hewett, F. M., Taylor, F. D. & Artuso, A. A. The Santa Monica Project: Evaluation of an engineered classroom design with emotionally disturbed children. *Exceptional Children*, 1969, *35*, 523-529.

2888 *O'Leary, K. D., Becker, W. C., Evans, M. B. & Saudargas, R. A. A token reinforcement program in a public school: A replication and systematic analysis. *Journal of Applied Behavior Analysis*, 1969, *2*, 3-13.

2889 *Brown, D. G. Behavior modification with children. *Mental Hygiene*, 1972, *56*, 22-30.

2890 Wahler, R. G. & Erickson, M. Child behavior therapy: A community program in Appalachia. *Behaviour Research and Therapy*, 1969, *7*, 71-78.

2891 Schwarz, M. L. & Hawkins, R. P. Application of delayed reinforcement procedures to the behavior of an elementary school child. *Journal of Applied Behavior Analysis*, 1970, *3*, 85-96.

2892 *Cantrell, R. P., Cantrell, M. L., Huddleston, C. M. & Wooldridge, R. L. Contingency contracting with school problems. *Journal of Applied Behavior Analysis*, 1969, *2*, 215-220.

2893 *Chan, A., Chin, A. & Mueller, D. J. An integrated approach to the modification of classroom failure and disruption: A case study. *Journal of School Psychology*, 1970, *8*, 114-121.

2894 *Haring, N. G. & Lovitt, T. C. Operant methodology and educational technology in special education. In N. G. Haring and R. L. Schiefelbusch (Eds.), *Methods in special education*. New York: McGraw-Hill, 1967. P. 12.

2895 Fargo, G. A., Behrns, C. & Nolen, P. (Eds.) *Behavior modification in the classroom*. Belmont, Calif.: Wadsworth, 1970.

2896 Axelrod, S. Token reinforcement programs in special classes. *Exceptional Children*, 1971, *37*, 371-379.

2897 Broden, M., Hall, R. V., Dunlap, A. & Clark, R. Effects of teacher attention and a token reinforcement system in a junior high school special education class. *Exceptional Children*, 1970, *36*, 341-349.

2898 Blom, G. E. A psychoanalytic viewpoint of behavior modification in clinical and educational settings. *Journal of the American Academy of Child Psychiatry*, 1972, *11*, 675-693.

2898.1 Ross, A. O. *Psychological disorders of children; a behavioral approach to theory, research, and therapy.* New York: McGraw-Hill, 1974.

2898.2 Hewett, R. M. Educational programs for children with behavior disorders. In H. C. Quay & J. S. Werry (Eds.), *Psychopathological disorders of childhood.* New York: Wiley, 1972. Pp. 388-413.

2898.3 Rutter, M. & Sussenwein, F. A developmental and behavioral approach to the treatment of preschool autistic children. *Journal of Autism and Childhood Schizophrenia,* 1971, *1,* 376-397.

2898.4 Ney, P. G., Palvesky, A. E. & Markely, J. Relative effectiveness of operant conditioning and play therapy in childhood schizophrenia. *Journal of Autism and Childhood Schizophrenia,* 1971, *1,* 337-349.

2898.5 Risley, T. R. & Baer, D. M. Operant behavior modification: The deliberate development of behavior. In B. M. Caldwell & H. N. Ricciuti (Eds.), *Review of child development research.* Vol. 3. *Child development and social policy.* Chicago: University of Chicago Press, 1973. Pp. 283-330.

2898.6 Ney, P. G. Effect of contingent and non-contingent reinforcement on the behavior of an autistic child. *Journal of Autism and Childhood Schizophrenia,* 1973, *3,* 115-127.

XX. PHARMACOTHERAPY OF CHILDREN

HISTORICAL AND THEORETICAL ISSUES IN DRUG RESEARCH

2899 Fish, B. Methodology in child psychopharmacology. In D. H. Efron, et al. (Eds.), *Psychopharmacology, a review of progress, 1957-1967.* Washington: U. S. Govt. Print. Off., 1969. Pp. 989-1001. (U. S. Public Health Service publication no. 1836)

2900 *Kornetsky, C. Psychoactive drugs in the immature organism. *Psychopharmacologia,* 1970, *17,* 105-136.

2901 Zrull, J. P., Westman, J. C. Arthur, B. & Rice, D. L. An evaluation of methodology used in the study of psychoactive drugs for children. *Journal of the American Academy of Child Psychiatry,* 1966, *5,* 284-291.

2902 Fish, B. Problems of diagnosis and the definition of comparable groups: A neglected issue in drug research with children. *American Journal of Psychiatry,* 1969, *125,* 900-908.

2903 *Benson, W. M. Symposium on "some current research methods and results with special reference to the central nervous system": Pharmacological approach. *American Journal of Mental Deficiency,* 1960, *65,* 172-181.

2904 Minde, K. K. & Weiss, G. C. The assessment of drug effects in children as compared to adults. *Journal of* the *American Academy of Child Psychiatry*, 1970, *9*, 124-133.

2905 Bender, L. & Cottington, F. The use of amphetamine sulfate (Benzedrine) in child psychiatry. *American Journal of Psychiatry*, 1942, *99*, 116-121.

2906 Bradley, C. The behavior of children receiving Benzedrine. *American Journal of Psychiatry*, 1937, *94*, 577-585.

2907 Cytryn, L., Gilbert, A. & Eisenberg, L. The effectiveness of tranquilizing drugs plus supportive psychotherapy in treating behavior disorders of children: A double-blind study of eighty outpatients. *American Journal of Orthopsychiatry*, 1960, *30*, 113-128.

2908 Eisenberg, L, Gilbert, A., Cytryn, L. & Molling, P. A. The effectiveness of psychotherapy alone and in conjunction with perphenazine or placebo in the treatment of neurotic and hyperkinetic children. *American Journal of Psychiatry*, 1961, *117*, 1088-1093.

2909 *Fish, B. Drug therapy in child psychiatry: Pharmacological aspects. *Comprehensive Psychiatry*, 1960, *1*, 212-227.

2910 *Eisenberg, L., et al. A psychopharmacologic experiment in a training school for delinquent boys: Methods, problems, findings. *American Journal of Orthopsychiatry*, 1963, *33*, 431-447.

2911 Freedman, A. M., Effron, A. S. & Bender, L. Pharmacotherapy in children with psychiatric illness. *Journal of Nervous and Mental Disease*, 1955, *122*, 479-486.

2912 Fish, B. & Shapiro, T. A typology of children's psychiatric disorders. I. Its application to a controlled evaluation of treatment. *Journal of the American Academy of Child Psychiatry*, 1965, *4*, 32-52.

2913 *Fish, B. The "one child, one drug" myth of stimulants in hyperkinesis: Importance of diagnostic categories in evaluating treatment. *Archives of General Psychiatry*, 1971, *25*, 193-203.

2914 *Freeman, R. D. Drug effects on learning in children: A selective review of the past thirty years. *Journal of Special Education*, 1966, *1*, 17-44.

2914.1 Boullin, D. J. & O'Brien, R. A. Uptake and loss of ^{14}C-dopamine by platelets from children with infantile autism. *Journal of Autism and Childhood Schizophrenia*, 1972, *2*, 67-74.

MAJOR TRANQUILIZERS/Phenothiazine Controlled Studies

2915 *Fish, B., Shapiro, T. & Campbell, M. Long-term prognosis and the response of schizophrenic children to drug therapy: A controlled study of trifluoperazine. *American Journal of Psychiatry*, 1966, *123*, 32-39.

2916 *Freed, H. & Peifer, C. A. Some considerations on the use of chlorpromazine in a child psychiatry clinic. *Journal of Clinical and Experimental Psychopathology and Quarterly Review of Psychiatry and Neurology*, 1956, *17*, 164-169.

2917 Hunt, B. R., Frank, T. & Krush, T. P. Chlorpromazine in the treatment of severe emotional disorders of children. *American Journal of Diseases of Children*, 1956, *91*, 268-277.

2918 *Fish, B. Drug use in psychiatric disorders of children. *American Journal of Psychiatry*, 1968, *124*(no. 8 Supplement), 31-36.

2919 *Shaw, C. R., Lockett, H. J., Lucas, A. R., Lamontagne, C. H. & Grimm, F. Tranquilizer drugs in the treatment of emotionally disturbed children: I. Inpatients in a residential treatment center. *Journal of the American Academy of Child Psychiatry*, 1963, *2*, 725-742.

2920 Miksztal, M. W. Chlorpromazine (Thorazine) and reserpine in residential treatment of neuropsychiatric disorders in children. *Journal of Nervous and Mental Disease*, 1956, *123*, 477-479.

2921 *Kenny, T. J., Badie, D. & Baldwin, R. W. The effectiveness of a new drug, mesoridazine, and chlorpromazine with behavior problems in children. *Journal of Nervous and Mental Disease*, 1968, *147*, 316-321.

2922 *Eisenberg, L., Gilbert, A., Cytryn, L. & Molling, P. A. The effectiveness of psychotherapy alone and in conjunction with perphenazine or placebo in the treatment of neurotic and hyperkinetic children. *American Journal of Psychiatry*, 1961, *117*, 1088-1093.

2923 *Tarjan, G., Lowery, V. E. & Wright, S. W. Use of chlorpromazine in two hundred seventy-eight mentally deficient patients. *American Journal of Diseases of Children*, 1957, *94*, 294-300.

2924 *Schulman, J. L. & Clarinda, S. M. The effect of promazine on the activity level of retarded children. *Pediatrics*, 1964, *33*, 271-275.

2925 *LaVeck, G. D. & Buckley, P. The use of psychopharmacologic agents in retarded children with behavior disorders. *Journal of Chronic Diseases*, 1961, *13*, 174-183.

2926 Craft, M. Tranquilizers in mental deficiency: Chlorpromazine. *Journal of Mental Deficiency Research*, 1957, *1*, 91-95.

2927 Smith, S. W. Trifluoperazine in children and adolescents with marked behavior problems. *American Journal of Psychiatry*, 1965, *122*, 702-703.

2928 Morton-Gore, N. Combined tranquillisation in the treatment of adolescents exhibiting the schizophrenic syndrome. *Journal of Mental Subnormality*, 1964, *10*, 53-62.

2929 *Werry, J. S., Weiss, G., Douglas, V. & Martin, J. Studies on the hyperactive child. III: The effect of chlorpromazine upon behavior and learning ability. *Journal* *of the American Academy of Child Psychiatry*, 1966, *5*, 292-312.

2930   Porteus, S. D. & Barclay, J. E. A further note on chlorpromazine: Maze reactions. *Journal of Consulting Psychology*, 1957, *21*, 297-299.

2931   Helper, M. M., Wilcott, R. C. & Garfield, S. L. Effects of chlorpromazine on learning and related processes in emotionally disturbed children. *Journal of Consulting Psychology*, 1963, *27*, 1-9.

2932   Ison, M. G. The effect of "Thorazine" on Wechsler scores. *American Journal of Mental Deficiency*, 1957, *62*, 543-547.

2933   *Molling, P. A., Lockner, A. W., Sauls, R. J. & Eisenberg, L. Committed delinquent boys: The impact of perphenazine and of placebo. *Archives of General Psychiatry*, 1962, *7*, 70-76.

2934   *Rettig, J. H. Chlorpromazine and Mysoline in the control of convulsive epilepsy in mentally deficient patients. *Journal of Nervous and Mental Disease*, 1956, *124*, 607-611.

2935   Pauig, P. M., Deluca, M. A. & Osterheld, R. G. Thioridazine hydrochloride in the treatment of behavior disorders in epileptics. *American Journal of Psychiatry*, 1961, *117*, 832-833.

2936   Ilem, P. G. & Osterheld, R. G. Adjunctive therapy of refractory epilepsy with Prozine. *Diseases of the Nervous System*, 1960, *21*, 326-329.

2936.1   Engelhardt, D. M., Polizos, P., Waizer, J. & Hoffman, S. P. A double-blind comparison of fluphenazine and haloperidol in outpatient schizophrenic children. *Journal of Autism and Childhood Schizophrenia*, 1973, *3*, 115-127.

2936.2   Waizer, J., Polizos, P., Hoffman, S. P., Engelhardt, D. M. & Margolis, R. A. A single-blind evaluation of thiothixene with outpatient schizophrenic children. *Journal of Autism and Childhood Schizophrenia*, 1972, *2*, 378-386.

MAJOR TRANQUILIZERS/Non-Phenothiazine Controlled Studies

2937   *Cunningham, M. A., Pillai, V. & Rogers, W. J. B. Haloperidol in the treatment of children with severe behaviour disorders. *British Journal of Psychiatry*, 1968, *114*, 845-854.

2938   Harman, C. & Winn, D. A. Clinical experience with chlorprothixene in disturbed children: A comparative study. *International Journal of Neuropsychiatry*, 1966, *2*, 72-77.

2939   *Timberlake, W. H., Belmont, E. H. & Ogonik, J. The effect of reserpine in 200 mentally retarded children. *American Journal of Mental Deficiency*, 1957, *62*, 61-66.

2940   Noce, R. H., Williams, D. B. & Rapaport, W. Reserpine (Serpasil) in the management of the mentally ill and mentally retarded. *Journal of the American Medical Association,* 1954, *156,* 821-824.

2941   Graham, B. D., Rosenblum, S. & Callahan, R. J. Placebo-controlled study of reserpine in maladjusted retarded children. *American Journal of Diseases of Children,* 1958, *96,* 690-695.

2942   Carter, C. H. The effects of reserpine and methyl-phenidylacetate (Ritalin) in mental defectives, spastics, and epileptics. *Psychiatric Research Reports of the American Psychiatric Association,* 1956, *4,* 44-48.

2942.1 McAndrew, J. B., Case, Q. & Treffert, D. A. Effects of prolonged phenothiazine intake on psychotic and other hospitalized children. In S. Chess & A. Thomas (Eds.), *Annual progress in child psychiatry and child development: 1973.* New York: Brunner/Mazel, 1974. Pp. 619-635.

STIMULANTS AND ANTI-DEPRESSANTS/Stimulants

2943   Clements, S. D. *Minimal brain dysfunction in children; terminology and identification, phase one of three-phase project.* Washington, D.C.: U. S. Govt. Print. Off., 1966. (NINDB monograph no. 3) (Public Health Service publication, no. 1415)

2944   *Werry, J. S. Developmental hyperactivity. *Pediatric Clinics of North America,* 1968, *15,* 581-599.

2945   *Conners, C. K. Symptom patterns in hyperkinetic, neurotic, and normal children. *Child Development,* 1970, *41,* 667-682.

2946   Knobel, M., Wolman, M. B. & Mason, E. Hyperkinesis and organicity in children. *Archives of General Psychiatry,* 1959, *1,* 310-321.

2947   *Laufer, M. W. & Denhoff, E. Hyperkinetic behavior syndrome in children. *Journal of Pediatrics,* 1957, *50,* 463-474.

2948   Millichap, J. G. & Boldrey, E. E. Studies in hyperkinetic behavior. II. Laboratory and clinical evaluations of drug treatments. *Neurology,* 1967, *17,* 467-471.

2950   *Stevens, D. A., Boydstun, J. A., Dykman, R. A., Peters, J. E. & Sinton, D. W. Presumed minimal brain dysfunction in children: Relationship to performance on selected behavioral tests. *Archives of General Psychiatry,* 1967, *16,* 281-285.

2951   Stevens, J. R., Sachdev, K. & Milstein, V. Behavior disorders of childhood and the electroencephalogram. *Archives of Neurology,* 1968, *18,* 160-177.

2952   Lindsley, D. B. & Henry, C. E. The effect of drugs on behavior and the electroencephalograms of children with behavior disorders. *Psychosomatic Medicine,* 1942, *4,* 140-149.

2953   *Menkes, M. M., Rowe, J. S. & Menkes, J. H. A twenty-five year follow-up study on the hyperkinetic child with minimal brain dysfunction. *Pediatrics*, 1967, *39*, 393-399.

2954   *Zrull, J. P., Westman, J. C., Arthur, B. & Rice, D. L. A comparison of diazepam, d-amphetamine and placebo in the treatment of the hyperkinetic syndrome in children. *American Journal of Psychiatry*, 1964, *121*, 388-389.

2955   *Sprague, R. L., Barnes, K. R. & Werry, J. S. Methylphenidate and thioridazine: Learning, reaction time, activity, and classroom behavior in disturbed children. *American Journal of Orthopsychiatry*, 1970, *40*, 615-628.

2956   Millichap, J. G., Aymat, F., Sturgis, L. H., Larsen, K. W. & Egan, R. A. Hyperkinetic behavior and learning disorders: III. Battery of neuropsychological tests in controlled trial of methylphenidate. *American Journal of Diseases of Children*, 1968, *116*, 235-244.

2957   *Weiss, G., Werry, J., Minde, K., Douglas, V. & Sykes, D. Studies on the hyperactive child--V. The effects of dextroamphetamine and chlorpromazine on behaviour and intellectual functioning. *Journal of Child Psychology and Psychiatry and Allied Disciplines*, 1968, *9*, 145-156.

2958   *Conners, C. K. The effect of Dexedrine on rapid discrimination and motor control of hyperkinetic children under mild stress. *Journal of Nervous and Mental Disease*, 1966, *142*, 429-433.

2959   Bradley, C. & Greene, E. Psychometric performance of children receiving amphetamine (Benzedrine) sulfate. *American Journal of Psychiatry*, 1940, *97*, 388-394.

2960   *Bender, L. & Cottington, F. The use of amphetamine sulfate (Benzedrine) in child psychiatry. *American Journal of Psychiatry*, 1942, *99*, 116-121.

2961   *Conners, C. K. & Eisenberg, L. The effects of methylphenidate on symptomatology and learning in disturbed children. *American Journal of Psychiatry*, 1963, *120*, 458-464.

2962   Conners, C. K., Eisenberg, L. & Barcai, A. Effect of dextroamphetamine on children: Studies on subjects with learning disabilities and school behavior problems. *Archives of General Psychiatry*, 1967, *17*, 478-485.

2963   Bradley, C. The behavior of children receiving Benzedrine. *American Journal of Psychiatry*, 1937, *94*, 577-585.

2964   Knights, R. M. & Hinton, G. G. The effects of methylphenidate (Ritalin) on the motor skills and behavior of children with learning problems. *Journal of Nervous and Mental Disease*, 1969, *148*, 643-653.

2965   *Epstein, L. C., Lasagna, L., Connors, C. K. & Rodriguez, A. Correlation of dextroamphetamine excretion and drug response in hyperkinetic children. *Journal of Nervous and Mental Disease*, 1968, *146*, 136-146.

2966   *Creager, R. O. & Van Riper, C. The effect of methylphenidate on the verbal productivity of children with cerebral dysfunction. *Journal of Speech and Hearing Research*, 1967, *10*, 623-628.

2967   Geller, S. J. Comparison of a tranquilizer and a psychic
        energizer used in treatment of children with behavioral
        disorders. *Journal of the American Medical Association*,
        1960, *174*, 481-484.
2968   Jacobs, J. A controlled trial of Deaner and a placebo in
        mentally defective children. *British Journal of Clini-
        cal Practice*, 1965, *19*, 77-86.
2969   Bell, A. & Zubek, J. P. Effects of deanol on the intel-
        lectual performance of mental defectives. *Canadian
        Journal of Psychology*, 1961, *15*, 172-175.
2970   Kurland, A. A., Dorf, H. J., Michaux, M. H. & Goldberg,
        J. B. Cypenamine treatment of mentally retarded chil-
        dren. *Current Therapeutic Research*, 1967, *9*, 293-297.
2971   Barnett, C. D. & Lampert, R. Effects of Metrazol on in-
        tellectual functioning in defectives. *Psychological
        Reports*, 1957, *3*, 551-554.

STIMULANTS AND ANTI-DEPRESSANTS/Anti-Depressants

2972   *Frommer, E. A. Treatment of childhood depression with
        antidepressant drugs. *British Medical Journal*, 1967,
        1, no. 5542, 729-732.
2973   *Kurtis, L. B. Clinical study of the response to nortrip-
        tyline on autistic children. *International Journal of
        Neuropsychiatry*, 1966, *2*, 298-301.
2974   *Rapoport, J. Childhood behavior and learning problems
        treated with Imipramine. *International Journal of
        Neuropsychiatry*, 1965, *1*, 635-642.
2975   Splitter, S. R. & Kaufman, M. A new treatment for under-
        achieving adolescents: Psychotherapy combined with
        nortriptyline medication. *Psychosomatics*, 1966, *7*,
        171-174.
2976   Carter, C. H. Nortriptyline HCl as a tranquilizer for
        disturbed mentally retarded patients: A controlled
        study. *American Journal of the Medical Sciences*, 1966,
        251, 465-467.
2977   Davies, T. S. A monoamine oxidase inhibitor (Niamid) in
        the treatment of the mentally subnormal. *Journal of
        Mental Science*, 1961, *107*, 115-118.
2978   Smith, E. H. & Gonzalez, R. Nortriptyline hydrochloride
        in the treatment of enuresis in mentally retarded boys.
        American Journal of Mental Deficiency, 1967, *71*, 825-
        827.
2979   *Werry, J. S. & Cohrssen, J. Enuresis--an etiologic and
        therapeutic study. *Journal of Pediatrics*, 1965, *67*,
        423-431.
2980   Huessy, H. R. & Wright, A. L. The use of imipramine in
        children's behavior disorders. *Acta Paedopsychiatrica*,
        1970, *37*, 194-199.
2981   Fisher, G. W., Murray, F., Walley, M. R. & Kiloh, L. G.
        A controlled trial of imipramine in the treatment of

nocturnal enuresis in mentally subnormal patients. *American Journal of Mental Deficiency*, 1963, *67*, 536-538.

2982   *Poussaint, A. F. & Ditman, K. S.   A controlled study of imipramine (Tofranil) in the treatment of childhood enuresis. *Journal of Pediatrics*, 1965, *67*, 283-290.

MINOR TRANQUILIZERS

2983   *Effron, A. S. & Freedman, A. M.   The treatment of behavior disorders in children with Benadryl: A preliminary report. *Journal of Pediatrics*, 1953, *42*, 261-266.

2984   Segal, L. J. & Tansley, A. E.   A clinical trial with hydroxyzine (Atarax) on a group of maladjusted educationally subnormal children. *Journal of Mental Science*, 1957, *103*, 677-681.

2985   *Craft, M.   Tranquilizers in mental deficiency: Meprobamate. *Journal of Mental Deficiency*, 1958, *2*, 17-20.

2986   Craft, M.   Tranquillizers in mental deficiency: Hydroxyzine. *Journal of Mental Science*, 1957, *103*, 855-857.

2987   Pilkington, T. L.   Comparative effects of Librium and Taractan on behavior disorders of mentally retarded children. *Diseases of the Nervous System*, 1961, *22*, 573-575.

2988   Heaton-Ward, W. A.   Inference and suggestion in a clinical trial (Niamid in Mongolism). *Journal of Mental Science*, 1962, *108*, 865-870.

GLUTAMIC ACID, DILANTIN, ETC.

2989   *Looker, A. & Conners, C. K.   Diphenylhydantoin in children with severe temper tantrums. *Archives of General Psychiatry*, 1970, *23*, 80-89.

2990   Lefkowitz, M. M.   Effects of Diphenylhydantoin on disruptive behavior: Study of male delinquents. *Archives of General Psychiatry*, 1969, *20*, 643-651.

2991   *Pasamanick, B.   Anticonvulsant drug therapy of behavior problem children with abnormal electroencephalograms. *Archives of Neurology and Psychiatry*, 1951, *65*, 752-766.

2992   *Zimmerman, F. T. & Burgemeister, B. B.   A controlled experiment of glutamic acid therapy: First report summarizing thirteen years of study. *Archives of Neurology and Psychiatry*, 1959, *81*, 639-648.

2993   Vogel, W., Broverman, D. M., Draguns, J. G. & Klaiber, E. L.   The role of glutamic acid in cognitive behaviors. *Psychological Bulletin*, 1966, *65(6)*, 367-382.

2994   Lombard, J. P., Gilbert, J. G. & Donofrio, A. F.   The effects of glutamic acid upon the intelligence, social maturity and adjustment of a group of mentally retarded children. *American Journal of Mental Deficiency*, 1955, *60*, 122-132.

2995   Zimmerman, F. T. & Burgemeister, B. B.   Permanency of
        glutamic acid treatment. *Archives of Neurology and
        Psychiatry*, 1951, *65*, 291-298.
2996   Houze, M., Wilson, H. D., & Goodfellow, H. D. L.   Treat-
        ment of mental deficiency with alpha tocopherol. *Amer-
        ican Journal of Mental Deficiency*, 1964, *69*, 328-329.

PSYCHOTROPIC DRUG REVIEW ARTICLES

2997   Bradley, C.   Tranquilizing drugs in pediatrics. *Pediat-
        rics*, 1958, *21*, 325-336.
2998   Bender, L. & Faretra, G.   Organic therapy in pediatric
        psychiatry. *Diseases of the Nervous System*, 1961, *22*,
        110-111.
2999   *Lourie, R. S.   Psychoactive drugs in pediatrics. *Pediat-
        rics*, 1964, *34*, 691-693.
3000   Shaw, C. R. & Lucas, A. R.   Psychopharmacologic treatment.
        In *The psychiatric disorders of childhood*. (2nd ed.)
        New York: Appleton-Century-Crofts, 1970. Pp. 436-456.
3001   *Eisenberg, L.   Role of drugs in treating disturbed chil-
        dren. *Children*, 1964, *11*, 167-173.
3002   *Eveloff, H. H.   Psychopharmacologic agents in child psy-
        chiatry: A survey of the literature since 1960. *Ar-
        chives of General Psychiatry*, 1966, *14*, 472-481.
3004   *Conners, C. K. & Rothschild, G. H.   Drugs and learning in
        children in learning disorders. *Seattle Special Child
        Publications*, 1968, *3*, 191-224.
3005   *Freeman, R. D.   Drug effects on learning in children: A
        selective review of the past thirty years. *Journal of
        Special Education*, 1966, *1*, 17-44.
3006   *Cole, J. O.   The amphetamines in child psychiatry: A
        review. *Seminars in Psychiatry*, 1969, *1*, 174-178.
3007   Copeland, R.   A critical review: Psychopharmacological
        experimentation with the mentally retarded. In J. O.
        Smith & T. C. Lovitt (Eds.), *Selected papers: Medical
        aspects of mental retardation and neuromuscular dys-
        function*. Lawrence, Kansas: University of Kansas
        Press, 1965. Pp. 263-278.
3008   *Millichap, J. G.   Drugs in management of hyperkinetic and
        perceptually handicapped children. *Journal of the Amer-
        ican Medical Association*, 1968, *206*, 1527-1530.
3008.1 Campbell, M., Fish, B., Korein, J., Shapiro, T., Collins,
        P. & Koh, C.   Lithium and chlorpromazine: A controlled
        crossover study of hyperactive severely disturbed young
        children. *Journal of Autism and Childhood Schizophre-
        nia*, 1972, *2*, 234-263.

ARTICLES WITH IMPLICATIONS FOR TREATMENT, DIAGNOSIS, ETC.

3009   *Levy, S.   Post-encephalitic behavior disorder--A for-
        gotten entity: A report of 100 cases. *American Journal*

of Psychiatry, 1959, *115,* 1062-1067.
3010 *Knobel, M. Brief communications: The environmental 'antidrug' effect. *Psychiatry,* 1960, *23,* 403-407.
3011 Weiss, B. & Laties, V. G. Enhancement of human performance by caffeine and the amphetamines. *Pharmacological Reviews,* 1962, *14,* 1-36.
3012 Irwin, S. & Benuazizi, A. Pentylenetetrazol enhances memory function. *Science,* 1966, *152,* 100-102.
3013 Callaway, E. The influence of amobarbital (Amylobarbitone) and methamphetamine on the focus of attention. *Journal of Mental Science,* 1959, *105,* 382-392.
3014 Chapel, J. L., Brown, N. & Jenkins, R. L. Tourette's disease: Symptomatic relief with haloperidol. *American Journal of Psychiatry,* 1964, *121,* 608-610.
3015 Mautner, H. Drug therapy in cerebral palsy. *Archives of Pediatrics,* 1956, *73,* 351-381.
3015.1 Kolvin, I., Taunch, J., Currah, J., Garside, R. F., Nolan, J. & Shaw, W. B. Enuresis: A descriptive analysis and a controlled trial. *Developmental Medicine and Child Neurology,* 1972, *14,* 714-726.
3015.2 Winsberg, B. G., Bialer, I., Kupietz, S. & Tobias, J. Effects of imipramine and dextroamphetamine on behavior of neuropsychiatrically impaired children. *American Journal of Psychiatry,* 1972, *128,* 1425-1431.
3015.3 Campbell, M., Fish, B., Korein, J., Shapiro, T., Collins, P. & Koh, C. Lithium and chlorpromazine: A controlled crossover study of hyperactive severely disturbed young children. In S. Chess & A. Thomas (Eds.), *Annual progress in child psychiatry and child development: 1973.* New York: Brunner/Mazel, 1974. Pp. 589-618.

BOOKS

3016 Fisher, S. (Ed.) *Child research in psychopharmacology.* Springfield, Ill.: Thomas, 1959.
3017 Freed, H. *The chemistry and therapy of behavior disorders in children.* Springfield, Ill.: Thomas, 1962.
3018 Klein, D. F. & Davis, J. M. *Diagnosis and drug treatment of psychiatric disorders.* Baltimore: Williams & Wilkins, 1969.
3019 *Strauss, A. A. & Lehtinen, L. E. *Psychopathology and education of the brain-injured child.* New York: Grune & Stratton, 1947-55.
3019.1 *Pharmacotherapy of children.* Washington, D.C.: National Institute of Mental Health, 1973. (DHEW publication no. (HSM) 73-9002)

XXI.   RESIDENTIAL TREATMENT OF CHILDREN

VARIETIES OF RESIDENTIAL CARE

3020   *Robinson, J. F. The use of residence in psychiatric treatment with children. *American Journal of Psychiatry*, 1947, *103*, 814-817.

3021   *Alt, H. *Residential treatment for the disturbed child: Basic principles in planning and design of programs and facilities.* New York: International Universities Press, 1961.

3022   *Benjamin, A. & Weatherly, H. E. Hospital ward treatment of emotionally disturbed children. *American Journal of Orthopsychiatry*, 1947, *17*, 665-674.

3023   *Bloch, D. A. Residential treatment for disturbed children. *Nursing Outlook*, 1957, *5*, 636-638.

3024   *Berman, S. P. Some lessons learned in developing a residential treatment center. *Child Welfare*, 1961, *40*(4), 12-18.

3025   *Bettelheim, B. A psychiatric school. *Quarterly Journal of Child Behavior*, 1949, *1*, 86-95.

3026   *Fenichel, C., Freedman, A. M. & Klapper, Z. A day school for schizophrenic children. *American Journal of Orthopsychiatry*, 1960, *30*, 130-143.

3027   Bradley, C. Indications for residential treatment of children with severe neuropsychiatric problems. *American Journal of Orthopsychiatry*, 1949, *19*, 427-431.

3028   Lennhoff, F. G. *Exceptional children: Residential treatment of emotionally disturbed boys at Shotton Hall.* (2nd ed.) London: Allen & Unwin, 1966.

3029   *Pollack, M. & Goldfarb, W. Patterns of orientation in children in residential treatment for severe behavior disorders. *American Journal of Orthopsychiatry*, 1957, *27*, 538-552.

3030   *Adessa, S. & Laatsch, A. Extended residential treatment: Eighth-year anxiety. *Social Work*, 1965, *10*(4), 16-24.

3031   Finkelstein, H. The use of court commitment in the residential treatment of disturbed children. *Social Casework*, 1964, *45*, 605-609.

3032   Laybourne, P. C. & Miller, H. C. Pediatric hospitalization of psychiatric patients: Diagnostic and therapeutic implications. *American Journal of Orthopsychiatry*, 1962, *32*, 596-603.

3033   *LaVietes, R. L., Hulse, W. C. & Blau, A. A psychiatric day treatment center and school for young children and their parents. *American Journal of Orthopsychiatry*, 1960, *30*, 468-482.

3034   *Peck, H. B. The role of the psychiatric day hospital in a community mental health program: A group process approach. *American Journal of Orthopsychiatry*, 1963, *33*, 482-493.

3035   LaVietes, R. L., Cohen, R., Reens, R. & Ronall, R. Day treatment center and school: Seven years experience. *American Journal of Orthopsychiatry*, 1965, *35*, 160-169.

3036 *Newman, R. The way back: Extramural schooling as a transitional phase of residential therapy. *American Journal of Orthopsychiatry*, 1960, *30*, 588-598.

3037 Naughton, F. X. After-care: The treatment center's responsibility. *Child Welfare*, 1958, *37*(10), 7-10.

3038 Lesser, S. R. A nursery school for atypical children in a general psychiatric hospital. *Nervous Child*, 1952, *10*, 163-166.

3039 Pfeiffer, E. A modified nursery school program in a mental hospital. *American Journal of Orthopsychiatry*, 1959, *29*, 780-790.

3040 *Middleman, R. & Seever, F. Short-term camping for boys with behavior problems. *Social Work*, 1963, *8*(2), 88-95.

3041 *Gula, M. Group homes--New and differentiated tools in child welfare, delinquency, and mental health. *Child Welfare*, 1964, *43*, 393-397.

3042 *Freud, A. & Dann, S. An experiment in group upbringing. *Psychoanalytic Study of the Child*, 1951, *6*, 127-168. (*Writings*, vol. 4, Pp. 163-229)

3043 Gavrin, J. B. & Sacks, L. S. Growth potential of preschool-aged children in institutional care: A positive approach to a negative condition. *American Journal of Orthopsychiatry*, 1963, *33*, 399-408.

3044 Fildes, L. G. Hostels for children in need of psychiatric attention. *Mental Health* (London), 1944, *5*, 31-32.

3045 *Noshpitz, J. D. Youth pervades half-way house at NIMH. *Mental Hospitals*, 1959, *10*(5), 25-30.

3046 *Winnicott, D. W. Children's hostels in war and peace. *British Journal of Medical Psychology*, 1948, *21*, 175-180.

3047 Whiles, W. H. Treatment of maladjusted children in hostels. *Journal of Mental Science*, 1955, *101*, 404-412.

3048 *Williams, J. M. Children who break down in foster homes: A psychological study of patterns of personality growth in grossly deprived children. *Journal of Child Psychology and Psychiatry and Allied Disciplines*, 1961, *2*, 5-20.

3049 *Naughton, F. X. Foster home placement as an adjunct to residential treatment. *Social Casework*, 1957, *38*, 288-295.

USES OF THE MILIEU

3050 *Redl, F. The concept of a "therapeutic milieu." *American Journal of Orthopsychiatry*, 1959, *29*, 721-736.

3051 Lander, J. & Schulman, R. The impact of the therapeutic milieu on the disturbed personality. *Social Casework*, 1960, *41*, 227-234.

3052 *Bettelheim, B. & Sylvester, E. Milieu therapy: Indications and illustrations. *Psychoanalytic Review*, 1949, *36*, 54-68.

3053   *Goldsmith, J. M., Schulman, R. & Grossbard, H. Integrating clinical processes with planned living experiences. *American Journal of Orthopsychiatry*, 1954, *24*, 280-290.

3054   Benjamin, A. Environmental therapy. *Child Welfare*, 1961, *40*(5), 13-14.

3055   Bettelheim, B. & Sylvester, E. Therapeutic influence of the group on the individual. *American Journal of Orthopsychiatry*, 1947, *17*, 684-692.

3056   *Blum, A. Peer-group structure and a child's verbal accessibility in a treatment institution. *Social Service Review*, 1962, *36*, 385-395.

3057   Devereux, G. The social structure of the hospital as a factor in total therapy. *American Journal of Orthopsychiatry*, 1949, *19*, 492-500.

3058   Goldstein, I. M., Judas, I., Sutton, H. A. & Falstein, E. I. Adjustment patterns of leadership and defenses in a disturbed child group. *Archives of Neurology and Psychiatry*, 1957, *77*, 312-317.

3059   *Konopka, G. The role of residential treatment for children. Symposium, 1954. 4. The role of the group in residential treatment. *American Journal of Orthopsychiatry*, 1955, *25*, 679-684.

3060   *Henry, J. The culture of interpersonal relations in a therapeutic institution for emotionally disturbed children. *American Journal of Orthopsychiatry*, 1957, *27*, 725-734.

3061   Winnicott, D. W. & Britton, C. Residential management as treatment for difficult children. *Human Relations*, 1947, *1*, 87-97.

3062   *Maier, H. W. & Campbell, S. G. Childhood psychosis. 3. Routines: A pilot study of three selected routines and their impact upon the child in residential treatment. *American Journal of Orthopsychiatry*, 1957, *27*, 701-709.

3063   *Scher, J. M. The structured ward: Research method and hypothesis in a total treatment setting for schizophrenia. *American Journal of Orthopsychiatry*, 1958, *28*, 291-299.

3064   *Wenar, C. The therapeutic value of setting limits with inhibited children. *Journal of Nervous and Mental Disease*, 1957, *125*, 390-395.

3065   McNeil, E. B. & Morse, W. C. The institutional management of sex in emotionally disturbed children. *American Journal of Orthopsychiatry*, 1964, *34*, 115-124.

3066   Gair, D. S., Bullard, D. M., Jr. & Corwin, J. H. Residential treatment. Seclusion of children as a therapeutic ward practice. *American Journal of Orthopsychiatry*, 1965, *35*, 251-252.

3067   Freeman, R. V. Contaminants of permissiveness in hospital care. *American Journal of Psychiatry*, 1954, *111*, 52-54.

3068   Konopka, G. Implications of a changing residential treat-
        ment program. Workshop, 1960. *American Journal of
        Orthopsychiatry*, 1961, *31*, 17-39.
3069   Baxter, M. J. House council--An integral part of residen-
        tial treatment for disturbed children. *Catholic Chari-
        ties Review*, 1963, *47*(5), 13-19.
3070   Adessa, S. & Laatsch, A. Therapeutic use of visiting in
        residential treatment. *Child Welfare*, 1965, *44*, 245-
        251.
3071   *Rioch, D. McK. & Stanton, A. H. Milieu therapy. *Psychi-
        atry*, 1953, *16*, 65-72.
3071.1 Benedek, E. P. & Salguero, R. A summer day treatment
        service program. *Journal of the American Academy of
        Child Psychiatry*, 1973, *12*, 724-737.

THERAPEUTIC METHODS

3072   *Krug, O. The application of principles of child psycho-
        therapy in residential treatment. *American Journal of
        Psychiatry*, 1952, *108*, 695-700.
3073   *Escalona, S. K. Some considerations regarding psycho-
        therapy with psychotic children. *Bulletin of the Men-
        ninger Clinic*, 1948, *12*, 126-134.
3074   Szurek, S. A. Child therapy procedures. *Psychiatry*,
        1944, *7*, 9-14.
3075   *Fraiberg, S. Some aspects of residential casework with
        children. *Social Casework*, 1956, *37*, 159-167.
3076   *Frank, G. Joint interviewing in a residential treatment
        center. *Journal of Jewish Communal Service*, 1962, *38*,
        385-390.
3077   Greenwood, E. D. The role of residential treatment for
        children. Symposium, 1954. 6. The role of psycho-
        therapy in residential treatment. *American Journal of
        Orthopsychiatry*, 1955, *25*, 692-698.
3078   Krug, O., Hayward, H. & Crumpacker, B. Intensive resi-
        dential treatment of a nine-year-old girl with an ag-
        gressive behavior disorder, petit mal epilepsy and en-
        uresis. *American Journal of Orthopsychiatry*, 1952, *22*,
        405-427.
3079   Ekstein, R. Round table: Child schizophrenia. The
        space child's time machine: On "reconstruction" in the
        psychotherapeutic treatment of a schizophrenoid child.
        American Journal of Orthopsychiatry, 1954, *24*, 492-506.
3080   Wise, L. J., et al. Residential treatment of a ten-year-
        old boy: Problems in the differential diagnosis and
        treatment of marked destructive behavior. Workshop
        1952. In G. E. Gardner (Ed.), *Case studies in child-
        hood emotional disabilities*. Vol. 1. New York: Amer-
        ican Orthopsychiatric Association, 1953. Pp. 331-368.
3081   *Redl, F. The life space interview. Workshop, 1957. 1.
        Strategy and techniques of the life space interview.

American Journal of Orthopsychiatry, 1959, *29*, 1-18.

3082 *Whitaker, C. A. Ormsby Village: An experiment with forced psychotherapy in the rehabilitation of the delinquent adolescent. *Psychiatry*, 1946, *9*, 239-250.

3083 Wineman, D. The life-space interview. *Social Work*, 1959, *4*(1), 3-17.

3084 *Dittman, A. T. & Kitchener, H. L. The life space interview. Workshop, 1957. 2. Life space interviewing and individual play therapy: A comparison of techniques. *American Journal of Orthopsychiatry*, 1959, *29*, 19-26.

3085 Redl, F. New ways of ego support in residential treatment of disturbed children. *Bulletin of the Menninger Clinic*, 1949, *13*, 60-66.

3086 Gerard, M. W. & Overstreet, H. M. Technical modification in the treatment of a schizoid boy within a treatment institution. *American Journal of Orthopsychiatry*, 1953, *23*, 171-185.

3087 *Scheidlinger, S. Social group work in psychiatric residential settings. Panel, 1955. *American Journal of Orthopsychiatry*, 1956, *26*, 709-750.

3088 Stewart, K. K. & Axelrod, P. L. Group therapy on a children's psychiatric ward: Experiment combining group therapy with individual therapy and resident treatment. *American Journal of Orthopsychiatry*, 1947, *17*, 312-325.

3088.1 Treffert, D. A., McAndrew, J. B. & Dreifurst, P. An inpatient treatment program and outcome for 57 autistic and schizophrenic children. *Journal of Autism and Childhood Schizophrenia*, 1973, *3*, 138-153.

FAMILY INVOLVEMENT

3089 *Mandelbaum, A. Parent-child separation: Its significance to parents. *Social Work*, 1962, *7*(4), 26-34.

3090 Howells, J. G. Child-parent separation as a therapeutic procedure. *American Journal of Psychiatry*, 1963, *119*, 922-926.

3091 Lane, L. The natural parent in institutional child placement. *Journal of Jewish Communal Service*, 1957, *33*, 305-313.

3092 McCann, M., Berwald, C. D. & Eldridge, K. Work with parents in a residential treatment center. *Child Welfare*, 1961, *40*(3), 9-16.

3093 *Cohen, R. L., Charny, I. W. & Lembke, P. Parental expectations as a force in treatment: The identification of unconscious parental projections onto the children's psychiatric hospital. *Archives of General Psychiatry*, 1961, *4*, 471-478.

3094 *Fochios, S. E. The use of families and family members as therapeutic levers in the treatment of disturbed delinquent children. *Child Welfare*, 1965, *44*, 556-562.

3095 *Davies, I. J., et al. Therapy with a group of families in a psychiatric day center. *American Journal of Orthopsychiatry*, 1966, *36*, 134-146.

3096 *Szurek, S. A. The family and the staff in hospital psychiatric therapy of children. *American Journal of Orthopsychiatry*, 1951, *21*, 597-611.

3097 *Szurek, S. A. & Berlin, I. N. Elements of psychotherapeutics with the schizophrenic child and his parents. *Psychiatry*, 1956, *19*, 1-9.

3098 Polskin, S. Working with parents of mentally ill children in residential care. *Social Work*, 1961, *6*, 82-89.

3099 *Peck, H. B., Rabinovitch, R. D. & Cramer, J. B. A treatment program for parents of schizophrenic children. *American Journal of Orthopsychiatry*, 1949, *19*, 592-598.

3100 Reidy, J. J. Family treatment approaches. 1. An approach to family-centered treatment in a state institution. *American Journal of Orthopsychiatry*, 1962, *32*, 133-142.

3101 *Behrens, M. L. & Goldfarb, W. A study of patterns of interaction of families of schizophrenic children in residential treatment. *American Journal of Orthopsychiatry*, 1958, *28*, 300-312.

3102 Mayer, M. F. The parental figures in residential treatment. *Social Service Review*, 1960, *34*, 273-285.

THE STAFF

3103 *Hirschberg, J. C. & Mandelbaum, A. Problems of administration and supervision in an inpatient treatment center for children. *Bulletin of the Menninger Clinic*, 1957, *21*, 208-219.

3104 *Bloch, D. A. & Silber, E. The role of the administrator in relation to individual psychotherapy in a residential treatment setting. *American Journal of Orthopsychiatry*, 1957, *27*, 69-74.

3105 *Sheimo, S. L., Paynter, J. & Szurek, S. A. Problems of staff interaction with spontaneous group formations on a children's psychiatric ward. *American Journal of Orthopsychiatry*, 1949, *19*, 599-611.

3106 Szurek, S. A. Dynamics of staff interaction in hospital psychiatric treatment of children. *American Journal of Orthopsychiatry*, 1947, *17*, 652-664.

3107 *Bettelheim, B. & Wright, B. Staff development in a treatment institution. *American Journal of Orthopsychiatry*, 1955, *25*, 705-719.

3108 Berlin, I. N. & Christ, A. E. The unique role of the child psychiatry trainee on an inpatient or day care unit. *Journal of the American Academy of Child Psychiatry*, 1969, *8*, 247-258.

3109 Bowers, S. The social worker in a children's residential treatment program. *Social Casework*, 1957, *38*, 283-288.

3110 *Boatman, M. J., Paynter, J. & Parsons, C. Nursing in the psychiatric treatment of children--Panel, 1961. 3. Nursing in hospital psychiatric therapy for psychotic children. *American Journal of Orthopsychiatry*, 1962, *32*, 808-817.

3111   Sutton, H. A. Some nursing aspects of a children's psychiatric ward. *American Journal of Orthopsychiatry*, 1947, *17*, 675-683.

3112   Schrager, J. A focus for supervision of residential staff in a treatment institution. *Bulletin of the Menninger Clinic*, 1954, *18*, 64-71.

3113   *Schrager, J. Child care staff recording in a treatment institution. *Social Casework*, 1955, *36*, 74-81.

3114   Maier, H. W., Hilgeman, L. M., Shugart, G. & Loomis, E. A., Jr. The role of residential treatment for children. Symposium, 1954. 7. Supervision of child care workers in a residential treatment service. *American Journal of Orthopsychiatry*, 1955, *25*, 699-704.

3115   *Bettelheim, B. Training the child-care worker in a residential center. *American Journal of Orthopsychiatry*, 1966, *36*, 694-705.

3116   *Montalvo, B. & Pavlin, S. Faulty staff communications in a residential treatment center. *American Journal of Orthopsychiatry*, 1966, *36*, 706-711.

3117   *Rabkin, L., Weinberger, G. & Klein, A. What made Allen run? The process of communication in residential treatment. *Journal of the American Academy of Child Psychiatry*, 1966, *5*, 272-283.

3118   *Alt, H. Symposium, 1953. The education of emotionally disturbed children. 2. Responsibilities and qualifications of the child care worker. *American Journal of Orthopsychiatry*, 1953, *23*, 670-675.

3119   Berwald, J. F. Cottage parents in a treatment institution. *Child Welfare*, 1960, *39*(10), 7-10.

3120   *Robinson, J. F. The role of the resident professional worker. *American Journal of Orthopsychiatry*, 1949, *19*, 674-682.

3121   Matsushima, J. & Berwald, C. D. The group worker's contribution in residential treatment of a disturbed boy. *Social Service Review*, 1965, *39*, 300-309.

3122   *Wasserman, S. & Gitlin, P. Child care worker training experience: A coordinated effort between classroom and agency. *Child Welfare*, 1963, *42*, 392-398.

3123   Weinstein, M. Adaptive patterns and theoretical implications of the mother-complex housemother. *Mental Hygiene*, 1963, *47*, 622-631.

3124   Sheimo, S. L. Problems encountered in dealing with handicapped and emotionally disturbed children. *American Journal of Occupational Therapy*, 1949, *3*, 303-307.

3125   Schrager, J. Observations on the loss of a housemother. *Social Casework*, 1956, *37*, 120-126.

3126   *Zellner, S. K. Recreational therapy experiences with mentally ill children. *Mental Hospitals*, 1955, *6*(4), 4-5.

3127   Liebman, R. T. "S.O.R.T. Room" activities aid young
       patients. *Mental Hospitals*, 1955, *6*(2), 4-5.
3128   Sucgang, R. C. Orienting new students in a residential
       treatment institution. *Federal Probation*, 1955, *19*(4),
       24-31.
3129   *Edelman, A. M. Some observations on occupational therapy
       with disturbed children in a residential program. *American Journal of Occupational Therapy*, 1953, *7*, 113-117.
3130   *Forbing, S. E. The teaching of schizophrenic children.
       In S. A. Szurek, I. N. Berlin & M. J. Boatman (Eds.),
       Inpatient care for the psychotic child. Palo Alto,
       Calif.: Science & Behavior Books, 1971. Pp. 206-214.
3131   Douglas, K. B. The teacher's role in a children's psy-
       chiatric hospital unit. *Exceptional Children*, 1961,
       27, 246-251.
3132   *Razy, V. The value of dance and percussion in the treat-
       ment of emotionally disturbed children. *Social Case-
       work*, 1961, *42*, 501-505.
3133   Phelan, J. F. The role of the volunteer in a residential
       treatment school. *Federal Probation*, 1959, *23*(3), 13-
       20.
3134   *Christ, A. E. & Wagner, N. N. Residential treatment.
       Iatrogenic factors in residential treatment: The psy-
       chiatric team's contribution to continued psychopathol-
       ogy. *American Journal of Orthopsychiatry*, 1965, *35*,
       253-254.
3135   *McNeil, E. & Cohler, R. Adult aggression in the manage-
       ment of disturbed children. *Child Development*, 1958,
       29, 451-461.
3136   Gunning, S. V. & Holmes, T. H. Dance therapy with psy-
       chotic children: Definition and quantitative evalua-
       tion. *Archives of General Psychiatry*, 1973, *28*, 707-
       713.
3137   *Szurek, S. A., Berlin, I. N. & Boatman, M. J. (Eds.)
       Inpatient care for the psychotic child. Palo Alto,
       Calif.: Science & Behavior Books, 1971.

USE OF EDUCATION

3138   *Hirschberg, J. C. Symposium, 1953. The education of
       emotionally disturbed children. 4. The role of edu-
       cation in the treatment of emotionally disturbed child-
       ren through planned ego development. *American Journal
       of Orthopsychiatry*, 1953, *23*, 684-690.
3139   *Toussieng, P. W. The role of education in a residential
       treatment center for children. *Mental Hygiene*, 1961,
       45, 543-551.
3140   *LaVietes, R. The teacher's role in the education of the
       emotionally disturbed child. *American Journal of Or-
       thopsychiatry*, 1962, *32*, 854-862.
3141   *Newman, R. G. Conveying essential messages to the emo-

tionally disturbed child at school. *Exceptional Children*, 1961, *28*, 199-204.

3142 Rabinow, B. The role of residential treatment for children. Symposium, 1954. 5. The role of the school in dential treatment. *American Journal of Orthopsychiatry*, 1955, *25*, 685-691.

3143 *Cohen, R. S. Some childhood identity disturbances: Educational implementation of a psychiatric treatment plan. *Journal of the American Academy of Child Psychiatry*, 1964, *3*, 488-499.

3144 *Bernstein, M. Use of public school for children in residential treatment. *Child Welfare*, 1960, *39*(6), 18-24.

3145 Kitchener, H. L. The life space interview in the school setting--Workshop, 1961. 2. The life space interview in the differentiation of school in residential treatment. *American Journal of Orthopsychiatry*, 1963, *33*, 720-722.

CARE OF DELINQUENTS

3146 *Aichhorn, A. (1925) *Wayward youth*. New York: Viking Press, 1935.

3147 *Aichhorn, A. Some remarks on the psychic structure and social care of a certain type of female juvenile delinquents. *Psychoanalytic Study of the Child*, 1949, *3-4*, 439-448.

3148 Noshpitz, J. D. & Spielman, P. Diagnosis: Study of the differential characteristics of hyperaggressive children. *American Journal of Orthopsychiatry*, 1961, *31*, 111-122.

3149 *Szurek, S. A. Some impressions from clinical experience with delinquents. In K. R. Eissler (Ed.), *Searchlights on delinquency*. New York: International Universities Press, 1949. Pp. 115-127.

3150 Newman, R. G. The acting-out boy. *Exceptional Children*, 1956, *22*, 186-190.

3151 *Oberndorf, C. P. Psychotherapy in a resident children's group. In K. R. Eissler (Ed.), *Searchlights on delinquency*. New York: International Universities Press, 1949. Pp. 165-173.

3152 *Kaplan, D. M. & Goodrich, D. W. A formulation for interpersonal anger. *American Journal of Orthopsychiatry*, 1957, *27*, 387-395.

3153 *Hirschberg, R. The socialized delinquent: Concept, etiology, psychometric evaluation and institutional training. *Nervous Child*, 1947, *6*, 447-466.

3154 Goodrich, D. W. & Boomer, D. S. Some concepts about therapeutic interventions with hyperaggressive children. Part II. *Social Casework*, 1958, *39*, 286-292.

3155 Goodrich, D. W. & Boomer, D. S. Some concepts about therapeutic interventions with hyperaggressive children: Part I. *Social Casework*, 1958, *39*, 207-213.

3156 *Gordon, G. & Siegel, L. The evolution of a program of individual psychotherapy for children with aggressive acting-out disorders in a new residential treatment unit. *American Journal of Orthopsychiatry*, 1957, *27*, 59-68.

3157 *Kitchener, H., Sweet, B. & Citrin, E. Problems in the treatment of impulse disorder in children in a residential setting. *Psychiatry*, 1961, *24*, 347-354.

3158 Alt, H. & Grossbard, H. Professional issues in the institutional treatment of delinquent children. *American Journal of Orthopsychiatry*, 1949, *19*, 279-294.

3159 Goldsmith, J. M., Krohn, H., Ochroch, R. & Kagan, N. Changing the delinquent's concept of school. Workshop, 1956. *American Journal of Orthopsychiatry*, 1959, *29*, 249-265.

3160 Papanek, E. Re-education and treatment of juvenile delinquents. *American Journal of Psychotherapy*, 1958, *12*, 269-296.

3161 *Straight, B. & Werkman, S. L. Control problems in group therapy with aggressive adolescent boys in a mental hospital. *American Journal of Psychiatry*, 1958, *114*, 998-1001.

3162 Stranahan, M., Schwartzman, C. & Atkin, E. Group treatment for emotionally disturbed and potentially delinquent boys and girls. *American Journal of Orthopsychiatry*, 1957, *27*, 518-527.

3163 *Polsky, H. W. & Kohn, M. Participant observation in a delinquent subculture. *American Journal of Orthopsychiatry*, 1959, *29*, 737-751.

3164 Bond, R. J. The work camp as a resource for the treatment of delinquents--Workshop, 1961. 5. Work as a therapeutic medium in the treatment of delinquents. *American Journal of Orthopsychiatry*, 1962, *32*, 846-850.

3165 Duncan, M. Environmental therapy in a hostel for maladjusted children. *British Journal of Delinquency*, 1953, *3*, 248-268.

3166 Finkelstein, H. Confidentiality, control, and casework: The therapist's role in a residential treatment center. *Crime and Delinquency*, 1964, *10*, 60-66.

3167 *Gildea, M. C.-L. Psychiatric problems in training school for delinquent girls. *American Journal of Orthopsychiatry*, 1944, *14*, 128-135.

3168 *Eissler, R. S. Riots: Observation in a home for delinquent girls. *Psychoanalytic Study of the Child*, 1949, *3-4*, 449-460.

3169 *Mays, J. B. A study of a delinquent community. *British Journal of Delinquency*, 1952, *3*, 5-19.

3170 Craig, L. P. Reaching delinquents through cottage committees. *Children*, 1959, *6*, 129-134.

3171 Carpenter, K. S. Halfway houses for delinquent youth. *Children*, 1963, *10*, 224-229.

ADOLESCENTS

3172 *Warren, W. Inpatient treatment of adolescents with psychological illnesses. *Lancet*, 1952, *262*, 147-150.
3173 *Sobel, R. The contribution of psychoanalysis to the residential treatment of adolescents. In M. Heiman (Ed.), *Psychoanalysis and social work*. New York: International Universities Press, 1953. Pp. 242-260.
3174 Scofield, J. B. Adolescent treatment in an adult hospital. *American Journal of Orthopsychiatry*, 1962, *32*, 660-668.
3175 Warren, W. Treatment of youths with behaviour disorders in a psychiatric hospital. *British Journal of Delinquency*, 1953, *3*, 234-247.
3176 *Robinson, J. F. Psychotherapy of adolescents at school: Plus inpatient treatment level. In B. Balser (Ed.), *Psychotherapy of the adolescent*. New York: International Universities Press, 1957. Pp. 67-85.
3177 *Noshpitz, J. D. Opening phase in the psychotherapy of adolescents with character disorders. *Bulletin of the Menninger Clinic*, 1957, *21*, 153-164.
3178 Cameron, K., Bardon, D. T. & Mackeith, S. A. Symposium on the in-patient treatment of psychotic adolescents. *British Journal of Medical Psychology*, 1950, *23*, 107-118.
3179 Burton, A. C., Wallerstein, J. & Bernard, V. W. Dosoris-- An experimental study and treatment home for adolescent girls. *American Journal of Orthopsychiatry*, 1949, *19*, 683-696.
3180 Boyd, J. N. & Rondell, F. R. Psychotherapy of older adolescents using a residential facility. *American Journal of Orthopsychiatry*, 1964, *34*, 503-509.
3181 *Cameron, K. Group approach to inpatient adolescents. *American Journal of Psychiatry*, 1953, *109*, 657-661.
3182 Offer, D. & Barglow, P. Adolescent and young adult self-mutilation incidents in a general psychiatric hospital. *Archives of General Psychiatry*, 1960, *3*, 194-204.
3183 *Siegel, L. Case study of a thirteen-year-old fire-setter: A catalyst in the growing pains of a residential treatment unit. *American Journal of Orthopsychiatry*, 1957, *27*, 396-410.
3184 *Specht, R. & Glasser, B. A review of the literature on social work with hospitalized adolescents and their families. *Social Service Review*, 1963, *37*, 295-306.
3185 Scher, B. Specialized group care for adolescents. *Child Welfare*, 1958, *37*(2), 12-17.
3186 Levy, M. M. Outdoor group therapy with preadolescent boys. *Psychiatry*, 1950, *13*, 333-347.
3187 *Pfautz, H. W. The functions of day-care for disturbed adolescents. *Mental Hygiene*, 1962, *46*, 223-229.

CONSULTATION IN RESIDENTIAL CARE

3188 *Riley, M. J. Psychiatric consultation in residential treatment. Workshop, 1957. 4. The child care worker's view. *American Journal of Orthopsychiatry*, 1958, *28*, 283-288.

3189 *Wright, B. Psychiatric consultation in residential treatment. Workshop, 1957. 3. The psychologist's view. *American Journal of Orthopsychiatry*, 1958, *28*, 276-282.

3190 *Perkins, G. L. Psychiatric consultation in residential treatment. Workshop, 1957. 2. The consultant's view. *American Journal of Orthopsychiatry*, 1958, *28*, 266-275.

3191 *Bettelheim, B. Psychiatric consultation in residential treatment. Workshop, 1957. 1. The director's view. *American Journal of Orthopsychiatry*, 1958, *28*, 256-265.

EVALUATION AND RESEARCH

3192 *Henry, J. Types of institutional structure. *Psychiatry*, 1957, *20*, 47-60.

3193 *Dettelbach, M. H. The role of residential treatment for children. Symposium, 1954. 2. Criteria for agency referral of a child to a residential treatment center. *American Journal of Orthopsychiatry*, 1955, *25*, 669-674.

3194 *Gair, D. S. & Salomon, A. D. Diagnostic aspects of psychiatric hospitalization of children. *American Journal of Orthopsychiatry*, 1962, *32*, 445-461.

3195 Bamford, C. & Heinstein, M. Selecting patients at a preschool treatment center. *Journal of Psychiatric Social Work*, 1953, *22*, 189-194.

3196 *Allerhand, M. E., Weber, R. E. & Polansky, N. A. The Bellefaire Follow-up Study: Research objectives and method. *Child Welfare*, 1961, *40*(7), 7-13.

3197 *Fanshel, D., Hylton, L. & Borgatta, E. F. A study of behavior disorders of children in residential treatment centers. *Journal of Psychological Studies*, 1963, *14*, 1-23.

3198 *Goodrich, D. W. & Dittmann, A. T. Observing interactional behavior in residential treatment. *Archives of General Psychiatry*, 1960, *2*, 421-428.

3199 *Harrison, S. I. & Burks, H. L. Some aspects of grouping in a children's psychiatric hospital. *American Journal of Orthopsychiatry*, 1964, *34*, 148-152.

3200 Johnson, L. J. What we learn from the child's own psychology to guide treatment in a small institution. *National Conference of Social Work Proceedings*, 1938, *65*, 313-325.

3201 Matsushima, J. Some aspects of defining "success" in residential treatment. *Child Welfare*, 1965, *44*, 272-277.

3202 *Laffal, J., Sarason, I. G., Ameen, L. & Stern, A. Individuals in groups: A behavior rating technique. *International Journal of Social Psychiatry*, 1957, *2*, 254-262.

3203 *Polansky, N. A., Weiss, E. S. & Blum, A. Children's verbal accessibility as a function of content and personality. *American Journal of Orthopsychiatry*, 1961, *31*, 153-169.

3204 Rabinovitch, R. D. Observations on the differential study of severely disturbed children. *American Journal of Orthopsychiatry*, 1952, *22*, 230-236.

3205 *Raush, H. L. Observational research with emotionally disturbed children: Session I. Symposium, 1958. 3. On the locus of behavior--Observations in multiple settings within residential treatment. *American Journal of Orthopsychiatry*, 1959, *29*, 235-242.

3206 Rashkis, H. A. Cognitive restructuring: Why research is therapy. *Archives of General Psychiatry*, 1960, *2*, 612-621.

3207 Alt, H. The concept of success in residential treatment-- An administrator's view. *Child Welfare*, 1964, *43*, 423-426; 430.

3208 *Dittmann, A. T. Problems of reliability in observing and coding social interactions. *Journal of Consulting Psychology*, 1958, *22*, 430.

3209 Allerhand, M. E., et al. *Adaptation and adaptability: The Bellefaire follow-up study.* New York: Child Welfare League of America, 1966.

3210 *Johnson, J. L. & Rubin, E. Z. A school follow-up study of children discharged from a psychiatric hospital. *Exceptional Children*, 1964, *31*, 19-24.

3211 Glickman, E. The planned return of a placed child to own family. Workshop, 1953. *American Journal of Orthopsychiatry*, 1953, *23*, 834-847.

3212 *Kane, R. P. & Chambers, G. Improvement - Real or apparent? A seven year follow-up of children hospitalized and discharged from a residential setting. *American Journal of Psychiatry*, 1961, *117*, 1023-1027.

3213 *Newman, R. G. The assessment of progress in the treatment of hyperaggressive children with learning disturbances within a school setting. *American Journal of Orthopsychiatry*, 1959, *29*, 633-643.

3214 Rose, J. A. & Sonis, M. The use of separation as a diagnostic measure in the parent-child emotional crises. *American Journal of Psychiatry*, 1959, *116*, 409-415.

3215 Vinter, R. & Janowitz, M. Effective institutions for juvenile delinquents: A research statement. *Social Service Review*, 1959, *33*, 118-130.

3215.1 McConville, B. J. & Purohit, A. P. Classifying confusion: A study of results of inpatient treatment in a multidisciplinary children's center. *American Journal of Orthopsychiatry*, 1973, *43*, 411-417.

BOOKS

3216   *American Psychiatric Association. *Psychiatric inpatient treatment of children.* Washington: APA, 1957,

3217   *Bettelheim, B. *The empty fortress: Infantile autism and the birth of the self.* New York: Free Press, 1967.

3218   Bettelheim, B. *Truants from life.* Glencoe, Ill.: Free Press, 1955.

3219   *Cohen, F. J. *Children in trouble: An experiment in institutional child care.* New York: Norton, 1952.

3220   Deutsch, A. *Our rejected children.* Boston: Little, Brown, 1950.

3221   *Directory of Facilities for Mentally Ill Children in the United States.* New York: National Association for Mental Health, 1964.

3222   *Jones, M. S., et al. *The therapeutic community.* New York: Basic Books, 1953.

3223   *Konopka, G. *Group work in the institution: A modern challenge.* New York: Whiteside, Inc., and W. Morrow, 1954.

3224   Lewis, H. S. *Deprived children.* London: Oxford University Press, 1954.

3225   *Polsky, H. W. *Cottage six: The social system of delinquent boys in residential treatment.* New York: Russell Sage Foundation, 1962.

3226   *Caudill, W. A. *The psychiatric hospital as a small society.* Cambridge: Harvard University Press, 1958.

3227   Redl, F. & Wineman, D. *Children who hate.* Glencoe, Ill.: Free Press, 1951.

3228   Redl, F. & Wineman, D. *Controls from within.* Glencoe, Ill.: Free Press, 1952.

3229   Reid, J. H. & Hagan, H. R. *Residential treatment of emotionally disturbed children: A descriptive study.* New York: Child Welfare League of America, 1952.

3230   *Robertson, J. *Young children in hospitals.* (2nd ed.) London: Tavistock, 1970.

3231   *Robinson, J. F., et al. (Eds.) *Psychiatric inpatient treatment of children.* Washington: American Psychiatric Association, 1957.

3232   *Stanton, A. H. & Schwartz, M. S. *The mental hospital.* New York: Basic Books, 1954.

3233   *Szurek, S. A., Berlin, I. N. & Boatman, M. J. (Eds.) *Inpatient care for the psychotic child.* Palo Alto, Calif.: Science & Behavior Books, 1971.

3234   Weber, G. H. & Haberlein, B. J. *Residential treatment of emotionally disturbed children.* New York: Behavioral Publications, 1972.

3234.1 Rae-Grant, Q. & Moffat, P. J. *Children in Canada residential care.* Toronto: Leonard Crainford for the Canadian Mental Health Association, 1971.

3234.2 Bettelheim, B. *A home for the heart.* New York: Alfred A. Knopf, 1974.

PART IV

COMMUNITY PSYCHIATRY

XXII. COMMUNITY MENTAL HEALTH

HISTORICAL BACKGROUND

3235   *Coleman, J. V. Psychiatric consultation in case work
       agencies. *American Journal of Orthopsychiatry,* 1947,
       17, 533-539.
3236   *Rosenfeld, J. M. & Caplan, G. Techniques of staff con-
       sultation in an immigrant children's organization in
       Israel. *American Journal of Orthopsychiatry,* 1954,
       24, 42-62.
3237   *Garrett, A. The use of the consultant. Symposium, 1955.
       2. Psychiatric consultation. *American Journal of
       Orthopsychiatry,* 1956, *26,* 234-240.
3238   *Berlin, I. N. Learning mental health consultation: His-
       tory and problems. *Mental Hygiene,* 1964, *48,* 257-266.
3239   Covner, B. J. Principles for psychological consulting
       with client organizations. *Journal of Consulting Psy-
       chology,* 1947, *11,* 227-244.
3240   *Vaughan, W. T. Mental health for school children. *Chil-
       dren,* 1955, *2,* 203-207.
3241   Valenstein, A. F. Some principles of psychiatric con-
       sultation. *Social Casework,* 1955, *36,* 253-256.
3242   *Caplan, G. *An approach to community mental health.* New
       York: Grune & Stratton, 1961.
3243   Gildea, M. C.-L. *Community mental health.* Springfield,
       Ill.: Thomas, 1959.
3244   Lemkau, P. V. *Mental hygiene in public health.* (2nd ed.)
       New York: McGraw-Hill, 1955.
3244.1 Beck, R. White House Conferences on Children: An his-
       torical perspective. *Harvard Educational Review,* 1973,
       43, 653-668.
3244.2 Edelman, P. B. The Massachusetts Task Force reports:
       Advocacy for children. *Harvard Educational Review,*
       1973, *43,* 639-652.

EPIDEMIOLOGY

3245   *Cassel, J. Social class and mental disorders: An analy-
       sis of the limitations and potentialities of current
       epidemiological approaches. In K. S. Miller & C. M.
       Grigg (Eds.), *Mental health and the lower classes.*

271

Tallahassee: Florida State University, 1966. Pp. 42-53.

3246   *Gruenberg, E. M. & Leighton, A. H. Epidemiology and psychiatric training. In S. E. Goldston (Ed.) *Concepts of community psychiatry: A framework for training.* Bethesda, Md.: U.S. National Institute of Mental Health, 1965. Pp. 109-115.

3247   *Hoch, P. H. & Zubin, J. (Eds.) *Comparative epidemiology of the mental disorders.* New York: Grune & Stratton, 1961. (*Proceedings of the American Psychopathological Association,* 1961, *49.)*

3248   *Monroe, R. R., Klee, G. D. & Brody, E. B. Psychiatric epidemiology and mental health planning. *Psychiatric Research Reports of the American Psychiatric Association,* 1967, *22.*

3249   Plunkett, R. J. & Gordon, J. E. *Epidemiology and mental illness.* New York: Basic Books, 1960.

3250   Reid, D. D. *Epidemiologic methods in the study of mental disorders.* Geneva: World Health Organization, 1960. (Public health papers, no. 2)

3251   *Werner, E. E., Bierman, J. M. & French, F. E. *The children of Kauai.* Honolulu: University of Hawaii Press, 1971.

3252   *Birch, H. G. The problem of "brain damage" in children. In *Brain damage in children: The biological and social aspects.* Baltimore: Williams & Wilkins, 1964. Pp. 3-12.

3253   *Knobloch, H., Rider, R., Harper, P. & Pasamanick, B. Neuropsychiatric sequelae of prematurity: A longitudinal study. *Journal of the American Medical Association,* 1956, *161,* 581-585.

3254   *Pasamanick, B. & Knobloch, H. Brain behavior: Session II. Symposium, 1959. 2. Brain damage and reproductive casualty. *American Journal of Orthopsychiatry,* 1960, *30,* 298-305.

3255   *Birch, H. G. & Gussow, J. D. *Disadvantaged children: Health, nutrition, and school failure.* New York: Grune & Stratton, 1970.

3256   *Cravioto, J., DeLicardie, E. R. & Birch, H. G. Nutrition, growth and neurointegrative development: An experimental and ecologic study. *Pediatrics,* 1966, *38,* 319-372.

3257   *Scrimshaw, N. S., Guzman, M. A. & Gordon, J. E. Nutrition and infection field study in Guatemalan villages, 1959-1964. I. Study plan and experimental design. *Archives of Environmental Health,* 1967, *14,* 657-662.

3258   Stoch, M. B. & Smythe, P. M. Undernutrition during infancy, and subsequent brain growth and intellectual development. In N. S. Scrimshaw & J. E. Gordon (Eds.), *Malnutrition, learning, and behavior.* Cambridge: MIT Press, 1968. Pp. 278-289.

3259   Provence, S. A. & Lipton, R. C. *Infants in institutions.* New York: International Universities Press, 1963.

3260   *Joint Commission on Mental Health of Children. *Crisis in child mental health: Challenge for the 1970's.* New York: Harper & Row, 1970.
3261   Joint Commission on Mental Illness and Health. *Action for mental health.* New York: Basic Books, 1961.
3262   Srole, L., Langner, T. S., Michael, S. T., Opler, M. K. & Rennie, T. A. C. *The Midtown Manhattan study.* Vol. 1. *Mental health in the metropolis.* New York: McGraw-Hill, 1962.
3263   *Chase, A. *The biological imperatives: Health, politics, and human survival.* New York: Holt, Rinehart & Winston, 1971.
3264   Laing, R. D. & Esterson, A. *Sanity, madness and the family.* (2nd ed.) London: Tavistock, 1970.
3265   Blum, H. L. & Leonard, A. R. *Public administration--a public health viewpoint.* New York: Macmillan, 1963.
3265.1 Ward, A. J. Childhood psychopathology: A natural experiment in etiology. *Journal of the American Academy of Child Psychiatry,* 1974, *13,* 153-165.

COMMUNITY MENTAL HEALTH CENTERS/History

3266   *Joint Commission on Mental Illness and Health. *Action for mental health.* New York: Basic Books, 1961.
3267   *Porterfield, J. D. *Community health: Its needs and resources.* New York: Basic Books, 1966.
3268   Whittington, H. G. *Psychiatry in the American community.* New York: International Universities Press, 1966.
3269   *Caplan, G. *An approach to community mental health.* New York: Grune & Stratton, 1961.
3270   *Bindman, A. J. & Klebanoff, L. B. Administrative problems in establishing a community mental health program. *American Journal of Orthopsychiatry,* 1960, *30,* 696-711.
3271   *Klerman, G. L. Mental health and the urban crisis. *American Journal of Orthopsychiatry,* 1969, *39,* 818-826.
3272   Hume, P. B. Community psychiatry, social psychiatry, and community mental health work: Some inter-professional relationships in psychiatry and social work. *American Journal of Psychiatry,* 1964, *121,* 340-343.
3273   Bellak, L. (Ed.) *Handbook of community psychiatry and community mental health.* New York: Grune & Stratton, 1964.
3273.1 McGarry, A. L. & Kaplan, H. A. Overview: Current trends in mental health law. *American Journal of Psychiatry,* 1973, *130,* 621-630.

COMMUNITY MENTAL HEALTH CENTERS/Principles

3274　*Stretch, J. J. Community mental health: The evolution of a concept in social policy. *Community Mental Health Journal*, 1967, *3*, 5-12.

3275　*Whittington, H. G. Institutional lodgement of the comprehensive community mental health center. *American Journal of Public Health*, 1969, *59*, 451-458.

3276　Soddy, K. & Ahrenfeldt, R. H. (Eds.) *International study group on mental health perspectives, 1961.* Vol. 3. *Mental health in the service of the community.* London: Tavistock, 1965-67.

3277　Schwartz, M. S., Schwartz, C. G. & Field, M. G., et al. *Social approaches to mental patient care.* New York: Columbia University Press, 1964.

3278　*Leopold, R. L. Urban problems and the community mental health center: Multiple mandates, difficult choices. 1. Background and current status. *American Journal of Orthopsychiatry*, 1971, *41*, 144-149.

3279　Bloomberg, W. & Schmandt, H. J. *Power, poverty and urban policy.* Vol. 2. *Urban affairs annual reviews.* Beverly Hills: Sage Publications, 1968.

3280　Biddle, W. W. & Biddle, L. J. *The community development process; the rediscovery of local initiative.* New York: Holt, Rinehart & Winston, 1965.

3281　*Eisdorfer, C., Altrocchi, J. & Young, R. F. Principles of community mental health in a rural setting: The Halifax County Program. *Community Mental Health Journal*, 1968, *4*, 211-220.

3283　Marris, P. & Rein, M. *Dilemmas of social reform: Poverty and community action in the United States.* (2nd ed.) London: Routledge & Kegan Paul, 1972.

3284　*McNeil, J. N., Llewellyn, C. E., Jr. & McCollough, T. E. Community psychiatry and ethics. *American Journal of Orthopsychiatry*, 1970, *40*, 22-29.

3285　*Hume, P. B. General principles of community psychiatry. In S. Arieti (Ed.), *American handbook of psychiatry*. Vol. 3. New York: Basic Books, 1966. Pp. 515-541.

3286　*Greenbaum, M. Resignations among professional mental health leaders: A study of a mild epidemic. *Archives of General Psychiatry*, 1968, *19*, 266-280.

3287　*Berlin, I. N. Resistance to change in mental health professionals. *American Journal of Orthopsychiatry*, 1969, *39*, 109-115.

3288　Joint Commission on Mental Illness and Health. *Action for mental health.* New York: Basic Books, 1961.

3289　Cowen, E. L., Gardner, E. A. & Zax, M. *Emergent approaches to mental health problems.* New York: Appleton-Century-Crofts, 1967.

3290　Kubie, L. S. Pitfalls of community psychiatry. *Archives of General Psychiatry*, 1968, *18*, 257-266.

3291　Bertalanffy, L. von. *General system theory.* New York: G. Braziller, 1968.

COMMUNITY MENTAL HEALTH CENTERS/Programs

3292   *Freed, H. M. & Miller, L. Planning a community mental
        health program: A case history. *Community Mental
        Health Journal,* 1971, *7,* 107-117.
3293   *Black, B. J. Psychiatric rehabilitation in the community.
        In L. Bellak (Ed.), *Handbook of community psychiatry and
        community mental health.* New York: Grune & Stratton,
        1964. Pp. 248-264.
3294   *Huessy, H. R. (Ed.) *Mental health with limited resources:
        Yankee ingenuity in low-cost programs.* New York: Grune
        & Stratton, 1966.
3295   *Fishman, J. R. & McCormack, J. "Mental health without
        walls": Community mental health in the ghetto. *Ameri-
        can Journal of Psychiatry,* 1970, *126,* 1461-1467.
3296   *Inner city mental health services. *American Journal of
        Psychiatry,* 1970, *126,* 1430-1486.
3297   Lamb, H. R., Heath, D. & Downing, J. J. *Handbook of com-
        munity mental health practice.* San Francisco: Jossey-
        Bass, 1969.
3298   Bellak, L. (Ed.) *Handbook of community psychiatry and
        community mental health.* New York: Grune & Stratton,
        1964.
3299   *Caplan, G. The role of pediatricians in community mental
        health (with particular reference to the primary pre-
        vention of mental disorders in children). In L. Bellak
        (Ed.), *Handbook of community psychiatry and community
        mental health.* New York: Grune & Stratton, 1964.
        Pp. 287-299.
3300   *Glasscote, R. M., et al. *The community mental health
        center: An interim appraisal.* Washington: Joint In-
        formation Service of the American Psychiatric Associa-
        tion and the National Association for Mental Health,
        1969.
3301   Astrachan, B. M., Flynn, H. R., Geller, J. D. & Harvey,
        H. H. Systems approach to day hospitalization. *Ar-
        chives of General Psychiatry,* 1970, *22,* 550-559.
3302   Allan, W. S. *Rehabilitation: A community challenge.*
        New York: Wiley, 1958.
3303   Duhl, L. J. *The urban condition; people and policy in
        the metropolis.* New York: Basic Books, 1963.
3304   Roberts, L. M., Halleck, S. L. & Loeb, M. B. *Community
        psychiatry.* Madison: University of Wisconsin Press,
        1966.
3306   Sarason, S. B., Levine, M., Goldenberg, I., Cherlin, D.
        L. & Bennett, E. M. *Psychology in community settings:
        Clinical, educational, vocational, social aspects.*
        New York: Wiley, 1966.
3306.1 Serrano, A. C. & Gibson, G. Mental health services to
        the Mexican-American community in San Antonio, Texas.
        American Journal of Public Health, 1973, *63,* 1055-
        1057.

3306.2   Rogeness, G. A. & Bednar, R. A.   Teenage helper: A role
         in community mental health. *American Journal of Psy-
         chiatry*, 1973, *130*, 933-936.
3306.3   Gentry, J. T., Kaluzny, A. D., Veney, J. E. & Coulter, E.
         J. Provision of mental health services by community
         hospitals and health departments: A comparative analy-
         sis. *American Journal of Public Health*, 1973, *63*, 863-
         871.
3306.4   Schwebel, A. I., Kershaw, R., Reeve, S., Hartung, J. G.
         & Reeve, W. A community organization approach to im-
         plementation of comprehensive health planning. *American
         Journal of Public Health*, 1973, *63*, 675-680.
3306.5   Brodt, E. W. Urbanization and health planning: Challenge
         and opportunity for the American Indian community.
         American Journal of Public Health, 1973, *63*, 694-701.
3306.6   Allerhand, M. E. & Lake, G. New careerists in community
         psychology and mental health. In S. E. Golann & C.
         Eisdorfer (Eds.), *Handbook of community mental health*.
         New York: Appleton-Century-Crofts, 1972. Pp. 921-937.

COMMUNITY MENTAL HEALTH CENTERS/Programs/*SPECIAL SETTINGS*

3307   *Kellam, S. G. & Schiff, S. K. The Woodlawn Mental Health
       Center: A community mental health center model. *Social
       Service Review*, 1966, *40*, 255-263.
3308   *Kiesler, F. More than psychiatry: A rural program. In
       M. F. Shore & F. V. Mannino (Eds.), *Mental health and
       the community: Problems, programs, and strategies*.
       New York: Behavioral Publications, 1969. Pp. 103-120.
3309   Daniels, D. N. The community mental health center in the
       rural area: Is the present model appropriate? *American
       Journal of Psychiatry*, 1967, *124*(Suppl.), 32-36.
3310   Hladky, F. A psychiatric program in a rural mental health
       plan. In L. F. Duhl & R. L. Leopold (Eds.), *Mental
       health and urban social policy*. San Francisco: Jossey-
       Bass, 1968. Pp. 140-160.
3311   Looff, D. H. Appalachian public health nursing: Mental
       health component in eastern Kentucky. *Community Mental
       Health Journal*, 1969, *5*, 295-303.
3312   *Mahoney, S. C. & Hodges, A. Community mental health cen-
       ters in rural areas: Variations on a theme. *Mental
       Hygiene*, 1969, *53*, 484-487.
3313   *Stage, T. B. & Keast, T. J. A psychiatric service for
       Plains Indians. *Hospital and Community Psychiatry*,
       1966, *17*, 74-76.
3314   Williams, R. H. & Ozarin, L. D. (Eds.) *Community mental
       health: An international perspective*. San Francisco:
       Jossey-Bass, 1968.
3314.1 Nir, Y. & Cutler, R. The therapeutic utilization of the
       juvenile court. *American Journal of Psychiatry*, 1973,
       130, 1112-1117.

3314.2 Lewis, D. O., Balla, D. A., Sacks, H. L. & Jekel, J. F.
Psychotic symptomatology in a juvenile court clinic
population. *Journal of the American Academy of Child
Psychiatry*, 1973, *12*, 660-674.
3314.3 Jacobson, G. F. Emergency services in community mental
health. *American Journal of Public Health*, 1974, *64*,
124-127.
3314.4 Nelson, S. H., Batalden, P. B., Kraft, D. P. & Stoddard,
F. J. Preventive mental health programming for a non-
health agency. *American Journal of Psychiatry*, 1974,
131, 419-422.
3314.5 Chapman, L. S. The neighborhood health center foundation
for health care: A portend for the future or a necessity for survival? *American Journal of Public Health*,
1973, *63*, 841-845.
3314.6 Rhodes, W. C. & Gibbins, S. Community programming for
the behaviorally deviant child. In H. C. Quay & J. S.
Werry (Eds.), *Psychopathological disorders of childhood.*
New York: Wiley, 1972. Pp. 348-387.

COMMUNITY MENTAL HEALTH CENTERS/Community Involvement

3315 *Freed, H., Schroder, D. & Baker, B. Community participation in mental health services: A case of factional
control. In L. Miller (Ed.), *Mental health in rapid
social change.* Jerusalem: Jerusalem Academic Press,
1972. Pp. 97-109.
3316 *Foster, D. L. A psychiatrist looks at urban renewal.
Journal of the National Medical Association, 1970, *62*,
95-138.
3317 Epps, R., et al. *A community concern.* Springfield, Ill.:
C. C. Thomas, 1965.
3318 *Holder, H. D. Mental health and the search for new organizational strategies: A systems proposal. *Archives
of General Psychiatry*, 1969, *20*, 709-717.
3319 *Niebuhr, R. Without consensus there is no consent.
Center Magazine, 1971, *4*(4), 2-9.
3320 *Querido, A. The shaping of community mental health care.
British Journal of Psychiatry, 1968, *114*, 293-302.
3321 *Minuchin, S. The paraprofessional and the use of confrontation in the mental health field. *American Journal of Orthopsychiatry*, 1969, *39*, 722-729.
3322 *Reiff, R. & Riessman, F. The indigenous nonprofessional:
A strategy of change in community action and community
mental health programs. *Community Mental Health Journal
Monograph Series*, 1968, *1*, 1-32.
3323 Sizemore, B. Educational leadership for the black community. *Observer*, 1970, *7*(7), 10-11.
3324 Ellis, W. *White ethics and black power; The emergence
of the West Side Organization.* Chicago: Aldine, 1969.
3325 Hollowitz, E. & Riessman, F. The role of the indigenous

nonprofessional in a community mental health neighborhood service center program. *American Journal of Orthopsychiatry*, 1967, *37*, 766-778.

3326   Pearl, A. & Riessman, F. *New careers for the poor.* New
York: Free Press, 1965,

3327   Lifton, R. J. *Revolutionary immortality: Mao Tse-tung
and the Chinese cultural revolution.* New York: Random
House, 1968.

3328   Fabian, A. E. The disturbed child in the ghetto day care
center: The role of the psychiatric consultant. *Journal of the American Academy of Child Psychiatry*, 1972,
11, 467-491.

3329   *Schiff, S. K. Community accountability and mental health
services. *Mental Hygiene*, 1970, *54*, 205-214.

3330   Muhich, D. F., Hunter, W. F., Williams, R. I., Swanson, W.
G. & DeBellis, E. J. Community development through social psychiatry. *British Journal of Social Psychiatry*,
1967, *1*, 180-188.

3331   *Kellam, S. G. & Schiff, S. K. An urban community mental
health center. In L. F. Duhl & R. L. Leopold (Eds.),
Mental health and urban social policy. San Francisco:
Jossey-Bass, 1968. Pp. 112-138.

3331.1 Kellam, S. G., Branch, J. D., Agrawal, K. C. & Grabill,
M. E. Woodlawn Mental Health Center: An evolving
strategy for planning in community mental health. In
S. E. Golann & C. Eisdorfer (Eds.), *Handbook of community mental health.* New York: Appleton-Century-Crofts,
1972. Pp. 711-727.

3331.2 Martinez, C. Community mental health and the Chicano
movement. *American Journal of Orthopsychiatry*, 1973,
43, 595-601.

3331.3 Kirp, D. Student classification, public policy, and the
courts. *Harvard Educational Review*, 1974, *44*, 7-52.

3331.4 Mercer, J. R. A policy statement on assessment procedures and the rights of children. *Harvard Educational
Review*, 1974, *44*, 125-141.

3331.5 Rosenheim, M. K. The child and the law. In B. M. Caldwell & H. N. Ricciuti (Eds.), *Review of child development research.* Vol. 3. *Child development and social
policy.* Chicago: University of Chicago Press, 1973.
Pp. 509-555.

3331.6 Worsfold, V. L. A philosophical justification of children's rights. *Harvard Educational Review*, 1974, *44*,
142-157.

3331.7 Westman, J. C. The legal rights of adolescents from a
developmental perspective. In J. C. Schoolar (Ed.),
Current issues in adolescent psychiatry. New York:
Brunner/Mazel, 1973. Pp. 252-262.

COMMUNITY MENTAL HEALTH CENTERS/Child Psychiatry and Community
Mental Health Centers

3332   *Rexford, E. N. Children, child psychiatry, and our brave
        new world. *Archives of General Psychiatry*, 1969, *20*,
        25-37.
3333   Rosenblum, G. & Ottenstein, D. From child guidance to
        community mental health: Problems in transition. *Com-
        munity Mental Health Journal*, 1965, *1*, 276-283.
3334   *Harrison, S. I., McDermott, J. F., Schrager, J. & Shower-
        man, E. R. Social status and child psychiatric prac-
        tice: The influence of the clinician's socioeconomic
        origin. *American Journal of Psychiatry*, 1970, *127*,
        652-658.
3335   Hersch, C. Child guidance services to the poor. *Journal
        of the American Academy of Child Psychiatry*, 1968, *7*,
        223-241.
3336   *Rafferty, F. T. Child psychiatry service for a total
        population. *Journal of the American Academy of Child
        Psychiatry*, 1967, *6*, 295-308.
3337   *Hetznecker, W. & Forman, M. A. Community child psychi-
        atry: Evolution and direction. *American Journal of
        Orthopsychiatry*, 1971, *41*, 350-370.
3338   *Klebanoff, L. B. & Bindman, A. J. The organization and
        development of a community mental health program for
        children: A case study. *American Journal of Ortho-
        psychiatry*, 1962, *32*, 119-132.
3339   *Malone, C. A. Children. In H. Grunebaum (Ed.), *The
        practice of community mental health*. Boston: Little,
        Brown, 1970. Pp. 3-34.
3340   *Rafferty, F. T. The community is becoming. *American
        Journal of Orthopsychiatry*, 1966, *36*, 102-110.
3341   *Malone, C. A. Child psychiatric services for low socio-
        economic families. *Journal of the American Academy of
        Child Psychiatry*, 1967, *6*, 332-345.
3342   *Kluger, J. M. The uninsulated caseload in a neighborhood
        mental health center. *American Journal of Psychiatry*,
        1970, *126*, 1430-1436.
3343   Berlin, I. N. From confrontation to collaboration. *Amer-
        ican Journal of Orthopsychiatry*, 1970, *40*, 473-480.
3344   Joint Commission on Mental Health of Children. *Crisis
        in child mental health: Challenge for the 1970's*.
        New York: Harper & Row, 1970.
3345   Fine, P. An appraisal of child psychiatry in a community
        health project: Relevance as a function of social con-
        text. *Journal of the American Academy of Child Psychi-
        atry*, 1972, *11*, 279-293.
3346   Van Buskirk, D. Child psychiatric services delivered to
        the small community. *Journal of the American Academy
        of Child Psychiatry*, 1973, *12*, 247-261.
3346.1 Fine, P. Family networks and child psychiatry in a com-
        munity health project. *Journal of the American Academy
        of Child Psychiatry*, 1973, *12*, 675-689.

COMMUNITY MENTAL HEALTH CENTERS/Prevention/*GENERAL PRINCIPLES*

3347   *Carbonara, N. T. *Techniques for observing normal child
       behavior.* Pittsburgh: University of Pittsburgh Press,
       1961.
3348   Levy, D. M. *The demonstration clinic for the psychologi-
       cal study and treatment of mother and child in medical
       practice.* Springfield, Ill.: Thomas, 1959.
3349   *Bolman, W. M. An outline of preventive psychiatric pro-
       grams for children. *Archives of General Psychiatry,*
       1967, *17,* 5-8.
3350   *Caplan, G. & Grunebaum, H. Perspectives on primary pre-
       vention: A review. *Archives of General Psychiatry,*
       1967, *17,* 331-346.
3351   Klein, D. C. The prevention of mental illness. *Mental
       Hygiene,* 1961, *45,* 101-109.
3352   White, R. W. *Ego and reality in psychoanalytic theory;
       a proposal regarding independent ego energies.* New
       York: International Universities Press, 1963. [*Psy-
       chological Issues,* 3(3, Monograph 11)]
3353   Caplan, G. *Prevention of mental disorders in children;
       initial exploration.* New York: Basic Books, 1961.
3354   Caplan, G. Opportunities for school psychologists in the
       primary prevention of mental disorders in children.
       Mental Hygiene, 1963, *47,* 525-539.
3355   Harlow, H. F. & Zimmermann, R. R. Affectional responses
       in the infant monkey. *Science,* 1959, *130,* 421-432.
3356   *Klein, D. C. & Lindemann, E. Preventive intervention in
       individual and family crisis situations. In G. Caplan
       (Ed.), *Prevention of mental disorders in children.*
       New York: Basic Books, 1961. Pp. 283-306.
3357   *Waldfogel, S. & Gardner, G. E. Intervention in crises as
       a method of primary prevention. In G. Caplan (Ed.),
       Prevention of mental disorders in children. New York:
       Basic Books, 1961. Pp. 307-322.
3358   *Becker, D. & Margolin, F. How surviving parents handled
       their young children's adaptation to the crisis of loss.
       American Journal of Orthopsychiatry, 1967, *37,* 753-757.
3358.1 Ward, A. J. Childhood psychopathology: A natural ex-
       periment in etiology. *Journal of the American Academy
       of Child Psychiatry,* 1974, *13,* 153-165.

COMMUNITY MENTAL HEALTH CENTERS/Primary Prevention/*GENERAL ISSUES*

3359   *Bowlby, J. *Maternal care and mental health.* Geneva:
       World Health Organization, 1951. (Monograph series,
       no. 2)
3360   *Brown, B. S. Definition of mental health and disease.
       In A. M. Freedman & H. I. Kaplan (Eds.), *Comprehensive
       textbook of psychiatry.* Baltimore: Williams & Wilkins,
       1967. Pp. 1516-1520.

3361   *Lindemann, E. & Dawes, L. G. The use of psychoanalytic
        constructs in preventive psychiatry. *Psychoanalytic
        Study of the Child*, 1952, *7*, 429-448.
3362   *Bolman, W. M. & Westman, J. C. Prevention of mental dis-
        order: An overview of current programs. *American Jour-
        nal of Psychiatry*, 1967, *123*, 1058-1068.
3363   *Berlin, I. N. Prevention of mental and emotional dis-
        orders of childhood. In B. B. Wolman (Ed.), *Manual of
        child psychopathology*. New York: McGraw-Hill, 1972.
        Pp. 1088-1109.
3364   *Caplan, G. Recent trends in preventive child psychiatry.
        In G. Caplan (Ed.), *Emotional problems of early child-
        hood*. New York: Basic Books, 1955. Pp. 153-163.
3366   *Bower, E. M. The modification, mediation and utilization
        of stress during the school years. *American Journal of
        Orthopsychiatry*, 1964, *34*, 667-674.
3367   Berlin, I. N. Preventive aspects of mental health con-
        sultation to schools. *Mental Hygiene*, 1967, *51*, 34-40.
3368   Caplan, G. The role of the social worker in preventive
        psychiatry. *Medical Social Work*, 1955, *4*, 144-159.
3369   *Leon, R. L. Some implications for a preventive program
        for American Indians. *American Journal of Psychiatry*,
        1968, *125*, 232-236.
3369.1 Anthony, E. J. Primary prevention with school children.
        In H. H. Barten & L. Bellak (Eds.), *Progress in com-
        munity mental health*. Vol. 2. New York: Grune &
        Stratton, 1962. Pp. 131-158.

COMMUNITY MENTAL HEALTH/Primary Prevention/*MOTHER-CHILD RELATIONS*

3370   *Bibring, G. L., Dwyer, T. F., Huntington, D. S. & Valen-
        stein, A. F. A study of the psychological processes in
        pregnancy and of the earliest mother-child relationship.
        I. Some propositions and comments. *Psychoanalytic
        Study of the Child*, 1961, *16*, 9-24.
3371   *Schaefer, E. S. & Bayley, N. Maternal behavior, child be-
        havior, and their intercorrelations from infancy through
        adolescence. *Monographs of the Society for Research in
        Child Development*, 1963, *28*(3, Serial No. 87).
3372   Blank, M. Some maternal influences on infants' rates of
        sensorimotor development. *Journal of the American Acad-
        emy of Child Psychiatry*, 1964, *3*, 668-687.
3373   *Blodgett, F. M. Growth retardation related to maternal
        deprivation. In A. J. Solnit & S. A. Provence (Eds.),
        Modern perspectives in child development. New York:
        International Universities Press, 1963. Pp. 83-93.
3374   *Bullard, D. M., Glasser, H. H., Heagarty, M. C. & Pivchik,
        E. Failure to thrive in the "neglected" child. *Ameri-
        can Journal of Orthopsychiatry*, 1967, *37*, 680-690.
3375   *Ainsworth, M. D. The effects of maternal deprivation:
        A review of findings and controversy in the context of

research strategy. In World Health Organization, *Deprivation of maternal care: A reassessment of its effects*. Geneva: World Health Organization, 1962. Pp. 97-165. (Public health papers, no. 14)

3376 *Castello, D. Importanza del rapporto madre-figlio nell'immaturo ospedalizzato. *Minerva Pediatrica*, 1966, *18*, 331-336.

3377 *Robertson, J. Mothering as an influence on early development: A study of well-baby clinic records. *Psychoanalytic Study of the Child*, 1962, *17*, 245-264.

3378 Patton, R. G. & Gardner, L. I. *Growth failure in maternal deprivation*. Springfield, Ill.: Thomas, 1963.

3379 Birns, B. Individual differences in human neonates' responses to stimulation. *Child Development*, 1965, *36*, 249-256.

3380 *Escalona, S. K. & Leitch, M. *Early phases of personality development; a non-normative study of infant behavior*. Evanston, Ill.: Child Development Publications, 1953. [*Monographs of the Society for Research in Child Development*, 1952, *17*(1, Serial No. 54)]

3381 DeHirsch, K., Jansky, J. & Langford, W. S. Comparisons between prematurely and maturely born children at three age levels. *American Journal of Orthopsychiatry*, 1966, *36*, 616-628.

3382 *Leonard, M. F., Rhymes, J. P. & Solnit, A. J. Failure to thrive in infants. *American Journal of Diseases of Children*, 1966, *111*, 600-612.

3383 *Greenberg, N. H. Developmental effects of stimulation during early infancy: Some conceptual and methodological considerations. *Annals of the New York Academy of Sciences*, 1965, *118*, Art. 21, 831-859.

3384 *Korner, A. F. & Grobstein, R. Visual alertness as related to soothing in neonates: Implications for maternal stimulation and early deprivation. *Child Development*, 1966, *37*, 867-876.

3385 *Sayegh, Y. & Dennis, W. The effect of supplementary experiences upon the behavioral development of infants in institutions. *Child Development*, 1965, *36*, 81-90.

3386 Brim, O. G. *Education for child rearing*. New York: Russell Sage Foundation, 1959.

3386.1 Walder, L. O. & Cohen, S. I. Parents as agents of behavior change. In S. E. Golann & C. Eisdorfer (Eds.), *Handbook of community mental health*. New York: Appleton-Century-Crofts, 1972. Pp. 595-616.

3386.2 Levenstein, P., Kochman, A. & Roth, H. A. From laboratory to real world: Service delivery of the mother-child home program. *American Journal of Orthopsychiatry*, 1973, *43*, 72-78.

COMMUNITY MENTAL HEALTH CENTERS/Primary Prevention/*NUTRITION AND ORGANIC DISEASES*

3387   Birch, H. G. The problem of "brain damage" in children. In H. G. Birch (Ed.), *Brain damage in children: The biological and social aspects.* Baltimore: Williams & Wilkins, 1964. Pp. 3-12.

3388   *Scrimshaw, N. S. Infant malnutrition and adult learning. *Saturday Review*, 1968, *51*(11), 64-66.

3389   *Cravioto, J., DeLicardie, E. R. & Birch, H. G. Nutrition, growth and neurointegrative development: An experimental and ecologic study. *Pediatrics*, 1966, *38*, 319-372.

3390   Winick, M. Changes in nucleic acid and protein content of the human brain during growth. *Pediatric Research*, 1968, *2*, 352-355.

3391   Wohl, M. G. & Goodhart, R. S. (Eds.) *Modern nutrition in health and disease.* (3rd ed.) Philadelphia: Lea & Febiger, 1964.

3392   *Oppe, T. The emotional aspects of prematurity. *Cerebral Palsy Bulletin*, 1960, *2*, 233-237.

3393   *Wiener, G., Rider, R. V., Oppel, W. C., Fischer, L. K. & Harper, P. A. Correlates of low birth weight: Psychological status at six to seven years of age. *Pediatrics*, 1965, *35*, 434-444.

3394   *Thomas, A., et al. *Behavioral individuality in early childhood.* New York: New York University Press, 1963.

3395   Steward, A. H., Weiland, I. H., Leider, A. R., Mangham, C. A., Holmes, T. H. & Ripley, H. S. Excessive infant crying (colic) in relation to parent behavior. *American Journal of Psychiatry*, 1954, *110*, 687-694.

COMMUNITY MENTAL HEALTH CENTERS/Primary Prevention/*LEARNING AND SCHOOL EXPERIENCES*

3396   *Washington Association for Supervision and Curriculum Development. New views of intellectual development in early childhood education. In *Intellectual development.* Washington, D.C.: National Education Association, 1964.

3397   *Wender, P. H., Pedersen, F. A. & Waldrop, M. F. A longitudinal study of early social behavior and cognitive development. *American Journal of Orthopsychiatry*, 1967, *37*, 691-696.

3398   *White, R. W. Motivation reconsidered: The concept of competence. *Psychological Review*, 1959, *66*, 297-333.

3399   *Braun, S. J. The well baby clinic: Its prospects for building ego strength. *American Journal of Public Health*, 1965, *55*, 1889-1898.

3400   Biber, B. Schooling as an influence in developing healthy personality. In R. Kotinsky & H. L. Witmer (Eds.), *Community programs for mental health.* Cambridge: Harvard University Press, 1955. Pp. 158-221.

3401   *Bower, E. M.   Primary prevention in a school setting.   In
       G. Caplan (Ed.), *Prevention of mental disorders in
       children*.   New York: Basic Books, 1961.   Pp. 353-377.
3402   Westman, J. C., Rice, D. L. & Bermann, E.   Nursery school
       behavior and later school adjustment.   *American Journal
       of Orthopsychiatry*, 1967, *37*, 725-731.
3403   *Moore, T.   Difficulties of the ordinary child in adjusting
       to primary school.   *Journal of Child Psychology and Psy-
       chiatry and Allied Disciplines*, 1966, *7*, 17-38.
3404   *Zax, M. & Cowen, E. L.   Early identification and preven-
       tion of emotional disturbance in a public school.   In
       E. L. Cowen, E. A. Gardner & M. Zax (Eds.), *Emergent
       approaches to mental health problems*.   New York: Apple-
       ton-Century-Crofts, 1967.   Pp. 331-351.
3405   *Stennett, R. G.   Emotional handicap in the elementary
       years: Phase or disease?   *American Journal of Ortho-
       psychiatry*, 1966, *36*, 444-449.
3406   Zimiles, H.   Preventive aspects of school experience.
       In E. L. Cowen, E. A. Gardner & M. Zax (Eds.), *Emergent
       approaches to mental health problems*.   New York: Apple-
       ton-Century-Crofts, 1967.   Pp. 239-251.
3407   *Morgan, M. I. & Ojemann, R. H.   The effect of a learning
       program designed to assist youth in an understanding of
       behavior and its development.   *Child Development*, 1942,
       13, 181-194.
3408   Ojemann, R. H.   Investigations on the effects of teaching
       an understanding and appreciation of behavior dynamics.
       In G. Caplan (Ed.), *Prevention of mental disorders in
       children*.   New York: Basic Books, 1961.   Pp. 378-397.
3409   Lewis, W. W.   Project Re-Ed: Educational intervention in
       discordant child rearing systems.   In E. L. Cowen, E. A.
       Gardner & M. Zax (Eds.), *Emergent approaches to mental
       health problems*.   New York: Appleton-Century-Crofts,
       1967.   Pp. 352-368.
3410   Ambrosino, S.   A project in group education with parents
       of retarded children.   In *Casework papers*.   New York:
       Family Service Association of America, 1960.   Pp. 95-
       104.
3411   Berlin, I. N.   Consultation and special education.   In I.
       Philips (Ed.), *Prevention and treatment of mental re-
       tardation*.   New York: Basic Books, 1966.   Pp. 279-293.
3412   *Kellam, S. G. & Schiff, S. K.   Adaptation and mental ill-
       ness in the first-grade classrooms of an urban commu-
       nity.   *Psychiatric Research Reports of the American
       Psychiatric Association*, 1967, *21*, 79-91.
3412.1 Sapir, S. G. & Wilson, B.   A developmental scale to assist
       in the prevention of learning disability.   In S. G.
       Sapir & A. C. Nitzburg (Eds.), *Children with learning
       problems: Readings in a developmental-interaction ap-
       proach*.   New York: Brunner/Mazel, 1973.   Pp. 606-612.
3412.2 Murphy, L. B. & Chandler, C. A.   Building foundations
       for strength in the preschool years: Preventing devel-

opmental disturbances. In S. E. Golann & C. Eisdorfer
(Eds.), *Handbook of community mental health.* New York:
Appleton-Century-Crofts, 1972. Pp. 303-330.

3412.3 Bower, E. M. Education as a humanizing process and its
relationship to other humanizing processes. In S. E.
Golann & C. Eisdorfer (Eds.), *Handbook of community
mental health.* New York: Appleton-Century-Crofts,
1972. Pp. 37-49.

3412.4 Levine, M. & Graziano, A. M. Intervention programs in
elementary schools. In S. E. Golann & C. Eisdorfer
(Eds.), *Handbook of community mental health.* New York:
Appleton-Century-Crofts, 1972. Pp. 541-573.

3412.5 Trickett, E. J., Kelly, J. G. & Todd, D. M. The social
environment of the high school: Guidelines for individual change and organizational redevelopment. In S. E.
Golann & C. Eisdorfer (Eds.), *Handbook of community
mental health.* New York: Appleton-Century-Crofts,
1972. Pp. 331-406.

3412.6 Silver, A. A. & Hagin, R. A. Profile of a first grade:
A basis for preventive psychiatry. *Journal of the American Academy of Child Psychiatry,* 1972, *11,* 645-674.

COMMUNITY MENTAL HEALTH CENTERS/Primary Prevention/*ADOLESCENT
EXPERIENCES*

3413   *Siegel, E., Dillehay, R. & Fitzgerald, C. J. Role changes
within the child health conference: Attitudes and professional preparedness of public health nurses and physicians. *American Journal of Public Health,* 1965, *55,*
832-841.

3414   *Silber, E., Coelho, G. V., Murphey, E. B., Hamburg, D. A.,
Pearlin, L. I. & Rosenberg, M. Competent adolescents
coping with college decisions. *Archives of General Psychiatry,* 1961, *5,* 517-527.

3415   *Silber, E., Hamburg, D. A., Coelho, G. V., Murphey, E. B.,
Rosenberg, M. & Pearlin, L. I. Adaptive behavior in
competent adolescents: Coping with the anticipation of
college. *Archives of General Psychiatry,* 1961, *5,* 354-
365.

3416   *Kvaraceus, W. C. Forecasting delinquency: A three-year
experiment. *Exceptional Children,* 1961, *27,* 429-435.

3417   *Toby, J. An evaluation of early identification and intensive treatment programs for pre-delinquents. *Social Problems,* 1965, *13,* 160-175.

3418   *Abend, S. M., Kachalsky, H. & Greenberg, H. R. Reactions
of adolescents to short-term hospitalization. *American
Journal of Psychiatry,* 1968, *124,* 949-954.

COMMUNITY MENTAL HEALTH CENTERS/Secondary Prevention

3419   *Freud, A. *Normality and pathology in childhood: Assessments of development.* London: Hogarth Press, 1966. (Writings, vol. 6)

3420   *Hess, R. D. & Shipman, V. C. Early experience and the socialization of cognitive modes in children. *Child Development*, 1965, *36*, 869-886.

3421   Kagan, J., Moss, H. A. & Sigel, I. E. Psychological significance of styles of conceptualization. In J. C. Wright & J. Kagan (Eds.), Basic cognitive processes in children. *Monographs of the Society for Research in Child Development*, 1963, *28*(2, Serial No. 86), 73-112.

3422   *John, V. P. Mental health programs for the socially deprived, urban child--1962 Panel. 2. The intellectual development of slum children: Some preliminary findings. *American Journal of Orthopsychiatry*, 1963, *33*, 813-822.

3423   Crow, M. Preventive intervention through parent group education. *Social Casework*, 1967, *48*, 161-165.

3424   *Scott, J. P. Critical periods in behavioral development. *Science*, 1962, *138*, 949-958.

3425   *Skeels, H. M. Adult status of children with contrasting early life experiences: A follow-up study. *Monographs of the Society for Research in Child Development*, 1966, *31*(3, Serial No. 105).

3426   *Kubzansky, P. E. The effects of reduced environmental stimulation on human behavior: A review. In A. D. Biderman & H. Zimmer (Eds.), *The manipulation of human behavior.* New York: Wiley, 1961. Pp. 51-95.

3427   *Lidz, T. F. The marital relationship, family structure and personality development. In *Proceedings of the Third World Congress of Psychiatry, 1961.* Vol. 3. Montreal: University of Toronto Press, 1961-63. Pp. 117-120.

3428   *Pasamanick, B., Knobloch, H. & Lilienfeld, A. M. Socioeconomic status and some precursors of neuropsychiatric disorder. *American Journal of Orthopsychiatry*, 1956, *26*, 594-601.

3429   *Rutter, M., Birch, H. G., Thomas, A. & Chess, S. Temperamental characteristics in infancy and the later development of behavioural disorders. *British Journal of Psychiatry*, 1964. *110*, 651-661.

3430   Fried, M. Effects of social change on mental health. *American Journal of Orthopsychiatry*, 1964, *34*, 3-28.

3431   *Provence, S. A. & Lipton, R. C. *Infants in institutions.* New York: International Universities Press, 1963.

3432   Glueck, S. & Glueck, E. *Predicting delinquency and crime.* Cambridge: Harvard University Press, 1959.

3433   *Eisenberg, L. & Gruenberg, E. M. The current status of secondary prevention in child psychiatry. In A. J.

Bindman & A. D. Spiegel (Eds.), *Perspectives in community mental health.* Chicago: Aldine, 1969. Pp. 250-262.

3434 *Berlin, I. N. Secondary prevention. In A. M. Freedman & H. I. Kaplan (Eds.), *Comprehensive textbook of psychiatry.* Baltimore: Williams & Wilkins, 1967. Pp. 1541-1548.

3435 *Bower, E. M. *Early identification of emotionally handicapped children in school.* (2nd ed.) Springfield, Ill.: C. C. Thomas, 1969.

3436 Brody, S. Preventive intervention in current problems of early childhood. In G. Caplan (Ed.), *Prevention of mental disorders in children.* New York: Basic Books, 1961. Pp. 168-191.

3437 Arsenian, J. Situational factors contributing to mental illness in the United States: A theoretical summary. *Mental Hygiene,* 1961, *45,* 194-206.

3438 Freeman, H. E. & Sherwood, C. C. Research in large-scale intervention programs. *Journal of Social Issues,* 1965, *21*(1), 11-28.

3439 Farberow, N. L. & Schneidman, E. S. (Eds.) *The cry for help.* New York: McGraw-Hill, 1961.

3440 Augenbraun, B., Reid, H. L. & Friedman, D. B. Brief intervention as a preventive force in disorders of early childhood. *American Journal of Orthopsychiatry,* 1967, *37,* 697-702.

3441 *Cary, A. C. & Reveal, M. T. Prevention and detection of emotional disturbances in preschool children. *American Journal of Orthopsychiatry,* 1967, *37,* 719-724.

3442 Cornely, P. B. & Bigman, S. K. Some considerations in changing health attitudes. *Children,* 1963, *10,* 23-28.

3443 *Mechanic, D. The concept of illness behavior. *Journal of Chronic Diseases,* 1962, *15,* 189-194.

3444 Eisenberg, L. The sins of the father: Urban decay and social pathology. *American Journal of Orthopsychiatry,* 1962, *32,* 5-17.

3445 *Furman, E. Treatment of under-fives by way of their parents. *Psychoanalytic Study of the Child,* 1957, *12,* 250-262.

3447 *Keller, S. Mental health programs for the socially deprived, urban child--1962 Panel. 3. The social world of the urban slum child: Some early findings. *American Journal of Orthopsychiatry,* 1963, *33,* 823-831.

3448 Newman, R. G. Conveying essential messages to the emotionally disturbed child at school. *Exceptional Children,* 1961, *28,* 199-204.

3449 Tasem, M., Augenbraun, B. & Brown, S. L. Family group interviewing with the preschool child and both parents. *Journal of the American Academy of Child Psychiatry,* 1965, *4,* 330-340.

3450 Townsend, E. H. The social worker in pediatric practice: An experiment. *American Journal of Diseases of Chil-*

dren, 1964, *107,* 77-83.

3451   Burks, H. L. & Harrison, S. I. Aggressive behavior as a
means of avoiding depression. *American Journal of Orthopsychiatry,* 1962, *32,* 416-422.

3452   Rahe, R. H., Meyer, M., Smith, M., Kjaer, G. & Holmes,
T. H. Social stress and illness onset. *Journal of
Psychosomatic Research,* 1964, *8,* 35-44.

3453   *Balser, B. H., Wacker, E., Gratwick, M., Mumford, R. S.,
Clinton, W. & Balser, P. Predicting mental disturbance
in early adolescence. *American Journal of Psychiatry,*
1965, *121*(Suppl.), xi-xix.

3454   Barger, B. The University of Florida mental health program. In B. Barger & E. E. Hall (Eds.), *Higher education and mental health.* Gainesville: University of
Florida, Mental health project, 1963. Pp. 27-46.

3455   Bruch, H. Psychological aspects of obesity. *Psychiatry,*
1947, *10,* 373-381.

3456   Eisenberg, L. If not now, when? *American Journal of
Orthopsychiatry,* 1962, *32,* 781-793.

3457   *Kenyon, F. E. Hypochondriasis: A survey of some historical, clinical and social aspects. *British Journal of
Medical Psychology,* 1965, *38,* 117-133.

3458   Glass, A. J. Observations upon the epidemiology of mental illness in troops during warfare. In *Symposium on
Preventive and Social Psychiatry,* Walter Reed Army Institute of Research, 1957. Washington: U.S. Govt.
Print. Off., 1958. Pp. 185-198.

3459   Philips, I. (Ed.) *Prevention and treatment of mental retardation.* New York: Basic Books, 1966.

3460   *Guttmacher, A. F. Unwanted pregnancy: A challenge to
mental health. *Mental Hygiene,* 1967, *51,* 512-516.

3461   Leighton, D. C., Harding, J. S., Macklin, D. B., Macmillan, A. M. & Leighton, A. H. *The character of danger.*
New York: Basic Books, 1963. (Stirling County study
of psychiatric disorder and sociocultural environment,
vol. 3)

3462   Srole, L., Langner, T. S., Michael, S. T., Opler, M. K. &
Rennie, T. A. C. *The Midtown Manhattan study.* Vol. 1.
Mental health in the metropolis. New York: McGraw-
Hill, 1962.

3463   *Silver, A. A. & Hagin, R. A. Profile of a first grade:
A basis for preventive psychiatry. *Journal of the
American Academy of Child Psychiatry,* 1972, *11,* 645-
674.

3464   *Schiff, S. K. & Kellam, S. G. A community-wide mental
health program of prevention and early treatment in
first grade. *Psychiatric Research Reports of the American Psychiatric Association,* 1967, *21,* 92-102.

3464.1 Chess, S. & Thomas, A. Differences in outcome with early
intervention in children with behavior disorders. In
M. Roff, L. N. Robins & M. Pollack (Eds.), *Life history
research in psychopathology.* Vol. 2. Minneapolis:
University of Minnesota Press, 1972. Pp. 35-46.

COMMUNITY MENTAL HEALTH CENTERS/Tertiary Prevention

3465   Berlin, I. N. An early-warning system for detecting
        childhood problems. *Medical Insight,* 1969, *1,* 11-15.
3466   Deutscher, I. The social causes of social problems: From
        suicide to delinquency. In E. H. Mizruchi (Ed.), *The
        substance of sociology; codes, conduct, and conse-
        quences.* New York: Appleton-Century-Crofts, 1967.
        Pp. 247-258.
3467   *Caplan, G., Mason, E. A. & Kaplan, D. M. Four studies of
        crisis in parents of prematures. *Community Mental
        Health Journal,* 1965, *1,* 149-161.
3468   *Prugh, D. G. & Harlow, R. G. "Masked deprivation" in in-
        fants and young children. *World Health Organization
        Public Health Papers,* 1962, *14,* 9-29.
3469   Coleman, R. W. & Provence, S. Environmental retardation
        (hospitalism) in infants living in families. *Pediat-
        rics,* 1957, *19,* 285-292.
3470   *Green, M. & Solnit, A. J. Reactions to the threatened
        loss of a child: A vulnerable child syndrome. Pedi-
        atric management of the dying child, part III. *Pedi-
        atrics,* 1964, *34,* 58-66.
3471   *Mason, E. A. The hospitalized child--His emotional
        needs. *New England Journal of Medicine,* 1965, *272,*
        406-414.
3472   Prugh, D. G., Staub, E. M., Sands, H. H., Kirschbaum,
        R. M. & Lenihan, E. A. A study of the emotional re-
        actions of children and families to hospitalization
        and illness. *American Journal of Orthopsychiatry,*
        1953, *23,* 70-106.
3473   Mahler, M. S. On sadness and grief in infancy and child-
        hood. Loss and restoration of the symbiotic love ob-
        ject. *Psychoanalytic Study of the Child,* 1961, *16,*
        332-351.
3474   Engel, G. L. Is grief a disease? A challenge for medi-
        cal research. *Psychosomatic Medicine,* 1961, *23,* 18-22.
3475   *Lindemann, E. Symptomatology and management of acute
        grief. *American Journal of Psychiatry,* 1944, *101,* 141-
        148.
3476   *Milowe, I. D. & Lourie, R. S. 9. The child's role in the
        battered child syndrome. *Journal of Pediatrics,* 1964,
        65, 1079-1081.
3477   Schwartz, L. H., Snider, J. & Schwartz, J. E. Psychiatric
        case report of nutritional battering with implications
        for community agencies. *Community Mental Health Jour-
        nal,* 1967, *3,* 163-169.
3478   *Sperling, M. The neurotic child and his mother: A psy-
        choanalytic study. *American Journal of Orthopsychiatry,*
        1951, *21,* 351-362.
3479   *Berlin, I. N., Boatman, M. J., Sheimo, S. L. & Szurek, S.
        A. Adolescent alternation of anorexia and obesity.
        Workshop, 1950. *American Journal of Orthopsychiatry,*
        1951, *21,* 387-419.

3480   *Sperling, M. Mucous colitis associated with phobias.
       Psychoanalytic Quarterly, 1950, *19*, 318-326.
3481   Hobbs, D. B. & Osman, M. P. From prison to the community:
       A case study. *Crime and Delinquency*, 1967, *13*, 317-322.
3482   *Zetzel, E. R. Depression and the incapacity to bear it.
       In M. Schur (Ed.), *Drives, affects, behavior*. Vol. 2.
       New York: International Universities Press, 1965.
       Pp. 243-274.
3483   *Call, J. D. Prevention of autism in a young infant in a
       well-child conference. *Journal of the American Academy
       of Child Psychiatry*, 1963, *2*, 451-459.
3484   Weisman, A. D. & Hackett, T. P. Psychosis after eye sur-
       gery: Establishment of a specific doctor-patient re-
       lation in the prevention and treatment of "black-patch
       delirium". *New England Journal of Medicine*, 1958, *258*,
       1284-1289.
3485   White, R. W. The experience of efficacy in schizophrenia.
       Psychiatry, 1965, *28*, 199-211.

COMMUNITY MENTAL HEALTH CENTERS/Evaluation

3486   *Suchman, E. A. *Evaluative research: Principles and
       practice in public service & social action programs.*
       New York: Russell Sage Foundation, 1967.
3487   *Zusman, J. & Ross, E. R. R. Evaluation of the quality
       of mental health services. *Archives of General Psy-
       chiatry*, 1969, *20*, 352-357.
3488   *Schuman, L. M. *Research methodology and potential in
       community health and preventive medicine.* New York:
       New York Academy of Sciences, 1968. (*Annals of the
       New York Academy of Sciences*, 1962, *107*, Art. 2, 471-
       808)
3489   *Gruenberg, E. M. (Ed.) *Evaluating the effectiveness of
       mental health services.* New York: Milbank Memorial
       Fund, 1966.
3490   Selltiz, C., et al. *Research methods in social rela-
       tions.* New York: Holt, 1959.
3491   Hyman, H. H., Wright, C. R. & Hopkins, T. K. *Application
       of methods of evaluation; four studies of the encamp-
       ment for citizenship.* Berkeley: University of Cali-
       fornia Press, 1962.
3492   Group for the Advancement of Psychiatry. Committee on
       Research. *Psychiatric research and the assessment of
       change.* GAP report, no. 63. New York: Group for the
       Advancement of Psychiatry, 1966.
3493   Bergen, B. J. Professional communities and the evalua-
       tion of demonstration projects in community mental
       health. *American Journal of Public Health*, 1965, *55*,
       1057-1066.
3494   *Loeb, M. B. Evaluation as accountability: A basis for
       resistance to planning for community mental health

services. In L. M. Roberts, N. S. Greenfield & M. H. Miller (Eds.), *Comprehensive mental health: The challenge of evaluation*. Madison: University of Wisconsin Press, 1968. Pp. 249-258.

3494.1 Goltz, B., Rusk, T. N. & Sternbach, R. A. A built-in evaluation system in a new community mental health program. *American Journal of Public Health*, 1973, *63*, 702-709.

3494.2 Cline, D. W., Rouzer, D. L. & Bransford, D. Goal-attainment scaling as a method for evaluating mental health programs. *American Journal of Psychiatry*, 1973, *130*, 105-108.

XXIII. MENTAL HEALTH CONSULTATION

GENERAL THEORY

3495 *Caplan, G. *The theory and practice of mental health consultation*. New York: Basic Books, 1970.

3496 *Ferguson, C. K. Concerning the nature of human systems and the consultant's role. *Journal of Applied Behavioral Science*, 1968, *4*, 179-193.

3497 *Argyris, C. Explorations in consulting--client relationships. *Human Organization*, 1961, *20*, 121-133.

3498 *Bowman, P. H. The role of the consultant as a motivator of action. *Mental Hygiene*, 1959, *43*, 105-110.

3499 Gibb, J. R. The role of the consultant. *Journal of Social Issues*, 1959, *15*(2), 1-4.

3500 Gilbert, R. Functions of the consultant. *Teachers College Record*, 1960, *61*, 177-187.

3501 *Lippitt, G. L. A study of the consultation process. *Journal of Social Issues*, 1959, *15*(2), 43-50.

3502 *Kidneigh, J. C. The philosophy of administrative process and the role of the consultant. *Public Health Nursing*, 1951, *43*, 474-478.

3503 Meehan, M. The administrative staff consultant as a resource to the school administrator for the improvement of interpersonal relations. *American Journal of Orthopsychiatry*, 1969, *39*, 286-288.

3504 *Lippitt, G. L. Organizational climate and individual growth: The consultative process at work. *Personnel Administration*, 1960, *23*(5), 12-19;43.

3505 Deloughery, G. L. & Gebbie, K. M. Categories of cases presented to mental health consultants by health agencies. *American Journal of Public Health*, 1973, *63*, 1048-1054.

PRINCIPLES/Characteristics

3506   *Caplan, G.   Types of mental health consultation. *American Journal of Orthopsychiatry*, 1963, *33*, 470-481.
3507   *Brockbank, R.   Aspects of mental health consultation. *Archives of General Psychiatry*, 1968, *18*, 267-275.
3508   *Berlin, I. N.   Mental health consultation for school social workers: A conceptual model. *Community Mental Health Journal*, 1969, *5*, 280-288.
3509   Abramovitz, A. B.   Methods and techniques of consultation. *American Journal of Orthopsychiatry*, 1958, *28*, 126-133.
3510   *Haylett, C. H. & Rapoport, L.   Mental health consultation. In L. Bellak (Ed.), *Handbook of community psychiatry and community mental health*. New York: Grune & Stratton, 1964. Pp. 319-339.
3511   Kazanjian, V., Stein, S. & Winberg, W. L.   An introduction to mental health consultation. *Public Health Monographs*, 1962, *69*, 1-13.
3512   Mendel, W. M. & Solomon, P. (Eds.)   *The psychiatric consultation*. New York: Grune & Stratton, 1968.
3513   *Robbins, P. R. & Spencer, E. C.   A study of the consultation process. *Psychiatry*, 1968, *31*, 362-368.
3514   *Bindman, A. J.   Mental health consultation: Theory and practice. *Journal of Consulting Psychology*, 1959, *23*, 473-482.
3515   *Gorman, J. F.   Some characteristics of consultation. In L. Rapoport (Ed.), *Consultation in social work practice*. New York: National Association of Social Workers, 1963. Pp. 21-31.
3516   Glidewell, J. C.   The entry problem in consultation. *Journal of Social Issues*, 1959, *15*(2), 51-59.
3517   *Jarvis, P. E. & Nelson, S. E.   Familiarization: A vital step in mental health consultation. *Community Mental Health Journal*, 1967, *3*, 343-348.
3518   *Berlin, I. N.   Transference and countertransference in community psychiatry. *Archives of General Psychiatry*, 1966, *15*, 165-172.
3519   Hollister, W. G.   Some administrative aspects of consultation. *American Journal of Orthopsychiatry*, 1962, *32*, 224-225.
3520   *Klein, D. C.   Consultation processes as a method of improving teaching. *Boston University. Human Relations Center, Research Reports and Technical Notes*, 1964, *69*.
3521   *Mannino, F. V.   Developing consultation relationships with community agents. *Mental Hygiene*, 1964, *48*, 356-362.
3522   *Libo, L. M. & Griffith, C. R.   Developing mental health programs in areas lacking professional facilities: The community consultant approach in New Mexico. *Community Mental Health Journal*, 1966, *2*, 163-169.
3523   Adams, P. L.   Techniques for pediatric consultation. In J. J. Schwab, *Handbook of psychiatric consultation*.

New York: Appleton-Century-Crofts, 1968. Pp. 107-123.
3524   *Caplan, G. *The theory and practice of mental health con-
       sultation.* New York: Basic Books, 1970.
3525   Levy, D. M. *The demonstration clinic for the psychologi-
       cal study and treatment of mother and child in medical
       practice.* Springfield, Ill.: Thomas, 1959.

PRINCIPLES/Training

3526   Caplan, G. An approach to the education of community
       mental health specialists. *Mental Hygiene,* 1959, *43,*
       268-280.
3527   Barnes, R. H., Busse, E. W. & Bressler, B. The training
       of psychiatric residents in consultative skills. *Jour-
       nal of Medical Education,* 1957, *32,* 124-130.
3528   *Berlin, I. N. Learning mental health consultation: His-
       tory and problems. *Mental Hygiene,* 1964, *48,* 257-266.
3529   *Bernard, V. W. Roles and functions of child psychiatrists
       in social and community psychiatry: Implications for
       training. *Journal of the American Academy of Child
       Psychiatry,* 1964, *3,* 165-176.
3530   *Caplan, G. Problems of training in mental health consulta-
       tion. In S. E. Goldston (Ed.), *Concepts of community psy-
       chiatry: A framework for training.* Bethesda, Md.: U. S.
       National Institute of Mental Health, 1965. Pp. 91-108.
3531   Hume, P. B. Principles and practice of community psychi-
       atry: The role and training of the specialist in com-
       munity psychiatry. In L. Bellak (Ed.), *Handbook of
       community psychiatry and community mental health.* New
       York: Grune & Stratton, 1964. Pp. 65-81.
3532   *Leon, R. L. A participant-directed experience as a method
       of psychiatric teaching and consultation. *Mental Hy-
       giene,* 1960, *44,* 375-381.
3533   *Parker, B. The value of supervision in training psychia-
       trists for mental health consultation. *Mental Hygiene,*
       1961, *45,* 94-100.
3534   *vonFelsinger, J. M. & Klein, D. C. Professional training
       for the mental health field. *Mental Hygiene,* 1962, *46,*
       203-217.
3535   *Rogawski, A. S. Teaching consultation techniques in a
       community agency. In W. M. Mendel & P. Solomon (Eds.),
       The psychiatric consultation. New York: Grune & Strat-
       ton, 1968. Pp. 65-85.
3536   Adams, R. S. & Weinick, H. M. Consultation: An inservice
       training program for the school. *Journal of the Ameri-
       can Academy of Child Psychiatry,* 1966, *5,* 479-489.
3537   Schiff, S. K. & Turner, D. T. The Woodlawn School Mental
       Health Training Program: A community-based university
       graduate course. *Journal of School Psychology,* 1971,
       9, 292-302.
3538   Berken, G. & Eisdorfer, C. Closed ranks in microcosm:

Pitfalls of a training experience in community consultation. *Community Mental Health Journal,* 1970, *6,* 101-109.

PRINCIPLES/Evaluation

3539   *Eisenberg, L. An evaluation of psychiatric consultation service for a public agency. *American Journal of Public Health,* 1958, *48,* 742-749.
3540   *Weinberg, W. L. *Describing and evaluating mental health consultation sessions by the use of a rating scale.* Doctoral dissertation, California School of Professional Psychology, July, 1971.
3541   Balser, B. H., et al. Further report on experimental evaluation of mental hygiene techniques in school and community. *American Journal of Psychiatry,* 1957, *113,* 733-739.
3542   Eisdorfer, C. & Batton, L. The mental health consultant as seen by his consultees. *Community Mental Health Journal,* 1972, *8,* 171-177.
3543   Singh, R. K. J., Kazanjian, V. & Weinberg, W. L. *A study of the process and outcome of consultee centered case consultation. Research project: San Mateo County, Calif.* Berkeley: Mental Health Service and Community Psychiatry and Mental Health Administrative Center, 1967.

METHODS/General

3544   *Griffith, C. R. & Libo, L. M. *Mental health consultants: Agents of community change.* San Francisco: Jossey-Bass, 1968.

METHODS/Schools

3545   *Caplan, G. Mental health consultation in schools. In *Elements of a community mental health program.* New York: Milbank Memorial Fund, 1956. Pp. 77-85.
3546   *Berlin, I. N. Some learning experiences as psychiatric consultant in the schools. *Mental Hygiene,* 1956, *40,* 215-236.
3547   *Berkovitz, I. H. Mental health consultation to school personnel: Attitudes of school administrators and consultant priorities. *Journal of School Health,* 1970, *40,* 348-354.
3548   *Bonkowski, R. J. Mental health consultation and operation head start. *American Psychologist,* 1968, *23,* 769-773.
3549   *Parker, B. Some observations on psychiatric consultation

with nursery school teachers. *Mental Hygiene,* 1962,
46, 559-566.

3550   Perkins, K. J. Consultation service to public schools by
a mental-health team. *Mental Hygiene,* 1953, *37,* 585-
595.

3551   *Minde, K. K. & Werry, J. S. Intensive psychiatric teacher
counseling in a low socioeconomic area: A controlled
evaluation. *American Journal of Orthopsychiatry,* 1969,
39, 595-608.

3552   Hirschowitz, R. G. Psychiatric consultation in the
schools: Socio-cultural perspectives. *Mental Hygiene,*
1966, *50,* 218-225.

3554   *Berlin, I. N. Mental health consultation in schools as
a means of communicating mental health principles.
Journal of the American Academy of Child Psychiatry,
1962, *1,* 671-680.

3555   Berlin, I. N. Mental health consultation in schools:
Who can do it, and why. *Community Mental Health Journal,* 1965, *1,* 19-22.

3556   Berlin, I. N. School child guidance services: Retrospect
and prospect. *Psychology in the Schools,* 1966, *3,*
229-236.

3557   Altman, M. A child psychiatrist steps into the classroom:
Report of a training experience. *Journal of the American Academy of Child Psychiatry,* 1972, *11,* 231-242.

METHODS/Courts

3558   Malmquist, C. P. Dilemmas of the juvenile court. *Journal
of the American Academy of Child Psychiatry,* 1967, *6,*
723-748.

3559   Lindeman, F. T. & McIntyre, D. M. (Eds.) *The mentally
disabled and the law.* Chicago: University of Chicago
Press, 1961.

3560   *Gianascol, A. J. Psychiatry and the juvenile court:
Patterns of collaboration and the use of compulsory
psychotherapy. In S. A. Szurek & I. N. Berlin (Eds.),
The antisocial child: His family and his community.
Palo Alto, Calif.: Science & Behavior Books, 1969.
Pp. 149-159.

3561   *Susselman, S. Interrelationship of the correctional
worker, the offender, and the legal structure. In S.
A. Szurek & I. N. Berlin (Eds.), *The antisocial child:
His family and his community.* Palo Alto, Calif.:
Science & Behavior Books, 1969. Pp. 134-148.

3562   *Berlin, I. N. Mental health consultation with a juvenile
probation department. *Crime and Delinquency,* 1964, *10,*
67-73.

3563   Gibson, R. W. The psychiatric consultant and the juvenile court. *Mental Hygiene,* 1954, *38,* 462-467.

3564   *Elkins, A. M. & Papanek, G. O. Consultation with the

police: An example of community psychiatry practice.
American Journal of Psychiatry, 1966, *123*, 531-535.
3565 *Goldin, G. D. The psychiatrist as a court consultant:
A challenge to community psychiatry. *Community Mental
Health Journal*, 1967, *3*, 396-398.
3566 Berlin, I. N. & Szurek, S. A. (Eds.) *The antisocial
child: His family and his community.* Palo Alto,
Calif.: Science & Behavior Books, 1969. (*Clinical
approaches to problems of childhood.* Vol. 4)
3566.1 Shah, S. A. The criminal justice system. In S. E. Golann
& C. Eisdorfer (Eds.), *Handbook of community mental
health.* New York: Appleton-Century-Crofts, 1972.
Pp. 73-105.
3566.2 Beran, N. & Dinitz, S. An empirical study of the psychiatric probation-commitment procedure. *American
Journal of Orthopsychiatry*, 1973, *43*, 660-669.
3566.3 Lewis, D. O., Balla, D. A., Sacks, H. L. & Jekel, J. F.
Psychotic symptomatology in a juvenile court clinic
population. *Journal of the American Academy of Child
Psychiatry*, 1973, *12*, 660-674.

METHODS/Social Agencies

3567 *Coleman, J. V. The contribution of the psychiatrist to
the social worker and to the client. *Mental Hygiene*,
1953, *37*, 249-258.
3568 Maddux, J. F. Psychiatric consultation in a public welfare agency. *American Journal of Orthopsychiatry*,
1950, *20*, 754-764.
3569 *Rapoport, L. (Ed.) *Consultation in social work practice.*
New York: National Association of Social Workers, 1963.
3570 Thompson, W. C. Psychiatric consultation in social a-
gencies. *Child Welfare*, 1957, *36*(9), 1-3.
3571 *Berlin, I. N. Mental health consultation for school social workers: A conceptual model. *Community Mental
Health Journal*, 1969, *5*, 280-288.
3572 Bernard, V. W. Psychiatric consultation in the social
agency. *Child Welfare*, 1954, *33*(9), 3-8.
3573 *Coleman, J. V. Mental health consultation to agencies
protecting family life. In *Elements of a community
mental health program.* New York: Milbank Memorial
Fund, 1956. Pp. 69-76.
3575 Decker, J. H. & Itzin, F. An experience in consultation
in public assistance. *Social Casework*, 1956, *37*, 327-
334.
3576 Mercer, M. E. Mental health consultation to child health
protecting agencies. In *Elements of a community mental
health program.* New York: Milbank Memorial Fund,
1956. Pp. 47-56.
3578 *Chwast, J. Mental health consultation with street gang
workers. In W. C. Reckless & C. L. Newman (Eds.),

Interdisciplinary problems in criminology: Papers of the American Society of Criminology. 1964. Columbus: Ohio State University, 1965. Pp. 13-21.

3579   Forstenzer, H. M. Consultation and mental health programs. *American Journal of Public Health,* 1961, *51,* 1280-1285.

3580   *Davis, W. E. Psychiatric consultation--The agency viewpoint. *Child Welfare,* 1957, *36*(9), 4-9.

3581   *Spencer, E. C. & Croley, H. T. Administrative consultation. In L. Rapoport (Ed.), *Consultation in social work practice.* New York: National Association of Social Workers, 1963. Pp. 51-68.

METHODS/Public Health

3582   *Parker, B. *Psychiatric consultation for nonpsychiatric professional workers; a concept of group consultation developed from a training program for nurses.* Washington, D.C.: U.S. Dept. of Health, Education, and Welfare, Public Health Service, 1958. (Public health monograph no. 53)

3583   *Maddux, J. F. Consultation in public health. *American Journal of Public Health,* 1955, *45,* 1424-1430.

3584   *Farley, B. C. Individual mental health consultation with public health nurses. In L. Rapoport (Ed.), *Consultation in social work practice.* New York: National Association of Social Workers, 1963. Pp. 99-116.

3585   Howell, R. W. Mental health consultation to public health nurses. In *Elements of a community mental health program.* New York: Milbank Memorial Fund, 1956. Pp. 57-68.

3586   Mouw, M. L. & Haylett, C. H. Mental health consultation in a public health nursing service. *American Journal of Nursing,* 1967, *67,* 1447-1450.

3587   *Rieman, D. W. Group mental health consultation with public health nurses. In L. Rapoport (Ed.), *Consultation in social work practice.* New York: National Association of Social Workers, 1963. Pp. 85-98.

3588   Blumberg, A. A nurse consultant's responsibility and problems. *American Journal of Nursing,* 1956, *56,* 606-608.

3589   *Wodinsky, A. Psychiatric consultation with nurses on a leukemia service. *Mental Hygiene,* 1964, *48,* 282-287.

3590   *Stringer, L. A. Consultation: Some expectations, principles, and skills. *Social Work,* 1961, *6,* 85-90.

METHODS/Special Programs

3591 *Parker, B. Some observations on psychiatric consultation with nursery school teachers. *Mental Hygiene*, 1962, *46*, 559-566.
3592 *Perkins, G. L. Psychiatric consultation in residential treatment. Workshop, 1957. 2. The consultant's view. *American Journal of Orthopsychiatry*, 1958, *28*, 266-275.
3593 *Berlin, I. N. Consultation and special education. In I. Philips (Ed.), *Prevention and treatment of mental retardation*. New York: Basic Books, 1966. Pp. 279-293.
3594 Mumford, E., Brown, F. & Kaufman, M. R. A hospital-based school mental health project. *American Journal of Psychiatry*, 1971, *127*, 920-924.
3595 *Schowalter, J. E. & Solnit, A. J. Child psychiatry consultation in a general hospital emergency room. *Journal of the American Academy of Child Psychiatry*, 1966, *5*, 534-551.
3596 Mannino, F. V. Developing consultation relationships with community agents. *Mental Hygiene*, 1964, *48*, 356-362.
3597 *Libo, L. M. Multiple functions for psychologists in community consultation. *American Psychologist*, 1966, *21*, 530-534.
3598 *Maddux, J. F. Psychiatric consultation in a rural setting. *American Journal of Orthopsychiatry*, 1953, *23*, 775-784.
3599 *Kinzie, J. D., Shore, J. H. & Pattison, E. M. Anatomy of psychiatric consultation to rural Indians. *Community Mental Health Journal*, 1972, *8*, 196-207.
3600 Bindman, A. J. The psychologist as a mental health consultant. *Journal of Psychiatric Nursing*, 1964, *2*, 367-380.

METHODS/Group Consultation

3601 *Altrocchi, J., Spielberger, C. D. & Eisdorfer, C. Mental health consultation with groups. *Community Mental Health Journal*, 1965, *1*, 127-134.
3602 *Kevin, D. Use of the group method in consultation. In L. Rapoport (Ed.), *Consultation in social work practice* New York: National Association of Social Workers, 1963. Pp. 69-84.
3603 *Mackey, R. A. & Hassler, F. R. Group consultation with school personnel. *Mental Hygiene*, 1966, *50*, 416-420.
3604 *Rowitch, J. Group consultation with school personnel. *Hospital and Community Psychiatry*, 1968, *19*, 261-266.
3605 *Bradford, L. P. The use of psychodrama for group consultants. *Sociatry*, 1947, *1*, 192-197.
3606 Gibb, J. R. & Lippitt, R. Consulting with groups and

organizations. *Journal of Social Issues,* 1959, *15*(2), 1-74.

3607 *Kysar, J. E. The community psychiatrist and large organizations. *Mental Hygiene,* 1968, *52,* 210-217.

3608 *Cartwright, D. & Zander, A. (Eds.) *Group dynamics: Research and theory.* (3rd ed.) New York: Harper & Row, 1968.

3609 *Blumberg, A. A selected annotated bibliography on the consultant relationship with groups. *Journal of Social Issues,* 1959, *15*(2), 68-74.

XXIV. CRISIS INTERVENTION AND BRIEF THERAPY

CRISIS INTERVENTION

3610 *Rapoport, L. The state of crisis: Some theoretical considerations. *Social Service Review,* 1962, *36,* 211-217.

3611 *Cadden, V. Crisis in the family. In G. Caplan (Ed.), *Principles of preventive psychiatry.* New York: Basic Books, 1964. Pp. 288-296.

3612 *Fantl, B. Preventive intervention. *Social Work,* 1962, *7,* 41-47.

3613 *Karp, H. N. & Karls, J. M. Combining crisis therapy and mental health consultation. *Archives of General Psychiatry,* 1966, *14,* 536-542.

3614 *Berlin, I. N. Crisis intervention and short-term therapy: An approach in a child-psychiatric clinic. *Journal of the American Academy of Child Psychiatry,* 1970, *9,* 595-606.

3615 Stein, M. The function of ambiguity in child crises. *Journal of the American Academy of Child Psychiatry,* 1970, *9,* 462-476.

3616 *Klein, D. C. & Lindemann, E. Preventive intervention in individual and family crisis situations. In G. Caplan (Ed.), *Prevention of mental disorders in children.* New York: Basic Books, 1961. Pp. 283-306.

3617 Beck, A. T., Sethi, B. B. & Tuthill, R. W. Childhood bereavement and adult depression. *Archives of General Psychiatry,* 1963, *9,* 295-302.

3618 *Lindemann, E. Symptomatology and management of acute grief. *American Journal of Psychiatry,* 1944, *101,* 141-148.

3619 *Caplan, G. Patterns of parental response to the crisis of premature birth: A preliminary approach to modifying the mental-health outcome. *Psychiatry,* 1960, *23,* 365-374.

3620 Kaplan, D. M. & Mason, E. A. Maternal reactions to premature birth viewed as an acute emotional disorder. *American Journal of Orthopsychiatry,* 1960, *30,* 539-547.

3621 *Parad, H. J. *Crisis intervention: Selected readings.* New York: Family Service Association of America, 1965.

3622   *Strickler, M. Applying crisis theory in a community
       clinic. *Social Casework*, 1965, *46*, 150-154.
3623   Meerloo, J. A. M. First aid in acute panic states. *Amer-
       ican Journal of Psychotherapy*, 1951, *5*, 367-371.
3624   *Meerloo, J. A. M. Emergency psychotherapy and mental
       first aid. *Journal of Nervous and Mental Disease*,
       1956, *124*, 535-545.
3625   *Rosenthal, H. R. Emergency psychotherapy: A crucial
       need. *Psychoanalytic Review*, 1965, *52*, 446-459.
3626   Wayne, G. J. & Koegler, R. R. (Eds.) *Emergency psychi-
       atry and brief therapy*. Boston: Little, Brown, 1966.

BRIEF THERAPY

3627   *Jacobsen, G. F., et al. The scope and practice of an
       early-access brief treatment psychiatric center. *Amer-
       ican Journal of Psychiatry*, 1965, *121*, 1176-1182.
3628   *Kalis, B. L., Harris, M. R., Prestwood, A. R. & Freeman,
       E. H. Precipitating stress as a focus in psychotherapy.
       Archives of General Psychiatry, 1961, *5*, 219-226.
3629   Castelnuovo-Tedesco, P. *The twenty-minute hour*. Boston:
       Little, Brown, 1965.
3630   Gillman, R. D. Brief psychotherapy: A psychoanalytic
       view. *American Journal of Psychiatry*, 1965, *122*, 601-
       611.
3631   *Proskauer, S. Some technical issues in time-limited
       psychotherapy with children. *Journal of the American
       Academy of Child Psychiatry*, 1969, *8*, 154-169.
3632   *McGuire, M. T. The process of short-term insight psy-
       chotherapy. II: Content, expectations and structure.
       Journal of Nervous and Mental Disease, 1965, *141*, 219-
       230.
3633   Baum, O. E. & Felzer, S. B. Activity in initial inter-
       views with lower-class patients. *Archives of General
       Psychiatry*, 1964, *10*, 345-353.
3634   Bonstedt, T. Psychotherapy in a public psychiatric clin-
       ic: An attempt at "adjustment". *Psychiatric Quar-
       terly*, 1965, *39*, 1-15.
3635   Phillips, E. L. & Wiener, D. N. *Short-term psychotherapy
       and structured behavior change*. New York: McGraw-
       Hill, 1966.
3636   Shaw, R., Blumenfeld, H. & Senf, R. A short-term treat-
       ment program in a child guidance clinic. *Social Work*,
       1968, *13*, 81-90.
3637   Cain, A. C. & Maupin, B. M. Interpretation within the
       metaphor. *Bulletin of the Menninger Clinic*, 1961, *25*,
       307-311.
3638   Melges, F. T. & Bowlby, J. Types of hopelessness in psy-
       chopathological process. *Archives of General Psychi-
       atry*, 1969, *20*, 690-699.

3639   *Minuchin, S. The use of an ecological framework in the
        treatment of a child. In E. Anthony & C. Koupernik
        (Eds.), *The child in his family.* New York: Wiley,
        1970. Pp. 41-57. (International Yearbook for Child
        Psychiatry and Allied Disciplines, vol. 1)
3640   *Sarvis, M. A., Dewees, S. & Johnson, R. F. A concept of
        ego-oriented psychotherapy. *Psychiatry,* 1959, *22,*
        277-287.
3641   Pattison, E. M. Treatment of alcoholic families with
        nurse home visits. *Family Process,* 1965, *4,* 75-94.
3641.1 Corbett, R. M. Health planning: Some legal and politi-
        cal implications of comprehensive health planning.
        American Journal of Public Health, 1974, *64,* 136-139.

PART V

TRAINING IN ADMINISTRATION AND RESEARCH

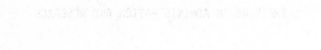

XXV. STAFF INTERACTION

STAFF PROBLEMS AND PATIENT DISORDER

3642   *Band, R. I. & Brody, E. B. Human elements of the thera-
       peutic community: A study of the attitudes of people
       upon whom patients must be dependent. *Archives of
       General Psychiatry*, 1962, *6*, 307-314.

3643   Devereux, G. The social structure of the hospital as a
       factor in total therapy. *American Journal of Ortho-
       psychiatry*, 1949, *19*, 492-500.

3644   *Rioch, D. McK. & Stanton, A. H. Milieu therapy. *Psychi-
       atry*, 1953, *16*, 65-72.

3645   *Schwartz, C. G., Schwartz, M. S. & Stanton, A. H. A
       study of need-fulfillment on a mental hospital ward.
       Psychiatry, 1951, *14*, 223-242.

3646   *Stanton, A. H. Staff relationships affect hospital at-
       mosphere. *Mental Hospitals*, 1957, *8*(2), 12-15.

3647   Stanton, A. H. & Schwartz, M. S. Medical opinion and the
       social context in the mental hospital. *Psychiatry*,
       1949, *12*, 243-249.

3648   Rosenhan, D. L. On being sane in insane places. *Science*,
       1973, *179*, 250-258.

3649   *Stanton, A. H. & Schwartz, M. S. The management of a
       type of institutional participation in mental illness.
       Psychiatry, 1949, *12*, 13-26.

3650   *Schwartz, M. S. & Will, G. T. Low morale and mutual with-
       drawal on a mental hospital ward. *Psychiatry*, 1953,
       16, 337-353.

3651   *Stanton, A. H. & Schwartz, M. S. Observations on dis-
       sociation as social participation. *Psychiatry*, 1949,
       12, 339-354.

3652   Schwartz, M. S. Patient demands in a mental hospital
       context. *Psychiatry*, 1957, *20*, 249-261.

3653   *Schwartz, M. S. & Stanton, A. H. A social psychological
       study of incontinence. *Psychiatry*, 1950, *13*, 399-416.

3654   Brandes, N. S. Some possible meanings of the hallway
       interview. *Journal of Nervous and Mental Disease*,
       1957, *125*, 564-569.

3655   *Rae-Grant, Q. A. F. & Marcuse, D. J. The hazards of
       teamwork. *American Journal of Orthopsychiatry*, 1968,
       38, 4-8.

3656   *Astrachan, B. M. & McKee, B. The impact of staff conflict
       on patient care and behaviour. *British Journal of Medi-
       cal Psychology*, 1965, *38*, 313-320.
3657   LaBarre, M. B. Dynamic factors in psychiatric team col-
       laboration. *British Journal of Medical Psychology*,
       1960, *33*, 53-60.
3658   *Brodey, W. M. & Hayden, M. Intrateam reactions: Their
       relation to the conflicts of the family in treatment.
       American Journal of Orthopsychiatry, 1957, *27*, 349-355.
3659   *Brody, E. M. & Weithorn, C. The need for refinements in
       the techniques of interdisciplinary hostility for social
       workers and psychologists. *American Journal of Ortho-
       psychiatry*, 1967, *37*, 797-799.

ROLE OF THE PSYCHIATRIC NURSE

3660   *Lewis, G. K. Nursing care on the ward level. *Mental
       Hospitals*, 1957, *8*(2), 30-33.
3661   Parloff, M. B. The impact of ward-milieu philosophies
       on nursing-role concepts. *Psychiatry*, 1960, *23*, 141-
       151.
3662   *Tudor, G. E. A sociopsychiatric nursing approach to in-
       tervention in a problem of mutual withdrawal on a mental
       hospital ward. *Psychiatry*, 1952, *15*, 193-217.
3663   Kalkman, M. E. What the psychiatric nurse should be edu-
       cated to do. *Psychiatric Quarterly. Supplement 1*,
       1952, *26*, 93-102.
3664   Weiss, M. O. *Attitudes in psychiatric nursing care.*
       New York: Putnam, 1954.
3665   *Stanton, A. H. & Schwartz, M. S. *The mental hospital.*
       New York: Basic Books, 1954.
3666   *Highley, B. L. & Norris, C. M. When a student dislikes
       a patient. *American Journal of Nursing*, 1957, *57*,
       1163-1166.

STAFF INTERACTION IN CHILDREN'S SETTINGS

3667   *Sheimo, S. L., Paynter, J. & Szurek, S. A. Problems of
       staff interaction with spontaneous group formations on
       a children's psychiatric ward. *American Journal of
       Orthopsychiatry*, 1949, *19*, 599-611.
3668   *Gordon, G. & Siegel, L. The evolution of a program of
       individual psychotherapy for children with aggressive
       acting-out disorders in a new residential treatment
       unit. *American Journal of Orthopsychiatry*, 1957, *27*,
       59-68.
3669   *Christ, A. E. & Wagner, N. N. Iatrogenic factors in resi-
       dential treatment: A problem in staff training. *Amer-
       ican Journal of Orthopsychiatry*, 1966, *36*, 725-729.
3670   *Szurek, S. A. & Berlin, I. N. The question of therapy

for the trainee in the psychiatric training program. *Journal of the American Academy of Child Psychiatry*, 1966, *5*, 155-165. (Also in S. A. Szurek & I. N. Berlin (Eds.), *Training in therapeutic work with children.* Palo Alto, Calif.: Science & Behavior Books, 1967. Pp. 243-252.)

3671 *Berlin, I. N., Boatman, M. J., Sheimo, S. L. & Szurek, S. A. Adolescent alternation of anorexia and obesity. Workshop, 1950. *American Journal of Orthopsychiatry*, 1951, *21*, 387-419.

3672 *Greenberg, H. A., Bettelheim, B., Perkins, G. L., Wright, B. & Riley, M. J. Psychiatric consultation in residential treatment. Workshop, 1957. *American Journal of Orthopsychiatry*, 1958, *28*, 256-290.

3673 *Sutton, H. A. Some nursing aspects of a children's psychiatric ward. *American Journal of Orthopsychiatry*, 1947, *17*, 675-683.

3674 Szurek, S. A., Johnson, A. & Falstein, E. Collaborative psychiatric therapy of parent-child problems. *American Journal of Orthopsychiatry*, 1942, *12*, 511-516.

3675 Schiele, H. & Harris, D. M. Dual therapy in residential treatment. *Child Welfare*, 1960, *39*(5), 10-13.

3676 Gilbertson, R. J. L. & Sutton, H. A children's psychiatric service. *American Journal of Nursing*, 1943, *43*, 570-572.

3677 Cutter, A. V. & Hallowitz, D. Different approaches to treatment of the child and the parents. *American Journal of Orthopsychiatry*, 1962, *32*, 152-158.

3677.1 Fine, M. J., Nesbitt, J. A. & Tyler, M. Analysis of a failing attempt at behavior modification. *Journal of Learning Disabilities*, 1974, *7*, 70-75.

3677.2 Tooley, K. The effects of treatment failure: Observations on the reactions of staff and children to the transferral of psychotic children. *Journal of the American Academy of Child Psychiatry*, 1972, *11*, 712-728.

XXVI. CLINICAL SUPERVISION OF THE TRAINEE IN GENERAL PSYCHIATRY AND CHILD PSYCHIATRY

PSYCHIATRIC TRAINING: PROBLEMS AND OPPORTUNITIES

3678 Leifer, R. The medical model as ideology. *International Journal of Psychiatry*, 1970-1971, *9*, 13-21.

3679 *Rudy, L. H. Psychiatric education: New challenges. *American Journal of Psychiatry*, 1971, *128*, 633-634.

3680 *Mariner, A. S. A critical look at professional education in the mental health field. *American Psychologist*, 1967, *22*, 271-281.

3681 *Rabkin, R. Affect as a social process. *American Journal of Psychiatry*, 1968, *125*, 773-779.

3682 Halleck, S. L. *The politics of therapy.* New York: Science House, 1971.

3683   Jason, H., Kagan, N., Werner, A., Elstein, A. S. & Thomas,
       J. B. New approaches to teaching basic interview skills
       to medical students. *American Journal of Psychiatry*,
       1971, *127*, 1404-1407.
3684   *Coker, R. E., Back, K. W., Donnelly, T. G. & Miller, N.
       Patterns of influence: Medical school faculty members
       and the values and specialty interests of medical stu-
       dents. *Journal of Medical Education*, 1960, *35*, 518-527.
3685   *Schlessinger, N., Muslin, H. L. & Baittle, M. Teaching
       and learning psychiatric observational skills. *Archives
       of General Psychiatry*, 1968, *18*, 549-552.
3686   *Engel, G. L. On the care and feeding of the faculty: A
       responsibility for students. *New England Journal of
       Medicine*, 1969, *281*, 351-355.
3687   *Miller, M. H., Fey, W. F. & Greenfield, N. S. The impli-
       cations of changing medical education for psychiatric
       training institutions. *American Journal of Psychiatry*,
       1970, *126*, 1127-1131.
3687.1 Daniels, R. S. Changing human service delivery systems:
       Their influences on psychiatric training. *American
       Journal of Psychiatry*, 1973, *130*, 1232-1236.
3688   *Raskin, D. E. Psychiatric training in the 70s--Toward a
       shift in emphasis. *American Journal of Psychiatry*,
       1972, *128*, 1129-1131.
3689   Plutchik, R., Conte, H. & Kandler, H. Variables related
       to the selection of psychiatric residents. *American
       Journal of Psychiatry*, 1971, *127*, 1503-1508.
3690   Riess, B. F. The selection and supervision of psycho-
       therapists. In N. P. Dellis & H. K. Stone (Eds.), *The
       training of psychotherapists; a multidisciplinary ap-
       proach*. Baton Rouge: Louisiana State University
       Press, 1960. Pp. 104-124.
3690.1 Goodman, G. Systematic selection of psychotherapeutic
       talent: Group assessment of interpersonal traits. In
       S. E. Golann & C. Eisdorfer (Eds.), *Handbook of com-
       munity mental health*. New York: Appleton-Century-
       Crofts, 1972. Pp. 939-954.
3691   *O'Connor, C. T. Peer group influences on the choice of a
       psychiatric viewpoint. *Archives of General Psychiatry*,
       1965, *13*, 429-431.
3692   Frayn, D. H. A relationship between rated ability and
       personality traits in psychotherapists. *American Jour-
       nal of Psychiatry*, 1968, *124*, 1232-1237.
3693   *Whitehorn, J. C. Education for uncertainty. *Perspectives
       in Biology and Medicine*, 1963, *7*, 118-123.
3694   Merklin, L. & Little, R. B. Beginning psychiatry train-
       ing syndrome. *American Journal of Psychiatry*, 1967,
       124, 193-197.
3695   *Ornstein, P. H. Sorcerer's apprentice: The initial
       phase of training and education in psychiatry. *Com-
       prehensive Psychiatry*, 1968, *9*, 293-315.
3696   *Halleck, S. L. & Woods, S. M. Emotional problems of

psychiatric residents. *Psychiatry*, 1962, *25*, 339-346.

3696.1 Burstein, A. G., Adams, R. L. & Giffen, M. B. Assessment
of suicidal risk by psychology and psychiatry trainees.
Archives of General Psychiatry, 1973, *29*, 792-793.

3697 *Allen, D. W., Houston, M. & McCarley, T. H. Resistances
to learning. *Journal of Medical Education*, 1958, *33*,
373-379.

3698 Lazerson, A. M. The learning alliance and its relation
to psychiatric teaching. *Psychiatry in Medicine*, 1972,
3, 81-91.

3699 Spiegel, J. P. Factors in the growth and development of
the psychotherapist. *Journal of the American Psychoanalytic Association*, 1956, *4*, 170-175.

3700 Burgum, M., Durkin, H., Gondor, L. H., Miller, S., Pfef-
fer, B. B. & Zucker, L. The therapeutic implications
of supervision. *American Journal of Orthopsychiatry*,
1959, *29*, 357-363.

3701 *Ornstein, P. H. & Kalthoff, R. J. Toward a conceptual
scheme for teaching clinical psychiatric evaluation.
Comprehensive Psychiatry, 1967, *8*, 404-426.

3702 *Marmor, J. The feeling of superiority: An occupational
hazard in the practice of psychotherapy. *American
Journal of Psychiatry*, 1953, *110*, 370-376.

3703 *Sharaf, M. R. & Levinson, D. J. The quest for omnipotence
in professional training: The case of the psychiatric
resident. *Psychiatry*, 1964, *27*, 135-149.

3704 Lewin, B. D. Education or the quest for omniscience.
Journal of the American Psychoanalytic Association,
1958, *6*, 389-412.

3705 Whitman, R. M., Kramer, M. & Baldridge, B. Experimental
study of supervision of psychotherapy. *Archives of
General Psychiatry*, 1963, *9*, 529-535.

3706 *Moulton, R. Views on the supervisory situation: Multiple dimensions in supervision. *Contemporary Psychoanalysis*, 1969, *5*, 146-150.

3707 *Moulton, R. My memories of being supervised. *Contemporary Psychoanalysis*, 1969, *5*, 151-157.

3708 *Castelnuovo-Tedesco, P. Psychiatric residents' appraisal
of psychiatric teaching in medical schools. *Comprehensive Psychiatry*, 1969, *10*, 475-481.

3709 Paidoussi, E. R. Varied experiences in supervision.
Contemporary Psychoanalysis, 1969, *5*, 163-168.

3710 *Kurtz, R. M. & Kaplan, M. L. Resident attitude development and the ideological commitment of the staff of
psychiatric training institutions. *Journal of Medical
Education*, 1968, *43*, 925-930.

3711 Miller, A. A. & Burstein, A. G. Professional development
in psychiatric residents: Assessment and facilitation.
Archives of General Psychiatry, 1969, *20*, 385-394.

3712 Escol, P. J. & Wood, H. P. Perception in residency training: Methods and problems. *American Journal of Psychiatry*, 1967, *124*, 187-193.

3713   *Kardener, S. H., Fuller, M., Mensh, I. N. & Forgy, E. W.
        The trainees' viewpoint of psychiatric residency. *American Journal of Psychiatry*, 1970, *126*, 1132-1138.
3713.1 Fried, F. E., Doherty, E. G. & Coyne, L. Psychiatric
        residents: A survey of training needs, satisfactions,
        and social attitudes. *American Journal of Psychiatry*,
        1973, *130*, 1342-1345.
3714   Wolberg, L. R. Supervision of the psychotherapeutic
        process. *American Journal of Psychotherapy*, 1951, *5*,
        147-171.
3715   Gaskill, H. S. & Norton, J. E. Observations on psychiat-
        ric residency training: Community psychiatry. *Ar-
        chives of General Psychiatry*, 1968, *18*, 7-15.
3715.1 Cohen, R. L. & Henderson, P. B. Experiences in the al-
        teration of sequence in child psychiatric training.
        Journal of the American Academy of Child Psychiatry,
        1973, *12*, 441-460.
3715.2 Benedek, E. P. Training the woman resident to be a psy-
        chiatrist. *American Journal of Psychiatry*, 1973, *130*,
        1131-1135.
3715.3 Raskin, D. E. Training psychiatrists in mental retarda-
        tion. *American Journal of Psychiatry*, 1972, *128*, 1443-
        1445.
3716   Holt, R. R. Personality growth in psychiatric residents.
        Archives of Neurology and Psychiatry, 1959, *81*, 203-215.
3717   *Sharaf, M. R. & Levinson, D. J. Patterns of ideology and
        role definition among psychiatric residents. In M.
        Greenblatt, D. J. Levinson, & R. H. Williams (Eds.),
        The patient and the mental hospital. Glencoe, Ill.:
        Free Press, 1957. Pp. 263-285.
3718   *Kogan, W. S., Boe, E. E., Gocka, E. F. & Johnson, M. H.
        Personality changes in psychiatric residents during
        training. *Journal of Psychology*, 1966, *62*, 229-240.
3719   *Erikson, E. H. The nature of clinical evidence. In D.
        Lerner (Ed.), *Evidence and inference.* Glencoe, Ill.:
        Free Press, 1959. Pp. 73-95.
3720   *Gardner, G. E. Training of clinical psychologists.
        Round table, 1951. 4. The development of the clinical
        attitude. *American Journal of Orthopsychiatry*, 1952,
        22, 162-169.
3721   *Fleming, J. Teaching the basic skills of psychotherapy.
        Archives of General Psychiatry, 1967, *16*, 416-426.
3722   *Woodmansey, A. C. Science and the training of psychia-
        trists. *British Journal of Psychiatry*, 1967, *113*,
        1035-1037.
3723   Brody, E. B. The development of the psychiatric resident
        as a therapist. In N. P. Dellis & H. K. Stone (Eds.),
        *The training of psychotherapists; a multidisciplinary
        approach.* Baton Rouge: Louisiana State University
        Press, 1960. Pp. 86-99.
3724   *Kubie, L. S. The retreat from patients: An unantici-
        pated penalty of the full-time system. *Archives of*

3725 *General Psychiatry*, 1971, *24*, 98-106.
3725 *Kahana, R. J. Psychotherapy: Models of the essential skill. In G. L. Bibring (Ed.), *The teaching of dynamic psychiatry: A reappraisal of the goals and techniques in the teaching of psychoanalytic psychiatry.* New York: International Universities Press, 1968. Pp. 87-103.
3726 *Klerman, G. L. The teaching of psychopharmacology in the psychiatric residency. *Comprehensive Psychiatry*, 1965, *6*, 255-264.
3727 Chien, C. P. & Appleton, W. S. The need for extensive reform in psychiatry teaching: An investigation in treatment, ideology and learning. In T. Rothman (Ed.), *Changing patterns in psychiatric care.* Los Angeles: Rush Research Foundation, 1970; New York: Crown, 1970. Pp. 267-278.
3728 Chessick, R. D. *How psychotherapy heals.* New York: Science House, 1969.
3729 Chessick, R. D. *Why psychotherapists fail.* New York: Science House, 1971.
3730 Henry, W. E., Sims, J. H. & Spray, S. L. *The fifth profession.* San Francisco: Jossey-Bass, 1971.
3730.1 Brenneis, C. B. & Laub, D. Current strains for mental health trainees. *American Journal of Psychiatry*, 1973, *130*, 41-45.
3730.2 Morrison, A. P., Shore, M. F. & Grobman, J. On the stresses of community psychiatry, and helping residents to survive them. *American Journal of Psychiatry*, 1973, *130*, 1237-1241.
3730.3 Yager, J. A survival guide for psychiatric residents. *Archives of General Psychiatry*, 1974, *30*, 494-499.
3730.4 Kline, F. M. How success nearly wrecked a residency experience. *American Journal of Psychiatry*, 1973, *130*, 1038-1040.
3730.5 Lazerson, A. M. Psychiatry residents as college teachers: An evaluation of a training for teaching program. *American Journal of Psychiatry*, 1973, *130*, 658-662.

PROBLEMS AND TECHNIQUES OF SUPERVISION

3731 *Ekstein, R. & Wallerstein, R. S. *The teaching and learning of psychotherapy.* New York: Basic Books, 1972.
3732 *Grotjahn, M. Problems and techniques of supervision. *Psychiatry*, 1955, *18*, 9-15.
3733 Rosenbaum, M. Problems in supervision of psychiatric residents in psychotherapy. *Archives of Neurology and Psychiatry*, 1953, *69*, 43-48.
3734 D'Zmura, T. L. The function of individual supervision. *International Psychiatry Clinics*, 1964, *1*(4), 377-387.
3735 Schwartz, D. A. Psychotherapy and supervisory focus. *Psychiatric Quarterly*, 1966, *40*, 692-701.
3736 Titchener, J. L. The epaminandos phenomenon. *American*

Journal of Psychiatry, 1965, *122*, 98-99.
3737   *Tischler, G. L. The beginning resident and supervision. *Archives of General Psychiatry*, 1968, *19*, 418-422.
3738   Wagner, F. F. Supervision of psychotherapy. *American Journal of Psychotherapy*, 1957, *11*, 759-768.
3739   Schuster, D. B. & Freeman, E. N. Supervision of the resident's initial interview. *Archives of General Psychiatry*, 1970, *23*, 516-523.
3740   Schlessinger, N. Supervision of psychotherapy: A critical review of the literature. *Archives of General Psychiatry*, 1966, *15*, 129-134.
3741   *Escoll, P. J. & Wood, H. P. Perception in residency training: Methods and problems. *American Journal of Psychiatry*, 1967, *124*, 187-193.
3742   *Worby, C. M. The first-year psychiatric resident and the professional identity crisis. *Mental Hygiene*, 1970, *54*, 374-377.
3743   Volkan, V. D. & Hawkins, D. R. The "fieldwork" method of teaching and learning clinical psychiatry. *Comprehensive Psychiatry*, 1971, *12*, 103-115.
3744   *Rice, D. G. & Thurrell, R. J. Teaching psychological evaluation to psychiatric residents: An area suited to bridging the theory-practice gap. *Archives of General Psychiatry*, 1968, *19*, 737-742.
3745   *Miller, A. A., Burstein, A. G. & Leider, R. J. Teaching and evaluation of diagnostic skills. *Archives of General Psychiatry*, 1971, *24*, 255-259.
3746   *Miller, A. A. & Burstein, A. G. Professional development in psychiatric residents: Assessment and facilitation. *Archives of General Psychiatry*, 1969, *20*, 385-394.
3747   *Kaplowitz, D. Teaching emphatic responsiveness in the supervisory process of psychotherapy. *American Journal of Psychotherapy*, 1967, *21*, 774-781.
3748   *Maltsberger, J. T. & Buie, D. H. The work of supervision. In E. V. Semrad, *Teaching psychotherapy of psychotic patients*. New York: Grune & Stratton, 1969. Pp. 65-91.
3749   *Grotjahn, M. The role of identification in psychiatric and psychoanalytic training. *Psychiatry*, 1949, *12*, 141-151.
3750   Hora, T. Contribution to the phenomenology of the supervisory process. *American Journal of Psychotherapy*, 1957, *11*, 769-773.
3751   *Bush, G. Transference, countertransference, and identification in supervision. *Contemporary Psychoanalysis*, 1969, *5*, 158-162.
3752   *Freud, S. (1912) The dynamics of transference. In *Standard Edition*, *12*, 97-108. London: Hogarth Press, 1958.
3753   *Chessick, R. D. How the resident and the supervisor disappoint each other. *American Journal of Psychotherapy*, 1971, *25*, 272-283.

3754   *Searles, H. F. The informational value of the supervisor's emotional experiences. *Psychiatry*, 1955, *18*,
135-146.
3755   Kolb, L. C. Consultation and psychotherapy. *Current
Psychiatric Therapies*, 1968, *8*, 1-10.
3756   *Emch, M. The social context of supervision. *International Journal of Psychoanalysis*, 1955, *36*, 298-306.
3757   Semrad, E. V. *Teaching psychotherapy of psychotic patients*. New York: Grune & Stratton, 1969.
3758   Holt, R. R. & Luborsky, L. B. *Personality patterns of
psychiatrists*. New York: Basic Books, 1958.
3758.1 Cleghorn, J. M. & Levin, S. Training family therapists
by setting learning objectives. *American Journal of
Orthopsychiatry*, 1973, *43*, 439-446.

SUPERVISION IN PSYCHOANALYTIC TRAINING

3759   *DeBell, D. E. A critical digest of the literature on
psychoanalytic supervision. *Journal of the American
Psychoanalytic Association*, 1963, *11*, 546-575.
3760   Fleming, J. & Benedek, T. F. *Psychoanalytic supervision*.
New York: Grune & Stratton, 1966.
3761   *Beckett, T. A candidate's reflections on the supervisory
process. *Contemporary Psychoanalysis*, 1969, *5*, 169-
179.
3762   *Marmor, J. Psychoanalytic therapy as an educational process: Common denominators in the therapeutic approaches
of different psychoanalytic "schools." *Science and Psychoanalysis*, 1962, *5*, 286-299.
3763   Blitzsten, N. L. & Fleming, J. What is supervisory analysis? *Bulletin of the Menninger Clinic*, 1953, *17*, 117-
129.
3764   *Dorn, R. M. Psychoanalysis and psychoanalytic education:
What kind of "journey"? *Psychoanalytic Forum*, 1969, *3*,
237-254.
3765   *Dewald, P. A. Learning problems in psychoanalytic supervision: Diagnosis and management. *Comprehensive Psychiatry*, 1969, *10*, 107-121.
3766   Arlow, J. A. The supervisory situation. *Journal of the
American Psychoanalytic Association*, 1963, *11*, 576-594.
3767   Kris, E. On some vicissitudes of insight in psycho-analysis. *International Journal of Psychoanalysis*, 1956,
37, 445-455.
3768   *Kramer, M. K. On the continuation of the analytic process
after psychoanalysis (a self-observation). *International Journal of Psychoanalysis*, 1959, *40*, 17-25.
3769   *Bernfeld, S. The facts of observation in psychoanalysis.
Journal of Psychology, 1941, *12*, 289-305.
3770   Benedek, T. Countertransference in the training analyst.
Bulletin of the Menninger Clinic, 1954, *18*, 12-16.
3771   *Ross, W. D. & Kapp, F. T. A technique for self-analysis

of countertransference: Use of the psychoanalyst's visual images in response to patient's dreams. *Journal of
the American Psychoanalytic Association*, 1962, *10*, 643-
657.
3772   Szasz, T. S. Psychoanalytic treatment as education. *Archives of General Psychiatry*, 1963, *9*, 46-52.
3773   Grotjahn, M. Present trends in psychoanalytic training.
In F. Alexander & H. Ross (Eds.), *Twenty years of psychoanalysis*. New York: Norton, 1953. Pp. 84-119.
3774   Mechanic, D. Medical sociology: A selective view. In
R. H. Coombs & C. E. Vincent (Eds.), *Psychosocial aspects of medical training*. Springfield, Ill.: Thomas,
1971. (*Medical Sociology: A selective view*. New
York: Free Press, 1968.)
3775   Coombs, R. H. & Vincent, C. E. (Eds.) *Psychosocial aspects of medical training*. Springfield, Ill.: Thomas,
1971.
3776   Arieti, S. Further training in psychotherapy. *American
Journal of Psychiatry*, 1968, *125*, 96-97.

SUPERVISION THROUGH PARTICIPATION, GROUPS AND USE OF VIDEO TAPES

3777   *Harrison, S. I. The psychotherapeutic function of the
orthopsychiatric team: Report of the committee on
psychotherapy. Panel, 1959. 5. Direct supervision
of the psychotherapist as a teaching method. *American
Journal of Orthopsychiatry*, 1960, *30*, 71-78.
3778   *Lewin, K. K. Psychiatric supervision by direct observation. *Journal of Medical Education*, 1966, *41*, 860-864.
3779   *Titchener, J. L., Robinson, J. & Woods, H. B. Observing
psychotherapy: An experience in faculty-resident relations. *Comprehensive Psychiatry*, 1968, *9*, 392-399.
3780   *Rosen, H. & Bartemeier, L. H. The psychiatric resident
as participant therapist. *American Journal of Psychiatry*, 1967, *123*, 1371-1378.
3781   Guiora, A. Z., Hammann, A., Mann, R. D. & Schmale, H. T.
The continuous case seminar. *Psychiatry*, 1967, *30*,
44-59.
3782   Volkan, V. D. & Hawkins, D. R. The "fieldwork" method of
teaching and learning clinical psychiatry. *Comprehensive Psychiatry*, 1971, *12*, 103-115.
3783   Muslin, H. L. & Carmichael, H. T. Exercises in self-
observation: A workshop for instructors in psychiatry.
American Journal of Psychiatry, 1967, *124*, 198-202.
3784   Zinberg, N. E. The psychiatrist as group observer:
Notes on training procedure in individual and group
psychotherapy. In *Psychiatry and medical practice in
a general hospital*. New York: International Universities Press, 1964. Pp. 322-336.
3785   *McGee, T. F. Supervision in group psychotherapy: A comparison of four approaches. *International Journal of*

Group Psychotherapy, 1968, *18*, 165-176.
3786   *Wilmer, H. A. Practical and theoretical aspects of videotape supervision in psychiatry. *Journal of Nervous and
Mental Disease*, 1967, *145*, 123-130.
3787   *Chodoff, P. Supervision of psychotherapy with videotape:
Pros and cons. *American Journal of Psychiatry*, 1972,
128, 819-823.
3788   *Froelich, R. E. Teaching psychotherapy to medical students through videotape simulation. In M. M. Berger
(Ed.) *Videotape techniques in psychiatric training and
treatment*. New York: Brunner/Mazel, 1970. Pp. 55-64.
3789   Wilmer, H. A. Television as participant recorder. *American Journal of Psychiatry*, 1968, *124*, 1157-1163.
3790   *Gladfelter, J. W. Videotape supervision of co-therapists.
In M. M. Berger (Ed.), *Videotape techniques in psychiatric training and treatment*. New York: Brunner/Mazel,
1970. Pp. 74-82.
3791   Schiff, S. B. & Reivich, R. Use of television as aid to
psychotherapy supervision. *Archives of General Psychiatry*, 1964, *10*, 84-88.
3792   *Gruenberg, P. B., Liston, E. H., Jr. & Wayne, G. J. Intensive supervision of psychotherapy with videotape recording. *American Journal of Psychotherapy*, 1969, *23*,
98-105. (Also in M. Berger (Ed.), *Videotape techniques
in psychiatric training and treatment*. New York: Brun-
ner/Mazel, 1970. Pp. 47-54.)
3793   Berger, M. M. (Ed.) *Videotape techniques in psychiatric
training and treatment*. New York: Brunner/Mazel, 1970.
3794   Miller, P. R. & Tupin, J. P. Multimedia teaching of introductory psychiatry. *American Journal of Psychiatry*,
1972, *128*, 1219-1223.
3795   *Stillman, R., Roth, W. T., Colby, K. M. & Rosenbaum, C. P.
An on-line computer system for initial psychiatric in-
ventory. *American Journal of Psychiatry*, 1969, *125*(7,
Suppl.), 8-11.
3796   Colby, K. M. Computer simulation of change in personal
belief systems. *Behavioral Science*, 1967, *12*, 248-253.
3797   *Hillman, R. G. The teaching of psychotherapy problems by
computer. *Archives of General Psychiatry*, 1971, *25*,
324-329.

SUPERVISION IN CHILD PSYCHIATRY

3798   *American Psychiatric Association. The special skills and
abilities of the child psychiatrist. In *Career training in child psychiatry*. Washington: APA, 1964.
Pp. 3-8.
3799   *American Psychiatric Association. Methods of training.
In *Career training in child psychiatry*. Washington:
APA, 1964. Pp. 125-148.
3800   *Szurek, S. A. Symposium, 1948. 7. Remarks on training

for psychotherapy. *American Journal of Orthopsychiatry*, 1949, *19*, 36-55. (Also in S. A. Szurek & I. N. Berlin (Eds.), *Training in therapeutic work with children*. Palo Alto, Calif.: Science & Behavior Books, 1967. Pp. 216-233.)

3801   *Hunter, D. Training in child psychotherapy at the Tavistock Clinic. *Journal of Child Psychology and Psychiatry and Allied Disciplines*, 1960, *1*, 87-93.

3802   *Berlin, I. N. Some implications of ego psychology for the supervisory process. In S. A. Szurek & I. N. Berlin (Eds.), *Training in therapeutic work with children*. Palo Alto, Calif.: Science & Behavior Books, 1967. Pp. 234-242. (*American Journal of Psychotherapy*, 1960, *14*, 536-544)

3803   *Szurek, S. A. & Berlin, I. N. The question of therapy for the trainee in the psychiatric training program. *Journal of the American Academy of Child Psychiatry*, 1966, *5*, 155-165. (Also in S. A. Szurek & I. N. Berlin (Eds.), *Training in therapeutic work with children*. Palo Alto, Calif.: Science & Behavior Books, 1967. Pp. 243-252.)

3804   Brunstetter, R. W. Status, role, and the function of supervision in the residential treatment center for children. *Journal of the American Academy of Child Psychiatry*, 1969, *8*, 259-271.

3805   Schrager, J. A focus for supervision of residential staff in a treatment institution. *Bulletin of the Menninger Clinic*, 1954, *18*, 64-71.

3806   *Noshpitz, J. D. Training the psychiatrist in residential treatment. *Journal of the American Academy of Child Psychiatry*, 1967, *6*, 25-37.

3807   Gardner, G. E. Problems of supervision and training in clinical psychology. Round table, 1952. 2. The supervision of psychotherapy. *American Journal of Orthopsychiatry*, 1953, *23*, 293-300.

3808   *Searles, H. F. The informational value of the supervisor's emotional experiences. *Psychiatry*, 1955, *18*, 135-146. (Also in H. F. Searles, *Collected papers on schizophrenia and related subjects*. London: Hogarth, 1965. Pp. 157-176.)

3809   *Fries, M. E. & Friedman, M. R. A method of organizing clinical data: A teaching aid for training residents in psychoanalytic psychotherapy. A preliminary report. *Journal of the Hillside Hospital*, 1960, *9*, 25-47.

3809.1 Lewis, M. Child psychiatry and medical education: Part I. Introductory phase. *Journal of the American Academy of Child Psychiatry*, 1973, *12*, 407-424.

3809.2 Erlich, F. M. Family therapy and training in child psychiatry. *Journal of the American Academy of Child Psychiatry*, 1973, *12*, 461-472.

XXVII. ADMINISTRATION

3810   *Ashby, E. The administrator: Bottleneck or pump?
       Daedalus, 1962, *91*, 264-278.
3811   *Parkinson, C. N. *Parkinson's law and other studies in
       administration*. Boston: Houghton, Mifflin, 1957.
3812   *Tappan, F. M. *Toward understanding administrators in the
       medical environment*. New York: Macmillan, 1968.
3813   *Worden, F. G. Psychotherapeutic aspects of authority.
       Psychiatry, 1951, *14*, 9-17.
3814   *Szurek, S. A. Emotional factors in the use of authority.
       In E. L. Ginsburg (Ed.), *Public health is people*. New
       York: Commonwealth Fund, 1950. Pp. 206-255. (Also in
       S. A. Szurek & I. N. Berlin (Eds.), *The antisocial child.
       His family and his community*. Palo Alto, Calif.:
       Science & Behavior Books, 1969. Pp. 48-61.
3815   *Technique of administration. *Lancet*, 1955, *269*, 768-769.
3816   *Beck, J. C., Macht, L. B., Levinson, D. J. & Strauss, M.
       A controlled experimental study of the therapist-admin-
       istrator split. *American Journal of Psychiatry*, 1967,
       124, 467-474.
3817   *Bloch, D. A. & Silber, E. The role of the administrator
       in relation to individual psychotherapy in a residential
       treatment setting. *American Journal of Orthopsychiatry*,
       1957, *27*, 69-74.
3818   *Hardy, O. B. Delegation: The administrator's challenge.
       Hospital Administration, 1970, *15*, 8-20.
3819   *Clark, D. H. Administrative therapy. In *Administrative
       therapy*. London: Tavistock, 1964. Pp. 47-75.
3820   *Clark, D. H. Positions for administrative therapy. In
       Administrative therapy. London: Tavistock, 1964.
       Pp. 76-102.
3821   *Clark, D. H. Administrative therapy and other skills.
       In *Administrative therapy*. London: Tavistock, 1964.
       Pp. 118-136.
3822   *Sonis, M. The administrative place of child psychiatry
       within a department of psychiatry of a school of medi-
       cine. In P. L. Adams,, H. H. Work & J. B. Cramer
       (Eds.), *Academic child psychiatry*. Gainesville, Fla.:
       Society of Professors of Child Psychiatry, 1970.
       Pp. 107-125.
3823   *Szurek, S. A. & Berlin, I. N. Teaching administration in
       the training of child psychiatrists. *Journal of the A-
       merican Academy of Child Psychiatry*, 1964, *3*, 551-560.
       (Also in S. A. Szurek & I. N. Berlin (Eds.), *Training
       in therapeutic work with children*. Palo Alto, Calif.:
       Science & Behavior Books, 1968. Pp. 276-284.)
3824   Barton, W. E. Administrative principles. In *Administra-
       tion in psychiatry*. Springfield, Ill.: Thomas, 1962.
       Pp. 349-363.
3825   Barton, W. E. The administrator. In *Administration in
       psychiatry*. Springfield, Ill.: Thomas, 1962. Pp. 420-
       433.

3826   Argyris, C. *Interpersonal competence and organizational effectiveness.* Homewood, Ill.: Dorsey Press, 1962.
3827   Weiland, I. H., et al. Task force administrative structure: A new approach to staff deployment. *Journal of the American Academy of Child Psychiatry,* 1973, *12,* 262-272.

XXVIII. RESEARCH IN CLINICAL CHILD PSYCHIATRY

RESEARCH METHODOLOGY/Scientific Method

3828   *Feinstein, A. R. *Clinical Judgment.* Baltimore: Williams & Wilkins, 1967.
3829   *American Psychiatric Association. Application of basic science techniques to psychiatric research. *Psychiatric Research Reports of the American Psychiatric Association,* 1956, *6.*
3830   *Holton, G. Scientific research and scholarship notes toward the design of proper scales. *Daedalus,* 1962, *91,* 362-399.
3831   *Schor, S. S. The double blind study. *Journal of the American Medical Association,* 1966, *195,* 1094.
3832   Ludwig, E. G. & Collette, J. C. Some misuses of health statistics. *Journal of the American Medical Association,* 1971, *216,* 493-499.
3833   *Rosenthal, R. & Reed, L. A longitudinal study of the effects of experimenter bias on the operant learning of laboratory rats. *Journal of Psychiatric Research,* 1964, *2,* 61-72.
3834   *Beecher, H. K. The powerful placebo. *Journal of the American Medical Association,* 1955, *159,* 1602-1606.
3835   Beecher, H. K. Surgery as placebo: A quantitative study of bias. *Journal of the American Medical Association,* 1961, *176,* 1102-1107.
3836   *Reichenbach, H. *The rise of scientific philosophy.* Berkeley: University of California Press, 1951.
3836.1 Fish, B. Research today or tragedy tomorrow. *American Journal of Psychiatry,* 1972, *128,* 1439-1440.

RESEARCH METHODOLOGY/Methodology in Psychiatry

3837   *Wolf, S. G. Considerations of research design. *Psychiatric Research Reports of the American Psychiatric Association,* 1960, *12,* 131-142.
3838   *Skinner, B. F. A case history in scientific method. *American Psychologist,* 1956, *11,* 221-233.
3839   *Szurek, S. A. & Philips, I. Clinical work and clinical research as scientific inquiry: Five conceptual barriers to clinical science. In *Clinical studies in childhood psychoses.* New York: Brunner/Mazel, 1973. Pp. 278-302.

3840   *Wilder, J. Basimetric approach to psychiatry. In S.
        Arieti (Ed.), *American handbook of psychiatry*. Vol. 3.
        New York: Basic Books, 1966. Pp. 333-343.
3841   *American Psychiatric Association. Approaches to the
        study of human personality. *Psychiatric Research Re-
        ports of the American Psychiatric Association*, 1955, *2*.
3842   *Benjamin, J. D. Directions and problems in psychiatric
        research. *Psychosomatic Medicine*, 1952, *14*, 1-9.
3843   Brosin, H. W. On discovery and experiment in psychiatry.
        American Journal of Psychiatry, 1955, *111*, 561-575.
3844   *Chassan, J. B. On the development of clinical statisti-
        cal systems for psychiatry. *Biometrics*, 1959, *15*,
        396-404.
3845   *Gluck, M. R. & LeGasse, A. A. Methodology and problems
        of clinical data collection and processing. *Journal of
        the American Academy of Child Psychiatry*, 1965, *4*,
        77-85.
3846   *Chassan, J. B. Population and sample: A major problem
        in psychiatric research. *American Journal of Orthopsy-
        chiatry*, 1970, *40*, 456-462.
3847   *Group for the Advancement of Psychiatry. Committee on
        Research. *Psychiatric research and the assessment of
        change*. GAP report, no. 63. New York: Group for the
        Advancement of Psychiatry, 1966.
3848   *Group for the Advancement of Psychiatry. Committee on
        Research. *Some observations on controls in psychiatric
        research*. GAP report, no. 42. New York: Group for
        the Advancement of Psychiatry, 1959.
3849   *Lessing, E. E. & Schilling, F. H. Relationship between
        treatment selection variables and treatment outcome in
        a child guidance clinic: An application of data-proc-
        essing methods. *Journal of the American Academy of
        Child Psychiatry*, 1966, *5*, 313-348.
3850   Chassan, J. B. On the unreliability of reliability and
        some other consequences of the assumption of probabil-
        istic patient-states. *Psychiatry*, 1957, *20*, 163-171.
3851   *Chassan, J. B. Statistical inference and the single
        case in clinical design. *Psychiatry*, 1960, *23*, 173-184.
3852   Chassan, J. B. Stochastic models of the single case as
        the basis of clinical research design. *Behavioral
        Science*, 1961, *6*, 42-50.
3853   Benjamin, J. D. Approaches to a dynamic theory of devel-
        opment. Round table, 1949. 2. Methodological con-
        siderations in the validation and elaboration of psy-
        choanalytical personality theory. *American Journal of
        Orthopsychiatry*, 1950, *20*, 139-156.
3854   *Escalona, S. K. Problems in psycho-analytic research.
        International Journal of Psychoanalysis, 1952, *33*,
        11-21.
3855   Kubie, L. S. Psychoanalysis as a basic science. In F.
        Alexander & H. Ross (Eds.), *Twenty years of psycho-
        analysis*. New York: Norton, 1953. Pp. 120-145. Dis-

cussions by J. D. Benjamin and T. M. French. Pp. 146-159.

3856　*Eiduson, B. T. & Ramsey, D. M. Pilot studies on decision-making in psychiatry. *Reiss-Davis Clinic Bulletin*, 1967, *4*, 115-129.

3857　*Flanagan, J. C. Evaluation and validation of research data in primary prevention. *American Journal of Orthopsychiatry*, 1971, *41*, 117-123.

3858　*Garmezy, N. Vulnerability research and the issue of primary prevention. *American Journal of Orthopsychiatry*, 1971, *41*, 101-116.

3859　Gardner, G. E. Clinical research in a child psychiatry setting. *American Journal of Orthopsychiatry*, 1956, *26*, 330-339.

3860　Henry, J. The study of families by naturalistic observation. In I. M. Cohen (Ed.), *Family structure, dynamics and therapy*. (*Psychiatric Research Reports of the American Psychiatric Association*, 1966, *20*, 95-104.)

3861　Scher, J. M. The structured ward: Research method and hypothesis in a total treatment setting for schizophrenia. *American Journal of Orthopsychiatry*, 1958, *28*, 291-299.

3862　Ruesch, J. The trouble with psychiatric research. *Archives of Neurology and Psychiatry*, 1957, *77*, 93-107.

3862.1　Mellsop, G. W. Psychiatric patients seen as children and adults: Childhood predictors of adult illness. In S. Chess & A. Thomas (Eds.), *Annual progress in child psychiatry and child development: 1973*. New York: Brunner/Mazel, 1974. Pp. 689-702.

RESEARCH METHODOLOGY/Research in Psychotherapy

3863　*Escalona, S. K. & Heider, G. M. *Prediction and outcome*. New York: Basic Books, 1959.

3864　*Kris, M. The use of prediction in a longitudinal study. *Psychoanalytic Study of the Child*, 1957, *12*, 175-189.

3865　*Rosenfeld, E., Frankel, N. & Esman, A. H. A model of criteria for evaluating progress in children undergoing psychotherapy. *Journal of the American Academy of Child Psychiatry*, 1969, *8*, 193-228.

3866　*Sargent, H. D. Intrapsychic change: Methodological problems in psychotherapy research. *Psychiatry*, 1961, *24*, 93-108.

3867　*Sager, C. J. The psychotherapist's continuous evaluation of his work. *Psychoanalytic Review*, 1957, *44*, 298-312.

3868　Wallerstein, R. S. The psychotherapy research project of the Menninger Foundation: An overview at the midway point. In L. A. Gottschalk & A. H. Auerbach (Eds.), *Methods of research in psychotherapy*. New York: Appleton-Century-Crofts, 1966. Pp. 500-516.

3869　Achenbach, T. M. & Lewis, M. A proposed model for

clinical research and its application to encopresis and enuresis. *Journal of the American Academy of Child Psychiatry*, 1971, *10*, 535-554.

RESEARCH METHODOLOGY/Training in Research

3870   *Reiser, M. F.   Research training for psychiatric residents: General problems. *Archives of General Psychiatry*, 1961, *4*, 237-246.
3871   *Anthony, E. J.   Research as an academic function of child psychiatry. *Archives of General Psychiatry*, 1969, *21*, 385-391.
3872   *Tarjan, G.   The administrator's responsibilities toward research. *Mental Hospitals*, 1964, *15*, 620-625.
3873   Hamburg, D. A.   Recent trends in psychiatric research training. *Archives of General Psychiatry*, 1961, *4*, 215-224.
3874   *Redlich, F. C.   Research atmospheres in departments of psychiatry. *Archives of General Psychiatry*, 1961, *4*, 225-236.

RESEARCH METHODOLOGY/Books

3875   *Langer, S.   *Philosophy in a new key: A study in the symbolism of reason, rite, and art*. (3rd ed.)   Cambridge, Mass.: Harvard University Press, 1957.
3876   *Young, J. Z.   *Doubt and certainty in science*. Oxford, England: Clarendon Press, 1951.
3877   *Dewey, J. & Bentley, A. F.   *Knowing and the known*. Boston: Beacon Press, 1949.
3878   *Burrow, T.   *Science and man's behavior*. New York: Philosophical Library, 1953.
3879   *Feinstein, A. R.   *Clinical judgment*. Baltimore: Williams & Wilkins, 1967.
3880   *Escalona, S. K. & Heider, G. M.   *Prediction and outcome*. New York: Basic Books, 1959.
3881   Holt, E. B.   *Animal drives and the learning process*. New York: Octagon, 1973.
3882   *Chassan, J. B.   Intensive design. In *Research design in clinical psychology and psychiatry*. New York: Appleton-Century-Crofts, 1967.   Pp. 180-216.
3883   Meehl, P. E.   *Clinical versus statistical prediction*. Minneapolis: University of Minnesota Press, 1954.
3884   Meltzoff, J. & Kornreich, M.   *Research in psychotherapy*. New York: Atherton Press, 1970.
3885   Krasner, L. & Ullmann, L. P.   *Research in behavior modification*. New York: Holt, Rinehart & Winston, 1965.

NORMATIVE AND EPIDEMIOLOGICAL STUDIES/Normative

3886   Pringle, M. L. (K), et al. *11,000 seven-year-olds: First report of the National Child Development Study (1958 Cohort).* London: Longmans, 1966.
3887   *Moore, T. Stress in normal childhood. *Human Relations,* 1969, *22,* 235-250.
3888   Roberts, J. & Baird, J. T., Jr. *Parent ratings of behavioral patterns of children: United States. (Vital and Health Statistics, Data from the National Health Survey,* Series 11, No. 108) Washington, D.C.: U. S. Govt. Print. Off., 1971. (DHEW publication no. (HSM) 72-1010)
3889   Rutter, M., Tizard, J. & Whitmore, K. (Eds.) *Education, health, and behaviour: Psychological and medical study of childhood development.* London: Longman, 1970.
3890   *Stennett, R. G. Emotional handicap in the elementary years: Phase or disease? *American Journal of Orthopsychiatry,* 1966, *36,* 444-449.
3891   Moore, T. W. Studying the growth of personality: A discussion of the uses of psychological data obtained in a longitudinal study of child development. *Vita Humana,* 1959, *2,* 65-87.
3892   Shepherd, M., Oppenheim, A. N. & Mitchell, S. *Childhood behaviour and mental health.* London: University of London Press, 1971.
3893   *Lapouse, R. & Monk, M. A. Behavior deviations in a representative sample of children: Variation by sex, age, race, social class and family size. *American Journal of Orthopsychiatry,* 1964, *34,* 436-446.
3894   *Steinhauer, P. D., Levine, S. V. & DaCosta, G. A. Where have all the children gone? Child psychiatric emergencies in a metropolitan area. *Canadian Psychiatric Association Journal,* 1971, *16,* 121-127.
3895   Walker, R. N. Body build and behavior in young children: I. Body build and nursery school teachers' ratings. *Monographs of the Society for Research in Child Development,* 1962, *27*(3, Serial No. 84).
3896   Walker, R. N. Body build and behavior in young children: II. Body build and parents' ratings. *Child Development,* 1963, *34,* 1-23.
3897   Mitchell, S. & Shepherd, M. A comparative study of children's behaviour at home and at school. *British Journal of Educational Psychology,* 1966, *36,* 248-254.
3898   Lurie, O. R. The emotional health of children in the family setting. *Community Mental Health Journal,* 1970, *6,* 229-235.
3899   *Hunter, E. C. Changes in teachers' attitudes toward children's behavior over the last thirty years. *Mental Hygiene,* 1957, *41,* 3-11.
3900   *Beilen, H. Teachers' and clinicians' attitudes toward the behavior problems of children: A reappraisal.

Child Development, 1959, *30*, 9-25.
3901 *Chess, S., Thomas, A. & Birch, H. G. Behavior problems revisited: Findings of an anterospective study. *Journal of the American Academy of Child Psychiatry*, 1967, *6*, 321-331.
3902 Boynton, P. L. & Wang, J. D. Relationship between children's play interests and their emotional stability. *Pedagogical Seminary and Journal of Genetic Psychology*, 1944, *64*, 119-127.
3903 *Croake, J. W. Fears of children. *Human Development*, 1969, *12*, 239-247.
3904 *Cramer, B. Some sex differences in children between three and seven. *Psychosocial Process*, 1970, *1*, 60-76.

NORMATIVE AND EPIDEMIOLOGICAL STUDIES/Epidemiology

3905 *Douglas, J. W. & Mulligan, D. G. Emotional adjustment and educational achievement: The preliminary results of a longitudinal study of a national sample of children. *Proceedings of the Royal Society of Medicine*, 1961, *54*, 885-891.
3906 *Langner, T. S., et al. Children of the city: Affluence, poverty, and mental health. In V. L. Allen (Ed.), *Psychological factors in poverty*. Chicago: Markham, 1970. Pp. 185-209.
3907 *Macfarlane, J. W., Allen, L. & Honzik, M. P. *A developmental study of the behavior problems of normal children between twenty-one months and fourteen years.* Berkeley: University of California Press, 1954.
3908 *Lapouse, R. The epidemiology of behavior disorders in children. *American Journal of Diseases of Children*, 1966, *111*, 594-599.
3909 *Ryle, A., Pond, D. A. & Hamilton, M. The prevalence and patterns of psychological disturbance in children of primary age. *Journal of Child Psychology and Psychiatry and Allied Disciplines*, 1965, *6*, 101-113.
3910 Huessy, H. R. & Gendron, R. M. Prevalence of the so-called hyperkinetic syndrome in public school children of Vermont. *Acta Paedopsychiatrica*, 1970, *37*, 243-248.
3911 Baldwin, J. A., Robertson, N. C. & Satin, D. G. The incidence of reported deviant behavior in children. *International Psychiatry Clinics*, 1971, *8*(3), 161-175.
3912 Chazan, M. & Jackson, S. Behaviour problems in the infant school. *Journal of Child Psychology and Psychiatry and Allied Disciplines*, 1971, *12*, 191-210.
3913 Brandon, S. Overactivity in childhood. *Journal of Psychosomatic Research*, 1971, *15*, 411-415.
3914 De-Nour, A. K., Moses, R., Rosenfeld, J. M. & Marcus, J. Psychopathology of children raised in the kibbutz: A critical review of the literature. *Israel Annals of Psychiatry and Related Disciplines*, 1971, *9*, 68-85.

3915   *Werry, J. S. & Quay, H. C. The prevalence of behavior
        symptoms in younger elementary school children. *American Journal of Orthopsychiatry*, 1971, *41*, 136-143.
3916   Sze, W. C. Social variables and their effect on psychiatric emergency situations among children. *Mental Hygiene*, 1971, *55*, 437-443.
3917   *Schechtman, A. Psychiatric symptoms observed in normal
        and disturbed children. *Journal of Clinical Psychology*, 1970, *26*, 38-41.
3918   *Rutter, M. & Graham, P. Psychiatric disorder in 10- and
        11-year-old children. *Proceedings of the Royal Society of Medicine*, 1966, *59*, 382-387.
3919   Stouffer, G. A. W. & Owens, J. Behavior problems of
        children as identified by today's teachers and compared
        with those reported by E. K. Wickman. *Journal of Educational Research*, 1955, *48*, 321-331.
3920   *Glidewell, J. C., Domke, H. R. & Kantor, M. B. Screening
        in schools for behavior disorders: Use of mothers' report of symptoms. *Journal of Educational Research*, 1963, *56*, 508-515.
3921   Mackie, J., Rafferty, F. T. & Maxwell, A. D. The diagnostic check point for community child psychiatry. *Psychiatric Research Reports of the American Psychiatric Association*, 1967, *22*, 171-192.
3922   Hare, E. H. & Shaw, G. K. *Mental health on a new housing
        estate; a comparative study of health in the two districts of Croydon*. London: Oxford University Press,
        1965. (Maudsley monographs, no. 12)
3923   *Shepherd, M., Oppenheim, A. N. & Mitchell, S. Childhood
        behaviour disorders and the child-guidance clinic: An
        epidemiological study. *Journal of Child Psychology and
        Psychiatry and Allied Disciplines*, 1966, *7*, 39-52.
3924   Brandon, S. An epidemiological study of eating disturbances. *Journal of Psychosomatic Research*, 1970, *14*,
        253-257.
3924.1 Fish, J. E. & Larr, C. J. A decade of change in drawings
        by black children. *American Journal of Psychiatry*,
        1972, *129*, 421-426.
3924.2 Straus, R. Current epidemiological research. *Psychiatric
        Annals*, 1973, *3*(10), 26-29.
3924.3 Conrad, R. D. & Kahn, M. W. An epidemiological study of
        suicide and attempted suicide among the Papago Indians.
        American Journal of Psychiatry, 1974, *131*, 69-72.
3924.4 Campion, E. & Tucker, G. A note on twin studies, schizophrenia and neurological impairment. *Archives of General Psychiatry*, 1973, *29*, 460-464.
3924.5 Dohrenwend, B. P. & Dohrenwend, B. S. Psychiatric epidemiology: An analysis of "true prevalence" studies. In
        S. E. Golann & C. Eisdorfer (Eds.), *Handbook of community mental health*. New York: Appleton-Century-Crofts,
        1972. Pp. 283-302.
3924.6 Ritvo, E. R., Cantwell, D., Johnson, E., Clements, M.,

Benbrook, F., Slagle, S., Kelley, P. & Ritz, M.   Social
class factors in autism. *Journal of Autism and Childhood Schizophrenia,* 1971, *1,* 297-310.

DESCRIPTION, NOSOLOGY AND CLASSIFICATION/Nosology and Classification

3925   *Veith, I. Psychiatric nosology: From Hippocrates to
Kraepelin. *American Journal of Psychiatry,* 1957, *114,*
385-391.
3926   Bahn, A. K. Need of a classification scheme for the psychosocial disorders. *Public Health Reports,* 1965, *80,*
79-82.
3927   Howells, J. G. *Nosology of psychiatry.* Ipswich, Eng.:
Society of Clinical Psychiatrists, 1970.
3928   Rutter, M., et al. A tri-axial classification of mental
disorders in childhood; an international study. *Journal of Child Psychology and Psychiatry and Applied
Disciplines,* 1969, *10,* 41-61. (WHO Seminar on Standardization of Psychiatric Diagnosis, Classification and
Mental Statistics, 3rd, Paris, 1967)
3929   *Miller, E. The problem of classification in child psychiatry (Some epidemiological considerations). In
Foundations of child psychiatry. Oxford: Pergamon,
1968. Pp. 251-269.
3930   Cameron, K. Symptom classification and diagnostic categories in child psychiatry. *Proceedings of the Third
World Congress of Psychiatry.* Vol. 1. Montreal: University of Toronto Press, 1961-63. Pp. 74-77.
3931   Kessler, J. W. Nosology in child psychopathology. In
H. E. Rie (Ed.), *Perspectives in child psychopathology.*
Chicago: Aldine-Atherton, 1971. Pp. 85-129.
3932   *Group for the Advancement of Psychiatry. Committee on
Child Psychiatry. *Psychopathological disorders in
childhood: Theoretical considerations and a proposed
classification.* GAP report, no. 62. New York: Group
for the Advancement of Psychiatry, 1966.
3934   *Bemporad, J. R., Pfeifer, C. M. & Bloom, W. Twelve
months' experience with the GAP classification of
childhood disorders. *American Journal of Psychiatry,*
1970, *127,* 658-664.
3935   *Fish, B. Limitations of the new nomenclature for children's disorders. *International Journal of Psychiatry,*
1969, *7,* 393-398.
3936   Lessing, E. E. & Zagorin, S. W. Dimensions of psychopathology in middle childhood as evaluated by three
symptom checklists. *Educational and Psychological
Measurement,* 1971, *31,* 175-198.
3937   Eysenck, H. J. & Eysenck, S. B. *Personality structure
and measurement.* London: Routledge & Kegan Paul,
1969.

3938   Kobayashi, S., Mizushima, K. & Shinohara, M. Clinical
        groupings of problem children based on symptoms and be-
        havior. *International Journal of Social Psychiatry*,
        1967, *13*, 206-215.
3939   *Fish, B. & Shapiro, T. A descriptive typology of chil-
        dren's psychiatric disorders: II. A behavioral classi-
        fication. *Psychiatric Research Reports of the American
        Psychiatric Association*, 1964, *18*, 75-86.
3940   *Wysocki, B. A. & Wysocki, A. C. Behavior symptoms as a
        basis for a new diagnostic classification of problem
        children. *Journal of Clinical Psychology*, 1970, *26*,
        41-45.
3941   *Wolff, S. Behavioural characteristics of primary school
        children referred to a psychiatric department. *British
        Journal of Psychiatry*, 1967, *113*, 885-893.
3942   Speer, D. C. Behavior Problem Checklist (Peterson-Quay):
        Base-line data from parents of child guidance and non-
        clinic children. *Journal of Consulting and Clinical
        Psychology*, 1971, *36*, 221-228.
3943   Jenkins, R. L. Classification of behavior problems in
        children. *American Journal of Psychiatry*, 1969, *125*,
        1032-1039.
3944   Stott, D. H. Classification of behavior disturbance a-
        mong school-age students: Principles, epidemiology and
        syndromes. *Psychology in the Schools*, 1971, *8*, 232-239.
3945   Rutter, M. Classification and categorization in child
        psychiatry. *Journal of Child Psychology and Psychiatry
        and Allied Disciplines*, 1965, *6*, 71-83.
3947   Anthony, E. J. The behavior disorders of childhood. In
        L. Carmichael, *Manual of child psychology*. Vol. 2.
        (3rd ed.) New York: Wiley, 1970. Pp. 667-764.
3948   Achenbach, T. M. The classification of children's psy-
        chiatric symptoms: A factor-analytic study. *Psycholog-
        ical Monographs*, 1966, *80*(7, Whole No. 615).
3949   Freeman, M. A reliability study of psychiatric diagnosis
        in childhood and adolescence. *Journal of Child Psychol-
        ogy and Psychiatry and Allied Disciplines*, 1971, *12*,
        43-54.
3950   *Eiduson, B. T., Johnson, T. C. & Rottenberg, D. Compara-
        tive studies of learning problems seen in five child
        clinics. *American Journal of Orthopsychiatry*, 1966,
        36, 829-839.
3951   Glidewell, J. C., Mensh, I. N. & Gildea, M. C. Behavior
        symptoms in children and degree of sickness. *American
        Journal of Psychiatry*, 1957, *114*, 47-53.
3952   Malmquist, C. P. Depressions in childhood and adoles-
        cence (First of two parts). *New England Journal of
        Medicine*, 1971, *284*, 887-893.
3953   Malmquist, C. P. Depressions in childhood and adoles-
        cence (Second of two parts). *New England Journal of
        Medicine*, 1971, *284*, 955-961.
3954   *Blom, G. E. & Whipple, B. A method of studying emotional

factors in children with rheumatoid arthritis. In L.
Jessner & E. Pavenstedt (Eds.), *Dynamic psychopathology
in childhood.* New York: Grune & Stratton, 1959.
Pp. 124-165.

3955 *Conners, C. K. Symptom patterns in hyperkinetic, neurotic, and normal children. *Child Development,* 1970, *41,*
667-682.

3956 *Fish, B. & Shapiro, T. A typology of children's psychiatric disorders: I. Its application to a controlled
evaluation of treatment. *Journal of the American Academy of Child Psychiatry,* 1965, *4,* 32-52.

3957 Haworth, M. R. & Menolascino, F. J. Video-tape observations of disturbed young children. *Journal of Clinical
Psychology,* 1967, *23,* 135-140.

3959 *Mensh, I. N., Kantor, M. B., Domke, H. R., Gildea, M. C.-
L. & Glidewell, J. C. Children's behavior symptoms and
their relationships to school adjustment, sex, and social class. *Journal of Social Issues,* 1959, *15*(1), 8-
15.

3960 *Quay, H. C., Morse, W. C. & Cutler, R. L. Personality
patterns of pupils in special classes for the emotionally disturbed. *Exceptional Children,* 1966, *32,* 297-
301.

3961 Paraskevopoulos, J. & McCarthy, J. M. Behavior patterns
of children with special learning disabilities. *Psychology in the Schools,* 1970, *7,* 42-46.

3962 *Tuckman, J. & Regan, R. A. Problems referred to children's outpatient psychiatric clinics. *Journal of
Health and Human Behavior,* 1966, *7,* 54-58.

3963 Allen, T. E. & Goodman, J. D. Home movies in child psy-
chodiagnostics: The unobserved observer. *Archives of
General Psychiatry,* 1966, *15,* 649-653.

3964 *Quay, H. C. & Quay, L. C. Behavior problems in early
adolescence. *Child Development,* 1965, *36,* 215-220.

3965 *Szasz, T. S. The problem of psychiatric nosology. *American Journal of Psychiatry,* 1957, *114,* 405-413.

3965.1 Freud, A. The symptomatology of childhood: A preliminary attempt at classification. *Psychoanalytic Study
of the Child,* 1970, *25,* 19-41.

DESCRIPTION, NOSOLOGY AND CLASSIFICATION/Record Keeping

3966 *Eiduson, B. T. Replacing traditional records by event
reports. *Hospital and Community Psychiatry,* 1966, *17,*
68-71.

3967 Eiduson, B. T., Brooks, S. H., Motto, R. L., Platz, A. &
Carmichael, R. New strategy for psychiatric research,
utilizing the psychiatric case history event system.
In N. S. Kline & E. Laska (Eds.), *Computers and elec-
tronic devices in psychiatry.* New York: Grune &
Stratton, 1968. Pp. 45-58.

FAMILIAL AND PARENTAL VARIABLES

3968   *Stout, I. W. & Langdon, G. A study of the home life of
       well adjusted children. *Journal of Educational Sociol-
       ogy*, 1950, *23*, 442-460.
3969   Zuckerman, M., Ribback, B. B., Monashkin, I. & Norton, J.
       A. Normative data and factor analysis on the parental
       attitude research instrument. *Journal of Consulting
       Psychology*, 1958, *22*, 165-171.
3970   *Anderson, L. M. Personality characteristics of parents
       of neurotic, aggressive, and normal preadolescent boys.
       Journal of Consulting and Clinical Psychology, 1969,
       33, 575-581.
3971   *Burchinal, L. G., Hawkes, G. R. & Gardner, B. The re-
       lationship between parental acceptance and adjustment
       of children. *Child Development*, 1957, *28*, 65-77.
3972   *Ainsworth, M. D. The effects of maternal deprivation:
       A review of findings and controversy in the context of
       research strategy. In *Deprivation of maternal care; a
       reassessment of its effects*. Geneva: World Health
       Organization, 1962. Pp. 97-165. (Public health papers,
       no. 14)
3973   *Yarrow, L. J. Maternal deprivation: Toward an empirical
       and conceptual re-evaluation. *Psychological Bulletin*,
       1961, *58*, 459-490.
3974   *Zuckerman, M., Barrett, B. H. & Bragiel, R. M. The paren-
       tal attitudes of parents of child guidance cases: I.
       Comparisons with normals, investigations of socioeco-
       nomic and family constellation factors, and relations
       to parents' reactions to the clinics. *Child Develop-
       ment*, 1960, *31*, 401-417.
3975   Murray, E. J., Seagull, A. & Geisinger, D. Motivational
       patterns in the families of adjusted and maladjusted
       boys. *Journal of Consulting and Clinical Psychology*,
       1969, *33*, 337-342.
3976   Ricci, C. S. Analysis of child-rearing attitudes of
       mothers of retarded, emotionally disturbed, and normal
       children. *American Journal of Mental Deficiency*, 1970,
       74, 756-761.
3977   Kogan, K. L. & Wimberger, H. C. Behavior transactions
       between disturbed children and their mothers. *Psycho-
       logical Reports*, 1971, *28*, 395-404.
3978   Burgental, D. E., Love, L. R., Kaswan, J. W. & April, C.
       Verbal-nonverbal conflict in parental messages to nor-
       mal and disturbed children. *Journal of Abnormal Psy-
       chology*, 1971, *77*, 6-10.
3979   Winder, C. L. & Rau, L. Parental attitudes associated
       with social deviance in preadolescent boys. *Journal of
       Abnormal and Social Psychology*, 1962, *64*, 418-424.
3980   Chafetz, M. E., Blane, H. T. & Hill, M. J. Children of
       alcoholics: Observations in a child guidance clinic.
       Quarterly Journal of Studies on Alcohol, 1971, *32*, 687-
       698.

3981   Tolor, A., Warren, M. & Weinick, H. M. Relation between
        parental interpersonal styles and their children's psy-
        chological distance. *Psychological Reports*, 1971, *29*,
        1263-1275.
3982   Morrison, J. R. & Stewart, M. A. A family study of the
        hyperactive child syndrome. *Biological Psychiatry*,
        1971, *3*, 189-195.
3983   Wolking, W. D., Dunteman, G. H. & Bailey, J. P. Multi-
        variate analyses of parents' MMPIs based on the psy-
        chiatric diagnoses of their children. *Journal of Con-
        sulting Psychology*, 1967, *31*, 521-524.
3984   Wolff, S. Social and family background of pre-school
        children with behaviour disorders attending a child
        guidance clinic. *Journal of Child Psychology and Psy-
        chiatry and Allied Disciplines*, 1961, *2*, 260-268.
3985   Abbe, A. E. Maternal attitudes toward child behavior and
        their relationship to the diagnostic category of the
        child. *Journal of Genetic Psychology*, 1958, *92*, 167-
        173.
3986   Wolff, S. & Acton, W. P. Characteristics of parents of
        disturbed children. *British Journal of Psychiatry*,
        1968, *114*, 593-601.
3987   Frankiel, R. V. *A review of research on parent influ-
        ences on child personality.* New York: Family Service
        Association of America, 1959.
3988   *Goldstein, K. M., Cary, G. L., Chorost, S. B. & Dalack,
        J. D. Family patterns and the school performance of
        emotionally disturbed boys. *Journal of Learning Dis-
        abilities*, 1970, *3*, 10-15.
3989   Guerney, B. G., Shapiro, E. B. & Stover, L. Parental
        perceptions of maladjusted children: Agreement between
        parents, and relation to mother-child interaction.
        Journal of Genetic Psychology, 1968, *113*, 215-225.
3990   *Curtis, J. L., Simon, M., Boykin, F. L. & Noe, E. R. Ob-
        servations on 29 multiproblem families. *American Jour-
        nal of Orthopsychiatry*, 1964, *34*, 510-516.
3991   *Beiser, H. R. Discrepancies in the symptomatology of
        parents and children. *Journal of the American Academy
        of Child Psychiatry*, 1964, *3*, 457-468.
3992   *Peterson, D. R., Becker, W. C., Shoemaker, D. J. , Luria,
        Z. & Hellmer, L. A. Child behavior problems and paren-
        tal attitudes. *Child Development*, 1961, *32*, 151-162.
3993   Rutter, M. *Children of sick parents; an environmental
        and psychiatric study.* London: Oxford University
        Press, 1966. (Maudsley monographs, no. 16)
3994   *Singer, M. T. & Wynne, L. C. Differentiating character-
        istics of parents of childhood schizophrenics, child-
        hood neurotics, and young adult schizophrenics. *Amer-
        ican Journal of Psychiatry*, 1963, *120*, 234-243.
3995   *Block, J. Parents of schizophrenic, neurotic, asthmatic,
        and congenitally ill children: A comparative study.
        Archives of General Psychiatry, 1969, *20*, 659-674.

3996   Rakoff, V., Sigal, J. J. & Sanders, S. S. Patterns of
        report on the hearing of parental voices by emotionally
        disturbed children. *Journal of Psychiatric Research,*
        1970, *8,* 43-50.
3997   Block, J., Patterson, V., Block, J. & Jackson, D. D. A
        study of the parents of schizophrenic and neurotic
        children. *Psychiatry,* 1958, *21,* 387-397.
3998   *Britton, R. S. Psychiatric disorders in the mothers of
        disturbed children. *Journal of Child Psychology and
        Psychiatry and Allied Disciplines,* 1969, *10,* 245-258.
3999   *Munro, A. Parent-child separation. Is it really a cause
        of psychiatric illness in adult life? *Archives of
        General Psychiatry,* 1969, *20,* 598-604.
4000   Davidson, P. O. & Schrag, A. R. The role of the father
        in guidance clinic consultations. *Journal of Psychol-
        ogy,* 1968, *68,* 249-256.
4001   *Biller, H. B. Father absence and the personality develop-
        ment of the male child. *Developmental Psychology,*
        1970, *2,* 181-201.
4002   *Herzog, E. & Sudia, C. E. Fatherless homes: A review of
        research. *Children,* 1968, *15,* 177-182.
4003   *Vogel, E. F. The marital relationship of parents of emo-
        tionally disturbed children: Polarization and isola-
        tion. *Psychiatry,* 1960, *23,* 1-12.
4004   Rutter, M. Parent-child separation: Psychological ef-
        fects on the children. *Journal of Child Psychology and
        Psychiatry and Allied Disciplines,* 1971, *12,* 233-260.
4005   Wardle, C. J. Two generations of broken homes in the gen-
        esis of conduct and behaviour disorders in childhood.
        British Medical Journal, 1961, *2,* no. 5248, 349-354.
4006   *Westman, J. C., Cline, D. W., Swift, W. J. & Kramer, D. A.
        Role of child psychiatry in divorce. *Archives of Gen-
        eral Psychiatry,* 1970, *23,* 416-420.
4006.1 Piers, E. V. Parent prediction of children's self-
        concepts. *Journal of Consulting and Clinical Psychol-
        ogy,* 1972, *38,* 428-433.
4006.2 Hetherington, E. M. & Martin, B. Family interaction and
        psychopathology in children. In H. C. Quay & J. S.
        Werry (Eds.), *Psychopathological disorders of childhood.*
        New York: Wiley, 1972. Pp. 30-82.
4006.3 Kaffman, M. Family conflict in the psychopathology of
        the kibbutz child. *Family Process,* 1972, *11,* 171-188.
4006.4 Wimberger, H. C. & Kogan, K. L. Status behaviors in
        mother-child dyads in normal and clinic subjects. *Psy-
        chological Reports,* 1972, *31,* 87-92.
4006.5 Kaplan, S. L. & Poznanski, E. Child psychiatric patients
        who share a bed with a parent. *Journal of the American
        Academy of Child Psychiatry,* 1974, *13,* 344-356.
4006.6 Allen, J., DeMyer, M. K., Norton, J. A., Pontius, W. &
        Yang, E. Intellectuality in parents of psychotic, sub-
        normal, and normal children. *Journal of Autism and
        Childhood Schizophrenia,* 1971, *1,* 311-326.

CHILD VARIABLES/Infant Indicators

4007   Fitti, R. M. & VanHauvaert, J. M. Emotional disturbances
       in the neo-natal period and early infancy. *Archives of*
       Pediatrics, 1960, *77*, 195-206.
4008   *Chess, S., Thomas, A., Rutter, M. & Birch, H. G. Inter-
       action of temperament and environment in the production
       of behavioral disturbances in children. *American Jour-*
       nal of Psychiatry, 1963, *120*, 142-147.
4009   *Shrader, W. K. & Leventhal, T. Birth order of children
       and parental report of problems. *Child Development*,
       1968, *39*, 1165-1175.
4010   *Ginott, H. G. & Lebo, D. Ecology of service. *Journal of*
       Consulting Psychology, 1963, *27*, 450-452.
4011   Lilienfeld, A. M., Pasamanick, B. & Rogers, M. Relation-
       ship between pregnancy experience and the development
       of certain neuropsychiatric disorders in childhood.
       American Journal of Public Health, 1955, *45*, 637-643.
4012   McNeil, T. F. & Wiegerink, R. Behavioral patterns and
       pregnancy and birth complication histories in psycho-
       logically disturbed children. *Journal of Nervous and*
       Mental Disease, 1971, *152*, 315-323.
4013   *McNeil, T. F., Wiegerink, R. & Dozier, J. E. Pregnancy
       and birth complications in the births of seriously, mod-
       erately, and mildly behaviorally disturbed children.
       Journal of Nervous and Mental Disease, 1970, *151*, 24-34.
4014   *Rothschild, B. F. Incubator isolation as a possible con-
       tributing factor to the high incidence of emotional dis-
       turbance among prematurely born persons. *Journal of*
       Genetic Psychology, 1967, *110*, 287-304.
4015   *Stott, D. H. Infantile illness and subsequent mental and
       emotional development. *Journal of Genetic Psychology*,
       1959, *94*, 233-251.
4015.1 Wohlwill, J. F. *The study of behavioral development*.
       New York: Academic Press, 1973.
4015.2 Rutter, M. *Maternal deprivation reassessed*. Baltimore,
       Md.: Penguin Books, 1972.
4015.3 Lewis, R., Charles, M. & Patwary, K. M. Relationships
       between birth weight and selected social, environmental
       and medical care factors. *American Journal of Public*
       Health, 1973, *63*, 973-981.
4015.4 Shopper, M. Twinning reaction in nontwin siblings. *Jour-*
       nal of the American Academy of Child Psychiatry, 1974,
       13, 300-318.
4015.5 Koluchova, J. Severe deprivation in twins: A case study.
       In S. Chess & A. Thomas (Eds.), *Annual progress in child*
       psychiatry and child development: 1973. New York:
       Brunner/Mazel, 1974. Pp. 448-458.

CHILD VARIABLES/Demographic Variables

4016   Bahn, A. K., Chandler, C. A. & Eisenberg, L. Diagnostic
       and demographic characteristics of patients seen in
       outpatient psychiatric clinics for an entire state
       (Maryland): Implications for the psychiatrist and the
       mental health program planner. *American Journal of
       Psychiatry*, 1961, *117*, 769-778.
4017   *Beach, A. W. & Beach, W. G. Family migratoriness and
       child behavior. *Sociology and Social Research*, 1937,
       21, 503-523.
4018   *Rosen, B. M., Bahn, A. K. & Kramer, M. Demographic and
       diagnostic characteristics of psychiatric clinic out-
       patients in the U.S.A., 1961. *American Journal of
       Orthopsychiatry*, 1964, *34*, 455-468.
4019   *Rosen, B. M., Wiener, J., Hench, C. L., Willner, S. G. &
       Bahn, A. K. A nationwide survey of outpatient psychi-
       atric clinic functions, intake policies and practices.
       American Journal of Psychiatry, 1966, *122*, 908-915.
4020   *Shechtman, A. Age patterns in children's psychiatric
       symptoms. *Child Development*, 1970, *41*, 683-693.
4021   *Speer, D. C., Fossum, M., Lippman, H. S., Schwartz, R. &
       Slocum, B. A comparison of middle- and lower-class
       families in treatment at a child guidance clinic. *Amer-
       ican Journal of Orthopsychiatry*, 1968, *38*, 814-822.
4022   Burchinal, L. G., Gardner, B. & Hawkes, G. R. Children's
       personality adjustment and the socio-economic status of
       their families. *Journal of Genetic Psychology*, 1958,
       92, 149-159.
4023   Hunt, R. G., Roach, J. L. & Gurrslin, O. Social-psycholog-
       ical factors and the psychiatric complaints of disturbed
       children. *Journal of Consulting Psychology*, 1960, *24*,
       194.
4024   *Harrison, S. I., McDermott, J. F., Wilson, P. T. &
       Schrager, J. Social class and mental illness in chil-
       dren: Choice of treatment. *Archives of General Psychi-
       atry*, 1965, *13*, 411-417.
4025   *McDermott, J. F., Harrison, S. I., Schrager, J. & Wilson,
       P. Social class and mental illness in children: Ob-
       servations of blue-collar families. *American Journal
       of Orthopsychiatry*, 1965, *35*, 500-508.
4026   *Hunt, R. G. Occupational status and the disposition of
       cases in a child guidance clinic. *International Journal
       of Social Psychiatry*, 1962, *8*, 199-210.
4027   *McDermott, J. F., Harrison, S. I., Schrager, J., Wilson,
       P., Killins, E., Lindy, J. & Waggoner, R. W. Social
       class and mental illness in children: The diagnosis of
       organicity and mental retardation. *Journal of the Amer-
       ican Academy of Child Psychiatry*, 1967, *6*, 309-320.
4028   Hunt, R. G. & Singer, J. H. Prevalences of religious
       groups in child-guidance clinics: Supplementary data.
       Journal of Consulting Psychology, 1965, *29*, 87-88.

4029   *Furman, S. S., Sweat, L. G. & Crocetti, G. M. Social
       class factors in the flow of children to outpatient
       psychiatric facilities. *American Journal of Public
       Health*, 1965, *55*, 385-392.
4029.1 Glidewell, J. C. A social psychology of mental health.
       In S. E. Golann & C. Eisdorfer (Eds.), *Handbook of com-
       munity mental health*. New York: Appleton-Century-
       Crofts, 1972. Pp. 211-246.
4029.2 Mills, R. C. & Kelly, J. G. Cultural adaptation and eco-
       logical analogies: Analysis of three Mexican villages.
       In S. E. Golann & C. Eisdorfer (Eds.), *Handbook of com-
       munity mental health*. New York: Appleton-Century-
       Crofts, 1972. Pp. 157-209.
4029.3 Goodwin, L. Middle-class misperceptions of the high life
       aspirations and strong work ethic held by the welfare
       poor. *American Journal of Orthopsychiatry*, 1973, *43*,
       554-564.

CHILD VARIABLES/Sex Differences

4030   *Beller, E. K. & Neubauer, P. B. Sex differences and
       symptom patterns in early childhood. *Journal of the
       American Academy of Child Psychiatry*, 1963, *2*, 417-433.
4031   *Gaddini, R. & Gaddini, E. Transitional objects and the
       process of individuation: A study in three different
       social groups. *Journal of the American Academy of
       Child Psychiatry*, 1970, *9*, 347-365.
4032   *Garai, J. E. Sex differences in mental health. *Genetic
       Psychology Monographs*, 1970, *81*, 123-142.
4033   *Bentzen, F. Sex ratios in learning and behavior dis-
       orders. *American Journal of Orthopsychiatry*, 1963, *33*,
       92-98.
4034   Mumpower, D. L. Sex ratios found in various types of
       referred exceptional children. *Exceptional Children*,
       1970, *36*, 621-622.
4034.1 Weintraub, W. & Aronson, H. Patients in psychoanalysis:
       Some findings related to sex and religion. *American
       Journal of Orthopsychiatry*, 1974, *44*, 102-108.

CHILD VARIABLES/Diagnostic Variables

4035   *Bahn, A. K., Chandler, C. A. & Eisenberg, L. Diagnostic
       characteristics related to services in psychiatric
       clinics for children. *Milbank Memorial Fund Quarterly*,
       1962, *40*, 289-318.
4036   Bagley, C. & Evan-Wong, L. Psychiatric disorder and
       adult and peer group rejection of the child's name.
       *Journal of Child Psychology and Psychiatry and Allied
       Disciplines*, 1970, *11*, 19-27.
4037   *Bucknam, F. G. & Reznikoff, M. Background factors and

symptom presentation in a child guidance clinic. *American Journal of Psychiatry,* 1960, *117,* 30-33.

4037.1   Churchill, D. W. & Bryson, C. Q. Looking and approach behavior of psychotic and normal children as a function of adult attention or preoccupation. In S. Chess & A. Thomas (Eds.), *Annual progress in child psychiatry and child development: 1973.* New York: Brunner/Mazel, 1974. Pp. 576-585.

4037.2   Ozer, M. N. & Richardson, H. B., Jr. The diagnostic evaluation of children with learning problems: A "process" approach. *Journal of Learning Disabilities,* 1974, *7,* 88-92.

4037.3   Forness, S. R. & Esveldt, K. Classroom observation of children referred to a child psychiatric clinic. *Journal of the American Academy of Child Psychiatry,* 1974, *13,* 335-343.

4037.4   DeMyer, M. K., Barton, S. & Norton, J. A. A comparison of adaptive, verbal, and motor profiles of psychotic and non-psychotic subnormal children. *Journal of Autism and Childhood Schizophrenia,* 1972, *2,* 359-377.

4037.5   DeMyer, M. K., Schwier, H., Bryson, C. Q., Solow, E. B. & Roeske, N. Free fatty acid response to insulin and glucose stimulation in schizophrenic, autistic, and emotionally disturbed children. *Journal of Autism and Childhood Schizophrenia,* 1971, *1,* 436-452.

4037.6   Goldstein, H. S. Internal controls in aggressive children from father-present and father-absent families. *Journal of Consulting and Clinical Psychology,* 1972, *39,* 512.

CHILD VARIABLES/Adoptive Children

4038   *Goodman, J. D., Silberstein, R. M. & Mandell, W. Adopted children brought to child psychiatric clinic. *Archives of General Psychiatry,* 1963, *9,* 451-456.

4038.1   Humphrey, M. & Ounsted, C. Adoptive families referred for psychiatric advice. I. The children. *British Journal of Psychiatry,* 1963, *109,* 599-608.

4038.2   Humphrey, M. & Ounsted, C. Adoptive families referred for psychiatric advice. II. The parents. *British Journal of Psychiatry,* 1964, *110,* 549-558.

4039   *Menlove, F. L. Aggressive symptoms in emotionally disturbed adopted children. *Child Development,* 1965, *36,* 519-532.

4040   Pringle, M. L. (K.) *Able misfits: A study of educational and behaviour difficulties of 103 very intelligent children (IQs 120-200).* Harlow: Longmans, 1970.

4040.1   Bohman, M. A study of adopted children, their background, environment and adjustment. In S. Chess & A. Thomas (Eds.), *Annual progress in child psychiatry and child development: 1973.* New York: Brunner/Mazel, 1974. Pp. 489-500.

CHILD VARIABLES/Learning Variables

4041   *Stringer, L. A.   Academic progress as an index of mental
        health. *Journal of Social Issues*, 1959, *15*(1), 16-29.
4042   Wolf, M. G.   Effects of emotional disturbance in child-
        hood on intelligence. *American Journal of Orthopsychi-
        atry*, 1965, *35*, 906-908.
4043   *Stott, D. H. & Wilson, D. M.   The prediction of early-
        adult criminality from school-age behaviour. *Inter-
        national Journal of Social Psychiatry*, 1968, *14*, 5-8.
4044   Graubard, P. S.   The relationship between academic a-
        chievement and behavior dimensions. *Exceptional Chil-
        dren*, 1971, *37*, 755-757.
4045   Kenny, T. J. & Clemmens, R. L.   Medical and psychological
        correlates in children with learning disabilities.
        Journal of Pediatrics, 1971, *78*, 273-277.
4046   *Harbin, A. L., Sklar, C. L. & Trautman, E. M.   A study of
        imitative learning in emotionally disturbed and normal
        children. *Nursing Research*, 1969, *18*, 160-164.
4046.1 Tizard, B., Cooperman, O., Joseph, A. & Tizard, J.   En-
        vironmental effects on language development: A study
        of young children in long-stay residential nurseries.
        In S. Chess & A. Thomas (Eds.), *Annual progress in child
        psychiatry and child development: 1973*. New York:
        Brunner/Mazel, 1974. Pp. 705-728.
4046.2 Matheny, A. P., Jr. & Dolan, A. B.   A twin study of genet-
        ic influences in reading achievement. *Journal of Learn-
        ing Disabilities*, 1974, *7*, 99-102.
4046.3 Hermelin, B.   Locating events in space and time: Experi-
        ments with autistic, blind, and deaf children. *Journal
        of Autism and Childhood Schizophrenia*, 1972, *2*, 288-298.
4046.4 Barcai, A., Umbarger, C., Pierce, T. W. & Chamberlain, P.
        A comparison of three group approaches to under-achiev-
        ing children. *American Journal of Orthopsychiatry*,
        1973, *43*, 133-141.
4046.5 Mnookin, R. H.   Foster care: In whose best interest?
        Harvard Educational Review, 1973, *43*, 599-638.

CHILD VARIABLES/Accident Proneness

4047   *Manheimer, D. I. & Mellinger, G. D.   Personality charac-
        teristics of the child accident repeater. *Child Devel-
        opment*, 1967, *38*, 491-513.
4048   Matheny, A. P., Brown, A. M. & Wilson, R. S.   Behavioral
        antecedents of accidental injuries in early childhood:
        A study of twins. *Journal of Pediatrics*, 1971, *79*,
        122-124.
4049   *Graffagnino, P. N., Boelhouwer, C. & Reznikoff, M.   An
        organic factor in patients of a child psychiatric clin-
        ic: Data from the early interviews and the electro-
        encephalogram. *Journal of the American Academy of Child*

Psychiatry, 1968, *7*, 618-638.

4049.1 Husband, P. & Hinton, P. E. Families of children with repeated accidents. *Archives of Disease in Childhood*, 1962, *47*, 396-400.

VALIDITY AND RELIABILITY OF ANAMNESTIC DATA

4050 *Yarrow, M. R., Campbell, J. D. & Burton, R. V. Recollections of childhood: A study of the restrospective method. *Monographs of the Society for Research in Child Development*, 1970, *35*(5, Serial No. 138).

4051 *Mednick, S. A. & Shaffer, J. B. P. Mothers' retrospective reports in child-rearing research. *American Journal of Orthopsychiatry*, 1963, *33*, 457-461.

4052 *Chess, S., Thomas, A. & Birch, H. G. Distortions in developmental reporting made by parents of behaviorally disturbed children. *Journal of the American Academy of Child Psychiatry*, 1966, *5*, 226-234.

4053 *Brekstad, A. Factors influencing the reliability of anamnestic recall. *Child Development*, 1966, *37*, 603-612.

4054 *Cotler, S. & Shoemaker, D. J. The accuracy of mothers' reports. *Journal of Genetic Psychology*, 1969, *114*, 97-107.

4055 Chess, S., Thomas, A., Birch, H. G. & Hertzig, M. Implications of a longitudinal study of child development for child psychiatry. *American Journal of Psychiatry*, 1960, *117*, 434-441.

4056 Hefner, L. T. & Mednick, S. A. Reliability of developmental histories. *Pediatric Digest*, 1969, *11*, 28-39.

4057 Robbins, L. C. The accuracy of parental recall of aspects of child development and of child rearing practices. *Journal of Abnormal and Social Psychology*, 1963, *66*, 261-270.

PSYCHOLOGICAL TESTING AND TEST DATA

4058 *Woody, R. H. Diagnosis of behavioral problem children: Mental abilities and achievement. *Journal of School Psychology*, 1968, *6*, 111-116.

4059 Lessing, E. E., Zagorin, S. W. & Nelson, D. WISC subtest and IQ score correlates of father absence. *Journal of Genetic Psychology*, 1970, *117*, 181-195.

4060 *Frankenburg, W. K., Goldstein, A. D. & Camp, B. W. The revised Denver Developmental Screening Test: Its accuracy as a screening instrument. *Journal of Pediatrics*, 1971, *79*, 988-995.

4061 Frankenburg, W. K., Camp, B. W. & Van Natta, P. A. Validity of the Denver Developmental Screening Test. *Child Development*, 1971, *42*, 475-485.

4062   Salfield, D. J. The usefulness of the Rorschach test for diagnosis, prognosis and epicrisis, mainly in child guidance treatment. *Journal of Mental Science*, 1951, *97*, 84-89.

4063   *Kessler, J. W. & Wolfenstein, C. M. A comparison of Rorschach retests with behavior changes in a group of emotionally disturbed children. *American Journal of Orthopsychiatry*, 1953, *23*, 740-754.

4064   *Sopchak, A. L. Anxiety indicators on the draw-a-person test for clinic and nonclinic boys and their parents. *Journal of Psychology*, 1970, *76*, 251-260.

4065   Burns, R. C. & Kaufman, S. H. *Kinetic family drawings*. New York: Brunner/Mazel, 1970.

4066   DiLeo, J. H. *Young children and their drawings*. New York: Brunner/Mazel, 1970.

4067   *Goodenough, F. L. & Harris, D. B. Studies in the psychology of children's drawings: II. 1928-1949. *Psychological Bulletin*, 1950. *47*, 369-433.

4067.1 Silver, A. A. Diagnostic value of three drawing tests for children. In S. G. Sapir & A. C. Nitzburg (Eds.), *Children with learning problems: Readings in a developmental-interaction approach*. New York: Brunner/Mazel, 1973. Pp. 586-605.

4068   *Engel, M. & Raine, W. J. A method for the measurement of the self-concept of children in the third grade. *Journal of Genetic Psychology*, 1963, *102*, 125-137.

4069   Eysenck, H. J. & Prell, D. B. A note on the differentiation of normal and neurotic children by means of objective tests. *Journal of Clinical Psychology*, 1952, *8*, 202-204.

4070   *Lessing, E. E., Pribyl, M. K. & Patek, D. J. Disturbed children's attitudes toward parents and peers as revealed by sentence completions. *Journal of Child Psychology and Psychiatry and Allied Disciplines*, 1966, *7*, 209-223.

4071   *Sines, J. O., Pauker, J. D., Sines, L. K. & Owen, D. R. Identification of clinically relevant dimensions of children's behavior. *Journal of Consulting and Clinical Psychology*, 1969, *33*, 728-734.

4072   Lessing, E. E. & Smouse, A. D. Use of the Children's Personality Questionnaire in differentiating between normal and disturbed children. *Educational and Psychological Measurement*, 1967, *27*, 657-669.

4072.1 Wolf, E. G., Wenar, C. & Ruttenberg, B. A. A comparison of personality variables in autistic and mentally retarded children. *Journal of Autism and Childhood Schizophrenia*, 1972, *2*, 92-108.

4073   Frostig, M., Lefever, D. W. & Whittlesey, J. R. B. A developmental test of visual perception for evaluating normal and neurologically handicapped children. *Perceptual and Motor Skills*, 1961, *12*, 383-394.

4073.1 Black, F. W. Achievement test performance of high and low perceiving learning disabled children. *Journal of Learning Disabilities,* 1974, *7,* 178-182.

4074   Ayres, A. J. Tactile functions: Their relation to hyperactive and perceptual motor behavior. *American Journal of Occupational Therapy,* 1964, *18,* 6-11.

4074.1 Coy, M. N. The Bender Visual-Motor Gestalt Test as a predictor of academic achievement. *Journal of Learning Disabilities,* 1974, *7,* 317-319.

4075   *Tymchuk, A. J., Knights, R. M. & Hinton, G. C. Neuropsychological test results of children with brain lesions, abnormal EEGs, and normal EEGs. *Canadian Journal of Behavioural Science,* 1970, *2,* 322-329.

4075.1 O'Leary, K. D. The assessment of psychopathology in children. In H. C. Quay & J. S. Werry (Eds.), *Psychopathological disorders of childhood.* New York: Wiley, 1972. Pp. 234-272.

4075.2 Register, M. & L'Abate, L. The clinical usefulness of an objective nonverbal personality test for children. *Psychology in the Schools,* 1972, *9,* 378-387.

4075.3 McIntosh, W. J. The use of a Wechsler subtest ratio as an index of brain damage in children. *Journal of Learning Disabilities,* 1974, *7,* 161-163.

4075.4 Colligan, R. C. Psychometric deficits related to perinatal stress. *Journal of Learning Disabilities,* 1974, *7,* 154-160.

CLINIC POPULATIONS-SERVED AND UNSERVED

4076   *Gordon, S. Are we seeing the right patients? Child guidance intake: The sacred cow. *American Journal of Orthopsychiatry,* 1965, *35,* 131-137.

4076.1 Joint Commission on Mental Health of Children. *The mental health of children; services, research, and manpower; reports of Task Forces IV and V and the report of the Committee on Clinical Issues by the Joint Commission on Mental Health of Children.* New York: Harper & Row, 1973.

4077   *Livingstone, J. B., et al. A new multidisciplinary child clinic: Description of a research study and a report of clinical results. *Journal of the American Academy of Child Psychiatry,* 1970, *9,* 688-706.

4078   Goldensohn, S. S., Fink, R. & Shapiro, S. The delivery of mental health services to children in a prepaid medical care program. *American Journal of Psychiatry,* 1971, *127,* 1357-1362.

4079   Phillips, E. L. Some features of child guidance clinic practice in the U.S.A. *Journal of Clinical Psychology,* 1957, *13,* 42-44.

4080   Solnit, A. J. Who deserves child psychiatry? A study in priorities. *Journal of the American Academy of Child Psychiatry,* 1966, *5,* 1-16.

4081   *Ables, B. S. & Newton, J. R. The diagnostic evaluation
       on a child psychiatry outpatient service from the per-
       spectives of parents and staff. *Journal of Clinical
       Psychology*, 1970, *26*, 384-386.
4082   *Adams, P. L. & McDonald, N. F. Clinical cooling out of
       poor people. *American Journal of Orthopsychiatry*,
       1968, *38*, 457-463.
4083   *Hersch, C. Child guidance services to the poor. *Journal
       of the American Academy of Child Psychiatry*, 1968, *7*,
       223-241.
4084   *Malone, C. A. Child psychiatric services for low socio-
       economic families. *Journal of the American Academy of
       Child Psychiatry*, 1967, *6*, 332-345.
4085   *Spurlock, J. & Cohen, R. S. Should the poor get none?
       Journal of the American Academy of Child Psychiatry,
       1969, *8*, 16-35.
4086   *Kurtz, R. M., Weech, A. A., Jr. & Dizenhuz, I. M. Deci-
       sion-making as to type of treatment in a child psychia-
       try clinic. *American Journal of Orthopsychiatry*, 1970,
       40, 795-805.
4087   L'Abate, L. The effect of paternal failure to partici-
       pate during the referral of child psychiatric patients.
       Journal of Clinical Psychology, 1960, *16*, 407-408.

CLINIC POPULATIONS-SERVED AND UNSERVED/Termination of Treatment

4088   *Magder, D. & Werry, J. S. Defection from a treatment
       waiting list in a child psychiatric clinic. *Journal
       of the American Academy of Child Psychiatry*, 1966, *5*,
       706-720.
4089   *Cohen, R. L. & Richardson, C. H. A retrospective study
       of case attrition in a child psychiatric clinic. *So-
       cial Psychiatry*, 1970, *5*, 77-83.
4090   *Williams, R. & Pollack, R. H. Some nonpsychological
       variables in therapy defection in a child-guidance
       clinic. *Journal of Psychology*, 1964, *58*, 145-155.
4091   *Cole, J. K. & Magnussen, M. G. Family situation factors
       related to remainers and terminators of treatment.
       Psychotherapy: Theory, Research and Practice, 1967, *4*,
       107-109.
4092   Eiduson, B. T. Retreat from help. *American Journal of
       Orthopsychiatry*, 1968, *38*, 910-921.
4093   Lichtenberg, P., Kohrman, R. & Macgregor, H. *Motivation
       for child psychiatry treatment.* New York: Russell &
       Russell, 1960.
4094   Levitt, E. E. Parents' reasons for defection from treat-
       ment at a child guidance clinic. *Mental Hygiene*, 1958,
       42, 521-524.

RESEARCH IN CLINICAL SERVICES/Measurement Methods/*METHODOLOGY*

4095   *Macfarlane, J. W. Studies in child guidance. I. Meth-
       odology of data collection and organization. *Monographs
       of the Society for Research in Child Development,* 1938,
       3(6, Serial No. 19).
4096   *Gluck, M. R. & LeGasse, A. A. Methodology and problems of
       clinical data collection and processing. *Journal of the
       American Academy of Child Psychiatry,* 1965, *4,* 77-85.
4097   *Schachter, F. F., Cooper, A. & Gordet, R. A method for
       assessing personality development for follow-up evalu-
       ations of the preschool child. *Monographs of the Soci-
       ety for Research in Child Development,* 1968, *33*(3, Seri-
       al No. 119).
4098   Beller, E. K. *Clinical process: The assessment of data
       in childhood personality disorders.* New York: Free
       Press of Glencoe, 1962.
4099   *Vasey, I. T. Developing a data storage and retrieval
       system. *Social Casework,* 1968, *49,* 414-417.
4100   *Lapouse, R., Monk, M. A. & Street, E. A method for use
       in epidemiologic studies of behavior disorders in chil-
       dren. *American Journal of Public Health,* 1964, *54,*
       207-222.
4101   *Andrew, G. An investigation of methods for follow-up of
       child-guidance clinic cases. *Social Service Review,*
       1957, *31,* 74-80.
4102   *Douglas, J. W. B. Discussion. In E. H. Hare & J. K.
       Wing (Eds.), *Psychiatric epidemiology.* London: Oxford
       University Press, 1970. Pp. 86-89.
4103   *Rutter, M. & Graham, P. The reliability and validity of
       the psychiatric assessment of the child: I. Interview
       with the child. *British Journal of Psychiatry,* 1968,
       114, 563-579.
4103.1 Zigler, E. & Yando, R. Outerdirectedness and imitative
       behavior of institutionalized and noninstitutionalized
       younger and older children. In S. Chess & A. Thomas
       (Eds.), *Annual progress in child psychiatry and child
       development: 1973.* New York: Brunner/Mazel, 1974.
       Pp. 729-742.

RESEARCH IN CLINICAL SERVICES/Measurement Methods

4104   Spivack, G. & Swift, M. S. The Devereux Elementary
       School Rating Scales: A study of the nature and or-
       ganization of achievement related to disturbed class-
       room behavior. *Journal of Special Education,* 1966, *1,*
       71-90.
4105   *Ross, A. O., Lacey, H. M. & Parton, D. A. The develop-
       ment of a behavior checklist for boys. *Child Develop-
       ment,* 1965, *36,* 1013-1027.
4106   *Wimberger, H. C. & Gregory, R. J. A behavior checklist

for use in child psychiatry clinics. *Journal of the American Academy of Child Psychiatry*, 1968, *7*, 677-688.

4107   *Richman, N. & Graham, P. J.   A behavioural screening questionnaire for use with three-year-old children. Preliminary findings. *Journal of Child Psychology and Psychiatry and Allied Disciplines*, 1971, *12*, 5-33.

4108   Alderton, H. R.   The children's pathology index as a predictor of follow-up adjustment. *Canadian Psychiatric Association Journal*, 1970, *15*, 289-294.

4109   *Goldberg, F. H., Lesser, S. R. & Schulman, R.   A conceptual approach and guide to formulating goals in child guidance treatment. *American Journal of Orthopsychiatry*, 1966, *36*, 125-133.

4110   Gould, R. F.   Psychiatric clinic services for children. II. Research strategy and possibilities. *Social Service Review*, 1956, *30*, 289-299.

4111   Pasamanick, B.   A study design for the evaluation of the efficacy of guidance in the childhood behavior disorders. *Psychiatric Quarterly*, 1956, *30*, 494-503.

4112   *Rosenfeld, E., Frankel, N. & Esman, A. H.   A model of criteria for evaluating progress in children undergoing psychotherapy. *Journal of the American Academy of Child Psychiatry*, 1969, *8*, 193-228.

4113   *Seeman, J., Barry, E. & Ellinwood, C.   Personality integration as a criterion of therapy outcome. *Psychotherapy: Theory, Research and Practice*, 1963, *1*, 14-16.

4114   Walker, R. N.   A scale for parents' ratings: Some ipsative and normative correlations. *Genetic Psychology Monographs*, 1968, *77*, 95-133.

4115   *Graham, P. & Rutter, M.   The reliability and validity of the psychiatric assessment of the child: II. Interview with the parent. *British Journal of Psychiatry*, 1968, *114*, 581-592.

4116   *Becker, W. C., Peterson, D. R., Luria, Z., Shoemaker, D. J. & Hellmer, L. A.   Relations of factors derived from parent interview ratings to behavior problems of five-year-olds. *Child Development*, 1962, *33*, 509-535.

4117   Guerney, B. G., Burton, J., Silverberg, D. & Shapiro, E. Use of adult responses to codify children's behavior in a play situation. *Perceptual and Motor Skills*, 1965, *20*, 614-616.

4118   Miller, L. C.   Q-sort agreement among observers of children. *American Journal of Orthopsychiatry*, 1964, *34*, 71-75.

4119   Eisenberg, L., Landowne, E. J., Wilner, D. M. & Imber, S. D.   The use of teacher ratings in a mental health study: A method for measuring the effectiveness of a therapeutic nursery program. *American Journal of Public Health*, 1962, *52*, 18-28.

4120   *Rutter, M.   A children's behaviour questionnaire for completion by teachers: Preliminary findings. *Journal of Child Psychology and Psychiatry and Allied Disciplines*, 1967, *8*, 1-11.

4121   *Guerney, B. G., Stover, L. & DeMeritt, S.   A measurement of empathy in parent-child interaction. *Journal of Genetic Psychology*, 1968, *112*, 49-55.

4122   *Drechsler, R. J. & Shapiro, M. I.   A procedure for direct observation of family interaction in a child guidance clinic. *Psychiatry*, 1961, *24*, 163-170.

4123   *Elbert, S., Rosman, B., Minuchin, S. & Guerney, B.   A method for the clinical study of family interaction. *American Journal of Orthopsychiatry*, 1964, *34*, 885-894.

4124   *Kogan, K. L. & Wimberger, H. C.   Behavior transactions between disturbed children and their mothers. *Psychological Reports*, 1971, *28*, 395-404.

4125   Bijou, S. W., Peterson, R. F. & Ault, M. H.   A method to integrate descriptive and experimental field studies at the level of data and empirical concepts. *Journal of Applied Behavior Analysis*, 1968, *1*, 175-191.

4126   *Conners, C. K.   A teacher rating scale for use in drug studies with children. *American Journal of Psychiatry*, 1969, *126*, 884-888.

4127   *Lebo, D.   The present status of research on nondirective play therapy. *Journal of Consulting Psychology*, 1953, *17*, 177-183.

4128   *Levin, H. & Wardwell, E.   The research uses of doll play. *Psychological Bulletin*, 1962, *59*, 27-56.

4129   Michael, C. M. & Houck, F. C.   Use of the Glueck prediction scale in identification of potential delinquents. *Corrective Psychiatry and Journal of Social Therapy*, 1965, *11*, 66-71.

4129.1   Kohn, M. & Rosman, B. L.   Prediction of intellectual achievement from preschool social-emotional functioning. *Developmental Psychology*, 1972, *6*, 445-452.

4129.2   Kohn, M. & Rosman, B. L.   A social competence scale and symptom checklist for the preschool child: Factor dimensions, their cross-instrument generality, and longitudinal persistence. *Developmental Psychology*, 1972, *6*, 430-444.

4129.3   Leighton, D. C.   Measuring stress levels in school children as a program-monitoring device. *American Journal of Public Health*, 1972, *62*, 799-806.

4129.4   Miller, L. C., Hampe, E., Barrett, C. L. & Noble, H.   Test-retest reliability of parent ratings of children's deviant behavior. *Psychological Reports*, 1972, *31*, 249-250.

4129.5   Saunders, B. T.   A procedure for the screening, identification, and diagnosis of emotionally disturbed children in the rural elementary school. *Psychology in the Schools*, 1972, *9*, 159-164.

4129.6   Wright, L., Truax, C. B. & Mitchell, K. M.   Reliability of process ratings of psychotherapy with children. *Journal of Clinical Psychology*, 1972, *28*, 232-234.

4129.7   Kupietz, S., Bialer, I. & Winsberg, B. G.   A behavior rating scale for assessing improvement in behaviorally deviant children: A preliminary investigation. *American Journal of Psychiatry*, 1972, *128*, 1432-1435.

RESEARCH IN CLINICAL SERVICES/Therapist Variables

4130   Beiser, H. R. Personality characteristics of child analysts: A comparative study of child analyst students and other students as analysts of adults. *Journal of the American Psychoanalytic Association*, 1971, *19*, 654-669.

4131   *Amble, B. R., Kelly, F. J., Fredericks, M. & Dingman, P. Assessment of patients by psychotherapists. *American Journal of Orthopsychiatry*, 1968, *38*, 476-481.

4132   *Harrison, S. I., McDermott, J. F., Schrager, J. & Showerman, E. R. Social status and child psychiatric practice: The influence of the clinician's socioeconomic origin. *American Journal of Psychiatry*, 1970, *127*, 652-658.

4133   *Sobel, R. The child's role in therapy: A comparison of the child's sick role in treatment as seen by four disciplines. *Journal of the American Academy of Child Psychiatry*, 1967, *6*, 655-662.

4134   *Stoffer, D. L. Investigation of positive behavioral change as a function of genuineness, nonpossessive warmth, and empathic understanding. *Journal of Educational Research*, 1970, *63*, 225-228.

4135   *Cowden, J. E. & Pacht, A. R. Relationship of selected psychosocial variables to prognostic judgments. *Journal of Consulting and Clinical Psychology*, 1969, *33*, 254-256.

4136   *Amble, B. R. & Moore, R. The influence of a set on the evaluation of psychotherapy. *American Journal of Orthopsychiatry*, 1966, *36*, 50-56.

4137   *Rabkin, L. Y. Sources of strain in the treatment of disturbed children and their families. *Mental Hygiene*, 1965, *49*, 544-549.

4137.1 Rieger, N. I. & Devries, A. G. The child mental health specialist: A new profession. *American Journal of Orthopsychiatry*, 1974, *44*, 150-158.

RESEARCH IN CLINICAL SERVICES/Follow-up and Treatment Outcome

4138   Clarizio, H. Stability of deviant behavior through time. *Mental Hygiene*, 1968, *52*, 288-293.

4139   *Heinicke, C. M. & Goldman, A. Research on psychotherapy with children: A review and suggestions for further study. *American Journal of Orthopsychiatry*, 1960, *30*, 483-494.

4140   *Lessing, E. E. & Schilling, F. H. Relationship between treatment selection variables and treatment outcome in a child guidance clinic: An application of data-processing methods. *Journal of the American Academy of Child Psychiatry*, 1966, *5*, 313-348.

4141 *D'Angelo, R. Y. & Walsh, J. F. An evaluation of various therapy approaches with lower socioeconomic-group children. *Journal of Psychology*, 1967, *67*, 59-64.

4142 *Robins, L. N. Follow-up studies investigating childhood disorders. In E. H. Hare & J. K. Wing (Eds.), *Psychiatric epidemiology*. London: Oxford University Press, 1970. Pp. 29-68.

4143 Fleming, P. & Ricks, D. F. Emotions of children before schizophrenia and before character disorder. In M. Roff & D. F. Ricks (Eds.), *Life history research in psychopathology*. Minneapolis: University of Minnesota Press, 1970. Pp. 240-264.

4144 *Sindberg, R. M. A fifteen-year follow-up study of community guidance clinic clients. *Community Mental Health Journal*, 1970, *6*, 319-324.

4145 *Zax, M., Cowen, E. L., Rappaport, J., Beach, D. R. & Laird, J. D. Follow-up study of children identified early as emotionally disturbed. *Journal of Consulting and Clinical Psychology*, 1968, *32*, 369-374.

4146 *Westman, J. C., Rice, D. L. & Bermann, E. Nursery school behavior and later school adjustment. *American Journal of Orthopsychiatry*, 1967, *37*, 725-731.

4147 Glavin, J. P., Quay, H. C. & Werry, J. S. Behavioral and academic gains of conduct problem children in different classroom settings. *Exceptional Children*, 1971, *37*, 441-446.

4148 *Richardson, C. H. & Cohen, R. L. A follow-up of a sample of child psychiatry clinic dropouts. *Mental Hygiene*, 1968, *52*, 535-541.

4149 *Westman, J. C., Ferguson, B. B. & Wolman, R. N. School career adjustment patterns of children using mental health services. *American Journal of Orthopsychiatry*, 1968, *38*, 659-665.

4150 Maberly, A. & Sturge, B. After-results of child guidance: A follow-up of 500 children treated at the Tavistock Clinic, 1921-34. *British Medical Journal*, 1939, *1*, 1130-1134.

4151 *Zold, A. C. & Speer, D. C. Follow-up study of child guidance clinic patients by means of the Behavior Problem Checklist. *Journal of Clinical Psychology*, 1971, *27*, 519-524.

4152 *Weiss, G., Minde, K., Werry, J. S., Douglas, V. & Nemeth, E. Studies on the hyperactive child. VIII: Five year follow-up. *Archives of General Psychiatry*, 1971, *24*, 409-414.

4153 Rutter, M. Psycho-social disorders in childhood, and their outcome in adult life. *Journal of the Royal College of Physicians of London*, 1970, *4*, 211-218.

4154 Fish, B. Evaluation of psychiatric therapies in children.

Proceedings of the American Psychopathological Association, 1964, *52*, 202-220.

4155 Cunningham, J. M., Westerman, H. H. & Fischhoff, J. A follow-up study of patients seen in a psychiatric clinic for children. *American Journal of Orthopsychiatry*, 1956, *26*, 602-612.

4156 Hardcastle, D. H. A follow-up study of one hundred cases made for the Department of Psychological Medicine, Guy's Hospital. *Journal of Mental Science*, 1934, *80*, 536-549.

4157 Gluck, M. R., Tanner, M. M., Sullivan, D. F. & Erickson, P. A. Follow-up evaluation of 55 child guidance cases. *Behaviour Research and Therapy*, 1964, *2*, 131-134.

4158 Levitt, E. E., Beiser, H. R. & Robertson, R. E. A follow-up evaluation of cases treated at a community child guidance clinic. *American Journal of Orthopsychiatry*, 1959, *29*, 337-347.

4158.1 Jay, J. & Birney, R. C. Research findings on the kibbutz adolescent: A response to Bettelheim. *American Journal of Orthopsychiatry*, 1973, *43*, 347-354.

4158.2 DeMyer, M. K., Barton, S., DeMyer, W. E., Norton, J. A., Allen, J. & Steele, R. Prognosis in autism: A follow-up study. *Journal of Autism and Childhood Schizophrenia*, 1973, *3*, 199-246.

4158.3 Shore, M. F. & Massimo, J. L. After ten years: A follow-up study of comprehensive vocationally oriented psychotherapy. *American Journal of Orthopsychiatry*, 1973, *43*, 128-132.

4158.4 Grinker, R. R. & Werble, B. Mentally healthy young men (homoclites) 14 years later. *Archives of General Psychiatry*, 1974, *30*, 701-704.

4158.5 Klein, Z. E. *Research in the child psychiatric and child guidance clinics; a bibliography (1923-1970)*. Also Supplements 1 and 2. Chicago: University of Chicago, 1971.

PART VI

TEXTBOOKS OF CHILD PSYCHIATRY

4159   Arieti, S. (Ed.) Childhood and adolescence. In *American handbook of psychiatry*. (2nd ed.) Vol. 2. New York: Basic Books, 1974. Pp. 3-385.

4160   Barker, P. A. *Basic child psychiatry*. New York: Science House, 1971.

4161   Chess, S. *An introduction to child psychiatry*. (2nd ed.) New York: Grune & Stratton, 1969.

4162   Engel, G. L. *Psychological development in health and disease*. Philadelphia: Saunders, 1962.

4163   Finch, S. M. *Fundamentals of child psychiatry*. New York: Norton, 1960.

4164   Freedman, A. M. & Kaplan, H. I. (Eds.) Child psychiatry. In *Comprehensive textbook of psychiatry*. Baltimore: Williams & Wilkins, 1967. Pp. 1311-1496.

4165   Goodman, J. D. & Sours, J. A. *The child mental status examination*. New York: Basic Books, 1967.

4166   Haworth, M. R. (Ed.) *Child psychotherapy*. New York: Basic Books, 1964.

4167   Harrison, S. I. & McDermott, J. F. (Eds.) *Childhood psychopathology*. New York: International Universities Press, 1972.

4168   Howells, J. G. (Ed.) *Modern perspectives in adolescent psychiatry*. Edinburgh: Oliver & Boyd, 1971.

4169   Howells, J. G. (Ed.) *Modern perspectives in international child psychiatry*. Edinburgh: Oliver & Boyd, 1969.

4170   Kanner, L. *Child Psychiatry*. (4th ed.) Springfield, Ill.: C. C. Thomas, 1972.

4171   Kessler, J. W. *Psychopathology of childhood*. Englewood Cliffs, N.J.: Prentice-Hall, 1966.

4172   Lippman, H. S. *Treatment of the child in emotional conflict*. (2nd ed.) New York: Blakiston, 1962.

4173   Liebman, S. (Ed.) *Emotional problems of childhood*. Philadelphia: Lippincott, 1958.

4174   Shaw, C. R. & Lucas, A. R. *The psychiatric disorders of childhood*. (2nd ed.) New York: Appleton-Century-Crofts, 1970.

4175   Simmons, J. E. *Psychiatric examination of children*. Philadelphia: Lea & Febiger, 1969.

4176   Soddy, K. *Clinical child psychiatry*. London: Bailliere, Tindall & Cox, 1960.

4177   Wolman, B. B. (Ed.) *Manual of child psychopathology.* New York: McGraw-Hill, 1972.

4178   Yalom, I. D. *The theory and practice of group psychotherapy.* New York: Basic Books, 1970.

PART VII

CREATIVITY

CREATIVITY

THEORETICAL ASPECTS OF CREATIVITY

4179   *White, R. W. (Ed.) *The study of lives.* New York:
        Atherton Press, 1963.
4180   *Barron, F. The disposition toward originality. *Journal
        of Abnormal and Social Psychology,* 1955, *51,* 478-485.
4181   *Merleau-Ponty, M. *Sense and non-sense.* Evanston, Ill.:
        Northwestern University Press, 1964.
4182   *Barron, F. *Creativity and psychological health.* Prince-
        ton, N.J.: Van Nostrand, 1963.
4183   *Smith, E. E. & White, H. L. Wit, creativity, and sarcasm.
        Journal of Applied Psychology, 1965, *49,* 131-134.
4184   *Adelson, J. Creativity and the dream. *Merrill-Palmer
        Quarterly,* 1960, *6,* 92-97.
4185   *Anderson, C. C. A cognitive theory of the nonintellective
        correlates of originality. *Behavioral Science,* 1966,
        11, 284-294.
4186   *Bergson, H. *The creative mind.* New York: Wisdom Li-
        brary, 1946.
4187   *Koestler, A. *The act of creation.* New York: Macmillan,
        1964.
4188   *Cronbach, L. J. Review of J. W. Getzels and P. W. Jack-
        son, *Creativity and intelligence.* *American Journal of
        Sociology,* 1962, *68,* 278-279.
4189   Guilford, J. P. Creativity: Yesterday, today, and to-
        morrow. *Journal of Creative Behavior,* 1967, *1,* 3-14(a).
4190   Ghiselin, B. (Ed.) *The creative process.* New York:
        Mentor, 1955.
4191   *Hamilton, J. W. Object loss, dreaming, and creativity:
        The poetry of John Keats. *Psychoanalytic Study of the
        Child,* 1969, *24,* 488-531.
4192   *Kris, E. *Psychoanalytic explorations in art.* New York:
        International Universities Press, 1952.
4193   *Read, R. *Icon and idea: The function of art in the
        development of human consciousness.* Cambridge, Mass.:
        Harvard University Press, 1955.
4194   *Robbins, M. D. On the psychology of artistic creativity.
        Psychoanalytic Study of the Child, 1969, *24,* 227-232.
4195   *Robbins. M. D. On the psychology of artistic creativity.
        Psychoanalytic Study of the Child, 1969, *24,* 233-241.
4196   *Robbins, M. D. On the psychology of artistic creativity.
        Psychoanalytic Study of the Child, 1969, *24,* 241-251.

4197   Drevdahl, J. E. & Cattell, R. B. Personality and crea-
       tivity in artists and writers. *Journal of Clinical
       Psychology,* 1958, *14,* 107-111.
4198   *Rosenblum, W. Teaching photography. *Aperture,* 1956,
       4(3), 87-91.
4199   *Taylor, C. W. (Ed.) *Creativity: Progress and potential.*
       New York: McGraw-Hill, 1964.
4200   *Knapp, R. H. & Goodrich, H. B. *Origins of American sci-
       entists.* Chicago: University of Chicago Press, 1952.
4201   *Roe, A. *The making of a scientist.* New York: Dodd,
       Mead, 1953.
4202   Andrews, F. M. Factors affecting the manifestation of
       creative ability by scientists. *Journal of Personality,*
       1965, *13,* 140-152.
4203   *Stein, M. K. & Heinze, S. J. *Creativity and the individ-
       ual: Summaries of selected literature in psychology
       and psychiatry.* Glencoe, Ill.: Free Press, 1960.
4204   *Taylor, C. W., Smith, W. R. & Ghiselin, B. The creative
       and other contributions of one sample of research sci-
       entists. In C. W. Taylor & F. Barron (Eds.), *Scientific
       creativity: Its recognition and development.* New York:
       Wiley, 1963. Pp. 53-76.
4205   *Taylor, C. W. & Barron, F. (Eds.) *Scientific creativity:
       Its recognition and development.* New York: Wiley,
       1963.
4206   Roe, A. A psychological study of eminent psychologists
       and anthropologists, and a comparison with biological
       and physical scientists. *Psychological Monographs,*
       1953, *67*(2, Whole No. 352).

DEVELOPMENTAL/Child Related

4207   White, R. W. Ego and reality in psychoanalytic theory.
       Psychological Issues, 1963, *3*(3, Whole No. 11).
4208   *White, R. W. Motivation reconsidered: The concept of
       competence. *Psychological Review,* 1959, *66,* 297-333.
4209   Teeter, B., Rouzer, D. L. & Rosen, E. Development of a
       dimension of cognitive motivation: Preference for
       widely known information. *Child Development,* 1964,
       35, 1105-1111.
4210   *Ward, W. C. Creativity in young children. *Child Develop-
       ment,* 1968, *39,* 737-754.
4211   Wallach, M. A. & Kogan, N. *Modes of thinking in young
       children: A study of the creativity-intelligence dis-
       tinction.* New York: Holt, Rinehart & Winston, 1965.
4212   *Wallach, M. A. & Kogan, N. A new look at the creativity-
       intelligence distinction. In J. P. Hill & J. Shelton
       (Eds.), *Readings in adolescent development and behav-
       ior.* Englewood Cliffs, N.J.: Prentice-Hall, 1971.
4213   *Wallach, M. A. Creativity and the expression of possi-

bilities. In J. Kagan (Ed.), *Creativity and learning.*
Boston: Houghton Mifflin, 1967. Pp. 36-57.

4214 *Getzels, J. W. & Jackson, P. W. *Creativity and intelligence: Explorations with gifted students.* New York:
Wiley, 1962.

4215 *Lieberman, J. N. Playfulness and divergent thinking: An
investigation of their relationship at the kindergarten
level. *Journal of Genetic Psychology,* 1965, *107,* 219-
224.

4216 *Torrance, E. P. & Myers, R. E. *Teaching gifted elementary pupils how to do research.* Minneapolis: Percep-
tive Publishing, 1962.

4217 Sutton-Smith, B. Piaget on play: A critique. *Psychological Review,* 1966, *73,* 104-110.

4218 Piaget, J. *Play, dreams and imitation in childhood.*
New York: Norton, 1962.

4219 *Nagera, H. The concepts of structure and structuraliza-
tion: Psychoanalytic usage and implications for a
theory of learning and creativity. *Psychoanalytic
Study of the Child,* 1967, *22,* 93-102.

4220 *Nagera, H. The concepts of structure and structuraliza-
tion: Psychoanalytic usage and implications for a
theory of learning and creativity. *Psychoanalytic
Study of the Child,* 1967, *22,* 77-86.

4221 Torrance, E. P. Factors affecting creative thinking in
children: An interim research report. *Merrill-Palmer
Quarterly,* 1967, *7,* 171-180.

4222 Sutton-Smith, B. & Rosenberg, B. G. Manifest anxiety and
game preferences in children. *Child Development,* 1960,
31, 307-311.

4223 Flescher, I. Anxiety and achievement of intellectually
gifted and creatively gifted children. *Journal of Psychology,* 1963, *56,* 251-268.

4224 Flavell, J. H., Cooper, A. & Loiselle, R. H. Effect of
the number of preutilization functions on functional
fixedness in problem solving. *Psychological Reports,*
1958, *4,* 343-350.

4225 *Berlin, I. N. Aspects of creativity and the learning
process. *American Imago,* 1960, *17,* 83-99.

4226 Becher, B. A. A cross-sectional and longitudinal study
of the effect of education on free association responses. *Journal of Genetic Psychology,* 1960, *97,*
23-28.

4227 *Jones, R. M. *Fantasy and feeling in education.* New
York: New York University Press, 1968.

4228 *Yamamoto, K. Relationships between creative thinking
abilities of teachers and achievement and adjustment
of pupils. *Journal of Experimental Education,* 1963,
32, 3-25.

4229 *Gall, M. & Mendelsohn, G. A. Effects of facilitating
techniques and subject-experimenter interaction on
creative problem solving. *Journal of Personality and*

Social Psychology, 1967 *5*, 211-216.
4230 *Guilford, J. P. Creative abilities in the arts. *Psychological Review*, 1957, *64*, 110-118.
4231 *Thorndike, R. L. The measurement of creativity. *Teachers College Record*, 1963, *64*, 422-424.

DEVELOPMENTAL/Adolescents and Creativity

4232 *Piers, E. V. Adolescent creativity. In J. F. Adams (Ed.), *Understanding adolescence: Current development in adolescent psychology*. Boston: Allyn & Bacon, 1968. Pp. 159-182.
4233 Rivlin, L. G. Creativity and the self-attitudes and sociability of high school students. *Journal of Educational Psychology*, 1959, *50*, 147-152.
4234 *Mearns, H. *Creative power: The education of youth in the creative arts*. New York: Dover Publications, 1958.
4235 *Clark, C. M., Veldman, D. J. & Thorpe, J. S. Convergent and divergent thinking abilities of talented adolescents. *Journal of Educational Psychology*, 1965, *56*, 157-163.
4236 Davis, G. A. Training creativity in adolescence: A discussion of strategy. In R. E. Grinder (Ed.), *Studies in adolescence*. (2nd ed.) New York: Macmillan, 1969. Pp. 538-545.
4237 Maltzman, I. On the training of originality. *Psychological Review*, 1960, *67*, 229-242.
4238 Maddi, S. R. Motivational aspects of creativity. *Journal of Personality*, 1965, *33*, 330-347.

DEVELOPMENTAL/Adult Creativity

4239 *Guilford, J. P. Traits of creativity. In H. H. Anderson (Ed.), *Creativity and its cultivation*. New York: Harper, 1959. Pp. 142-161.
4240 Chambers, J. A. Relating personality and biographical factors to scientific creativity. *Psychological Monographs*, 1964, *78*(7, Whole No. 584).
4241 *Dennis, W. Age and productivity among scientists. *Science*, 1956, *123*, 724-725.
4242 *Mednick, S. A. & Mednick, M. T. An associationistic view of creative thinking. In C. W. Taylor (Ed.), *Widening horizons in creativity*. New York: Wiley, 1964. Pp. 54-68.
4243 Mendelsohn, G. A. & Griswold, B. B. Differential use of incidental stimuli in problem solving as a function of creativity. *Journal of Abnormal and Social Psychology*, 1964, *68*, 431-436.
4244 *Bayley, N. & Oden, M. H. The maintenance of intellectual

ability in gifted adults. *Journal of Gerontology,* 1955, *10,* 91-107.

4245   *Helson, R.   Personality of women with imaginative and artistic interests: The role of masculinity, originality, and other characteristics in their creativity. *Journal of Personality,* 1966, *34,* 1-25.

4246   *Feldhusen, J. F., Denny, T. & Condon, C. F.   Anxiety, divergent thinking, and achievement. *Journal of Educational Psychology,* 1965, *56,* 40-45.

4247   *Faris, R. E. L.   Review of J. W. Getzels & P. W. Jackson, *Creativity and intelligence. American Sociological Review,* 1962, *27,* 558-559.

4248   *Sarnoff, I.   Some psychological problems of the incipient artist. *Mental Hygiene,* 1956, *40,* 375-383.

4249   Mednick, S. A.   The associative basis of the creative process. *Psychological Review,* 1962, *69,* 220-232.

4250   *May, R.   The artist and the neurotic.   In *Love and will.* New York: Dell, 1969.   Pp. 20-23.

4251   Goldstein, M. J. & Palmer, J. O.   *The experience of anxiety.*   New York: Oxford University Press, 1963.

4252   Jones, R. M.   *Ego synthesis in dreams.*   Cambridge, Mass.: Schenkman, 1962.

4253   Barron, F.   The disposition towards originality.   In C. W. Taylor & F. Barron (Eds.), *Scientific creativity: Its recognition and development.*   New York: Wiley, 1963.   Pp. 139-152.

4254   *Cattell, R. B. & Drevdahl, J. E.   A comparison of the personality profile (16 P.F.) of eminent researchers with that of eminent teachers and administrators, and of the general population. *British Journal of Psychology,* 1955, *46,* 248-261.

4255   Boersma, F. J. & O'Bryan, K.   An investigation of the relationship between creativity and intelligence under two conditions of testing. *Journal of Personality,* 1968, *36,* 341-348.

4256   Stark, S.   Rorschach movement, fantastic daydreaming, and Freud's concept of primary process: Interpretive commentary. *Perceptual and Motor Skills,* 1966, *22,* 523-532.

4257   Hitschmann, E.   *Great men psychoanalytic studies.*   New York: International Universities Press, 1956.

FILMS

SOURCES OF FILMS

With Abbreviations as used on the Following Pages

B   Bellefaire
            22001 Fairmount Boulevard
            Cleveland, Ohio   44118

C   Cinevie, Inc.
            5429 South Dorchester Avenue
            Chicago, Illinois   60615

CDMH   California Department of Mental Hygiene
            Mental Health Film Library
            1320 "K" Street
            Sacramento, California   91405

CFC   Concord Film Council
            Nacton Inswich
            Suffolk, England

CFS   Creative Film Society
            14558 Valerio Street
            Van Nuys, California   91405

CHP   Chelsea House Publishers
            70 West 40th Street
            New York, New York   10018

CL   Charles Lyman
            1907 North Bissell Street
            Chicago, Illinois   60614

CMC   Center for Mass Communication
            440 West 110th Street
            New York, New York   10025

CSDPH   California State Department of Public Health
            Film Library
            2151 Berkeley Way, Berkeley, California   94704

CTW   Children's Television Workshop
            1865 Broadway
            New York, New York   10023

361

EBF   Encyclopedia Britannica Films
                425 North Michigan Avenue
                Chicago, Illinois 60611

EDC   EDC Film Library
                Educational Development Center
                39 Chapel Street
                Newton, Massachusetts 02160

EFVA   Education Foundation for Visual Aids
                33 Queen Anne Street
                London W 1, England

FF   Franciscan Films
                P.O. Box 6116
                San Francisco, California 94101

GP   Geigy Pharmaceuticals
                P.O. Box 430
                Yonkers, New York 10702

HF   Hallmark Films
                1511 East North Avenue
                Baltimore, Maryland 21213

IDEA   I/D/E/A, Information Services Division
                P.O. Box 446
                Melbourne, Florida 32901

IU   Indiana University
                Audio-Visual Center
                Bloomington, Indiana 47401

NCRY   National Commission on Resources for Youth
                36 West 44th Street
                New York, New York 10036

NFBC   National Film Board of Canada
                680 Fifth Avenue
                New York, New York 10019

NMA   National Medical Audiovisual
                Center Annex,
                Station K
                Atlanta, Georgia 30324

NYU   New York University, Film Library
                26 Washington Place
                New York, New York 10003

OSU Ohio State University
Department of Photography and Cinema
Film Distribution Supervisor
156 West 19th Avenue
Columbus, Ohio   43210

PCR Psychological Cinema Register
Audio-Visual Services
Pennsylvania State University
University Park, Pennsylvania   16802

PE Perennial Education, Inc.
1825 Willow Road
P.O. Box 236
Northfield, Illinois   60093

PW Pre-Schooler's Workshop
Attention: Mrs. Judith Bloch
38 Old Country Road
Garden City, New York   11530

SCIS Science Curriculum Improvement Study
University of California
Lawrence Hall of Science
Berkeley, California   94720

SFP Stanley R. Frager Productions
1326 Yale Street
Santa Monica, California   90404

SKF Smith Kline and French Laboratories
Medical Film Center
1500 Spring Garden Street
Philadelphia, Pennsylvania   19130

SLFP S-L Film Productions
5126 Hartwick Street
Los Angeles, California   90041

SP Sandoz Pharmaceuticals
Route 10
East Hanover, New Jersey   07936

TCP Technology for Children Project
Department of Education
Division of Vocational Education
225 West State Street
Trenton, New Jersey   08625

TLF Time-Life Films
4 West 16 Street
New York, New York   10003

UCEMC   University of California, Extension Media Center
Berkeley, California 94720

UI   University of Illinois
Division of University Extension
Visual Aids Service
Champaign, Illinois 61822

UW   University of Wisconsin
Division of Mental Hygiene
School of Social Work
Madison, Wisconsin 53706

VN   Video Nursing, Inc.
2645 Girard Avenue
Evanston, Illinois 60201

W   Wedico Films
267 West 25th Street
New York, New York 10001

FILMS

ANIMAL STUDIES RELATED TO UNDERSTANDING CHILD BEHAVIOR

Constitutional and Environmental Interactions in Rearing Four Breeds of Dogs. (19 min.) Illustrates procedures and find-ings of experiment in which inbred strains of basenjis, Shetland sheepdogs, beagles, and wire-haired terriers are raised in either "indulged" or "disciplined" fashion follow-ing weaning at 3 weeks of age. A test is administered at 8 weeks in which a bowl of meat is placed on the floor and the puppy is punished each time he eats from it. Experimen-ter then leaves the room and observing through a one-way glass, records the time elapsed before the puppy again eats. The results demonstrate the interaction of constitutional type (breed) and mode of rearing. Similarly, observations in the follow-up period indicate that there are lasting ef-fects of early experience which are unique for each breed. D. G. Freedman, 1962. *PCR-2124K*.

Animal War--Animal Peace. (28 min.) Comparisons drawn between animal and human societies. In both, conflict between ag-gression and fear exists, as does proclaiming and defending of territorial rights. However, animals resolve disputes with minimum of bloodshed, whereas man often fights to death. Why? Examples of species resolving conflicts in-clude stickleback fish, gulls, and squirrel monkeys; reaches the conclusion that a better understanding of animals may lead to better understanding of man. McGraw-Hill Text-Films, 1968. *PCR-31434*.

Social Reaction in Imprinted Ducklings. (21 min.) Newly hatched ducklings when first exposed to moving stimulus, often form filial attachment (i.e., imprint) to it in much the same fashion that other ducklings imprint to their biological mother. Shows the effects of sequence of experimental pro-cedures in which newly hatched ducklings were first imprint-ed to moving stimulus (a plastic milk bottle mounted over a model train engine) and then taught to peck a pole, using presentation of moving stimulus as sole response - contin-gent (reinforcing) event. Illustrates (1) duckling's ini-tial reaction to apparatus and to imprinting stimulus (2) duckling's tendencies to follow imprinted stimulus (3) man-ner in which presentation and withdrawal of imprinted stim-

365

ulus controls duckling's distress calls (4) procedure of
shaping the duckling to peck the pole (5) manner in which
calls are emitted when stimulus presentation is determined
by duckling's own behavior (via learned peck responses)
(6) effects of failing to present stimulus when pecks occur
(i.e., extinction), and (7) comparison between effects of
presenting moving stimulus to imprinted versus experimentally naive ducklings. H. Hoffman. The Pennsylvania State
University, 1968. *PCR-2180K.*

Imprinting. (37 min.) Formation of early social attachments and
their biological importance. Black-necked swans and bar-
nacle geese seen in family social behavior, then with members of another species and with an inanimate object. Laboratory imprinting shows effects of age, rearing conditions,
and the characteristics of the imprinting stimulus. Rotating
light functions both as imprinting and reinforcing stimulus.
Appleton-Century-Croft (E.P. Reese and P. Bateson), 1968.
PCR-40127.

*Ape and Child Series: Pt. I.-Some Behavior Characteristics of
Human and Chimpanzee Infants in the Same Environment* (19
min. No S). *Pt. II-Comparative Tests on a Human and a Chim-
panzee Infant of Approximately the Same Age* (18 min. No S).
*Pt. III-Experiments Upon a Human and a Chimpanzee Infant
After 6 Months in the Same Environment* (18 min. No S).
*Pt. IV-Some General Reactions of a Human and a Chimpanzee
Infant After 6 Months of the Same Environment* (17 min. No S).
*Pt. V-Facial Expressions of a Human and Chimpanzee Infant
Following Taste Stimuli* (9 min. No S). *PCR.*

Mechanical Interest and Ability in a Home Raised Chimpanzee.
Hayes and Hayes. *I. Survey - 8 mo.-6 yrs.* Use of Tools
(17 min. No S). *II. Survey - 9 mo.-6 yrs.* Learning Re
Water and Fire (17 min. No S). *III. Survey - 9 mo.-6 yrs.*
Mechanical Objects (16 min. No S). *IV. Survey.* Self Care
and Eating and Toileting (18 min. No S). *PCR.*

Imitation in a Home Raised Chimpanzee. (17 min. No S). Hayes
and Hayes. *PCR.*

Motivation and Reward in Learning. (15 min.) N. E. Miller and
G. Hart. *NYU.*

Experimentally Produced "Social Problem" in Rats. (11 min. No S)
Social problem created by placing three rats in Skinner box
with lever some distance from food trough. At first any rat
pressing lever finds food eaten by others. Violent fighting
over empty trough ensues. Finally one rat discovers way to
obtain food for all three by depressing lever several times.
With this rat as worker and other two as parasites, "class
society has emerged". O. H. Mowrer, 1939. *PCR-28.*

Competition and Dominance in Rats. O. W. Mower, et al. (13 min. No S). *PCR.*

Animal Studies in Social Modification of Organically Motivated Behavior. O. H. Mowrer. (12 min. No S). *PCR.*

Effect of Infantile Feeding Frustration on Adult Hoarding in White Rats. (15 min. No S) J. McV. Hunt, et al. *PCR.*

Dynamics of an Experimental Neurosis. J. H. Masserman. *Pt. I- Conditioned Feeding Behavior and Induction of Experimental Neurosis in Cats.* (21 min. No S) *Pt. II-Effects of Environmental Frustrations and Intensification of Conflict in Neurotic Cats.* (16 min. No S) *Pt. III-Experimental Diminution of Neurotic Behavior in Cats.* (19 min. No S) *Pt. IV- Active Participation in Establishing More Satisfactory Adjustment.* (20 min. No S) *PCR.*

Experimental Masochism. (10 min. No S) J. H. Masserman. *PCR.*

Dynamics of Competition in Cats: Intercat Relations in a Manipulative Feeding Situation. J. H. Masserman. (15 min. No S) *PCR.*

Dominance, Neurosis, and Aggression in Cats. (30 min.) J. H. Masserman and P. W. Silver. *PCR.*

Experiment # 6 - Childhood of the Chimpanzee. (30 min.) W. Mason. Contrasts and comparisons between the behavioral characteristics of the human and chimpanzee infant. Physical similarities, intelligence, need for clinging. National Educational Television: Delta Primate Research Center, 1967. *PCR-31225.*

Mother Love. (26 min.) Dr. Harry F. Harlow, past President of the APA studies the infant-mother relationship in new-born rhesus monkeys. Dr. Harlow tests their reactions to a variety of unusual and inanimate mother substitutes which he calls "mother surrogates", in order to find the key to the bond between mother and child and to understand the effects of denial and maternal love. He demonstrates through these unusual experiments that the single most important factor is body contact, holding and nestling, and further concludes that deprivation of this can cause deep emotional disturbances, even death. From TV Program "Conquest", CBS. *NYU.*

Social Behavior of Rhesus Monkeys. (26 min.) C. R. Carpenter, 1947. *PCR.*

Sexual Behavior of Laboratory Monkeys. (30 min.) Dept. of
Health, Education and Welfare. *PCR.*

*The Effects of Delayed Auditory Feedback on Normal and Deviant
Rhesus Behavior.* (18 min.) M. Woolf and J. H. Masserman.
Illustrates research on effect of delayed auditory feedback.
Begins with demonstrations of effect on human subject when
voice of individual reading a passage is fed back through
earphones with a delay of a quarter of a second. Then a
series of experiments is shown involving delayed auditory
feedback to young rhesus monkeys, some of which are mater-
nally and socially deprived while others are normal. Animals are conditioned to vocalize for a prescribed period of
time to illuminate series of lights sequentially for a
banana pellet. Animals are then subjected to delayed feedback of their auditory responses. Results are discussed in
terms of biodynamic postulating that unexpected feedback
from an uncontrollable universe leads to apprehension or
anxiety. *PCR-2181K.*

*Behavior of the Macaques of Japan: The Macaca Fuscata of the
Takasakiyama and Koshima Colonies.* (28 min.) Ecological
and behavioral study of primate colonies indigenous to
Japan. Three provisionized groups of the Takasakiyama
colony have fairly distinct territorial ranges but rotate
use of common feeding ground and temple grove. Social
organization is reflected in spatial distribution patterns.
Communication by sentinel tree signaling regulates inter-
group and intragroup actions. Mother-infant conditioning
through positive and negative reinforcements, adaptive
learning, and grooming as a conditioning activity shown.
Animals in Koshima Island colony transmit learned behavior
of washing potatoes and separating wheat from sand to infants and juveniles. Pennsylvania State University, 1969.
PCR-2184K.

Experimental Neuroses in Monkeys. J. H. Masserman and C. Pechtel
(19 min. No S). *PCR.*

Miss Goodall and the Wild Chimpanzees. (28 min.) Story of a 26-
year-old English woman and her adventures in East Africa
where she observed and lived with wild chimpanzees. Rein-
forces the belief that the complete understanding of the
behavior of chimpanzees will eventually bring man to a
better understanding of himself. Edited from National
Geographic Society version. Britannica Educational Corporation, 1968. *PCR-31269.*

Bleeding Hearts and Bone Breakers. (45 min.) John Hurrell
Crook, British anthropologist, studies social organization
of Gelada Baboons in their natural state in the mountains
of Ethiopia. Baboons are seen playing, eating, grooming,

mating, and avoiding conflict. Mystery of broken bones traced to the lammergeier, a large bird of prey. Time-Life Films, 1967. *PCR-40116*.

Chacma Baboons (Papio Ursinus): Ecology and Behavior. (20 min.) Study of a well organized group photographed in the Cape Point Nature Reserve, Cape of Good Hope. Reports information collected by Professor Hall during 153 days of systematic observations: Interactions of the baboons with food plants and coastal organisms in the rugged coastal environment. A single isolated group of baboons consisting of about twenty-eight animals is described in terms of the actions and reactions of males, females, and young. Examples depicted of test situations of animals under free ranging conditions. Descriptions of the gestural and vocal communications systems as well as the different modalities of behavior such as feeding, play, grooming, and aggressive actions. Range of group described. K. Hall and C. Carpenter, Pennsylvania State University, 1967. *PCR-2167*.

Baboon Social Organization. (17 min.) Analyzes the troop as a compact social unit, the nature of the interdependence of its members and its close relation to baboon ecology. Baboon Social Life Series, University of California. *NYU*.

Baboon Ecology. (21 min.) Ecological principles at work among the average baboon troop filmed in the Royal Nairobi National al Park in Kenya. Baboon Social Life Series, University of California. *NYU*.

Baboon Behavior. (31 min.) Describes aspects of baboon life fostering social cohesion between various ages and sexes that compose the troop. Baboon Social Life Series, University of California. *NYU*.

CHILD DEVELOPMENT/Physical Development

Genetics and Behavior. (16 min.) J. Antonitis and J. P. Scott, 1953. *PCR*.

Embryology of Human Behavior. (31 min.) Medical Audio-Visual Institute of the Association of American Medical Colleges, 1951. *CDMH*.

Life Begins. An overall view of Dr. Arnold Gesell's work at the Yale University Clinic of Child Development. The film is a photographic record of the patterns of normal development of infants from birth to eighteen months. Interesting use is made of the technique of showing two pictures at once on the screen, illustrating different stages of growth of one child or contrasting reactions of different infants to similar

situations. The children are shown in typical routines of
sleeping, bathing, eating, playing, with Dr. Gesell pointing
out similarities, differences and characteristic reactions
of the infants to test situations. *EBF, NYU.*

Life With Baby. (18 min.) How children grow mentally and physically has been diligently charted during the past 35 years
by a group of specialists working under the direction of Dr.
Arnold Gesell at the Yale University Clinic of Child Development. They have been able to establish definite standards
of development for children up to six years of age. Many of
these findings are illustrated in this film with candid-
camera sequences photographed through a one-way vision dome.
Non-technical in character, the picture aims at a better
understanding of the young child by adults and older children. March of Time. *NYU.*

Principles of Development. (17 min.) Outlines the fundamentals
of growth and change from early infancy and develops basic
principles. (1) Development follows a pattern that is
continuous, orderly, progressive, and predictable. (2)
Within this developmental process there is considerable
correlation between types of development, e.g., physical
growth affects motor development--the baby's back is erect
before he can stand; often, one type of development waits
for another--if the baby concentrates on walking he may
learn no new words for some months. (3) Development goes
from general to specific responses; at first the baby responds to all food before he learns that he prefers certain
ones. (4) Most children follow the same pattern. (5) Each
stage of the pattern has its own characteristic traits. (6)
All development is the result of maturation and learning:
the interrelation of these two is the key to all child
training. McGraw-Hill. *NYU.*

Expressive Movements (Affectomotor Patterns) in Infancy. Bela
Mittelmann, et al. (42 min.) *NYU.*

Motility in Parent-Child Relationships. (40 min. No S). The
second film in Dr. Mittelmann's series on motility is focused on its important role in the development of interpersonal relationships in the first year and a half of life.
Reciprocity between parent and child involving modes of motility, is the main theme of this film. Maturational aspects
are considered under three headings: (1) the prepersonal
phase--up to about 3 months, when humans are important only
because they supply flexibly the basic wants of the infant
(2) the general personal phase--roughly three to 8 months
when people as such are important to the baby (3) the specific personal phase--when the child recognizes familiar
people, notably the mother, and is shy or anxious with
strangers. The newborn infant's motility, at first random

activity or reactions to distress, soon includes vigorous
manifestations of pleasure. These merge into aggressive
behavior and are related to the developments of adaptive
patterns of locomotion and manipulation. The film shows how
the parents' active response to the baby's motor behavior
results in social interchange. Of interest to college and
professional groups in the areas of child development,
psychology, nursing, pediatrics, as well as community organizations, especially parents' groups. *NYU.*

*Sleep of Babies, The: Spontaneous Cyclical Phenomena During
Neonate Sleep.* D. Coleman and J. G. Minard. (30 min.)
Records observable behavior of three to five-day-old infants
during sleep by means of normal speed,slowed motion, speeded
motion, and stop motion cinephotography. Illustrates methods
of classifying and recording various types of behavior during
sleep including body movements, rapid eye movements, respira-
tion, and brain activity. Shows rhythmic patterns of activity which are possible indicators of maturational changes.
University of Pittsburgh, 1970. *PCR-2226.*

Study in Human Development: Part I: Six to Thirty Weeks. (19
min. No S) Presents boy at six, twelve, seventeen, twenty-
one, twenty-five and thirty weeks of age. At each stage
child's reactions shown to objects including cup, spoon and
blocks. Supine, prone, and sitting (with support) postures
demonstrated. Sequence at twenty-one weeks shows rolling
from back to stomach, early patterns of crawling and feeding.
Last two age levels show later development of manipulation,
response to soundmaking objects, and improvements in postural
and locomotor activities. H. D. Behrens, 1946. *PCR-90.*

*Study in Human Development: Part II: Forty-two Weeks to Fifteen
Months.* (17 min. No S) Records at forty-two weeks, twelve
months, and fifteen months of age. Emphasis given to gross
motor development and to perceptual-manipulatory reactions
to objects including cup, spoon, bell, hoop, ball, and mirror. Child pulls up, stands, crawls, mounts stairs, and
exhibits walking readiness. At one year of age he is given
simple tests for fine manipulation, imitation, and stair
climbing. Development of motor skills further demonstrated
for fifteen month stage, and early interactions with another
child described photographically. H. D. Behrens, 1946.
PCR-91.

*Study in Human Development: Part III: Nineteen Months to Two
Years and Eight Months.* (19 min. No S) Emphasizes continued gross and fine motor development and beginnings of
cooperative play. Stages shown are nineteen, twenty-four
and thirty-two months. At nineteen months boy imitates
building block tower, drinks by holding glass with both
hands, and throws ball. Exhibits handedness. Play is non-

cooperative. At two years boy walks up stairs but shows hesitation and caution about descending. Marks on paper, but no patterns made. Great increment in motor development, but play still essentially individualistic. Child draws patterns and crude "man" at thirty-two months. Plays more cooperatively with other children, uses wide variety of toys and play equipment. H. D. Behrens, 1946. *PCR-92.*

Study in Human Development: Part IV: Three Years to Five Years. (18 min. No S) At third year socially interdependent play, development of skill in drawing, and typical motor coordination demonstrated. Fourth year brings finer coordination, greater ability in drawing and rudimentary musical skills; application of performance tests for intelligence shown at this level. During fifth year boy enrolls in kindergarten and begins characteristic social play activities. H. D. Behrens, 1948. *PCR-92-A.*

Study of Twins: Part I. (17 min. No S) Series presents growth and development of identical twin boys; deals primarily with responses to everyday informal situations; stresses differences between developing twins. Present part illustrates motor growth in infancy, especially differences in rate of development among various parts of body; emphasizes cephalocaudal pattern. Sequences provided at fourteen, twenty-two, twenty-eight, and forty weeks. H. D. Behrens, 1947. *PCR-97-A.*

Study of Twins: Part II. (17 min. No S) Demonstrates twins at 12, 15, 18, and 21 months. Shows getting up, standing, and walking stages; also amount of independent play and cooperative play. H. D. Behrens, 1947. *PCR-97-B.*

Study of Twins: Part III. (18 min. No S) Records behavior at 24, 28, and 32 months. Shows amicable but independent play, and rapidity of development of motor skills and of larger muscles. H. D. Behrens, 1949. *PCR-97-C.*

Study of Twins: Part IV. (19 min. No S) Sequences at ages 3, 4, and 5 years illustrate increasingly cooperative play and improved muscular coordination. Shows ultimate self-sufficiency in such activities as eating, washing teeth, and playing. H. D. Behrens, 1951. *PCR-97-D.*

Abby's First Two Years: A Backward Look. (30 min.) Usually past development of a child tends to be absorbed into his present behavior and we lose sight of the transformations that occur. By viewing Abby's developmental sequence backwards, from age 2 years to 2 months we see the physical and behavioral changes of infancy as they drop out. We trace Abby's relations with adults and children, play patterns, eating, bathing, locomotion, prehension, self-awareness and affectivity. *NYU.*

Betty Tells Her Story. (Normal Development). (20 min.) Liane
Brandon, 1972. *New Day Films*, 267 West 25th Street, New
York, NY. 10001.

*Eight Infants: Tension Manifestations in Response to Perceptual
Stimulation.* (42 min. No S) The behavior of eight infants,
18 to 25 weeks of age, was systematically examined before and
after prolonged perceptual stimulation of the kind to which
they are frequently exposed when shown toys, played with
vigorously by siblings and visiting relatives, included in
family events, etc. The film shows the infant's behavior
before, during, and after such stimulation. S. Escalona and
Mary Leitch. *NYU.*

*Grasping. Film Studies of the Psychoanalytic Research Project
on Problems in Infancy Series.* (20 min. No S) An experimental study in motion pictures of the development of the
grasping pattern. Grasping develops as a sequence in which
motor skills interact progressively with the everwidening
radius of the unfolding of the psyche. Grasping proper is an
intentional act. Its earliest predecessor in the development is the clutching reflex, a purely motor pattern present
at birth and shown in the first pictures. A learning process
adapts this motor pattern to purposeful use. Between grasping proper and clutching reflex there is also a motor difference shown in the film: the clutching reflex takes place
with unopposed thumb, grasping with opposed thumb. Mastery
of grasping is achieved when the infant uses the neuromuscu-
lar pattern adequately to exploit environmental facilities
to gratify its needs. This development takes all of the
first year. R. Spitz. *NYU.*

Imitation: Part I. Gestural. Part II. Vocal. (35 min.) The
development of gestural and vocal imitation. I. C. Uzgiris
and J. McV. Hunt. *NYU.*

CHILD DEVELOPMENT/Cognitive Development

*Birth and the First Fifteen Minutes of Life. Film Studies of
the Psychoanalytic Research Project on Problems in Infancy
Series.* (10 min. No S) Shows the birth of a baby and its
reactions to stimuli presented within the first fifteen
minutes after birth. The first feeding twenty-four hours
later is shown. A second baby with contrasting reactions to
the same stimuli is presented. *NYU.*

Learning and Growth. (11 min.) Shows principles of learning in
children 24 to 48 weeks old. Encyclopaedia Britannica Films.
A. Gesell, 1935. *PCR-136.7-11.*

Classification (Piaget's Developmental Theory). (17 min.)
Children shown at several developmental stages responding to
tasks designed by Piaget and Inhelder. Each task highlights
a different mental operation essential to classification,
such as multiple classification, class inclusion, and heir-
archial classification. Davidson Films. *NYU. PCR-21269.*

Piaget's Developmental Theory: Classification. (17 min.) The
second in a series of filmed observations of children illustrating the developmental theory of Jean Piaget, the famed
Swiss child psychologist. Shows children at several developmental stages responding to tasks designed by Piaget and
Inhelder. Each task highlights a different mental operation
essential to classification, such as multiple classification,
class inclusion, and hierarchial classification. Davidson
Films. *NYU.*

Piaget's Developmental Theory: Conservation. (28 min.) Children between the ages of five and 12 are presented in individual interviews using the standard procedures developed in
Geneva, Switzerland. The tasks involve conservation of
quantity, length, area, and volume. The characteristics of
thought from preoperational to formal are identified. Tests
are given and anlyzed by Dr. Robert Karplus, Prof. of Phy-
sics at the University of California and Dr. Celia Standler,
Prof. of Education and Child Development at the University of
Illinois. Davidson Films. *NYU.*

Learning in Infants. (28 min.) A laboratory experimental approach to the study of several behavioral processes during
infancy; neonatal olfactory adaptation; control of neonatal
sucking by classical conditioning and intra-oral stimulation
conjugate social reinforcement with four and eight month-
olds; discrimination learning in the first and second years;
and reinforcement schedule control with toddlers. Brown
University (H. Kaye, L. P. Lipsitt, & P. Weisberg), 1967.
PCR-30992.

Object Permanence. (40 min.) The development of visual pursuit
and the permanence of objects. I. C. Uzgiris and J. McV.
Hunt. *NYU.*

Operational Causality. (20 min.) The development of pragmatic
causal sequences. I. C. Uzgiris and J. McV. Hunt. *NYU.*

*Behavior of Animals and Human Infants in Response to a Visual
Cliff.* (15 min.) A comparative study of depth discrimina-
tion by young animals and human infants. R. D. Walk and
E. J. Gibson, 1959. *PCR-2095.*

Growth of Infant Behavior: Early Stages. (11 min.) Traces rapid growth of early infant behavior patterns. Contrasts typical infant reactions at various ages by technique allowing study of two different pictures simultaneously on the screen. Animated diagrams clarify characteristics of psychological growth. Encyclopaedia Britannica Educational Corporation. A. Gesell, 1934. *PCR-136.7-36.*

Focus on Behavior: Learning About Learning. (30 min.) Exploration of ways in which psychologists are developing new testing methods for measuring and increasing human capabilities. Dr. Lloyd Humphreys demonstrates development of tests for choosing pilots in World War II. Dr. James Gallagher shows methods being used to develop productive creative thinking in the modern day classroom. National Educational Television, 1963. *PCR-30292.*

Focus on Behavior: A World to Perceive. (29 min.) Research of Drs. Herman Witkin, Eleanor Gibson, and Richard Walk demonstrates the role of perception in handling and processing information from the environment, and the way in which our personalities affect our perception. National Educational Television, 1963. *PCR-30296.*

Development of Means. (35 min.) The development of means for achieving desired environmental events. I. C. Uzgiris and J. McV. Hunt. *NYU.*

Understanding Children's Play. (11 min.) Suggests that adults can understand and help children through observation in their use of play materials. By watching and listening to children at play, adults can gain a better understanding of children and find ways of helping each child to mature in his own way. Caroline Zachry Institute. *NYU.*

The Child at Play. (18 min.) The picture opens with a group of adults seating themselves in the observation section of a one-way vision room. The therapist is arranging toys in the special playroom. The first sequence presents Judy, a 3-year old, as she plays with different toys and chats with the unseen therapist. In the second sequence, she is shown in the playroom with a group of other children of various ages; all the children are strangers to each other except two brothers. Here her activity and responses are quite different. In the third sequence she is in the playroom with a little friend. *NYU.*

California Project Talent: 14 Evaluation. (29 min.) Development of critical appreciation through a study of the fundamental forms of music. Application of Jerome Bruner's description of the stages of learning in the Process of Education to the development of critical appreciation. Acme Film

Labs., 1967. *PCR-31213.*

Discovering Individual Differences. Elementary School Teacher Education Series. (25 min.) This film uses the same five cases described in "Each Child is Different" to demonstrate how Ms. Smith got to know and understand each child and adapted her teaching program to meet their individual needs. Through observation, records, talks with other teachers and with parents, consultations, and testing out methods that her head and heart suggested, Ms. Smith was able to work out class projects that provided learning opportunities for every member of her class. McGraw-Hill. *NYU.*

Each Child is Different. Elementary School Teacher Education Series. (17 min.) The opening day of school. Five children, representing a cross-section of Ms. Smith's fifth-grade class, are presented to illustrate what the good teacher must come to know about each individual child if she is to adapt her teaching program to his needs and abilities. Robert, socially adjusted and secure in his family life, is mechanically inclined and physically capable; he is a poor reader. Ruth, tired, listless and neglected looking, keeps house and takes care of her baby brother in addition to her schoolwork. Mark is a natural leader, superior in ability and intelligence. Elizabeth is withdrawn, sullen, a victim of frequent quarrels between her parents; John, small for his age, is a misfit at home and in school. How Ms. Smith proceeds to find out these and other facts about her fifth graders is the subject of the film. McGraw-Hill. *NYU.*

Developmental Characteristics of Preadolescents. Elementary School Teacher Education Series. (18 min.) As the child grows toward maturity, says this film successive states of development are apparent. Each stage has a distinctive pattern of behavior. An understanding of these patterns is essential if the teacher is to provide effective teaching experience for the children in her class. To reveal the behavior patterns characteristic of eight and nine year-olds, two children are shown in relation to each other, to their parents, and with other children. These children are intolerant, self-centered. McGraw-Hill. *NYU.*

Growing Up Safely. (25 min.) How major sources of childhood accidents can be prevented by relating accident protection to the child's level of development. *NYU.*

CHILD DEVELOPMENT/Social Development

Social Development. (16 min.) McGraw-Hill, 1950. *CSDPH, PCR, NYU.*

Development of Individual Differences. Psychology Series.
(13 min.) No two individuals are alike. Differences result
from both heredity and environment. This film reviews and
illustrates what is known and generally accepted about the
relative influence of these two factors. In general, it is
concluded, heredity sets very broad limiting conditions to
behavior, but within those limits the effects of environment
can be regarded as decisive. In the area of environment a
comparison is drawn between two brothers four years apart in
age. The film shows how environment can account for many
differences between the boys as well as for certain similarities. We are shown a second home next door where a very
different set of behavior patterns is being developed in a
child in another type of family environment. The film indicates that there are three principal ways in which family
resemblances in behavior are handed on from generation to
generation: opportunity through shared environment, direct
interaction between family members, and social expectancy.
McGraw-Hill. *NYU.*

Learning to Learn in Infancy. (30 min.) This film stresses the
essential role of curiosity and exploration in learning, and
points to the kinds of experience that cultivate and stimulate an eager approach to the world. It also points out the
cumulative nature of learning. Ways are suggested in which
adults can help infants make approaches, differentiate
between objects, and develop the earliest communication
skills. Vassar College for Project Head Start. *NYU.*

Person to Person in Infancy. (22 min.) This film stresses the
importance of the human relationships between infant and
adult, and shows that in group care as well as at home there
can be a considerable range of warmth and adequacy of relationship. The impact of this relationship on the infant's
readiness and eagerness for new experience are suggested.
Vassar College for Project Head Start. *NYU.*

Sibling Rivalries and Parents. Child Development Series. (11
min.) In any family one encounters a certain amount of
rivalry among brothers and sisters, a rivalry for attention,
esteem, and love. This film describes the reasons for this
rivalry, the varied manifestations of it, and means for
holding natural frictions to a minimum. It answers such
questions as: Should parents forbid quarreling? Is it better to reason a child out of anger? Will training children
to separate feelings from action help curb home quarrels?
What can the family council do for this problem? This film
shows that friction is a normal human trait. McGraw-Hill.
NYU.

Sibling Relations and Personality. Child Development Series.
(22 min.) In a series of case studies this film describes
the relationships a child has with his brothers and sisters
throughout developmental years. These relationships are an
important factor in shaping personality. The film explores
personality influences on the oldest child of a large family,
the middle child, the girl who has been reared to be the
model child, the girl who feels that her parents would have
preferred a boy. Here, too, are studies of differences in
siblings: the boy whose brother is more talented, the girl
whose sister is prettier and more popular, and the boy who
feels his grandparents prefer his sister. *NYU.*

*The Terrible Two's and the Trusting Three's. Ages and Stages
Series.* (22 min.) Examines the growing years between two
and four. At the beginning the camera is trained on a nursery school play yard where the "terrible two's" are seen in
action, pushing and pulling, climbing and crawling in seemingly aimless activity. The two-year-old's constant activity
may seem undirected to adults but through it the youngster
is learning. When discipline is necessary it comes best in
the form of distraction for reasoning is beyond understanding. Curiosity can be channeled by providing toys that stimulate creative imagination--modeling clay, crayons, functional blocks. At three the parallel play of the two gives way
to a primary form of organized play. His activities have
become more purposeful--he now models a definite shape from
clay and no longer merely takes pleasure in handling it. He
is very conscious of social approval and desirous of winning
it at home. National Film Board of Canada. *NYU.*

Two and Three-Year Olds in Nursery School. (37 min.) What
children are like while learning and growing. We see the
skill, the effort and the delight with which two-year-olds
go about their daily affairs in nursery school. Teachers
offer help by setting understandable limits as well as by
giving support and encouragement. Part I of " A Long Time
to Grow" series. *NYU.*

Frustrating Fours and Fascinating Fives. Ages and Stages Series.
(22 min.) A study of the behavior of four and five-year-old
children at home and at nursery school. Young Roddy presents
typical examples of the actions of a child at these ages as
the film follows his development and that of his classmates.
We are shown the vacillation between infantile helplessness
and vigorous self-assertion at four, the development of
independence and the beginnings of cooperation at five.
The film gives advice and encouragement to parents, teachers,
and other adults interested in the development of children
at this age level. Crawley Films, Ltd., for the National
Film Board of Canada. *NYU.*

From Sociable Six to Noisy Nine. Ages and Stages Series.
(22 min.) Illustrates the behavior that may normally be
expected in children in the six to nine age group. Sociable
Six is represented by Betty Arden. Peter Arden portrays
the behavior characteristic of seven and eight year olds.
National Film Board of Canada. *NYU.*

Six, Seven, and Eight-Year Olds--Society of Children. (30 min.)
Depicts the middle years of childhood, with strong allegiance
to the group, declaration of independence from adults and the
cleavage of the sexes. How children acquire formal and informal skills and knowledge applicable to later stages of
development. Part III of "A Long Time to Grow" series. *NYU.*

From Ten to Twelve. Ages and Stages Series. (28 min.) Describes the general characteristics of boys and girls from
ten to twelve. Children of these ages have a wide range
physically and in personality. The film begins by describing five boys, age ten to eleven. In general, they may be
characterized by a messy appearance, much noise, and the use
of strong language. At twelve, boys are somewhat neater and
better organized. A group of girls is described who vary in
size, as the boys, and are characterized by a great deal of
talk that is frequently catty, cruel and critical but which
reveals their keen awareness of human relations. National
Film Board of Canada. *NYU.*

Children Growing Up With Other People. (30 min.) A story of
children in their relationship to parents and friends. We
see the child's development from its early and involuntary
dependence to an increasing self-reliance, tempered by
membership in its group. British Information Services. *NYU.*

Children as People. (35 min.) *Polymorph Films,* 331 Newbury
Street, Boston, Mass.

And So They Grow. (28 min.) This film study of a group of
typical nine year-olds in a year-round play program at
Manhattan's P.S. 125 was produced by the Play School's
Association by means of a grant from the Good Neighbor Federation. We observe these children in actual play situations
over a year-round period. At first shy and hesitant, the
children gradually acquire a sense of belonging, an identification with the group, and an intense interest in their
projects and games. The film stresses (1) the universality
of play and its meaning to children of school age; (2) the
value of good adult leadership and (3) the importance of
good play programs in all communities. *NYU.*

Palmour Street. (27 min.) Shows the influence that parents have
on the mental and emotional development of their children.
The simple incidents of the picture are not much different

from the day-to-day experiences of the leading actors, a Negro family: father, mother, and four young children. It presents the problems that are common in the daily lives of families everywhere. Southern Education Film Production Service, University of Georgia. *NYU*.

Pizza Pizza Daddy-O. (18 min.) A group of young black girls playing singing games on a Los Angeles playground. The film provides a folkloric record of eight of these games. *UCEMC*.

Sean. (15 min.) Sean is a 4-year-old boy who lives in the Haight Ashbury district of San Francisco. The film, an interview with him intercut with silent footage of his environment, provides a keen insight into the way he perceives the world. *CFS*.

CHILD DEVELOPMENT/Affective Development

Some Basic Differences in Newborn Infants During the Lying-In Period. Film Studies on Integrated Development Series. (23 min. No S) Actual records of children from the moment of birth, showing distinct individual differences in activity and in reactions to presentation, removal, and restoration of objects of gratification. The importance for the child's total development of the mother's emotional adjustment to her newborn child is emphasized by an analysis of three contrasting maternal attitudes during nursing. Distribution limited to professional groups. *NYU*.

Genesis of Emotions. Film Studies of the Psychoanalytic Research Project on Problems in Infancy Series. (30 min. No S) Starting with children two weeks old, this picture shows how, from an unspecific beginning in which the only discernible emotion is one of negative excitation, the child develops interest for the human being by the end of the first month. The differentiation of the first positive emotions from this interest is shown with the aid of the smiling response in children ranging from two to six months. Experiments show the factors operative in the smiling response. The differentiation of the negative emotion is shown in the four-months-old child. The negative emotion's preponderant role between the eighth and the tenth month, during which it leads the development of the other emotions, is shown, as well as its role in the process of environmental discrimination. The last part of the film demonstrates the wide gamut of emotions the child has already developed at the end of its first year. Distribution limited to professional groups. *NYU*.

Expressive Movements (Affectomotor Patterns) in Infancy. (42
   min. No S)   Shows the development of expressive movements in
   healthy infants during the first year of life.   Distinctive
   "affectomotor patterns" tend to emerge successively, marked
   changed usually occurring the third and eighth months.
   "Infants cry and smile with their whole bodies."   The patterns are described with attention to individual variations
   which seem to be inborn.   A secondary theme, reaching its
   climax in the final section of the film, is the relationship
   of these expressive patterns to the development of adaptive
   patterns of manipulation, locomotion, etc., and to interpersonal relations.   Parents respond to the distress of the
   infant and, after the third month, to its manifestations of
   pleasure.   Thus the infant's expressive movements are a form
   of communication and contribute significantly to the mother-
   child relationship. *NYU.*

*Smile of the Baby, The.   Film Studies of the Psychoanalytic
   Research Project on Problems in Infancy Series.*   (30 min.)
   An experimental study, this film shows the first stage of
   the infant's response to the human being in babies two to
   six months old from a group of 115 unselected children.   A
   number of experiments with babies who smile at faces, masks,
   and movement are shown.   Some babies do not smile, such as
   a rejected child in the presence of his mother.   Mothers are
   shown feeding babies, bathing, and dressing them.   The film
   indicates that the love of the parents creates a special
   atmosphere about the baby which he associates with pleasure,
   play, food, and relief from discomfort.   His security, satis-
   faction and happiness coincide with the presence of the
   mother, and her love gives him a positive attitude toward
   society, making him a friendly, socially secure human being.
   NYU.

*Development of the Smile and Fear of Strangers in the First Year
   of Life.*   (22 min.)   Development of smile and of fear of
   strangers during the first year of life in identical and
   fraternal trwins.   Identical twins show greater concordance.
   Infants become more selective, smiling only at familiar
   persons.   Strangers are probably first persons to elicit
   fear.   Similarity of twins' fear of strangers is shown.   D.
   G. Freedman, The Langley Porter Neuropsychiatric Institute,
   1963. *PCR-2140.*

*The Smiling Response.   Film Studies of the Psychoanalytic
   Research Project on Problems in Infancy Series.*   (20 min.
   No S)   An excerpt from the film "The Smile of the Baby"
   which presents only the experimental part of the film.   Useful for graduate classes in psychology and psychiatry. *NYU.*

Children's Emotions.   Child Development Series.   (22 min.)   Discusses the major emotions of childhood: curiosity, fear,

anger, jealousy, and joy. Narrator points out the principal
characteristics of children's emotions as intense, frequently
of short duration, and resulting in a wide variety of behavior responses. The film examines the major causes of fear at
different age levels ("suddenness" of any kind, loud noises)
and cautions that fear is natural but must not be allowed
to become a habit. McGraw-Hill. *NYU.*

*Two Children: Contrasting Aspects of Personality Development.
Film Studies on Integrated Development Series.* (20 min.
No S) Shows differences in the way two children establish
homeostatic equilibrium during the lying-in period, and the
influence of the congenital activity type in predisposing
to--not causing--a certain developmental sequence during the
period from birth to 8 years in regard to parent-child relationship, psychosexual development, ego development, defense
mechanisms, and predisposition to pathology. Since every
condition is overdetermined, it must be remembered that the
congenital activity type is one of many etiological factors
in personality development. Not available in the NY area.
Distribution limited to professional groups. *NYU.*

He Acts His Age. Ages and Stages Series. (13 min.) Describes
the activities of children at different age levels and suggests that such activities are a gauge of emotional and
mental development. Crawley Films, Ltd., for the National
Film Board of Canada. *NYU.*

Children's Play. Child Development Series. (27 min.) Play is
a dynamic factor in a child's development and a necessary
requirement for good health. The film shows how play dif-
fers at each age level and describes some different forms of
play such as spontaneous, make-believe, and constructuve
play. It then goes on to emphasize the need for play time,
ample space for play both indoors and out of doors, and
proper equipment, as well as games that are geared to the
child's ability. All these factors are important considerations for parents. McGraw-Hill. *NYU.*

Children's Fantasies. Child Development Series. (21 min.) To
children all fantasies, useful or destructive, are real.
This film explores the reasons for a child's fantasies and
explains how they develop, as well as how the child may be
affected by them. Beginning with the problem of excessive
daydreaming, the film discusses such common problems as how
should Santa Claus be presented, what to do about imaginary
friends, why some children imagine that they are adopted,
how to combat fear of the dark. The film also points up the
effect of parental discipline, television, comic books, and
fairy tales on such fantasies. Fantasy or daydreaming is
seen as a pasttime that can be either an escape from reality
or, when properly channeled, an impetus to artistic, creative

living. McGraw-Hill. *NYU.*

The World of Three. (28 min.) How the presence of a new sibling leads to disturbed feelings and disruptive behavior on
the part of its three year-old brother. *NYU.*

Finger Painting. (22 min. No S) An introduction to finger
paints emphasizing their value for understanding the "language of behavior". Nine children's characteristic approaches to creative opportunities give cues to the understanding
of personality and to interpretation of behavior. *NYU.*

The Metooshow. A series of films for and about children aged
three to six. Produced in Association with the Erikson
Institute for Early Education. *Three Prong Television Productions, Inc.,* 1525 East 53rd Street, Chicago, Illinois,
60615.

The Normal Child. (25 min.) Shows Karl, a 6 year-old boy,
interacting normally and positively with his environment.
He responds to gratifications, frustrations and challenges
offered in psychiatric interview situation, in a realistic
flexible manner. Shows how he handles affect, his capacity
for imagination and play, and his constructive use of relationship with examiner. Pennsylvania State University, 1967.
PCR-2171.

Focus on Behavior: The Conscience of a Child. (30 min.) Psychologists study growth and development of personality and
emotional behavior in children in the laboratory of Dr.
Robert Sears at Stanford University. National Educational
Television, 1963. *PCR-30289.*

Feeling of Rejection, The. Mental Mechanisms Series. (28 min.)
Produced for the Mental Health Division of the Dept. of
National Health and Welfare of Canada. This is the case
history of a young woman who learned in childhood not to
risk disapproval by taking independent action. The film
shows the harmful effects of her inability to engage in
normal competition and analyzed the cause of her trouble.
We see her childhood relationship with her parents and the
factors that contributed to her later development. Therapy
methods are briefly shown that help the girl to face and
examine her problems and finally to break away from the
habit of blind obedience established early in life. *NYU.*

Feeling of Hostility, The. Mental Mechanisms Series. (27 min.)
Produced for the Mental Health Division of the Dept. of
National Health and Welfare of Canada, this film is concerned
with the problem of Clare, outwardly a successful, attractive
young woman. Sure of herself in her job, but insecure and
constrained in her personal relationships, Clare has built

her life around the only thing that has never hurt her and
has always won her praise--her intellectual capacity. We
follow her development as a child from the point at which
she experiences her first profound disappointment in the
loss of her father. The pattern of her development is one
in which the feeling of hurt is followed by strong resentment, which in turn fosters a determination to win at least
respect and admiration if not love. The mechanism of her
success is her feeling of hostility, unconsciously working
to make her so successful that she will never need the love
she finds so hard to give or accept. *NYU.*

Early Expressionists. (15 min.) Two to four year-old children
recording their spontaneous and rhythmic movements with
varying art media. Filmed at the Golden Gate Nursery School
in San Francisco. *Modern Talking Picture Service, Inc.,*
1212 Avenue of the Americas, New York, N. Y. 10036.

*Wishes, Lies, and Dreams: Kenneth Koch Teaching Children to
Write Poetry.* (29 min.) The poet Kenneth Koch teaching
poetry writing to a class of elementary school students in
New York. He gives them assignments such as writing poems
based on their feelings about a piece of music or based on
using the names of rivers. The children respond with very
inventive and original poems. *National Endowment for the
Arts,* GSA Building, 19th & F Streets N. W., Washington, D. C.

Bing Bang Boom. (24 min.) A novel approach to the teaching of
music to children, filmed in a Toronto classroom. Composer-
conductor R. Murray Schafer has seventh grade music students
listen to the sounds around them and within them. From such
exercises, the children develop an awareness of rhythm and
musical phrasing and then go on to try their own composition.
NFBC.

Balloons: Aggressions and Destruction Games. (17 min.) Demonstration of a projective play technique for the study of aggression and destruction in young children, showing how
children between four and five years of age respond to a
graduated series of opportunities to break balloons. One
child enjoys a happy-go-lucky approach, and the other shows
a strong resistance to an inferable impulse to break balloons. *NYU.*

Being Me. (13 min.) A creative dance class for nine girls,
aged 8 to 13, conducted by Hilda Mullin at the Pasadena
Art Museum. The girls' spontaneous movements, evolved in a
series of explorations, reveal the total physical, mental and
emotional involvement of the dancers. Each child follows her
own body rhythm, not one that is superimposed or prescribed.
University of California, Extension Media Center, Berkeley,
California 94720.

Frustration Play Techniques. (35 min.) A demonstration of projective play techniques developed by the late Eugene Lerner. *Part I: Ego-Blocking Games.* How several children respond to a series of games involving intrusions, prohibitions and competitions. *Part II: Frustration and Hostility Games.* How each of several children responds to a series of frustrations and interruptions in his use of attractive toys. Each toy is removed and a dull stick is substituted, providing a play level parallel to life's boring and interfering routines. *NYU.*

When Should Grownups Stop Fights? (15 min.) When fights and conflicts occur in nursery schools, the teacher must decide whether to intervene. Such decisions require that a teacher be understanding and a skilled, sympathetic observer. Incidents are repeated so that they may be shown before and after discussion without rewinding. *NYU.*

CHILD DEVELOPMENT/Mother-Child Interaction

Mother Love. Film Studies of the Psychoanalytic Research Project on Problems in Infancy Series. (20 min. No S) The first part of this film shows the social relations of Johnny to his mother beginning with the first day of life in the feeding situation. The first feeding is shown, and the mother's attitude toward Johnny is illustrated. Later stages of the development of a close relationship between Johnny and his mother are presented during the nursing situation. The continuation of these relations after weaning and their shifting pattern is shown again in the feeding situation. The influence of the birth of a sibling three years later and the mother's way of dealing with the new situation are presented. In the second part of the film the loss of mother love is shown in another child. The child's happy behavior so long as she is enjoying her mother's care is described, followed by unhappiness after separation from her mother. Similar stages are shown in three other children. The behavior of these children at the approach of a stranger is presented. In contrast, the film ends by showing Johnny, the first child shown, whose relations with his mother have been constantly happy ones, in free and boisterous interchanges with a complete stranger. Distribution limited to professional groups. *NYU.*

Emotional Ties in Infancy. (12 min.) The film shows the importance of strong emotional ties between infant and adult by comparing four 8 to 10 month old infants: a home-raised girl with strong attachment to her mother; a child in an institution who is equally attached to his nurse; another institutional baby who is indiscriminate in his attachment to any adult; still another institutional baby who has formed no attachment and appears withdrawn and uninterested in his surroundings. Vassar College for Project Head Start. *NYU*.

Study in Maternal Attitudes, A. (30 min.) Describes the Attitude Study Project developed and conducted by David M. Levy, M. D., at the Kips Bay Health Center, NYC Dept. of Health. The purpose of this project is to make the study and treatment of the emotional life of children and mothers an integral part of pediatrics and the health supervision of infants and children. Portions of seven interviews with mothers and children are shown. Skillful questioning by the interviewers elicits discussion of such parental problems as thumbsucking, in-laws, sibling rivalry, relief of tension, etc. The New York Fund for Children. *NYU*.

Baby Meets His Parents. No. 1 in the Series on Personality Development. (11 min.) This film states that we are all different not only because of hereditary factors but because we have been treated differently in early life. The shaping of the baby's personality is determined largely by the manner in which his early needs are met. *NYU*.

How Babies Learn. (35 min.) Describes some of the important developmental advances made by babies during the first year of life. All types of infant learning are subiect to the influence of the kind of interpersonal **and physical** environment in which the baby lives. Special attention is given to the importance of the mother-child relationship in enabling children to profit from their learning encounters with the environment. Part of a research project concerned with infant learning and patterns of family care. Bettye M. Caldwell and Julius B. Richmond. *NYU*.

Mother-Infant Interaction: Forms of Feeding at Six Weeks. Mother-Infant Interaction Series. (49 min.) Dr. Sylvia Brody. Shows seven basic types of maternal behavior, criteria for each type and influences upon the infant's psychological development. 1968. *NYU*.

Resemblances in Expressive Behavior. Mother-Infant Interaction Series. Dr. Sylvia Brody. Shows a variety of examples of mother-infant interaction in which particular modes of maternal behavior have been repeatedly available to the infant's experience during feeding. The typical interaction of each pair suggests that the expressive behavior of the infant is derived to an important extent, from the maternal behavior. *NYU*.

Feeding and Function Pleasure in the First Year of Life. Mother-Infant Interaction Series. (42 min.) Dr. Sylvia Brody. Presents relationships between types of maternal behavior and maturity of function pleasure of infants. One mother and infant pair from each of 7 maternal types is shown. Selections from the feeding scenes of each pair at 6 weeks, 6 months, and 1 year are followed by parts of the infant's psychological test performance at age 1. *NYU*.

Mother-Infant Interaction: Forms of Feeding at Six Months. Mother-Infant Interaction Series. (42 min.) Dr. Sylvia Brody. Demonstrates eight types of interaction with special attention to relationships between infantile experience at feeding and tension tolerance. *NYU*.

Mother-Infant Interaction: Forms of Feeding at One Year. Mother-Infant Interaction Series. (39 min.) A study of mother-infant relationships during feeding at the age of one year. Dr. Sylvia Brody. *NYU*.

Maternal Behavior and the Infant's Object Cathexis in the First Year. Mother-Infant Interaction Series. (41 min.) Shows relationship between the way an infant is mothered as exemplified by the way he is fed, and the quality, quantity and stability of his investment in the outer world of objects at 1 year. *NYU*.

Shaping the Personality: The Role of Mother-Child Relations in Infancy. Film Studies of the Psychoanalytic Research Project on Problems of Infancy Series. (20 min. No S) Illustrates forms of mother-child relations and their influence on the child. A brief anamnesis of the mother's pregnancy is confronted with her behavior during breast feeding in an attempt to present the biological and psychological factors which will decide the future attitude of the mother to her child. Five mothers, breast feeding their children, are successively shown. The first, patient, loving, and secure; the second, outgoing with mild anxiety; the third, concerned but without hostility; the fourth, rejecting and hostile toward the child; the fifth, hostile to an unwanted child. The behavior of the mothers in feeding and play situations is shown to be an expression of their conscious or unconscious wishes of what their children should be like. Five children are shown. Each is followed by a catamnesis of the further development of the child, showing how much the child's personality is a product of the mother's wishes and how much it molds itself to the picture she has of him. Distribution limited to professional groups. *NYU*.

Helping the Child to Accept the Do's. (11 min.) No. 2 in the Series on Personality Development. The film states that we are all different due not only to heredity factors but also due to the environment in which we grow. The "do's" consist of the rules for living to which children learn to conform in our society and which help shape the emerging personality. *NYU*.

Helping the Child to Face the Don'ts. (11 min.) No. 3 in the Series on Personality Development. This film shows that personality is shaped in children by conforming to the "don't" imposed by parents and the society in which we live. *NYU.*

Let Your Child Help You. Parent-Child Relations in the Early Years Series. (11 min.) Shows how very young children may help at home and thus achieve a sense of accomplishment and responsibility as well as increase of skills. Dishwashing, setting the tea table, helping prepare food, and laundering are shown with small children participating actively. The father's role in this connection is shown briefly. *NYU.*

Visit Through Saturday. (14 min.) A narrative that deals with the father-son relationship revealing a young boy's eagerness to discover the world. *NYU.*

CHILD DEVELOPMENT/Parenting, Developmental Issues and Problems

Of Skates and Elephants. (15 min.) Father-child relations and parental discipline. M.G.M. *PCR.*

Counseling With Parents: Interview III. (35 min.) Parents and teacher discuss the question of sensitivity in children and their reaction to criticism and discipline. Chico State College: Western Regional Center. Interprofessional Research Commission on Pupil Personnel Services, 1967. *PCR-2169.*

Bright Side, The. (23 min.) Stresses that being a parent is not primarily a problem, but is essentially a source of pleasure, and indicates that the anxiety of parents can hurt the children they are trying to help. Day-to-day enjoyment of family living by parents can provide the best emotional climate in which children can grow into happy, well-adjusted people. Mental Health Film Board. *NYU.*

Borderline. (27 min.) This story of a teen-age girl who is on the "borderline" between useful citizenship and delinquency points up some of the problems of emotional adjustment confronting many adolescents in their striving toward maturity. In its treatment of an adolescent who gets out of her parents' control, this film also deals provocatively with two common parental problems, how late is "too late" for a date and guidance versus discipline for the teenager. National Film Board of Canada. *NYU.*

Parent to Child About Sex. (31 min.) Shows teachers how to teach children important facts and wholesome attitudes about sex in a simple, direct fashion. Frederick J. Margolis, M.D.

and Rex Fleming. *PE*.

Childbirth: The Great Adventure. (20 min.) Two major emphases are found in this film: first, pregnancy and childbirth can be understood and enjoyed; second, the husband is given a meaningful and supportive role throughout. Morris Gold, M.D. *PE*.

Love is for the Byrds. (28 min.) The need for understanding and effective communication--especially in marriage--is forcibly demonstrated in this story about Tom and Donna Byrd, a young married couple. Brigham Young University. *PE*.

SOCIO-CULTURAL ASPECTS OF CHILD PSYCHIATRY/Cultural Differences in Child Rearing

Balinese Family. Character Formation in Different Cultures Series. (17 min.) A study of a Balinese family showing the way in which father and mother treat the three youngest children--the lap baby, the knee baby, and the child nurse. *NYU*.

Bathing Babies in Three Cultures. Character Formation in Different Cultures Series. (9 min.) A comparative series of sequences showing the interplay between mother and child in three different settings--bathing in the Sepik River in New Guinea, in a modern American bathroom, and in a mountain village of Bali in Indonesia. Gregory Bateson and Margaret Mead, 1954. *NYU*.

Karba's First Years. Character Formation in Different Cultures Series. (19 min.) A series of scenes in the life of a Balinese child, beginning with a seven-month birthday cere-monial, showing Karba's relationships to parents, aunts and uncles, child-nurse, and other children, as he is suckled, taught to walk and to dance, teased and titillated. Illus-trates the process by which a Balinese Child's responsiveness is muted as parents stimulate and themselves fail to respond. Gregory Bateson and Margaret Mead. *NYU*.

Childhood Rivalry in Bali and New Guinea. Character Formation in Different Cultures Series. (17 min.) A series of scenes in which children of the same age in the two cultures respond to: the mother attending to another baby, the ear piercing of a younger sibling, and the experimental presentation of a doll. Where the Balinese mother handles sibling rivalry by theatrical teasing of her own child through conspicuous attention to other babies, the Iatmul mother, even when nursing a newborn infant, makes every effort to keep her own child from feeling jealous. Gregory Bateson and Margaret Mead. *NYU*.

Trance and Dance in Bali. Character Formation in Different Cultures Series. (20 min.) The Balinese ceremonial dance drama in which the never-ending struggle between the witch and the dragon, the death dealing and the life protecting, is played out to the accompaniment of comic interludes and violent trance seizures. Balinese music forms a background for the narration. Gregory Bateson and Margaret Mead. *NYU.*

First Days in the Life of a New Guinea Baby. Character Formation in Different Cultures Series. (19 min.) A series of scenes beginning immediately after birth and before the cord is cut, showing the way the newborn child is fed by a wet nurse, bathed, anointed with earth, and carried, with special emphasis on the infant's readiness to respond. Gregory Bateson and Margaret Mead. *NYU.*

Three Grandmothers. (28 min.) Three grandmothers in three different parts of the world, namely, Nigeria, Canada, and Brazil. Although their roles and circumstances vary, they share certain similarities. Those shown in the film have led full, active lives, learned wisdom and compassion, know sorrow and loneliness, and find consolation in their children and grandchildren. Cultural differences, including customs, religions, and mores, are shown that affect the roles of these women. National Film Board of Canada. *NYU.*

Four Families. (60 min.) A novel venture into international understanding. Focuses on a child's upbringing in each of four countries and its relationship to distinctive national characteristics. Family life in India and France is examined in Part I. Japan and Canada are the subject of Part II. The center of attention in each case is a year-old baby in the family of a farmer of average means. The film reveals marked differences in such details of daily life as feeding and bathing the baby and in attitudes toward child training, dispensing rewards or punishments, and religious observance. Dr. Margaret Mead summarizes the more typical national characteristics. Canadian Broadcasting Company. *NYU.*

Family Life of the Navaho Indians. Film Studies on Integrated Development Series. (31 min. No S) Taken in western New Mexico among Indians who have retained much of their original culture, this film highlights some of the ways in which the Navaho child develops into a typical Navaho adult. The use of a culture so different from our own serves to focus attention on the basic fact that how one learns follows universal laws while what one learns is determined by the specific culture. It also helps us to view objectively certain daily experiences in our own culture otherwise taken for granted. M. Fries, C. Kluckhohn, and P. Woolf. *NYU.*

Forgotten Village. (67 min.) The story of the struggle in the life of the small Mexican village community of Santiago between traditional ignorance and superstition and the new ways of science. Juan Diego, a young man of the village, and the schoolmaster endeavor to save their village from a colitis epidemic due to a poisoned well. The community, under the influence of Trini, the "Wise Woman", places every obstacle in the way of the visiting medical unit which has come as a result of Juan's trip alone to the city. The film has been called a minor masterpiece. Brandon Films. *NYU.*

Peiping Family. (21 min.) Julien Bryan and William James. *NYU.*

SOCIO-CULTURAL ASPECTS OF CHILD PSYCHIATRY/Poverty and Discrimination: Effects on Children

Portrait of a Disadvantaged Child: Tommy Knight. (16 min.) A day in the life of a slum child, Tommy Knight. His fatigue after a restless night is only one of the factors affecting his ability to learn. The film shows the contrasting home life in which two equally disadvantaged children live, revealing other factors that play a role in causing such children to become academic failures. The necessity for improved methods of communication between teacher and child is indicated. McGraw-Hill. *NYU.*

The Jungle. Ghetto kids. *Churchill Films,* 622 N. Robertson Street, Los Angeles, California.

Portrait of the Inner City. (17 min.) Examines the streets, schools, and living quarters of the inner-city slums of a large, but nameless urban community in the US. The film views the area from the viewpoint of young people growing up in this environment, including young Tommy Knight and the inhabitants who serve as models for the growing boy. Shown are some of the techniques of communication between the school and the community that have been used successfully by Dr. Samuel Shepard in St. Louis. McGraw-Hill. *NYU.*

This is the Home of Mrs. Levant Graham. (15 min.) Made in cinemaverite style, provides a glimpse of the household life of an inner city black family. A young voice introduces some of the people who live in the house and their friends. Shows the relationships between Mrs. Graham and all the others. *New Thing Art and Architecture Center,* 1811 Columbia Road N.W., Washington, D.C.

Riff '65. (12 min.) A subtle, poetic documentary of an American Indian boy living in Harlem. Provides a sensitive, tough, but poignant look at a pitifully alienated youngster. *NYU.*

Roots of Happiness. (25 min.) This film is about family life, stressing the role of the father. Although filmed in Puerto Rico, it carries a message that is applicable to families everywhere. It dramatizes the contrast between a family where the father respects and loves his wife and children and a family environment in which each person has dignity and an opportunity to be himself. With English or Spanish sound tract. Mental Health Film Board. *NYU.*

Song for my Sister. (45 min.) A sociological study of the alienated concerning a "teeny-bopper" and her brother in their wanderings through New York City. *NYU.*

The Victims. (51 min.) Prejudice and child development. Westinghouse Broadcasting Company and Anti-defamation League of B'nai B'rith, 1966. *Anti-defamation League,* 315 Lexington Avenue, New York, N. Y. 10021.

Everybody's Prejudiced. (22 min.) Everybody? Well, there is prejudice and prejudice, from the man who rejects eggs because experience tells him to, to the man who dislikes his neighbors for no reason at all. Offers examples of prejudice that everyone will recognize and wish to discuss. They are all found ready at hand in a six-unit apartment dwelling and range all the way from simple prejudgment (deciding without knowing all the facts) to the emotional bias of the bigot. *NYU.*

Crisis in Levittown. (31 min.) This film is made up largely of interviews with men and women who live in Levittown, Pennsylvania, recorded just after the outbreak of violence that occurred when a Negro family moved into the all-while community of 60,000. These interviews reflect prejudice against minority groups as well as tolerance, irrational fears as well as a willingness to adapt to a changed situation, and, in short, describe a cross section of opinion in an American town dealing with interracial integration in the community. *NYU.*

Can We Immunize Against Prejudice? (7 min.) An animated film narrated by Eddie Albert and designed by Leo Leonni showing how three families try in entirely different ways to raise their children free of prejudice. *NYU.*

Desk for Billie, A. (57 min.) The story of Billie, whose migrant parents traveled incessantly in search of work. Billie's childhood was spent on dusty roads, in tents, and with makeshift meals eaten out of doors. From adult conversations she learned that "real" children went to school and that schools in America were free to all. She and her sister arranged to be sent to school whenever the family stopped for a time. Teachers helped her to overcome her school deficiencies, to make friends, and to improve her appearance. National Education Association. *NYU*.

Christmas in Appalachia. (29 min.) On a tour of the abandoned coal-mining community of Whiteburg, Ky., we are shown the stark poverty and hopelessness of the one million persons living in the desolation of Appalachia. Broken remnants of buildings serve as homes for children who have little prospects of gaining any education. CBS-TV News. *NYU*.

Take a Running Start. (17 min.) Portrays a Headstart program in Appalachian West Virginia. The groups meet at different homes in the community. The Headstart leaders are seen encouraging the children to learn on their own. *Screenscope, Inc.*, 3518 P Street N.W., Washington, D.C.   20007.

Appalachia: Rich Land, Poor People. (59 min.) Jack Willis for NET Journal, 1968. *NET Film Service*, Audio-Visual Center, Indiana University, Bloomington, Indiana   47401.

Phyllis and Terry. (36 min.) Two teenage Negro girls create a portrait of what it is like growing up in a slum, living in a ghetto. An image evolves of unrealistic hope and deep-seated despair. Eugene and Carol Marner. *PE*.

Derrick. (25 min.) Depicted are the pitiful conditions in urban public schools and the chaos, indifference, anger, boredom, desperation, and unhappiness which results. It is apparent that the run-down schools are part of the larger problem of the run-down neighborhoods. Candid scenes, taken in classrooms by the teacher-producers of the film, are juxtaposed with motion picture footage of a black boy named Derrick--walking, skipping, and running his way through the deteriorated ghetto neighborhood. The film provides an incentive and challenge to teachers, prospective teachers, parents--all concerned people--to correct and change the existing state of urban schools. Free Circle. *PE*.

SOCIO-CULTURAL ASPECTS OF CHILD PSYCHIATRY/Socio-Cultural Factors and Behavior

Obedience. (45 min.) Subjects of a Yale University Experiment on obedience to authority are instructed to administer electric shocks of increasing severity to another person. *NYU*.

Mrs. Case. (14 min.) A subjective view of a single parent attempting to bring up her children in an impoverished area of Montreal. *NFBC*.

Children of Change. (31 min.) Dramatizes the special stresses and strains placed on children whose mothers work outside

the home and on the mothers who must adjust to two full-time
jobs. Mental Health Film Board. *NYU.*

The Neglected. (35 min.) A frank portrayal of families whose
children have come under the protection of community author-
ities as a result of abuse or neglect. It reveals that
through the insight and skill of the caseworker, immature,
abusive, and even retarded or emotionally unstable human
beings can be helped to achieve acceptable standards of
parenthood. The operation of child protective services is
shown in detail, stressing the role of the supervisory personnel and the relationship between the supervisor and the
caseworker. Mental Health Film Board. *NYU.*

War of the Eggs. (27 min.) This 1972 NCFR award-winning film
dissects the anatomy of a modern American marriage. A young
couple quarrel bitterly. As a result, their two-year-old son
begins to cry hysterically. This enrages the wife who shoves
him down the stairs, badly injuring him. While the child
undergoes emergency surgery, a staff psychiatrist tries to
help. Painfully, husband and wife open to each other,
accept responsibility for their battered child, and turn
outside themselves for help. Paulist Productions. *PE.*

The Teddy Bear Years. (25 min.) A week of "live-in" type
shooting at a child welfare agency produces impressive
coverage of the life of an orphan. WKYC-TV. *PE.*

NEUROTIC DISORDERS

Preface to a Life. (30 min.) Sun Dial Films for National Institute of Mental Health, 1950. *CDMH, PCR, NYU.*

Play and Personality. (44 min.) This film is a record, photographed over a period of ten months, of the play of a group
of preschool children. The mothers of these children are
being treated in hospital by psychotherapy for severe neurotic problems. The children themselves are living in the
hospital with their mothers. The film is particularly
concerned with two boys, aged 2 and 4 years. It attempts to
show how their anxieties about themselves and their parents
are revealed in play, and how the nature of these anxieties
seems to be related to their mother's own difficulties. As
the film progresses it shows how a child tries to master his
fears and feelings in play and how it may be important for
an understanding adult to observe him closely on such occa-
sions. Although the film attempts to make some suggestions
about the meaning and value of play, the film is essentially
a record of children's experiences from which the audience
may draw their own conclusions. Cassel Hospital at Richmond,
Surrey, England. *NYU.*

Meeting the Emotional Needs of Childhood. (30 min.) Department of Child Study, Vassar, 1947. *CDMH, PCR, NYU.*

Shyness. (23 min.) Shyness in children, its causes, and how this problem may be dealt with through a greater understanding by parents and teachers. From a description of the lonely existence of a typically shy adult, the film turns to a study of three children: Anna, shy but wistfully wanting association with others; Jimmy, whose excessive timidity is really a symptom of profound emotional disturbance; Robert, aloof but happily independent. Studying their condition, a psychiatrist from the Child Guidance Clinic reveals that confidence-destroying demands of parents have predisposed the children to shyness. Together, teacher, psychiatrist, and parents bring about a change in the children's attitudes. *NYU.*

Anxiety: Its Phenomenology in the First Year of Life. Film Studies of the Psychoanalytic Research Project on Problems in Infancy Series. (20 min. No S) The phenomenology of anxiety from birth to the end of the first year is presented on the basis of behavioristic observation of its manifestations. *NYU.*

This is Robert: A Study of Personality Growth in a Preschool Child. (75 min.) L. Langmuir, T. Stone, and J. Bucher, 1942. *PCR, NYU.*

Problem Children. (20 min.) Ohio State Division of Mental Health, 1947. *CDMH, PCR, NYU.*

Don't Be Afraid. (12 min.) Encyclopedia Britannica Films, 1953. *PCR.*

Afraid of School. (28 min.) Six year-old Tommy will not go to school. Parents seek help at a children's hospital and are referred to a psychiatrist, who understands that Tommy is obsessed with terrors of death and dying. His family has been through a series of tragic events. Counseling with the parents and treatment for Tommy finally bring him to accept school. *PCR-31224.*

The Neurotic Child. (28 min.) Depicts Alan, a 7 year-old boy diagnosed as a psychoneurotic, in clinical interview situation. Shows the defensive mechanisms involved in his struggle to relate to the world as he perceives it. Illustrates reactions to reality testing, attitudes toward father, and fantasy portrayal related to relative sizes of boy and his father. Demonstrates aggressive feelings inhibited by fear of reprisal. Pennsylvania State University, 1968. *PCR-2174.*

Overcoming Fear. (13 min.) Water phobia. Coronet Films. *PCR.*

The Lonely Night. (62 min.) Mental Health Film Board, 1952. *CDMH, NYU.*

Don't Get Angry. (12 min.) Encyclopedia Britannica Films, 1953. *CDMH.*

Your Children's Sleep. (22 min.) British Information Service, 1947. *CDMH, NYU.*

Why Won't Tommy Eat? (17 min.) Canadian Film Board, 1948. *CSDPH, NYU.*

Psychological Implications of Behavior During the Clinical Visit. (20 min. No S) M. E. Fries and P. J. Woolf. *NYU.*

The Search: New Hope for Stutters. (25 min.) Young America Films. Columbia Broadcasting System TV, 1955. *PCR.*

Report on Donald. (20 min.) University of Minnesota Speech Clinic. *PCR.*

Stuttering From the Horse's Mouth. (33 min.) State University of Iowa Speech Clinic. *PCR.*

Face of Youth. (28 min.) Bureau of Visual Instruction, University of Wisconsin, 1951. *CDMH, NYU.*

Character Neurosis with Depressive and Compulsive Trends in the Making: A Life History of Mary from Birth to Fifteen Years. Film Studies on Integrated Growth Series. (40 min. No S) Shows how a child with superior biological capacity and an active congenital-activity type develops a neurosis through interaction with those in her environment. The film follows Mary's total development from birth to fifteen years, illustrating how the so-called average child--in a family that society considers normal--may never be referred for needed psychiatric treatment. *NYU.*

Anna N. Life History from Birth to Fifteen Years. The Development of Emotional Problems in a Child Reared in a Neurotic Environment. Film Studies on Integrated Development Series. (60 min. No S) Shows a child of superior intelligence, in mediocre health at birth which is overcome by the age of about 2. Her constitutional mode of adjusting in infancy, as shown by her quiet to moderately active congenital-activity type, is seen in her behavior. The interaction of her hereditary endowment with her neurotic parents, grandparents and sister results in a personality difficult to categorize. More of her psychodynamics are revealed by unconscious material obtained through interviews, controlled play tests, play and

Rorschachs. *NYU.*

Boys in Conflict. (72 min.) The feature film in the Guidance
Camp Series. A college student experiences a summer at
Wediko, caring for nine boys who exhibit a variety of emotional problems. During the course of the summer, both the
counselor, Steve and the boys in his cabin undergo changes
in dealing with their emotional problems. *Center for Mass
Communication,* 440 West 110th Street, New York, N. Y.   10025.

Angry Boy. (33 min.) Affiliated Film Producers, Michigan Mental
Health Authority, 1951. *CDMH, PCR.*

PSYCHOPHYSIOLOGIC DISORDERS

Neurological Examination of the Newborn. (30 min.) Normal and
abnormal responses to a series of tests. Wexler Film Productions: Dept. of HEW, NIH, 1960. *PCR-30350.*

Neurological Examination of the One-Year-Old. (30 min.) Standards of examination of infants at one year. Normal and
abnormal responses to tests. Wexler Film Productions: Dept.
of HEW, NIH, 1960. *PCR-30351.*

Stress. (11 min.) McGraw-Hill Films and Hans Selye, 1955. *CDMH,
NYU.*

Stress and the Adaptation Syndrome. (35 min.) Hans Selye, 1955.
Charles Pfizer and Co., 630 Flushing Avenue, Brooklyn, N.Y.

Somatic Consequences of Emotional Starvation in Infants. (30 min.
No S) *NYU.*

The Brain and Behavior. (22 min.) McGraw-Hill. *NYU, PCR.*

Epidemic Encephalitis. (31 min.) *NYU.*

Visual Perception. (19 min.) Demonstrations used at the Perception Center at Princeton University showing the effects of
some of our assumptions on what we "see". Educational
Testing Service, 1959. *PCR-152-5.*

Visual Perception and Failure to Learn. (20 min.) Effects of
visual perceptual disabilities upon the performance and
behavior of children. Good visual perception is not dependent upon good eyesight, but upon the brain's ability to
interpret the incoming visual stimuli. Use of the Marianne
Frostig Developmental Test of Visual Perception. Churchill
Films, 1966. *PCR-20772.*

School Day, A: Study of a Visually Handicapped Child. (24 min.) Shows how a nine-year-old girl functions adaptively in a neighborhood school with her sighted peers. *NYU.*

Pay Attention. (27 min.) Some emotional and educational problems of the child who is moderately or severely hard of hearing, and suggested ways in which parents, teachers and specialists can help. Follows selected preschool, school age and high school children and indicates a variety of problems and remedial techniques. *NYU.*

Epileptic Seizure Patterns. (25 min.) Original art work used to show historical aspects of epilepsy and various types of epileptic seizures in actual patients. Shows and explains electroencephalograph tracing in a normal man and uses a split frame technique to compare normal tracings with those of grand mal, petite mal, automatism, myoclonic, psychomotor, and mixed adversive-grand mal patients. Synchronous sound gives audio as well as visual characteristics of the seizures shown. Indiana University, 1963. *PCR-31395.* (Color version *PCR-31007)*

Deficiency in Finger Schema (Finger Agnosia and Acalculia). (14 min. No S) Demonstration of 2 cases of finger agnosia, inability to localize fingers which have been touched, among subjects having special difficulties in field of arithmetic. Authors, psychiatrist, and psychologist respectively, have made this demonstration from larger study showing that finger agnosia seems to be connected with disabilities in simple processes of arithmetical calculation. A. Strauss and H. Werner, 1938. *PCR-512.*

Focus on Behavior: The Brain and Behavior. (30 min.) Mechanisms of the brain which control our behavior. Dr. Donald B. Lindsley and Dr. Horace W. Magoun demonstrate the way in which electrical activity in the brain gives us information about man's behavior. National Educational Television, 1963. *PCR-30290.*

Electroencephalogram. (15 min. No S) Preliminary scenes show external appearance of EEG amplifiers, continuous-paper kymograph, magnetic ink styluses, and construction of electrodes. Method of attaching scalp electrodes and construction of shielded room shown. Last 200 feet of film presents encephalograms: normal alpha and beta, epileptic, brain tumor, disturbance in paresis, recovery patterns after fever treatment, and records of schizophrenics and behavior problems. Some parts of this film are out-of-date, but much is still useful. A.E. Bennett and P.T. Cash, 1941. *PCR-515.*

Effects of Various Drugs on Emotional Mimetic Reactions of Hypothalamus and Cerebral Cortex of the Cat. (20 min. No S) *PCR.*

Psychosomatic Conditions--Obesity. The Disordered Mind Series.
(28 min.) This 13-year-old girl is unhappy because she is
fat. She is fat because eating helps to relieve her feelings
of frustration over a lack of communication between herself
and her mother. The girl's parents also receive treatment,
and after several months, the family is made aware of the
relationship between the girl's unmet emotional needs and
her overeating. They learn to communicate more effectively
with one another. Dr. V. Rakoff is the psychiatrist who
treats the girl and her family. The discussant is Dr. Henry
Kravitz. Contemporary Films. *NYU.*

CHILDREN IN THE HOSPITAL AND DEATH AND DYING

Going to the Hospital with Mother. (45 min.) The greatest
single cause of distress in young children in hospitals is
not illness or pain but separation from the mother. The
young child is normally intensely attached to his mother,
and if going to hospital means losing her care (which it
usually does), he commonly reacts with acute distress and
disturbed behavior. Even after a brief hospital stay such
behavior may persist for weeks, months, or even longer.
James Robertson, Tavistock Institute of Human Relations,
Child Development Research Unit. *NYU.* (Guide to the Film
published by Tavistock Publications, London, 1963)

John: An Infant in the Hospital. J. Robertson, 1969. *NYU.*

Two Year-Old Goes to the Hospital, A. (50 min.) This film was
produced by Dr. James Robertson as part of a research project
on "The Effects of Personality Development of Separation from
the Mother in Early Childhood", at the Tavistock Clinic in
London, which is part of the British National Health Service.
The film describes the behavior of a child, two years and
five months old, during 8 days in a hospital ward in which
conditions and nursing care are good by contemporary standards. As the subject of research is the effect of maternal
deprivation upon the capacity for relationships, the film
shows how the child is when alone, how she treats nurses,
and how she behaves toward her parents when they visit. This
film was made by procedures devised to minimize the subjective element, which is unavoidable in written descriptions of
human behavior, and it is presented without interpretation.
The aim is to provide an objective record that, being visual,
gives the viewer a close approximation to direct observation
and permits the child's behavior, and environment within
which it occurs, to be examined as often as desired for the
stury of detail. *NYU.*

Two Year-Old Goes to the Hospital, A. (30 min.) (Abridged Version) In the new version, which is for general release, much

of the research detail of the original has been omitted,
leaving a pure narrative which is true not only of the
British child shown but of young children everywhere for
whom going to the hospital means leaving the care of the
mother. Recommended to teachers and to community groups
seeking to study the problem of young children in hospitals
with view of pressing for improved facilities in local hospitals. *NYU.* (Guide to the Film published by Tavistock
Publications, London, 1953a)

Jane: Aged 17 months in Foster Care for 10 Days. (37 min.)
Young Children in Brief Separation Series. Because she
developed a strong attachment to her foster mother, it is
weeks before Jane can give her up following reunion with her
mother. *NYU.*

Kate: A Two Year-Old in Foster Care. (33 min.) Young Children
in Brief Separation Series. During a stay of 27 days Kate
revealed lowered frustration tolerance, increasing disappointment and conflict of feeling about her absent parents.
NYU.

Separations and Reunions: Parts I-IV. (35 min.) Documents
reactions of four children age fourteen to twenty months,
hospitalized for from five to 24 days. In these separations
from parents, complicated by illnesses, the following behavior is noted: apathy, withdrawal, self-comforting, acute
misery, dull unresponsiveness, and varying responses to play
with nurses. At reunion hostility and resentment are combined with joy and relief. In time, after reunion, normal
behavior returns. Frequency of visits by parents and "living
in" by one mother help alleviate anxiety. Showing restricted
to appropriate professional groups. H. Lowenstein and D.
MacCarthy. The Pennsylvania State University, 1968. *PCR-
2222.*

Robin, Peter and Darryl: Three to the Hospital. (53 min.)
Illustrates the effect of maternal separation and the reactions of three children to hospitalization. *NYU.*

Children in the Hospital. (44 min.) A record on film of the
spontaneous activity of children on the wards at Boston City
Hospital. It illustrates types of emotional responses of
four to eight-year-olds to the stress of hospitalization,
illness, and separation. A picture of hospital life as the
child sees it, the film includes its noises, its joys, and
its isolation. There is evidence of the varying defense
mechanisms that children use, as well as types of supportive
help that one child can give another and which various adults
in contact with children can offer. *NYU.*

John 17 Months: Nine Days in a Residential Nursery. (45 min.)
John is admitted to a residential nursery while his mother
is in the hospital. However, the system of group care does
not allow any of his nurses to substitute for the absent
mother. The severity of John's distress is not recognized
until a late stage. When on the ninth day John's mother
finally returns, he does not readily accept her and struggles to get out of her arms. *NYU.*

The Day Hospital. (22 min.) Dr. Joshua Bierer, a prominent
English psychiatrist, takes the audience on an informative
tour of Malborough Day Hospital, located in a quiet residential section of London. Patients live "out"--though not
necessarily in their own homes--and come to this large
Edwardian house for such therapies as individual counseling,
activity therapy, electroshock, chemotherapy, and group
therapy. TV Reporters International, London. *NYU.*

LEARNING AND LEARNING DISTURBANCES

What Does it Need to Grow? (29 min.) The setting for the film
is provided by preschool programs conducted at the University
of California Child Study Center in Berkeley. The teachers
respect the children's individual ideas and interests. A
companion film to "My Art is Me". *UCEMC.*

Setting the Stage for Learning. (22 min.) A filmed experiment
in which a group of nursery-school youngsters are urged to
play in a sandbox containing only sand. The debacle is
contrasted with a number of familiar behavioral situations
that lead to beneficial learning experiences. Churchill
Films. *NYU.*

Children Learning by Experience. (40 min.) British Ministry of
Information, 1948. *CDMH, PCR, NYU.*

Starting Nursery School: Patterns of Beginning. (23 min.)
Shows child's gradual introduction to nursery school without
the sudden stress of abrupt separation from mother. Of
especial value for nursery school and kindergarten staffs,
parent groups and students of early childhood education. *NYU.*

My Own Yard to Play In. (9 min.) Received citation at Venice
Festival. Brief and simple film showing resourcefulness of
children playing in a large city. *NYU.*

*Nursery School Child-Mother Interaction: Three Head Start Chil-
dren and Their Mothers.* (41 min.) In the first part three
Negro mothers are shown alone with their four year-old boys;
two of the children are "difficult" and the third well
adjusted. Emphasizes the mother's influence and child's

attachment to her. Then we are shown three children in their
Head Start school emphasizing social attitudes with scenes
of mealtime behavior, preferred activities and goal pursuit.
Differences in interaction patterns and maternal attitudes
can be observed. *NYU.*

From Cradle to Classroom: Part I. (25 min.) Shows how preschool education is having remarkable success in teaching
the very young. New processes can start the education of
children as early as 12 or 13 months: toys and association
drills for younger groups, reading and logic for 2, 3 and 4
year-old groups. Discussion of controversies caused by
early education. CBS, 21st Century Series. McGraw-Hill
Text Films, 1968. *PCR-31535.*

From Cradle to Classroom: Part II. (26 min.) Ibid. *PCR-31536.*

Head Start to Confidence. Head Start Training Series, Vassar.
(17 min.) Shows how teachers may overcome apathy, fear and
hesitance of disadvantaged preschool children and instill
self-confidence. *NYU.*

Organizing Free Play. Head Start Training Series, Vassar.
(22 min.) Shows that free play in the nursery school should
offer a variety of carefully prepared activities, not regi-
mented uniformity or chaos. *NYU.*

Discipline and Self-Control. Head Start Training Series, Vassar.
(24 min.) Suggests how to prevent discipline problems in
nursery school and how to deal with them when they arise.
NYU.

A Chance for Change. (39 min.) Describes a Head Start Nursery
school center in Mississippi that was built and operated by
Negro parents who had little schooling and no previous exposure to educational theories and practices. Concentrates on
everyday activities in the playground, classroom, at meals,
and on nature walks during an 8 week session. Child Development Group of Mississippi. *NYU.*

Blocks--A Material for Creative Play. (16 min.) Campus Films
Productions. *PCR.*

Hello Up There! (9 min.) Children's drawings, paintings, and
comments are used to create an expressive film illustrating
the way youngsters see--and feel about-- the adult world.
Children give voice and form to emotions of jealousy, anger,
hurt--and love--in a world where one is so small that he
must cry "Hello, up there!" even to be noticed. *NYU.*

Their First Teachers. (10 min.) City College of New York. *PCR.*

Four and Five Year-Olds in School. (37 min.) Fours are seen as masters of a familiar world of activities and interests; fives, while continuing many of these activities, are beginning to enter the world of older children, a more formalized, enlarging world. Part II of "A Long Time to Grow" series. *NYU.*

Primary Education in England. (17 min.) Shows the British infant school, an experiment in nongraded education in the early years of a child's life. Made at one of the leading infant schools in England. The children perform plays which they wrote themselves, make music with instruments supplied by nature, and learn math by charting egg production from their class-managed chicken coops. *IDEA.*

Westfield Infant School (Two Days in May). *EDC.*

Medbourne Primary School (Four Days in May). *EDC.*

Don't Tell Me--I'll Find Out. (22 1/2 min.) Classroom demonstrations of an elementary school science curriculum project based on the "discovery" approach. First graders observe and discuss organisms and their interactions; second graders study the life cycles of plants and animals; and third graders discover the interdependence of organisms. *SCIS.*

Design for Learning. (20 min.) Shows the Technology for Children Project sponsored by the New Jersey Board of Education. The classroom is open and children of different ages work together. The emphasis is on problem solving. The children make storybooks, musical instruments, and other things. They observe demonstrations and go on field trips. *TCP.*

Here I Am. (28 min.) The teachers in this film work with withdrawn preschool children over a period of months to show the changes which take place in the children. *CL.*

Learning is Searching. (30 min.) This film shows children learning about tools; it is concerned with a liberal elementary school curriculum, methods of learning and how children can be freed to search for knowledge. The children's needs and interests, delicate reminders of age limitations and exciting indications of their potentialities, are integral parts of the film. *NYU.*

My Art is Me. (21 min.) An experimental preschool program at the University of California Child Study Center in Berkeley. The film demonstrates how an art program can relate to the whole curriculum. A companion film to "What Does It Need to Grow?" *UCEMC.*

What Makes Man Human? (15 min.) Jerome Bruner as theoretician and Mrs. Thalia Kitulakis as practitioner (fifth grade teacher), examine the pros and cons of the Bruner curriculum, "Man: A Course of Study". *CHP.*

They Can Do It. (34 min.) Children in a Philadelphia first grade class become involved with individual prjects and work at their own pace. Shows them changing over a period of months. *EDC.*

A Time for Learning. (38 min.) In urban and suburban schools, fifth grade teachers and students work and study with the Bruner curriculum, following the life patterns and cycles of gulls, fish, baboons, and Eskimos, in an effort to understand themselves and their environment. *CHP.*

Cloud 9. (25 min.) Filmed in the Cardozo Model School District in Washington, D.C., during a 3-week period following the death of Martin Luther King. The young black children in three fifth grade classes express their feelings about Dr. King's death, and the burning and rioting which occurred in Washington afterwards. *EDC.*

A Lesson on Change. (12 min.) An elementary school teacher's spontaneous explanation to her class of Dr. Martin Luther King's death and the social changes for which he gave his life. *OSU.*

Mrs. Ryan's Drama Class. (35 min.) An experiment in freewheeling dramatic expression for a class of 8 to 12 year-old boys and girls in a Toronto public school. Under the unobtrusive direction of their teacher, Mrs. Ryan, they invent their own dramas, then act them out, progressing in skill and confidence to the point where they stage their own play for the rest of the school. *NFBC.*

Summerhill. (28 min.) A visit to Summerhill, a school without fixed rules, where no one studies except as he wishes and where each student is his own master. A co-educational boarding school, Summerhill was founded 45 years ago by A. S. Neill. In the film, Neill explains his objectives. *NFBC.*

Meeting Emotional Needs in Childhood: The Groundwork of Democracy. (32 min.) Methods of meeting the child's needs for acceptance, security and independence; suggests that how these needs of seven to ten year-olds are met makes a difference for democratic citizenship. *NYU.*

Children Learning by Experience. (40 min.) A film about children playing and working together in natural surroundings. Sequences are devoted to the urge to learn, practicing simple skills, understanding the world about them, learning at second hand, and learning through play and imagination. *NYU.*

Children Dance. (14 min.) Boys and girls from kindergarten through third grade through dance improvisations which express and explore space, time, force, and imagery feelings, moods, and ideas. Filmed during regularly scheduled "dance times" at inner city and suburban classrooms in metropolitan Washington, D.C. *UCEMC.*

Chance at the Beginning, A. (28 min.) Demonstrates that preschool training, particularly for children from educationally limited environments provides a sound foundation for the development of each child's potential throughout the school years. Actual scenes were filmed in a Harlem school where an experiment in preschool training is under way. *NYU.*

Pre-Kindergarten Program--New Haven, A. (30 min.) Camera Visits to Preschools for Disadvantaged Children Series, Vassar. A preschool located in a gymnasium of a neighborhood recreation center; the school and all equipment must be removed after 3 p.m. *NYU.*

Los Nietos Kindergarten--Camera Visit. (25 min.) Camera Visits to Preschools for Disadvantaged Children Series, Vassar. A public school kindergarten in a predominately Mexican-American Neighborhood. *NYU.*

Vassar College Nursery School. (35 min.) Camera Visits to Preschools for Disadvantaged Children Series, Vassar. Shows a program meeting two afternoons a week, for disadvantaged children, using facilities of a well-equipped nursery school. *NYU.*

Who Will Teach Your Child? (24 min.) National Film Board of Canada, 1948. *CDMH, NYU.*

Bright Boy, Bad Scholar. (28 min.) Repeated failure in an unfriendly environment causes children to develop emotional difficulties and learning problems. This film document of such a child indicates that children can be taught if their problems are recognized early enough and if special help is provided. *NYU.*

Best of Sesame Street Revisited. (30 min.) Selections from the best of the "Sesame Street" programs. Included are several sequences on counting and an introduction to basic geometric shapes. *CTW.*

Battling Brook Primary School (Four Days in September). *EDC.*

Acquisition of Language by a Speechless Child. (17 min.) An 8 year-old boy who has never used words is demonstrated responding accurately to oral instructions which require the understanding of prepositions, varieties of adjectives, and complicated syntax. Some family, birth, developmental, medical, and psychometric information is presented. He was born with multiple anomalies (ptosis, strabismus, cleft lip, clubfeet), but the speech difficulty is "not due to any peripheral motor or anatomic defects". Brief recordings of spontaneous and imitative vocalizations are played. His "perfect understanding of English" is offered as evidence against the assumption that "development of understanding is dependent upon simultaneous development of speaking". Showings restricted to appropriate groups in the professions. *PCR-2125K.*

And So They Live. (25 min.) This is one of two films produced by the Educational Film Institute of New York University in cooperation with the University of Kentucky to document the gap between the everyday needs of the community and the actual instruction in the schools of this particular rural area. This film shows the tragic poverty of the land in a rural southern community; the lack of proper diet, housing and sanitation; and the need for better adaptation of the school program to the problems of the community. *NYU.*

Access to Learning. (20 min.) Documents the efforts of four elementary school teachers in the Columbus, Ohio, public schools to provide their students with opportunities to strengthen their powers of thought. The program is based on the belief that the teacher who consistently provides the child with opportunities to develop skill in thinking provides him with access to learning. *OSU.*

A Search for Learning. (14 min.) The use of innovative teaching techniques, the discovery method and various classroom strategies for individualizing learning opportunities. *NYU.*

Image in a Mirror. (9 min.) Critical Moments in Teaching Series. Working with an elementary school child lacking in self-confidence. *NYU.*

Children Without. (29 min.) A moving commentary on the current problem in education involving the disadvantaged child. Shown is the inner city, the slums, occupied largely by the rural dispossessed. The story centers around one such child and the school that is adapting to change conditions in the community, which, in turn, demands of teachers a fresh approach to changing needs. The principal indicates some of the methods employed to educate children whose parents have become indifferent or apathetic concerning the value of education. *NYU.*

Why Can't Jimmy Read?   (18 min.)   Syracuse University, 1950. *PCR*.

Skippy and the Three R's.   (29 min.)   National Education Association, 1953.   *PCR, NYU*.

Oral Language: A Breakthrough to Reading.   (28 min.)   Describes a 6-week language development project in the Columbus, Ohio, public schools, where four teachers used their special skills in music, art, physical education and language to develop each child's ability to communicate.   *OSU*.

Incitement to Reading.   (37 min.)   A candid documentary of a combined first and second grade of a liberal school learning to read by an approach that stresses beginners' curiosity and enthusiasm rather than the mechanics of reading. The essence lies in repeatedly living significant experiences, reliving the experiences in words and seeing the words translated into written symbols.   *NYU*.

A Child Who Cheats.   (10 min.)   Critical Moments in Teaching Series. Handling a problem of cheating in an elementary classroom.   *NYU*.

How's School, Enrique?   (18 min.)   Depicts some of the environmental and educational problems which face young Mexican-Americans. Two teachers are featured in the film. One speaks Spanish and is excited by her subject matter and students; the other is teacher-oriented and expects the students to fail.   *SFP*.

Why Some Children Don't Learn.   (26 min.)   Excerpts from four interviews reveal some of the causes and consequences of resistance to learning and illustrate a counseling approach. To learn in a regular school, a student must see and hear, attend and comprehend. The origins of resistant behavior are varied: in some cases minor sensory defects lead to failure, frustration and the avoidance of school tasks: in others, familial conflicts interfere with the ability to attend to classwork; or previous absence or inattention or preschool cultural impoverishment make comprehension too difficult. Research findings are graphically presented to show the possibilities for change in resistant behavior and underachievement; and the interviews with three adolescents and one mother suggest the counselor's role. M. Schwebel and B. Schwebel for the New York State Counselors Association and New York State Board of Regents.   *NYU*.

This is Robert.   (45 min.)   This now classical longitudinal study traces the growth of Robert--an aggressive, but appealing child--from nursery school at two to public school at seven. First released in 1943, the film has been re-edited and

abridged in 1970 without changing the essential content.
This abridgement replaces the original 80 minute version
hereafter available only by special request. *NYU*.

PROBLEMS OF ADOLESCENCE

The Invention of the Adolescent. (28 min.) From the past, when
distinction between childhood and adulthood were not as fine-
ly drawn as they are today, this film traces the development
of the adolescent and shows some of the real problems of
this age. It notes that it was the defense of the young, the
protection afforded by reformers and educators, that created
the generation gap so evident today. *NYU*.

Developmental Characteristics of Preadolescents. (18 min.)
Herbert Kerkow, 1954. *CDMH, NYU*.

Farewell to Childhood. (23 min.) Susan Stewart is a normal
teenager, full of the swift emotions typical of adolescence.
She wants independence and the privileges of adulthood while
at the same time she fears them. She stumbles in uncertainty
yet believes only she could possibly be "right". The film
catches her moods--of rebellion and trust, self-pity, and
idealism. *MHFB, NYU*.

The Teens. (28 min.) National Film Board. *NYU*.

Age of Turmoil. Adolescent Development Series. (20 min.) This
film is concerned with early adolescence--a period approximately from age 13 to 15 years. It focuses on the behavior
that reflects the emotional turmoil of this age group. *NYU*.

Social Development. Child Development Series. (16 min.) The
film offers an analysis of social behavior at different age
levels and the reasons underlying the changes in behavior
patterns as the child develops. The infant is the passive
bystander in the social scene; the preschool child is aggressive in his play activities and plays cooperatively with
others of his age group only after several years of learning.
Points out development from the stage where the sexes and
ages mix indiscriminately to the point where children begin
to pick members of their own sex as playmates, to seek out
the natural leader for their groups. All these patterns mix,
and overlap, but at different age levels there is a definite
organization of children's social behavior. The film goes on
to the emotional conflicts that come with the gang age, when
home and family are no longer the center of the child's
world. It stresses the point that while the child must meet
and solve each problem as he reaches that level of growth and
development, guidance from understanding adults can make the
adjustment infinitely easier and smoother. McGraw-Hill. *NYU*.

Emotional Maturity. Adolescent Development Series. (20 min.)
Dramatizes the immature behavior of a high school boy and
shows some of the consequences when an adolescent fails to
channel his emotions into positive actions and feelings.
Dave has been "going steady" with Jill who rejects him for
Jimmy, a football star. Angry and frustrated Dave is re-
venged by slashing a tire on Jimmy's car. Scenes with his
parents reveal that they have treated Dave as a child and
have set up standards that are too high for him to reach.
The film asks how Dave's emotional instability could have
been prevented. *NYU.*

Social Acceptability. Adolescent Development Series. (20 min.)
The story of a high school girl who fails to be accepted by
a popular school clique illustrates the correlation between
social acceptability and the successful adjustment and happiness of the average adolescent. The film emphasizes the
responsibility of parents to provide adolescents with guidance in the social skills and opportunities to put these
skills into practice. Marion, who is shy and doesn't know
what to talk about in the company of her friends, is not
invited to a party. Scenes at home indicate that her mother
is afraid of Marion's friends and reluctant to entertain
them. Under pressure from the father, Marion's mother begins to realize that Marion needs guidance and help socially.
The film states that the degree of social acceptance tends
to affect personality. *NYU.*

Toward Emotional Maturity. Psychology for Living Series. (11
min.) What causes unreasoning emotion? Why is common sense
swept away in a moment of jealousy, fear or hatred? How can
the adolescent be prepared to understand and control his
emotions? These are a few of the questions explored in this
film. Sally Bronson, an average 18-year-old student, is
wondering, doubting, at times confused. Sally is faced with
a decision that deeply involves her feelings for both her
parents and a boy whom she likes very much. With Sally we
review several episodes in her past that reveal the violence
and at times destructive quality of strong emotions. In
these incidents Sally sees how she--and others--were robbed
of sensible values and left incapable of handling the situation. Her final decision is based on this realization.
McGraw-Hill. *NYU.*

Borderline. (27 min.) National Film Board. *NYU.*

Family Affair. (31 min.) Adolescent son's defiance of parents
reveals husband's resentment against wife's domination of
family affairs. Counsel from social caseworker helps in
solving family problems. International Film Bureau: Mental
Health Film Board, 1955. *PCR-2135.*

Youth Tutors Youth. (20 min.) Depicts a program, now used in over 200 school systems, where older students, aged 14-15, who themselves have been underachievers, tutor younger students in the second to sixth grades, most of whom have difficulties with reading or writing. The tutors use photography, making tapes, and writing stories to help the children improve their skills. *NCRY.*

Discipline During Adolescence. Adolescent Development Series. (16 min.) Takes up the question of how much discipline is good for adolescents. Results of both too little and too much parental control are dramatized in a typical family setting. Stevie is keeping very late hours, his schoolwork is suffering, and his parents are worried. His father advocates discipline but after a discussion with his wife, the decision is made to say nothing. The boy seems indifferent, is cocky and irresponsible. The father insists on handling the situation and cuts off Stevie's allowance. The boy sulks. The film ends by asking the audience to consider how this situation could have been handled more effectively. *NYU.*

What's A Nice Girl Like You Doing in a Place Like This? (11 min.) A sprightly, sophisticated short about a young man with a hallucination. Satirizing the use of cliche, the film winds up with an unexpected "splash". Department of Television, Motion Pictures, and Radio of NYU. *NYU.*

Who Cops Out? (10 min.) This film raises the question of the choices today's adolescents make when faced with the confusion and uncertainty of teen-age years. We meet five teen-agers; a pregnant girl who may be asked to leave school, a school dropout working in a gas station, a high school athlete, a scholastic achiever, a runaway drug user. Each describes his feeling and attempts to explain the reasons for his choice. *NYU.*

The People Next Door. (79 min.) Two families face an ordeal involving one daughter who has a bad LSD trip, her brother whose hippie appearance causes animosity and distrust from his father and the "respectable" boy next door who is discovered to be the pusher that furnished the drug. The girl's eventual commitment to a mental institution exemplified the tragic results of misusing drugs. CBS Playhouse Production. *NYU.*

No Reason to Stay. (28 min.) Reasons for school dropout from child's view. John Kemeny, National Film Board of Canada, 1966. *EBF.*

The Dropout. (29 min.) When the film opens, Joe has dropped out of school and is the envy of many former classmates because he has a job and a car. Through a series of flashbacks the viewer sees Joe's discontent with senior high school, his boredom in class, and the efforts made by his counselor to persuade him not to leave school. The audience soon realized that Joe's dislike of school began long before-- when he had reading problems in the fifth grade. *NYU*.

A Nice Kid Like You. (40 min.) Articulate college students speak with candor about some of their most important concerns: drugs, sex, political action, faculty and curriculum, their relationships with their peers, and the generation gap. Filmed at uninhibited dormitory bull sessions, breakfast conversations in middle-class homes, college dining commons, and kaffeeklatchs among suburban mothers. *NYU*.

I Walk Away in the Rain. Critical Moments in Teaching Series. (11 min.) The problem of motivating a highly capable adolescent making minimal effort. *NYU*.

Confrontation. (25 min.) A penetrating study of the student world of today demonstrating how young people are impatient with the processes of orderly change, of reasoning, of cooperation, and agreement. Filmed at Antioch College, we see a student meeting seething with passionate protests of current college policies in which a militant black appears as one of the most eloquent and extreme of their spokesmen. *NYU*.

A Far Cry from Yesterday. (20 min.) A realistic film about the common crisis of how an unwanted pregnancy can destroy a loving relationship. It is the story of a teenage student couple who, after having been married and tied down, look back at how they got involved. Shows couple in early stages of dating and physical involvement, which often lacks proper birth control practices. Laura's fear of pregnancy is ultimately confirmed and she faces a dilemma in making a personal decision. By following their fantasies about love and having a baby, instead of looking at the realities and difficulties of having a successful marriage as young parents, we find the couple in an angry, deteriorated partnership. The film ends with a shocking statistic that reflects the theme: "Seventy-five percent of sexually active teenagers do not use a birth control method"--U. S. Population Commission. Steven Dreben. *PE*.

Phoebe: Story of a Premarital Pregnancy. (31 min.) A sensitive, yet powerful study of a young girl's love affair and her reactions at finding herself pregnant. National Film Board of Canada. *NFBC, PE*.

Your Amazing Mind. (15 min.) A new approach to the drug problem...a concept that makes young people THINK! This film not only shows the dangers of the most commonly misused drugs but, more importantly, establishes the fact that our minds are our most valuable possessions. Film asks the question--"Why take a chance with anything that might hurt your most valuable possession?" Especially created for grades five through eight. Higgins. *PE*.

Human Growth. (20 min.) Creates instructional atmosphere that permits the subject of human sex to be discussed in the classroom without embarrassment or tension by presenting the biological facts as a natural part of human growth and development. Introductory sequences in the home and classroom precede the main part of the film, an animated presentation of the elementary facts of human growth and reproduction in simple, diagrammatic style. Concepts presented include: differences between boys and girls in rate of physical and sexual maturation, glands which control physical and sexual activity, male and female sex organs, menstruation, fertilization, pregnancy and birth. In final classroom scene children raise questions for teacher to answer. Wexler Film Productions. *PE*.

DELINQUENCY, ANTI-SOCIAL, IMPULSIVE AGGRESSIVE DISORDERS

Street Corner Research. (30 min.) A record of the initial contact and first interview of an experimental program to prevent juvenile delinquency, in which the psychologist or social worker actively seeks out his client. Dr. Ralph Schwitzgebel, a psychologist approaches two boys in Harvard Square and offers to pay them if they agree to take part in his project. The camera then focuses on the first interview where the boys are surprisingly frank and reveal significant material. *NYU*.

Criminal is Born. (22 min.) Metro Goldwyn Mayer, 1938. *PCR*.

Who's Delinquent? (16 min.) Shows a typical American town in which occurs an incident involving two boys who steal a car and nearly kill the local policeman. The city editor of the town's newspaper sets out to discover the causes of juvenile delinquency in the area. His reporters discover that delinquency usually begins at home but that the whole town bears the responsibility. The probation officer is not equipped to handle youthful offenders, the judge does not have time to guide them, schools are over-crowded, playgrounds are not sufficient, and taverns attract many youngsters. The film ends with the townspeople meeting in an effort to solve the problem. *NYU*.

Beginnings of Conscience. *Sociology Series*. (16 min.) The social conscience of James Bryce, the adult, is traced back to his socialization as a child. From incidents at home and in school, Jimmy Bryce learns from his parents, teachers, and schoolmates what is right and what is wrong. *NYU.*

Problem Children. (20 min.) A film about two children, Roy and Jimmy, in the 7th grade of an American public school who present special problems for the teacher. Roy is active, athletic, but restive, a show-off, and a bully. Jimmy is shy, lacking in self-confidence, passive, and pushed around. The techniques employed in helping these children, the family background, and the relationship between school and home are shown. The film makes the plea that there are problem children because there are problem homes, schools, and communities. Ohio State Mental Hygiene Service. *NYU.*

A Chance to Live. (19 min.) March of Time. *NYU.*

Hard Brought Up. (40 min.) When a child is caught in an act of delinquency and brought into court, a wise judge looks behind the act itself and tries to handle the case in the way that offers the best chance for rehabilitation. To help him, he may use the services of the local public welfare agency. This film deals with the story of two young boys who get into trouble and shows how they are helped by the child welfare worker assigned to their case. As the camera follows this worker through her activities on behalf of the court, the boys, their parents, and the community, the entire organization and facilities of child welfare services are revealed. All the characters are portrayed by citizens of Jackson, Mississippi. *NYU.*

Children on Trial. (52 min.) A study of delinquency and its treatment in the British approved schools. The story is concerned with a boy, Fred, and a girl, Shirley, and the conditions that led to their being placed by the courts in schools where a rehabilitation program had been established. Activities of the program are shown, including vocational training, classroom instruction, work on the farm, etc. The dramatic treatment of the story is enhanced by excellent photography and a high quality of acting on the part of the central character. *NYU.*

Angry Boy. (33 min.) The problem of hidden hostility in a child that is expressed finally in terms of stealing. Through the help of a child guidance clinic this hostility is traced back to the source in the home life of the child where a good and well-intentioned mother has been taking out her hostility toward her mother and her husband in an overprotective attitude toward the child. The film then develops dramatically as it describes the process in which the child is helped by guidance personnel. But no techniques are used that might not be available to any understanding parents. *NYU.*

The Aggressive Child. (28 min.) Documents the case of an intelligent six year-old who fights constantly; through counseling we learn that this behavior actually masks deep seated fears. He receives play therapy from a psychiatrist, who also counsels his parents. After seven months' treatment he expresses his feelings more directly, and the parents are more skilled in handling him. *NYU.*

Boy With a Knife. (15 min.) Laslo Benedektor, Los Angeles. Community Chest, 1955. *CDMH.*

The High Wall. (32 min.) An outbreak on the South Side between teen-age gangs lands two boys, Tom Gregory and Peter Zenwicz, in the hospital. Psychiatrist Dr. Nordhoff (Irving Pichel), with the aid of a social caseworker, reconstructs the background facts. Anti-Defamation League. *NYU.*

The Quiet One. (67 min.) Film Documents, Inc., 1948. *CDMH, PCR, NYU.*

Psychopath. (30 min.) Case history of an anti-social personality, a psychopath, whose criminal tendencies constituted a threat to the community. H.B. Durost and H.E. Lehmann, Verdun Protestant Hospital, 1961. *PCR-2121.*

Borderline. (30 min.) Midnight consultation of teen-ager and psychologist in home for delinquent girls is followed by flashbacks revealing development of inmate's problems. Mother in her first visit is led to realize that her behavior may have contributed to daughter's problem. McGraw-Hill Text Films, 1957. *PCR-136.73-8.*

Alcoholism. (22 min.) Encyclopedia Britannica Films, 1952. *CDMH, NYU.*

Hide and Seek. (14 min.) A dramatic and hard-hitting film on drug addiction that portrays the anguish and despair of a teen-ager who has been caught by the habit and can't shake it. Shows how he relives his initiation to drugs, and the subsequent alienation from family and friends, his helplessness in relation to the drug, the desperate realization of the life he has unwittingly committed himself to. The events depicted are actual experiences, and the dialogue was written and narrated by an addict. *NYU.*

Monkey on the Back. (30 min.) National Film Board of Canada, 1956. *PCR-616.86-6.*

Speedscene: The Problem of Amphetamine Abuse. (17 min.) Richard S. Scott, 1970. *Bailey Film Associates,* 11559 Santa Monica Boulevard, Los Angeles, California   90025.

Bruce. (26 min.) This film provides a portrait of a 13 year-old boy at Camp Wediko who lacks control of his impulses. He is seen in a variety of situations during the summer. His behavior includes fighting, threats of running away, and talking to individual counselors. *CMC*.

Girl in Danger. (28 min.) Documents the case of a pre-delinquent girl of 13 who behaves emotionally as a six year-old. In a psychiatric hospital she undergoes individual counseling, group therapy, and takes special classes; her parents also receive counseling. After six months' treatment she appears capable of handling her problems with more maturity and control. *NYU*.

Randy. (27 min.) Portrays an 11 year-old boy, more seriously disturbed than most of those at Camp Wediko. Randy's beguiling but inconsistent behavior makes his care difficult. *CMC*.

The Cry for Help. (33 min.) A training film for police officers and law enforcement agencies designed to develop a feeling of concern and understanding in handling the suicidal person. Presents some of the major causes of suicide and the early manifestations of such behavior. *NYU*.

The Law: How Effective Is It? (36 min.) Tom Burrows, for KCET-TV. *NET Film Service,* Indiana University, Bloomington, Indiana 47401.

Troubled Campers. (18 min.) Montage of footage of disturbed children attending Camp Wediko. Underlines some of the dimensions of emotional handicaps and encourages discussion about prevention, treatment, rehabilitation, and education. Professional audiences. 1971. *W*.

Johnny. (32 min.) A nine year-old boy with a history of aggressive behavior attempts to gain more control of his feelings and better ways to communicate. He tests staff with hyperactive and erratic behavior. Several of his frequent tantrums are faithfully reported on film and illustrate problems in the management of this type of disturbance. Professional audiences. *W*.

Facing Up To Vandalism. (16 min.) Three groups of junior high schoolers, **inner** city, suburbia and rural discuss their personal involvement in vandalism. We learn about the "fun and games" attitude, revenge, relief of boredom. The film is designed to stimulate classroom discussion. It is now known that such self-examination among peers immediately lessens vandalism appreciably and sharply curtails destructive behavior in many young people. Weisenborn. *PE*.

PSYCHOSES IN CHILDHOOD

The Natural History of Psychotic Illness in Childhood. (19 min.) Describes the evolution of a psychotic child from infancy to adolescence. The change from normal to abnormal is shown by photographic material made available by the father of the child. The "behavior day" of a psychotic child is fully documented. Institute of Psychiatry, London. *NYU.*

Diagnosis of Childhood Schizophrenia. (35 min.) Traces the step-by-step procedure of screening clinical data in order to establish the diagnosis of childhood schizophrenia. This process involves a review of the pertinent historical material, psychological test finding, and clinical observations, while noting the absence of significant medical, neurological, and laboratory test results. Differential diagnosis follows to rule out clinical syndromes with which childhood schizophrenia is commonly confused. The teamwork involved in the diagnostic effort is emphasized throughout. The film concludes with a therapeutic sequence which, in addition to pointing up some of the pathognomonic features that were presented, also demonstrates the clinical approach to the schizophrenic child. Brooklyn Juvenile Guidance Center. *NYU.*

Development of an Infantile Psychosis. (18 min.) Activities of a psychotic child in nursery school setting with scenes from his earlier childhood selected from family home movies. University of Washington, 1963. *PCR-20095.*

Maternal Deprivation in Young Children. (30 min.) Forms part of a collection of studies on deprivation of maternal care, subsidized by the Centre International de l'Enfance. This film is part of the record collected by a French research unit studying the effects of maternal deprivation in young children. The children studied are between one and two-and-a-half years old. All had been reared in institutions that had not provided for a stable and intimate relationship with one person. All had been displaced several times from institution to institution, sometimes from birth. Most of these children had reached a point where, because of their experiences of impersonal care they were seriously impaired in the capacity for human relationship. *NYU.*

Food and Maternal Deprivation. (20 min.) This is part of the record collected by the French research unit studying the effects of maternal deprivation on child development. The children studied are between ten months and four years old. They have lived in institutions since birth and have been displaced several times from one institution to another. As a consequence, all these children have experienced severe maternal deprivation. The film indicates that feeding diffi-

culties are often linked with maternal deprivation and that
the attitude of a child toward food is frequently an expression of his attitude toward adults willing to give him maternal care. Five typical attitudes are shown: namely, active
refusal, ambivalence, indiscriminate acceptance, excessive
intake, and autistic indifference. Professional audiences.
NYU.

Illustrations of Childhood Autism. (22 min.) Documents behavior
of autistic children at Stoke-Mandeville Hospital, England,
using slow and stop motion to emphasize symptoms: failure
to relate to another person, visual avoidance, inappropriate
motions, preoccupation with parts of the body or specific
objects and rhythmical movements of things or the body; makes
some visual comparisons with normal children. Also describes
symptoms of autism not documented in the film. Restricted to
appropriate professional groups. *PCR-2221.*

Clinical Aspects of Childhood Psychosis. (55 min. No S) Institute of Psychiatry, London. *NYU.*

Approach to Objects by Psychotic Children, The. (15 min. No S)
The film sets out to study the behavior of regressed psychotic children toward objects, judged from the general theoretical standpoint of Piaget. The searching, uncovering, reaching, and retrieving tendencies in these children are illustrated. The film ends with a depiction of mirror responses.
Institute of Psychiatry, London. *NYU.*

Autistic Syndrome I. (43 min.) Differences between a three year
old autistic child and her twin sister, changes in behavior
during one year's treatment. Autistic Syndrome Series, Holland. *NYU.*

Autistic Syndrome II. (42 min.) Studies episodes of increased
anxiety; exploring a pool, retreating to bed and destructive
games. Autistic Syndrome Series, Holland. *NYU.*

Autistic Syndrome III. (36 min.) The patient's activities
expand during her eighth year; she is happy and active and
development is progressing. Autistic Syndrome Series, Holland. *NYU.*

Autistic Syndrome IV. (43 min.) The child becomes preoccupied
with the therapist's clothes, receives medication and is
reunited with her sister. Autistic Syndrome Series, Holland.
NYU.

The Headbangers. (30 min.) A documentary studying a small group
of emotionally disturbed children who have injured themselves
through compulsive headbanging. In particular the film follows the progress of Jeanne, a 14 year-old who had blinded

herself in this way. Various treatment methods are combined to help Jeanne diminish her self-injury and become more tolerant of people. This is a unique study of a condition about which little is known and written. *NYU.*

A Time for Georgia. (15 min.) A film about a nursery-kindergarten for emotionally disturbed, schizophrenic, and autistic children in Nassau County, N.Y. The film focuses on one little girl, as she copes with the problems of learning and socializing. *PW.*

The Camarillo Story. (26 min.) Guild Films, 1956. *CDMH.*

The World Outside. (31 min.) A documentary which studies two autistic children and how they were prepared to function in a normal environment. Filmed at the Marianne Frostig School of Educational Therapy in Los Angeles. *SLFP.*

Shadows on the Mirror. (55 min.) Shows Step, Inc., a school in Chicago where the emotional problems of seriously disturbed children are treated. The many scenes showing teachers working with the children provide insight into the special techniques used at the school. *C.*

The Search for the Lost Self. (60 min.) A study of seriously disturbed children in an educational day care setting filmed over a 2-year period. Describes a unique methodology of personalized education tailored to the organic needs of the individual. *MLF Productions,* 267 W. 25th Street, New York, N.Y. 10001.

The Psychotic Child. (25 min.) Psychiatric examiner, through series of maneuvers, tries to engage Sidney, a 7 year-old boy, in variety of relationships. He actively resists by autistic defenses and ritualistic, compulsive behavior. Motor skills development is 2-3 year level, affective control is poor, reality testing is minimal. The examination includes a rather stressful situation, which elicits responses of rebellion and frustration as well as evidences of autistic behavior. Pennsylvania State University, 1967. *PCR-2172.*

Out of True. (41 min.) The story of a typical case of mental illness followed through to its conclusion, centers around Molly Slade who lives with her husband, two children, and mother-in-law, which finally takes expression in a suicide attempt. In the mental hospital Molly is given expert and sympathetic psychiatric treatment. Her doctor contrives by skillful questioning to establish the reason for her breakdown, which is seen as a subconscious association between her mother-in-law's presence in the home and Molly's memories of a childhood made unhappy by an overpowering mother. Final sequences show the complete restoration of her mental health and her confident return to her family. *NYU*.

Out of Darkness. (55 min.) This compelling and sensitive report on one woman's step-by-step recovery from mental illness was produced by CBS Public Affairs. It tells the story of a young woman, mute and withdrawn, who is admitted by California's Metropolitan State Hospital. For 2-1/2 months a concealed camera recorded her psychiatric sessions with Dr. Louis Cholden in his slow struggle to make contact with her. Finally, in a dramatic moment, her indifference fades, she smiles for the first time, and speaks the first word. *NYU*.

Child Behind the Wall. (35 min.) Smith Kline & French, 1956. *CDMH*.

Fragile Egos. (35 min.) Henry Morgenthau and WGBH for Social and Rehabilitation Service, Department of HEW, 1968. Vocational Rehabilitation Agency of each state or *Mr. Morgenthau, WGBH*, 125 Western Avenue, Boston, Mass. 02134.

Children in Search of a Self. (21 min.) Autistic children who are in treatment are shown. A variety of symptom patterns are discussed with an emphasis on the difficulties of these children in their relationships with other people. There is a good presentation of symptoms, but etiological and dynamic factors must be presented by the instructor who may use the film. *PCR-2115*.

Folie a Deaux. *Mental Symptoms Series*. (15 min.) A demonstration of symptoms in one of the less common forms of mental disease, folie a deaux, or induced insanity. Two patients, mother and daughter, are presented. The psychosis developed first in the daughter and was then communicated to the mother, who is very dependent upon and has a close emotional attachment to her child. The daughter expresses a number of grandiose delusions and delusions of persecution, which ideas the mother accepts as reality. *NYU*.

Breakdown. (40 min.) Ann, 23 years old, has always been a model daughter. From a quiet, clever, obedient child she has grown into a charming and responsible young woman, holding a good job in the office of a family friend. It is in the seemingly unexplainable deterioration in her work that we first see evidence of Ann's breakdown. Her employer is puzzled and seeks the advice of her family. At home Ann remains away from meals, sulks in her room, refuses to see her friends and is suspicious of all the food prepared in the house. *NYU*.

Asylum. (95 min.) Asylum is valuable as an adjunct to Dr. Laing's published writings, but also stands on its own as a penetrating and powerful document of human behavior. *Peter Robinson*, Suite 803, 43 West 16th Street, New York, N.Y. 10011.

Dehumanization and the Total Institution. (15 min.) Humorous animation shows how staff members, especially in mental institutions, can become so impersonal in their relations with patients as to be "dehumanizing". De, the chief cartoon character to whom the points are made, seems to be modeled after a bumbling detective in a television series. *NYU.*

Behavior Therapy With an Autistic Child. (42 min.) Demonstrates the systematic application of reinforcement in the form of candy for responsive behaviors by a 5-year-old autistic child. After an initial period in which the therapist responded warmly, but not contingently, the therapist would reward the child with candy for obeying his requests and for such desirable behavior as smiling or verbalizing. Although the entire action takes place within one session, there are noticeable behavior changes. An introduction and final summary statement bring the demonstration within the framework of current work in behavior therapy. L. Krasner and G. C. Davison, 1965. *NMA.*

Boy in the Doorway. (28 min.) Presents a withdrawn boy who comes to Bellefaire, a residential psychiatric treatment center for children. Focuses on the relationships, especially with his father, that are at the root of the boy's disturbance, and on the casework methods that are used at Bellefaire to help him. The total program of the center is quite clearly indicated. Film would be useful for professional people working with disturbed children, and for parent-teacher groups, with an experienced leader, trained in mental health. Cinecraft Productions, 1956. *B.*

Child Draw Nearer. (20 min.) Depicts advances made at a special school for teaching autistic children and shows how, in response to patient instruction, they begin to use language in a normal way. Bristol Films for Society for Autistic Children, 1965. *CFC.*

The Child with Severe Emotional Problems. (44 min.) Discusses differences between child and adult emotional problems, manifestations of symptoms at various ages, and role of psychiatric nurse and other staff members in caring for disturbed child. Discussion of nurse's role in prevention. Video Nursing, 1967. *VN.*

Childhood Schizophrenia. (42 min.) Presents different types of schizophrenia in a classroom setting, including numerous cases of infantile autism and symbiotic psychoses. Shows

patients in the nursery school classroom during recreational
therapy and while undergoing group occupational therapy.
Depicts the interpretive and interpersonal relationships of
the personnel and the patient, demonstrates how personnel
are challenged to develop new skills and means of breaking
barriers, and evaluates various forms of therapy. Sandoz
Pharmaceuticals. *SP.*

The Emotionally Disturbed Child. (55 min.) Defines types of
emotionally disturbed children, observes children in treatment, and comments on the use of behavior modification in
treatment programs. Robert Leff, Ph.D., Children's Treatment Center, Madison, Wis., 1969. *UW.*

Free Expression Painting in Child Psychiatry. (18 min.) Contrasts the normal child's painting with that of the mentally
disturbed child. Geigy Pharmaceuticals, 1966. *GP.*

The Mentally Ill: Treatment of Children. (29 min.) Story of
emotionally disturbed boy and his rehabilitation. Portrays
home situation which precipitated the boy's illness, his
reaction to it, and his antagonism toward the work which
leads him into juvenile delinquency. Shows how his commitment takes place, treatment he receives, eventual readjust-
ment and return home. Briefly describes prevalence and
causes of mental illness in children, and the prospect for
their rehabilitation. WCET-TV, 1960. *IU.*

Someday I'll Happy Be. (28 min.) Follows the progress of an
emotionally disturbed teenaged boy who is admitted to Bellefaire. Focuses on the work of treatment team, psychiatrist,
psychologist, caseworkers, special education teachers and
childcare workers. Fox Video Productions, 1967. *B.*

Warrendale. (100 min.) Describes Warrendale, a center for
emotionally disturbed children, and the treatment methods
used there. The children live in a family atmosphere and are
encouraged to express all of their feelings, even their most
violent and destructive ones. Allan King Associates for
Canadian Broadcasting Corp., 1967. *EFVA.*

Why They Can't Stay Home. (23 min.) Shows severe antisocial
behavior in emotionally disturbed children who required care
in a residential treatment center. *FF.*

MENTAL RETARDATION AND OTHER HANDICAPS

One in Every Hundred. (58 min.) Mental Retardation in community
mental health center (in two parts). *NET Film Services,*
Indiana University Audio-Visual Center, Bloomington, Indiana
47401.

Clinical Types of Mental Deficiency. (39 min. No S) *PCR.*

Feebleminded. (41 min.) N. O. Pearce, 1942. *PCR.*

Exceptional Children. (26 min.) Guild Films, 1956. *CDMH.*

Eternal Children. (30 min.) Presents an intimate study of the special problems of retarded children. Children who through heredity, brain injury, or various other causes are not equipped to keep pace in a competitive world--are they to be society's unwitting castaways? Gives a frank appraisal of the problem and shows care and training methods being evolved in special schools and institutions across Canada. *NYU.*

The Long Childhood of Timmy. (53 min.) A sensitive portrayal of a mentally retarded child making the transition from an optimal family setting to a residential training school. Timmy is a nine year-old mongoloid, the youngest of six children of a middle-income family. His parents are realistic about the limits of Timmy's educability, recognizing that they have done as much as circumstances permit in laying a foundation for more formal education which only a school can give. Upon his arrival at school, he is received by the superintendent who sympathetically and skillfully eases the pain of family separation. Timmy is shown undergoing ability testing and speech therapy, 2 aspects of a program designed to help him maximize his basic potential. ABC-TV. *NYU.*

In Need of Special Care. (35 min.) Made at a boarding school for 200 mentally handicapped and emotionally disturbed children in Aberdeen, Scotland. The children are helped to come to terms with their handicaps in order to lead comparatively full and useful lives as adults. *TLF.*

Care of the Young Retarded Child. (18 min.) Shows how the progress of the normal child is instructive in caring for the young retarded child. Stresses the importance of good child care and management and the value of early assessment of the infant to insure a proper feeding and training program. International Film Bureau, 1965. *PCR-20536.*

No Less Precious. (14 min.) National Association for Retarded Children, 1956. *CDMH.*

Somebody Waiting. (24 min.) What helps the mentally retarded? Hal Riney and Dick Snider, 1971. *Extension Media Center, University of California,* Berkeley, California   94720.

Tuesday's Child. (14 min.) National Film Board, 1955. *CDMH.*

Michael: A Mongoloid Child. (14 min.) Provides an intimate
study of a mongoloid teenager living on a farm in rural
England. Michael is a boy brimming with affection, playfulness, and captivating charm. He leads an ordinary family
life and, although he lives in a more limited way than the
normal fifteen-year-old, he appears to be happy. He has a
social life, makes friends of his own, and goes off and
visits them by himself. Michael's family and neighbors have
come to accept him on his own terms, recognizing that although his limitations prevent him from having the worries
of most youths of his age, neither does he have their pleas-
ures. British Film Institute. *NYU.*

Danny and Nicky. (56 min.) A comparison of the care and training of two mentally retarded mongoloid boys, one living at
home with brothers and sisters and attending a special neighborhood school and the other in a large institution for the
retarded. *NFBC.*

Show Me. (28 min.) Designed to promote the teaching of movement and rhythms to the mentally retarded and to convey the
need for these activities. Children enrolled in the Wood
County Retarded School (Ohio) are shown participating in
activities that stimulate exploration of the parts of the
body and attack coordination problems. The activities are
presented with no verbalization except "Show me". The passive, depressed child responds to this simple approach as
does the uninhibited, overexcited and anxious child. Universal. *NYU.*

Comprehensive Treatment in Mental Retardation. (34 min.) Smith
Kline & French. *SKF.*

In Touch: Movement for Mentally Handicapped Children. (25 min.)
In the first part of this film made by staff and students
from the National Association for Mental Health's Teacher
Training Course at Bristol, England, student-teachers explore
many ways in which movement can aid contact with children.
They also explore more sensitive, expressive, and dramatic
ways of relating to others. Later we see how students develop an awareness of themselves by discovering parts of their
bodies. Finally, each student works with a child partner.
NYU.

Aids for Teaching the Mentally Retarded. (39 min.) Series of
five films, available separately or combined on one reel.
NYU.

*Advanced Perceptual Training. Aids for Teaching the Mentally
Retarded Series.* (9 min.) Experiences are provided in the
third phase of this film series that aid the student in
making decisions and drawing conclusions. The child learns

to manipulate devices such as the slot box and electric
maze which are adjusted to his level of dexterity and can
be altered to challenge his increasing skill. *NYU.*

The Brain Damaged Child. (31 min.) Records interview between
psychiatrist and Bobby, a seven year-old boy with organic
brain damage. Through play with clay figures and discussion
shows such behavior phenomena as hyperactivity, poor motor
coordination, dependency relationship with mother, heightened
sibling rivalries and resentments, and resistance to pressure
to perform beyond capability. Brings out lack of ego defenses and uninhibited relatedness to interviewer. The
stress situation of the interview produces some overt responses which illustrate the above behavior more clearly.
Pennsylvania State University, 1968. *PCR-2173.*

The Growth and Development of a Multiply Handicapped Infant.
(10 min.) This is a longitudinal record of a profoundly
retarded blind infant's first three and one-half years of
life. Clinical examinations during the first year of life
are juxtaposed with a typical day at home at 22 months of
age. The family's decision to institutionalize the child is
shown, as is a visit from his mother when he is 42 months
old and a resident of the State School for the Retarded.
NYU.

Nursery School for the Blind. (20 min.) Home life is as important for the blind as for the normal child, but the problems
of the blind child are usually greater than parents can cope
with unaided. For this reason blind children are often sent
away from home into residential nurseries. The nursery
school shown in this film enables young blind children to
stay at home by supplementing the care given by their par-
ents--by helping to make up for stages of development which
have been missed, by encouraging curiosity, and by keeping
up a continual verbal communication in order to facilitate
orientation and make up for missing visual contact. *NYU.*

Thursday's Children. (19 min.) The old nursery rhyme says,
"Thursday's child has far to go." The children of this
film are deaf--some were born so. They cannot learn to
speak as others do because they have never heard a word
spoken. "Without words, there can be no thoughts, only
feelings with nothing to join them together." This film is
the story of how a group of these children from four to
seven are led out of their world of silence by the devotion
and skill of their teachers. Academy Award winner for the
best documentary short subject, 1954. *NYU.*

Julia. (10 min.) Working with a child handicapped by hearing
impairment. *NYU.*

Stress: Parents with a Handicapped Child. (30 min.) Depicts the impact which a child with à physical or mental disability has on a variety of families from different socio-economic backgrounds. We are afforded intimate glimpses into six households in Britain, with children in such conditions as mental retardation, schizophrenia, cerebral palsy, epilepsy, and muscular dystrophy. Particular causes of stress are examined as they affect any family with a handicapped child: the emotional strain on family life, the lack of adequate welfare and medical services, and the severe financial burden. *NYU.*

Like Other People. (37 min.) Deals with sexual, emotional and social needs of the mentally or physically handicapped. Two main characters, cerebral palsy patients, using their own words make a plea to humanity for the understanding that they are "real" people. At one point this is a poignant love story which will help us to understand that physically handicapped people share our emotions. Because their speech may be affected, cerebral palsy patients sometimes have a hard time communicating. There is a tendency to switch off the film, because it is sometimes difficult to understand. This fact reflects the attitude of society--only then it is people we are switching off and not a film. This film raises intense questions about the quality of life, about privacy, and about understanding "other people". (Didactic.) *PE.*

DIAGNOSIS AND PSYCHOTHERAPY

Psychogenic Diseases in Infancy: An Attempt at Their Classification. Film Studies of the Psychoanalytic Research Project on Problems in Infancy Series. (20 min. No S) In infants during the first year of life a series of clinical pictures can be distinguished, in the etiology of which psychological factors appear to be involved. This film illustrates a series of psychogenic diseases and attempts to relate the clinical picture with one of the etiological factors, namely, the infants' relationship with their mothers. The clinical pictures accordingly are divided into two categories: (1) those diseases in which the wrong kind of mother-child relation act, as it were, as a psychic toxin; these are called psychotoxic diseases; (2) those diseases in which the lack of sufficient mother-child relations result in a deficiency of emotional supplies for the infant;these are called emotional deficiency diseases. In the first part of the film examples of seven psychotoxic diseases are shown and, wherever possible, the corresponding maternal attitudes are presented or described. The diseases are: vomiting during the first months of life, coma in the newborn, three months' colic, atopic dermatitis, hypermotility, fecal play, aggressive hyperthymia. In the second part of the film the emotional deficiency diseases are illustrated by a number of cases. They are divided into (1) partial emotional deprivation (anaclitic depression) and (2) complete emotional depriva- tion (marasmus). The conclusion is drawn that the etiologi- cal factors underlying this classification are the quality of the mother-child relation in the psychotoxic diseases and the quantity of mother-child relations in the groups. *NYU.*

Psychological Hazards in Infancy. (22 min.) In group care and at home, the vital experiences and learning of infancy may be hampered by inadequate stimulation, insufficient warm attention from adults, or inappropriate handling which is not geared to changing developmental needs. The film shows both mild and severe psychological damage and suggests means of prevention. Vassar College for Project Head Start. *NYU.*

Grief: A Peril in Infancy. (23 min. No S) Describes the despondency which overwhelms a young infant when the mother is absent for at least three months. Comparisons in infant's behavior before and after the absence of mother indicates negative changes which may have permanent effect if mother fails to return. Close look at infants in an institution since birth and their slower development compared to an in- fant who had constant attention of a real mother. *PCR-20803.*

Fears of Children. (30 min.) A film about Paul, a normal five year-old and his well-intentioned parents. In a series of episodes it shows how Paul's fears--of the dark, of being alone, of new situations--are related to his feelings about his parents. The film points out that Paul's feelings are common to children of his age and may be accentuated when parents become either unduly protective or overly severe. *NYU.*

Facing Reality. Psychology for Living Series. (12 min.) A shadow screen is used to illustrate and explain some common defense mechanisms--rationalization projection, negativism-- and some typical escape mechanisms. Daydreaming, identifi- cation, suppression, and malingering are some common ways in which people try to escape from their duties, identities, and families. The major part of the film is taken up by the case-study of Mike Squires, a basically attractive boy, who has developed a strong negativist attitude. Mike has allowed his small failures, real or imagined to bother him until they have affected all his social contacts. *NYU.*

Overdependency. Mental Mechanisms Series. (32 min.) The film describes the case of Jimmy, an attractive young man, whose life is crippled by behavior patterns carried over from a too-dependent childhood. When the film opens, Jimmy is sick, but we learn that his illness has no physical cause. He finds it difficult to face and deal with the ordinary prob-

lems of life and takes frequent refuge in being comforted by
his wife and mother. In his conferences with a doctor,
Jimmy gradually retraces the patterns of his childhood,
begins to understand the emotional causes of his illness and
his own fear, and takes hold of life with new confidence.
NYU.

Rock-A-Bye Baby: A Group Projective Test for Children. (35 min.)
A filmed puppet show designed to elicit projective responses
of children from five to ten years of age. Taps areas of
sibling rivalry, aggressions, fears, guilt feelings, and
attitudes toward parents. Suggested uses: personality
research and diagnostic screening in schools and psychology
clinics. Designed for use with groups. Special manual
includes directions for administering the film and scoring
the protocols. Showing restricted to appropriate professional groups. M.R. Haworth and A.G. Woltmann. *PCR-2094.*

*Psychological Implications of Behavior During the Clinical Visit.
Film Studies on Integrated Development Series.* (20 min. No S)
Important clues to a child's emotional attitudes as seen from
its overt behavior during the clinic at the New York Infir-
mary for Women and Children. These clues are not intended to
offer a sequential case study of any one child or group of
children. The observer, however, will note many significant
differences in attitudes from contrasting behavior of
several children, while awaiting examination, during physical
and dental examinations, IQ tests, and at play. Distribution
limited to professional groups. *NYU.*

*An Exercise in the Differential Diagnosis of Psychiatric Syn-
dromes of Childhood.* (25 min.) A composite of excerpts from
four previously published films: The Normal Child, The
Neurotic Child, The Psychotic Child, The Brain Damaged Child.
Presents comparative data by which differences and similarities among four psychiatric syndromes seen in childhood can
be shown. It has been left relatively free of commentary to
permit most flexible use when it can be stopped between each
series of excerpts for discussion. Pennsylvania State University, 1970. *PCR-2229.*

Understanding Children's Drawings. (10 min.) Describes and
interprets the drawings of children from three to five years
old. Drawing for the three-year-old is a natural language,
a part of play, and at this time requires no teaching on the
part of teachers but only the use of materials. There is
rhythm and movement. The four-year-old is beginning to
organize lines into design, is more controlled. From now on
the drawings are more representative, and the child is trans-
lating his inner impressions freely. The film suggests that
he should not be urged to copy standard forms because his
ability springs from the freshness of his impressions, his

imaginative use of color, etc. *NYU*.

Looking For Me. (29 min.) Dance therapist Janet Adler narrates this filmed report on an unusual research project in which she investigated the therapeutic benefits of patterned movement in working with four types of pupils: Normal preschool children at the ages of four and five, emotionally disturbed children, two autistic children aged two and five, and a group of adult teachers. *NYU*.

Role Playing in Guidance. (14 min.) U.C.L.A., 1952. *CSDPH*.

Activity Group Therapy. (50 min.) Columbia University, 1950. *PCR*.

Psychotherapeutic Interviewing: Introduction. (11 min.) U.S. Veterans Administration. J.E. Finesinger & F. Powdermacher, 1949. *CSDPH, PCR*.

Psychotherapeutic Interviewing: A Method of Procedure. (31 min.) Ibid. *CSDPH, PCR*.

Psychotherapeutic Interviewing. Part 4. Non-Verbal Communication. (27 min.) U.S. Veterans Administration. *PCR*.

A Song for Michael. (22 min.) Despite ten years of treatment, fourteen year-old Michael had no spontaneous speech and had not developed concepts. His psychiatrist referred Michael to the center in the hope that his life-long attraction to music might provide a pathway to communication. Demonstrates how music is used as a functional tool to promote emotional and social growth as an adjunct to psychotherapy. Music Therapy Center, Creative Arts Rehabilitation Center, Inc., New York, 1966. *PCR-31228*.

This Year, Next Year, Sometime. (20 min.) Shows a modern alternative to placing children in a resident mental hospital. Children are placed in a day treatment center where they stay part time. Also includes an interview with Dr. Roth, a well-known psychiatrist who discusses the use of day treatment facilities for the mentally disturbed. Marlborough Day Hospital, London. *NYU*.

Beach Interview. (27 min.) Two boys at Wediko become upset and demand to leave camp. They discuss their problem with the head counselor who becomes the focus for their anger. In the course of this "life space interview", the boys, who are normally able to express their emotions only through action, succeed in verbalizing their resentment and discussing alternative ways of dealing with it. *CMC*.

A Problem of Acceptance. (47 min.) A condensation of a two-hour therapy session held with patients of the psychiatric ward of the University of Oregon Medical School. The theme is a psychodramatic exploration of a 17-year-old girl's attempt to deal with her problem of homosexuality as it affects herself, her family, and the psychotherapy group. *NYU.*

Boys in Conflict. (72 min.) This award winning film presents a college student's experiences as a counselor caring for 9 boys who exhibit a variety of emotional problems. It is intended to generate discussion about emotional and practical issues involved in the handling and treatment of such children. *Center for Mass Communications of Columbia University Press,* 440 West 110th Street, N.Y., N.Y. 10025.

Carol and Dr. Fischer. (45 min.) Interview between Dr. Fischer, consulting psychiatrist, and Carol, a young patient at Warrendale. A study of the process of self-awareness and ways a skillful and sensitive adult can help a child express and understand himself. During the session, conducted in the presence of staff members, Carol is led to confront her anger, sibling rivalry, disguised aggression, and early experiences of rejection and loss. This multi-level presentation is relevant in differing ways to psychiatrists, philosophers, educators, and parents. Grove Press, 1967. *PCR-50213.*

Broken Appointment. (30 min.) This is No. 1 in the Professional Education Series produced by the Mental Health Film Board. The film describes the experience of a young public health nurse, Susan Burke, who discovered that, in handling a case successfully, it was as important to understand a patient's feelings as to interpret physical symptoms. Ms. Burke is attached to a well-baby clinic and in the course of her work becomes involved with the case of Mrs. Peters, a miner's wife, who breaks an appointment at the clinic and is reluctant to come for treatment. *MHFB, NYU.*

The Deep Well. (36 min.) The work of social agencies who care for children in families where death, divorce, illness, and other factors have served to make a temporary adjustment necessary. This is the story of a small boy, Bobby, who has run away from home several times. His father is in a mental hospital; his mother works in addition to caring for Bobby and his sister, Sheila. Interviews between the mother and the social worker reveal that the mother is no longer able to care properly for the children. Bobby is sent to a school where he is helped to relate to children and adults, Sheila is placed temporarily in a foster home. The aim of the social agency is to make it possible for the family to be reunited eventually. Child Welfare League of America. *NYU.*

Aid to Families with Dependent Children. (18 min. each, 4 films) A four-part series designed specifically for training social workers in techniques of interviewing. Each of two interview studies contains two versions--a less effective and a more effective one--providing an object demonstration of the voices of client and worker. Shows how the interviewer's skills and attitudes affect the client and determine the success of the interview. *NYU.*

Dr. Erich Fromm, Part I. (45 min.) In an interview with Dr. Richard I. Evans, Dr. Fromm discusses productive and nonproductive character orientations in contemporary society, mechanisms of escape, and individuation. *NYU.*

Dr. Erich Fromm, Part II. (50 min.) This interview is focused on Dr. Fromm's approach to psychotherapy: theory and techniques, drug and group therapy, and plans for future work. *NYU.*

Dr. Ernest Jones. (30 min.) In an interview with Lionel Trilling, Dr. Jones discusses the last years of Freud and evaluates his contribution in the field of psychoanalysis and the effects of his work upon the areas of child study and parent-child relationships. Encyclopaedia Britannica Films, National Broadcasting Company, 1958. *PCR-921-48.*

Maslow and Self-Actualization: Part I--Honesty, Awareness. (30 min.) Dimensions of self-actualization; recent research and theory. Themes discussed are honesty and awareness. Honesty expressed in a sense of humor, social interest, and love. Awareness expressed in the efficient perception, freshness of appreciation, the peak experience, and ethical awareness. Psychological Films, 1969. *PCR-31543.*

Maslow and Self-Actualization: Part II--Freedom, Trust. (30 min.) Dimensions of self-actualization; recent research and theory. Themes discussed are freedom and trust. Freedom expressed in detachment, creativeness, and spontaneity. Trust expressed in a life mission, autonomy of culture and environment, and acceptance of human nature. Psychological Films, 1969. *PCR-31544.*

Sessions in Gestalt Therapy: Grief and Pseudo-Grief. (28 min.) Session with Frederick Perls. Two cases of what Freud termed "mourning labor" illustrated: one patient masks resentment while the other resolves the remainder of a mother fixation and achieves an increased degree of self-support and maturity. First example demonstrates utilization of humor to mobilize emotional involvement; second case illustrates therapist's need for detail in order to empty out a symptom completely. The Mediasync Corporation, 1970. *PCR-31525.*

Target Five. (48 min.) Reel 1: Virginia Satir, family therapist, in cooperation with Dr. Everett L. Shostrom, Director
of the Institute of Therapeutic Psychology, demonstrates the
four manipulative response forms. Reel 2: The three essential qualities of an actualizing relationship are presented:
hearing and listening, understanding, and mutual meaning.
Each of these is discussed in detail and demonstrated.
Psychological Films, 1967. *PCR-50212.*

The Need to Work. (24 min.) Describes successful industrial
therapy programs in two British hospitals; shows mental
patients performing a wide range of jobs. Discusses the
need for giving patient gainful work to do under conditions
which closely parallel those in industry and shows the
patients' responses to real work and adequate wages. Emphasizes that the aim of industrial therapy is to help patients
return to outside employment and normal community living.
Smith Kline and French, 1962. *SKF.*

Back Into the Sun. (30 min.) Illustrates treatment of mental
health problems at the day hospital of the Allan Memorial
Institute in Montreal, where patients not requiring full
hospitalization come for daytime treatment and return to
their homes at night. Presents case of a young matron under
severe emotional stress, pointing out how interviews with a
psychiatrist and group therapy sessions show her the root of
her trouble and set her on the path to overcoming her problem. National Film Board of Canada, 1956. *PCR.*

FAMILY DYNAMICS, SIMULTANEOUS PSYCHOTHERAPY AND FAMILY THERAPY

Trouble in the Family. (90 min.) Demonstrates the use of family
therapy to probe the root cause of a family's emotional problems and lack of communication. *NYU.*

The Things I Cannot Change. (55 min.) A look at a family in
trouble, seen from the inside. There is trouble with the
police, the begging for stale bread at the convent, the
birth of another child, and the father who explains his
family's predicament. This is the anatomy of poverty as
seen by a camera that became part of the family life for
several weeks. *NFBC.*

The Summer We Moved to Elm Street. (28 min.) Family stress
and alcoholism effects on the child. McGraw-Hill Films,
1967. *NFBC.*

*The Hillcrest Family: Studies in Human Communication; Assess-
ment Series: Assessment Interview 1.* (32 min.) This series
consists of four separate interviews of the Hillcrest family
by four psychiatrists. Each psychiatrist then discusses his

views on the dynamics of the family situation with a therapist who has been working with the family. The Hillcrest
family comprises a husband, wife and four children. Husband
and wife have been married previously, some of the children
are from the two former marriages, and one is from the present marriage. The family has sought psychiatric help because
of problems with the children. Interviewer: Nathan W.
Ackerman, M.D., Eastern Pennsylvania Psychiatric Institute,
Pennsylvania University, 1968. Showings restricted to appropriate professional groups. *PCR-2191K*.

*The Hillcrest Family: Studies in Human Communication; Assess-
ment Series: Assessment Interview 2*. (31 min.) Ibid.
Interviewer: Carl A. Whitaker, M. D., Eastern Pennsylvania
Psychiatric Institute, Pennsylvania State University, 1968.
Showings restricted to appropriate professional groups.
PCR-2189K.

*The Hillcrest Family: Studies in Human Communication; Assess-
ment Series: Assessment Interview 3*. (32 min.) Ibid.
Interviewer: Don Jackson, M. D., Eastern Pennsylvania
Psychiatric Institute, Pennsylvania State University, 1968.
Showing restricted to professional groups. *PCR-2193K*.

*The Hillcrest Family: Studies in Human Communication; Assess-
ment Series: Assessment Interview 4*. (29 min.) Interviewer: Murray Bowen, M.D., Eastern Pennsylvania Psychiatric
Institute, Pennsylvania State University, 1968. Showing
restricted to appropriate professional groups. *PCR-2195K*.

Total Family Treatment. (45 min.) Discusses family involvement
in the treatment problem. Points out the contribution of
cottage personnel, activity therapist, and social worker in
treatment. M. B. Fliegel, M.D., Children's Treatment Center,
Madison, Wisconsin, 1969. *UW*.

GROUP PSYCHOTHERAPY

Children of Synanon. (16 min.) About the Synanon School in
California which includes participation by the children in
encounter sessions using the "Synanon Game". Part was shot
by the children themselves. *SLFP*.

Broad Spectrum Behavior Therapy in a Group. (29 min.) Highlights some of the active behavioral methods which Dr. Arnold
Lazarus has applied to groups. Underscores the common
ground and points of departure between conventional group
psychotherapy and Lazarus' brand of group behavior therapy.
Four principle sequences depict Lazarus and his co-therapist,
Lawrence Kaiden, dealing with hostility in the group; employ-
ing behavioral rehearsal and modeling techniques; applying

group desensitization; and using assertive training to re-
place aggressive behavior. Overall framework is the broad
base of specific interpersonal skills and other social behaviors, rather than the stimulus-response models which have
become associated with "behavior therapy". Shows how application of certain behavioral procedures can enhance processes of group therapy. Eastern Pennsylvania Psychiatric
Institute, 1969. Showing restricted. *PCR-2187.*

The Actualization Group--Self-disclosure of the Therapist.
(39 min.) Originally presented on KHJ-TV in Los Angeles by
E. L. Shostrom, Ph.D., and Nancy W. Ferry, M.S.W. An au-
thentic, unrehearsed therapy or sensitivity group which
points up personality problems of some of its members. The
themes are (1) The Calculator: A Poker Player with Life,
(2) The Calculator and the Clinging Vine, (3) Self-disclosure of the Therapist, (4) A Magic Moment: A Peak Experience.
This is the sixth film in a series of seven. Psychological
Films, 1966. *PCR-40132.*

Autism's Lonely Children. (20 min.) Work with autistic children
being conducted by Dr. Frank Hewett of the Neuropsychiatric
School at UCLA. With a device called the "learning box",
Dr. Hewett is shown attempting to teach individual children
to talk and to identify objects for the first time. Hewett
concludes with a tentative statement about the possible effectiveness of his approach with other autistic children.
National Educational Television: Neuropsychiatric School
at UCLA, 1967. *PCR-31440.*

BEHAVIOR MODIFICATION

Controlling Behavior Through Reinforcement. (16 min.) McGraw-
Hill. *NYU.*

Reinforcement in Learning and Extinction. (8 min.) McGraw-
Hill. *NYU.*

Learning Discriminations and Skills. (19 min.) McGraw-Hill.
NYU.

Reinforcement Therapy. (45 min.) Experimental programs applying learning theory to treatment of mentally and emotionally
disturbed children and adults. *NYU.*

COMMUNITY MENTAL HEALTH

Nation's Mental Health. (18 min.) National Association Mental
Health. *PCR.*

Community Mental Health. (31 min.) Mental Health Film Board. *CDMH, NYU.*

The Bold New Approach. (62 min.) Photographed in ten locations in the United States and abroad, this film shows the multiple services that can be provided for troubled people of all ages by a comprehensive community mental health center. Stresses the continuity of care and relationships of various professions to each other. *MHFB, NYU.*

With No One to Help Us. (22 min.) Community psychology. *Modern Talking Picture Service, Inc.,* 1212 Avenue of the Americas, New York, New York 10036.

One Day a Week. (33 min.) Illustrates the actual experiences of a community psychiatrist on his visit to the Rodman Job Corps Center in New Bedford, Massachusetts, where he offers mental health consultation to the staff of the center. This film portrays one style of consultation and is intended to stimulate discussion by mental health personnel about roles and the training for them in the field of community psychiatry. *CMC, NYU.*

Storefront. (49 min.) The Neighborhood Service Center storefronts are a vital component of a community mental health program serving thousands of people in the ghettos of the South Bronx in New York City. To these centers people bring such problems as housing, family and community crises, delayed or marital problems, addiction, unemployment. The staff consists of indigenous nonprofessional workers who listen with the understanding of someone who has been there himself. This film describes their selection, training, and development into community mental health workers on the staff of a new Neighborhood Service Center. Lincoln Hospital Mental Health Service. *NYU.*

Mental Health Year. (49 min.) This visual survey of mental health over the world shows psychiatric treatment and facilities in 22 countries and emphasizes the contrast between modern therapeutic procedures and the restraint and confinement of the recent past. In reviewing new techniques in hospital operations, the film takes us to Japan, to France, to Iran--even to Equatorial Africa. Open hospitals, aftercare clinics, preventive and educational services are shown. Sequences describe a 24-hour emergency psychiatric service provided by the Amsterdam Department of Health; day-and-night psychiatric services at the Montreal General Hospital; child psychiatry in Israel; workshops in Australia; patients performing a classical Greek drama in Athens; group therapy in Japan; public education about mental health in the Philippines, Greece and Africa; the psychiatric department in a small town general hospital in the United States. *MHFB, NYU.*

Chain of Care. (38 min.) Shows actual patients in the various institutions that make up a coordinated statewide program of prevention, treatment, aftercare, and rehabilitation. The camera reveals the physical facilities, the professional skills, and the human understanding that are brought to bear at all stages of mental illness. Shown are the mental health clinic, the psychiatric service in the general hospital, the modern mental health hospital, and the aftercare center. *MHFB, NYU.*

Role of the Neighborhood Worker. Neighborhood Worker Training Series. (20 min.) The nature of the neighborhood worker's job and his key role in community programs. *NYU.*

A Family Affair. (33 min.) Family Service Association of America. *CDMH, CSDPH, NYU.*

Head of the House. (37 min.) World Federation of Mental Health. *CDMH, CSDPH, PCR.*

Resident Participation. Neighborhood Worker Training Series. (20 min.) Demonstrates the need for and results of effective resident participation. *NYU.*

Knowing Your Neighborhood. Neighborhood Worker Training Series. (20 min.) How the worker acquires knowledge of a neighborhood, its people and their problems. *NYU.*

The Secret Love of Sandra Blain. (28 min.) 1972 NCFR award-winning film shows, step by step, the progression into alcoholism of a wife and mother. We see how she, in her unrecognized illness, deceives her friends, her family, her physician and herself. The extent of the problem is indicated by recent statistics which reveal that half the nine million alcoholics in the U.S. are women! In its positive approach to the problem, the film focuses attention on the facilities and treatments available for the successful treatment and recovery of victims of the disease of alcoholism. Don Hoster. *PE.*

A Community Mental Health Center--The New Way. (10 min.) Stresses the need for community mental health centers. Demonstrates how these centers tie together mental health services such as emergency care, inpatient and outpatient care, partial hospitalization, consultation, and education. National Institute of Mental Health, 1966. *NMA.*

STAFF INTERACTION

Interstaff Communications. (42 min.) A condensation of a two-hour, spontaneous workshop session that demonstrates the use of psychodramatic technique to facilitate interstaff communications. The theme concerns the working through of a work-centered relationship problem between the psychiatrist in charge of a psychiatric unit at the University of Oregon Medical School and his chief resident. *NYU*.

TRAINING - RELATIONSHIP TO PATIENTS

Delayed Journey. (22 min.) Mental patients are brought from four State hospitals for a two-week summer camp. A rehabilitation therapist introduces a varied group of patients to activities ranging from spraying cobwebs to roasting marshmallows. Flashbacks show the steps the therapist took in choosing her career. Journeymen Productions, 1964. *HF*.

CLINICAL RESEARCH

California Project Talent: 4-Analysis. (29 min.) Development of scientific discovery, methodology, and investigation through a study of graphic representation of statistical information. Application of Benjamin Bloom's and others' Taxonomy of Education Objectives: Cognitive Domain to the study of mathematics. Depicts actual classroom situations. Acme Film Labs, 1967. *PCR-31203*.

California Project Talent: 5-Synthesis. (29 min.) Development of scientific discovery, methodology, and investigation through a study of graphic representation of statistical information. Application of Benjamin Bloom's and others' Taxonomy of Educational Objectives: Cognitive Domain to the study of mathematics. Depicts actual classroom situations. Acme Film Labs, 1967. *PCR-31204*.

California Project Talent: 6-Evaluation. (29 min.) Ibid. *PCR-31205*.

California Project Talent: 7-Cognition. (29 min.) Development of creative expression through a study of the literary element of characterization. Application of J. P. Guilford's "Structure of Intellect" to the development of creative expression. Depicts actual classroom situations. Acme Film Labs, 1967. *PCR-31206*.

California Project Talent: 8-Memory. (29 min.) Ibid. *PCR-31207*.

California Project Talent: 9-Convergent Thinking. (29 min.) Ibid. *PCR-31208*.

California Project Talent: 10-*Divergent Thinking.* (29 min.)
Ibid. *PCR-31209.*

California Project Talent: 11-*Evaluation.* (29 min.) Ibid.
PCR-31210.

California Project Talent: 12-*Acquisition.* (29 min.) Development of critical appreciation through a study of the fundamental forms of music. Application of Jerome Bruner's
description of the stages of learning in The Process of Education to the development of critical appreciation. Acme
Film Labs, 1967. *PCR-31211.*

California Project Talent: 13-*Transformation.* (29 min.) Ibid.
PCR-31212.

Focus on Behavior: The Chemistry *of Behavior.* (30 min.) Psychopharmacology, the study of the effect of psychoactive drugs
on behavior, as one of the newest and most promising areas
of psychology: Dr. Roger Russell shows some of the tests
being conducted to measure effect of drugs on behavior. Dr.
Sebastian Grossman demonstrates methods used to introduce
drugs in specific areas of the brain and shows their effect
upon behavior. National Educational Television, 1963.
PCR-30291.

The Brain and Behavior. Psychology Series. (22 min.) Demonstrates two ways by which we can study the function of different brain areas in human behavior. One method shown is
the artificial stimulation of different parts of the living
brain with an electrode and to observe the results. The
other method is to measure, by means of tests, the changes
in behavior following injuries in different areas of the
brain. *NYU.*

The Emotional Dilemma. (60 min.) Series: America's Crises.
Explores one of the most pressing concerns facing our nation
today--the growing number of Americans who have mental and
emotional problems and the limited facilities available to
them. Actress Vivian Vance sets the theme by describing her
own emotional problems and relating her experiences with a
nervous breakdown. Dr. Stanley F. Yolles, former Director
of the National Institute of Mental Health, points out the
immediate need to help millions of Americans who are emotionally disturbed, cites recent Federal legislation establishing community mental health centers, and describes the
government's long-range mental health goals. Interviews
psychologists, health center officials, and affected citizens who emphasize the problem of limited facilities and
offer possible solutions. NET Film Service, 1965. *IU.*

HISTORY

Dr. Pinel Unchains the Insane. (27 min.) Series: You Are
There. Reconstructs events of May 24, 1793, at an asylum
in Paris, as Dr. Philippe Pinel fights for humane treatment
of the mentally ill, who, until then, had been chained and
treated like dangerous animals. CBS Television, 1956. *UI*.

Early Treatment of the Mentally Ill. (29 min.) Outlines the
history of the treatment of insanity from earliest times
through the Middle Ages. Describes misapprehensions about
insanity, the ways ancient Romans and Greeks treated it,
and what happened to classical thought on the subject after
the fall of the Roman Empire. Shows influence of the Roman
Catholic Church and belief in angels, devils, and magic,
and methods used to cure insanity. WCET-TV, released by
NET Film Service, 1960. *IU*.

AUTHOR INDEX*

* Due to an error the authors in Early Intervention were omitted and are included at the end of the section.

439

Allen, C. E., *1776*
Allen, D. W., *3697*
Allen, F. H., *0020, 0022,*
  0067, 0116, 2415
Allen, J., *1897.2, 2661.2,*
  4006.6, 4158.2
Allen, J. R., *1457, 2310.1*
Allen, K. E., *2886*
Allen, L., *3907*
Allen, M. G., *0259.1, 0488.2*
Allen, T. E., *3963*
Allen, V. L., *3906*
Allentuck, S., *1545*
Allerhand, M. E., *3196, 3209,*
  3306.6
Allison, R., *2367*
Alpern, G. D., *1775, 1812,*
  1897.2, 2041, 2158.5
Alpert, A., *0522, 0579, 1939,*
  2042, 2075
Alpert, M., *1888*
Alpert, R., *0164, 0177*
Alt, H., *3021, 3118, 3158,*
  3207
Altman, M., *3557*
Altrocchi, J., *3281, 3601*
Amatruda, C. S., *0104*
Amble, B. R., *4131, 4136*
Ambrosino, S., *3410*
Ameen, L., *3202*
American Academy of Pediat-
  rics, *1061*
American Handbook of Psy-
  chiatry, *1431, 3285*
American Medical Associa-
  tion, *2226*
American Psychiatric Associ-
  ation, *3216, 3798, 3799,*
  3829, 3841
Ames, F., *1544*
Ames, L. B., *0761*
Amster, F., *2397*
Anders, T. F., *1000.9*
Andersen, I. N., *1976*
Anderson, C., *1646*
Anderson, C. C., *4185*
Anderson, D., *2784*
Anderson, H. H., *4239*
Anderson, J. E., *2802*
Anderson, L. M., *3970*

Anderson, L. S., *0803*
Andrew, G., *4101*
Andrews, F. M., *4202*
Andronico, M. P., *2537, 2591,*
  2592, 2595
Andry, R. G., *1509*
Angoff, K., *1118*
Anker, J. M., *2797*
Annell, A. L., *2079*
Ansbacher, H. L., *0680*
Anthony, E. J., *0048, 0052.1*
  0069, 0183, 0304, 0311.1,
  0312, 0353, 0392, 0556, 0589,
  0759, 0834, 0843, 0872, 0888,
  1143, 1144, 1145, 1160, 1188,
  1189, 1190, 1191, 1193, 1195,
  1198, 1202, 1209, 1230, 1236,
  1241, 1243, 1245, 1252, 1253,
  1254, 1258, 1259, 1260, 1261,
  1262, 1263, 1264, 1265, 1266,
  1268.1, 1400, 1611, 1867, 2057,
  2412.3, 2741, 2742, 2865, 2869,
  3369.1, 3639, 3871, 3947
Anthony, S., *1161*
Apley, J., *0923, 0926*
Aponte, J., *0690*
Aponte, J. F., *1001*
Appelbaum, M. I., *0066.1*
Appleton, W. S., *3727*
April, C., *3978*
Archer, M., *1660*
Archibald, D., *0944*
Arensdorf, A. M., *0052.4*
Argyris, C., *3497, 3826*
Aries, P., *0018.2, 1271, 1573,*
  2613
Arieti, S., *0958, 0974.1, 1340,*
  1431, 1479, 2117, 2209, 2646,
  3285, 3776, 4159
Arlow, J. A., *3766*
Armstrong, H. E., *2010*
Aronson, E., *0440, 2333*
Aronson, H., *4034.1*
Arsenian, J., *3437*
Arthur, B., *0644, 2901, 2954*
Artuso, A. A., *2887*
Ashby, E., *3810*
Ashenden, B., *2048.1*
Ashenden, B. J., *0810*
Ashton-Warner, S., *1291*

Clarke, A. D. B. *(cont.)*, *2215, 2247.1, 2344*
Clarke, A. M., *0573, 2186, 2215, 2231, 2247.1, 2344*
Clarke-Stewart, K. A., *0279.1*
Clausen, J. A., *0119, 1921*
Clayton, B. E., *2196.1*
Cleghorn, J. M., *3758.1*
Clement, P. W., *2519, 2520, 2783*
Clements, M., *3924.6*
Clements, S. D., *1012, 1013, 2943*
Clemmens, R. L., *4045*
Cline, D. W., *3494.2, 4006*
Cline, F. W., *1124.1*
Cloward, R. A., *2341*
Clower, C. G., *2830*
Coates, R. B., *2319.1*
Cobb, B., *1222*
Cobb, S., *0423, 2265*
Cobbs, P. M., *2299*
Coddington, R. D., *0660, 0800.1, 0800.2, 0903*
Coelho, G. V., *1378, 3414, 3415*
Coffey, H. S., *1963, 2800*
Cohen, D. J., *0219, 0259.1*
Cohen, F. J., *3219*
Cohen, H. J., *1897.1*
Cohen, I. M., *2654, 3860*
Cohen, J., *2298, 2348, 2349*
Cohen, M., *1538, 2348*
Cohen, M. I., *1602*
Cohen, R., *0606, 3035*
Cohen, R. L., *3093, 3715.1, 4089, 4148*
Cohen, R. S., *1985, 3143, 4085*
Cohen, S., *1328, 1860.2*
Cohen, S. I., *3386.1*
Cohen, W. J., *2314*
Cohler, R., *3135*
Cohrssen, J., *2979*
Coker, R. E., *3684*
Colby, K. M., *2033, 3795, 3796*
Cole, J. K., *4091*
Cole, J. O., *3006*
Cole, N., *2367*

Coleman, J. V., *0013, 3235, 3567, 3573*
Coleman, M., *1908*
Coleman, R. W., *1649, 3469*
Coleman, W. F., *1413.1*
Coles, R., *0120, 0121, 0122, 0760, 1579*
Collette, J. C., *3832*
Collier, J. G., *2534, 2807*
Colligan, R. C., *2012, 4075.4*
Collins, M. H., *1899.1*
Collins, P., *2027.1, 3008.1, 3015.3*
Collins, P. J., *1908.1*
Collomb, H., *0456.1, 1266*
Colm, H. N., *0600*
Colman, A. D., *0189*
Colodny, D., *2191*
Comly, H. H., *1090*
Comstock, G. A., *0437, 0438*
Conant, J. B., *2359*
Condon, C. F., *4246*
Conference on Economic Progress, *2313*
Connell, P. H., *2020, 2470*
Conners, C. K., *1032, 1033, 1037, 1038, 1039, 2945, 2958, 2961, 2962, 2965, 2989, 3004, 3955, 4126*
Connolly, K., *0233.5*
Connor, R., *0139*
Conrad, R. D., *3924.3*
Conte, H., *3689*
Cook, S. S., *1270.1*
Cooley, R. E., *1279.3*
Coolidge, J. C., *0609, 0613.2, 0864, 2566, 2763*
Coombs, J., *2138*
Coombs, R. H., *3774, 3775*
Cooper, A., *1967, 4097, 4224*
Cooper, I. S., *0995*
Cooper, M. M., *2539*
Cooperman, O., *4046.1*
Copeland, R., *3007*
Coppolillo, H. P., *1268.8, 2447*
Corbett, J. A., *2470*
Corbett, R. M., *3641.1*
Corbin, H. P. F., *0240*
Corcoran, J., *1000*
Corday, R. J., *1442*

Davis, J. M., *3018*
Davis, W. E., *3580*
Davison, G. C., *2517*
Dawes, L. G., *3361*
Day, R., *2148*
Dealy, M. N., *2084*
DeBell, D. E., *3759*
Debuskey, M., *0810*
Decarie, T. G., *0285.1*
Decker, J. H., *3575*
De Elejalde, F., *0753*
De Francis, V., *1709*
Defries, Z., *2451*
DeHirsch, K., *0101, 1339.1,*
1352.3, 1790, 3381
de la Burde, B., *0893.1*
de la Cruz, F. F., *1031.5,*
2213.2
DeLeeuw, L., *2269*
Delgado, R. A., *0558*
DeLicardie, E. R., *2132, 3256,*
3389
Dellis, N. P., *3690, 3723*
Deloria, V., *2306, 2307*
Deloughery, G. L., *3505*
Delsordo, J. D., *1680*
Deluca, M. A., *2935*
DeMeritt, S., *4121*
DeMyer, M. *1794, 1882*
DeMyer, M. K., *1712, 1774,*
1794, 1812, 1882, 1897,
1897.2, 1906, 2008, 2026,
2032, 2158.5, 2661.2,
4006.6, 4037.4, 4037.5,
4158.2
DeMyer, W. E., *2158.5,*
4158.2
Denhoff, E., *1018, 2484,*
2947
Dennis, W., *0461, 3385,*
4241
Denny, T., *4246*
De-Nour, A. K., *3914*
DeReuck, A. V. S., *0422, 0448,*
0487
DeSaix, C., *1643*
De Sanctis, S., *1737*
DesLauriers, A. M., *1742,*
1868, 2036
Despert, J. L., *0306, 0656,*

Despert, J. L. *(cont.), 0959,*
1721, 1727.1, 1743, 1795,
1805, 2420
Dettelbach, M. H., *3193*
Deutsch, A., *3220*
Deutsch, A. L., *2829*
Deutsch, C. P., *0141.4*
Deutsch, F., *0779, 0784, 1006*
Deutsch, H., *0330, 1450*
Deutsch, M., *0326, 0358, 2348, 2351*
Deutscher, I., *3466*
Devereux, G., *0488, 3057, 3643*
DeVito, E., *1908.1*
Devries, A. G., *4137.1*
Dewald, P. A., *3765*
Dewees, S., *3640*
Dewey, J., *3877*
Dewey, R., *0351*
Dibble, E., *0259.1*
Dicks, H. V., *2703*
Dieruf, W., *1015, 1025*
Dietiker, K. E., *0847*
Diggory, J. C., *1157*
DiLeo, J. H., *2447.1, 4066*
Dillehay, R., *3413*
Dine, M. S., *1624*
Dingman, P., *4131*
Dinitz, S., *3566.2*
Dinnage, R., *0182.1*
Directory of Facilities for
Mentally Ill Children in the
United States, *3221*
Ditman, K. S., *2982*
Dittmann, A. T., *3084, 3198, 3208*
Dizenhuz, I. M., *4086*
Dizmang, L. H., *0645, 1438.6*
Dobbing, J., *2145*
Doherty, E. G., *3713.1*
Dohrenwend, B. P., *3924.5*
Dohrenwend, B. S., *3924.5*
Doi, L. T., *0420*
Dolan, A. B., *4046.2*
Domke, H. R., *3920, 3959*
Donnelly, T. G., *3684*
Donofrio, A. F., *2994*
Dorf, H. J., *2970*
Dorfman, E., *2395*
Doris, J. L., *2243*
Dorn, R. M., *3764*
Dorsen, M. M., *1714*

Ekstein, R., *1312, 1329, 1713,*
1807, 1818, 1831, 1931,
1940, 1941, 1949, 1956,
1974, 1997, 2043, 2044,
2046, 2050, 2052, 2054,
2056, 2083, 2087, 2090,
2480, 3079, 3731
Elbert, S., *4123*
Eldridge, K., *3092*
Eldridge, R., *0995*
Elgar, S., *1987*
Elkind, D., *1282*
Elkins, A. M., *3564*
Elkisch, P., *1820, 1827,*
1836, 1979
Ellinwood, C., *4113*
Elliott, C. D., *2433*
Ellis, W., *3324*
Ellison, P., *1658*
Elmer, E., *1595, 1599, 1617,*
1634, 1635, 1656, 1658,
1670, 1697
Elonen, A. S., *2487*
Elstein, A. S., *3683*
Emch, M., *3756*
Emde, R. N., *0099.1, 0204.2,*
0237
Emerson, P. E., *0272*
Emerson, R., *0790*
Emmerich, W., *0054, 0073,*
0123, 2381
Emmons, E. B., *1395.5*
Engel, G. L., *0767, 0918,*
1007, 3474, 3686, 4162
Engel, M., *2597, 4068*
Engelhardt, D. M., *1048.7,*
1752.3, 2936.1, 2936.2
Engeln, R., *2523*
Engels, W. D., *0989*
Enright, J., *2884*
Epps, R., *3317*
Epstein, A. W., *0940*
Epstein, J., *2787*
Epstein, L. C., *2965*
Epstein, N., *2767, 2812*
Erickson, F. H., *1116*
Erickson, M., *2521, 2890*
Erickson, M. E., *1239*
Erickson, P. A., *4157*
Erikson, E. H., *0074, 0075,*

Erikson, E. H. *(cont.), 0153,*
0154, 0226, 0281, 0282, 0338,
0366, 0377, 0378, 0401, 0462,
0463, 0464, 0467, 0468, 0502,
0505, 0699, 1364, 1371, 1384,
1409, 1419, 1449, 1837, 2393,
2396, 2416, 2432.1, 2715,
2737, 3719
Erlich, F. M., *3809.2*
Ernhart, C. B., *2153*
Eron, L. D., *0400.1, 1759*
Ervin, F., *0940*
Ervin-Tripp, S., *0103, 1337*
Escalona, S. K., *1838, 2382,*
3073, 3380, 3854, 3863, 3880
Escoll, P., *2496*
Escoll, P. J., *1555, 2569,*
3712, 3741
Esman, A. H., *3865, 4112*
Esterson, A., *2710, 3264*
Esveldt, K., *4037.3*
Etemad, J. G., *2109, 2110*
Evans, A. E., *1211*
Evans, J., *0238, 0560*
Evans, M. A., *2002.1*
Evans, M. B., *2888*
Evan-Wong, L., *4036*
Evarts, C. M., *1666*
Eveloff, H. H., *3002*
Everett, P. M., *2886*
Eysenck, H. J., *2508, 3937, 4069*
Eysenck, S. B., *3937*

Fabian, A. A., *1946*
Fabian, A. E., *3328*
Fabri, P. J., *1257.4*
Fagin, C. M., *1096*
Falick, M. L., *1312, 1329*
Falstein, E., *3674*
Falstein, E. I., *0607, 0868,*
0986, 1485, 3058
Fanon, F., *0155*
Fanshel, D., *3197*
Fantl, B., *3612*
Farb, P., *2308*
Farberow, N. L., *3439*
Faretra, G., *2998*
Fargo, G. A., *2895*
Faris, R. E. L., *4247*
Farley, B. C., *3584*

Koch, H. L., *2277, 2283*
Kochman, A., *3386.2*
Kodman, F., *2846*
Koegler, R. R., *3626*
Koel, B. S., *1650*
Koestler, A., *4187*
Kogan, K. L., *2609.11, 2705, 2706.1, 3977, 4006.4, 4124*
Kogan, N., *4211, 4212*
Kogan, W. S., *3718*
Kogelschatz, J. L., *2343*
Koh, C., *2027.1, 3008.1, 3015.3*
Kohn, M., *2492, 3163, 4129.1, 4129.2*
Kohn, M. L., *1921, 2349*
Kohrman, R., *4093*
Kohut, H., *0542*
Kolansky, H., *0604, 2468.2, 2533.1*
Kolb, L. C., *3755*
Kolodny, R. L., *2790*
Koluchova, J., *4015.5*
Kolvin, I., *1749, 1750, 1864, 1896, 1926, 1927, 3015.1*
Konopka, G., *0360.1, 3059, 3068, 3223*
Koocher, G. P., *1257.5*
Kooi, K. A., *0946*
Koos, E. L., *2653*
Koper, A., *0066.4,*
Koppitz, E. M., *0362, 2440*
Korein, J., *3008.1, 3015.3*
Korkina, M. V., *1427*
Korn, S., *0248*
Korner, A. F., *0106, 0207, 0211.2, 2412.4, 2430.2, 2609.3, 3384*
Kornetsky, C., *2900*
Kornreich, M., *3884*
Korsch, B. M., *1072, 1268.7*
Kosc, L., *1027.2*
Kosier, K. P., *0140*
Kotinsky, R., *1304, 3400*
Kounin, J. S., *1325*
Koupernik, C., *0311.1, 0759, 0786, 1160, 1188, 1190, 1191, 1198, 1236, 1241, 1243, 1252, 1253, 1260, 1261, 1266 1268.1*
Kraft, D. P., *3314.4*

Kraft, I. A., *2764, 2766, 2817, 2821, 2826, 2853*
Kramer, D. A., *4006*
Kramer, M., *3705, 4018*
Kramer, M. K., *3768*
Kramer, S., *1847, 2412.5*
Krasner, L., *3885*
Kraus, P. E., *0327.1*
Kraus, R. F., *0059*
Krawiec, T. S., *0039*
Krech, D., *0060, 2139*
Kreitler, H., *0107*
Kreitler, S., *0107*
Krevelen, D. A. van, *1430*
Krieger, H. P., *2114*
Kringlen, E., *0683*
Kripke, S. S., *0855*
Kris, E., *0292, 0309, 0497 3767, 4192*
Kris, M., *3864*
Krohn, H., *3159*
Krolick, G., *0285.2*
Kronick, D., *2884.1*
Krown, S., *2042*
Krug, O., *1331, 1969, 3072, 3078*
Krug, R. S., *0068, 0117*
Krumboltz, J. D., *2834*
Krush, T. P., *2917*
Kubie, L. S., *3290, 3724, 3855*
Kubzansky, P. E., *3426*
Kuchar, E., *2002.1*
Kugel, R. B., *2193, 2194, 2195, 2196*
Kuhn, C. C., *0897*
Kuhn, D. Z., *0169*
Kulka, A., *0785*
Kuniholm, P., *0586*
Kupietz, S., *0800.4, 3015.2, 4129.7*
Kurland, A. A., *2970*
Kurlander, L. F., *2191*
Kurtis, L. B., *2973*
Kurtz, R. M., *3710, 4086*
Kushner, J. H., *1196*
Kutscher, A. H., *1183, 1234*
Kvaraceus, W. C., *3416*
Kysar, J. E., *1982, 1983, 3607*

Laatsch, A., *3030, 3070*
LaBarba, R. C., *0798*
LaBarre, M. B., *2288, 3657*
LaBarre, W., *0408*
L'Abate, L., *4075.2, 4087*
Lacey, H. M., *4105*
Lachenbruch, P. A., *1450.2*
Laffal, J., *3202*
LaFranchi, S., *1766*
Laing, R. D., *2710, 3264*
Lake, G., *3306.6*
Lakin, M., *0199*
Lamb, H. R., *3297*
Lamontagne, C. H., *2919*
Lampert, R., *2971*
Lander, J., *1499, 3051*
Landowne, E. J., *4119*
Landtman, B., *0836*
Lane, L., *3091*
Lane, P. A., *2493, 2585*
Lang, P., *1004*
Langdell, J. I., *1975*
Langdon, G., *0138, 1119, 3968*
Langee, H., *2602*
Langer, J., *0108*
Langer, S., *3875*
Langford, W. S., *1137, 1186.1, 3381*
Langner, T., *2330*
Langner, T. S., *2259, 3462, 3906*
Langsley, D. G., *2692, 2753*
Lansing, C., *1929, 1962, 1965, 2794, 2799*
Lapouse, R., *0332, 0333, 0546, 1756, 3893, 3908, 4100*
Larr, C. J., *3924.1*
Larsen, K. W., *2956*
Lasagna, L., *2965*
Laties, V. G., *3011*
Laub, D., *3730.1*
Laufer, M., *0380, 0533, 1263, 1428*
Laufer, M. W., *1018, 1715, 2484, 2947*
Laughy, L., *2523*
LaVeck, G. D., *2158.6, 2213.2, 2925*
LaVietes, R., *3033, 3035, 3140*

Lawrence, R. J., *1703*
Lawrie, R., *1134*
Laws, D. R., *2787*
Lax, R. F., *0577*
Laybourne, P. C., *0630, 0963, 3032*
Layman, E. M., *0557, 0893*
Lazarus, A. A., *2517, 2785*
Lazerson, A. M., *3698, 3730.5*
Lazure, D., *0018*
Leaverton, D. R., *1676*
Lebo, D., *2403, 2405, 2421, 2430, 2432, 2435, 4010, 4127*
Lebo, E., *2435*
Lebovici, S., *1264, 2822*
Lebovitz, P. S., *0736*
Lederer, W., *2410*
Lee, D., *1880*
Lee, E. S., *2336*
Lee, M. L., *2770*
Leff, R., *2513*
Lefford, A., *1027.1*
Lefkowitz, M. M., *0400.1, 2990*
LeGasse, A. A., *3845, 4096*
Legg, D. R., *1786*
Lehman, E., *0889*
Lehtinen, L. E., *3019*
Leibowitz, E., *2587*
Leibowitz, G., *2587*
Leichter, H. J., *2726*
Leider, A. R., *3395*
Leider, R. J., *3745*
Leiderman, P. H., *0212, 2836*
Leifer, R., *3678*
Leighton, A. H., *0414, 0419, 0422, 0442, 2250, 2323, 3246*
Leighton, D. C., *0441, 2324, 3461, 4129.3*
Leiken, S. J., *0842*
Leist, N., *0852*
Leitch, M., *3380*
Leitenberg, H., *0829.4*
Leler, H., *2726.1*
Lembke, P., *3093*
Lemkau, P. V., *3244*
Lendrum, B. L., *1128*
Lennhoff, F. G., *3028*
Leon, R. L., *3369, 3532*
Leonard, A. R., *3265*
Leonard, C. O., *2377.4*

Lipton, R. C. *(cont.)*, *1588*, *2174*, *3259*, *3431*
Lipton, S. D., *1081*
Lis, E. F., *1618*
Liss, E., *0011*, *1306*
Lister, J., *0243*
Liston, E. H., *3792*
Litin, E. M., *1489*, *1504*, *1506*
Little, R. B., *3694*
Littman, R. A., *2272*
Livingstone, J. B., *4077*
Llewellyn, C. E., *3284*
Llorens, L. A., *0702*
Lo, W. H., *0591*
Locke, H. J., *2623*
Lockett, H. J., *2919*
Lockhart, H. E., *0879*
Lockner, A. W., *2933*
Lockyer, L., *2096*, *2097*
Loeb, M. B., *3494*
Loesch, J. G., *0199*, *0200*
Loew, L. H., *1712*
Loewenstein, R. M., *0497*, *2384*, *2386*
Loftin, J., *1853*
Loiselle, R. H., *4224*
Lomas, P., *2716*
Lombard, J. P., *2994*
Long, N. J., *1324*
Long, R. T., *0805*, *0844*
Lonsdale, D., *1666*
Looff, D. H., *0794*, *2347*, *3311*
Looker, A., *2989*
Loomis, E. A., *1829*, *1843*, *2417.1*, *2427.1*, *3114*
Loomis, W. G., *1687*
Lorand, S., *1443*
Lord, J. P., *2661.6*
Lordi, W. M., *1912*
Lorenz, K., *2417*
Lott, G. M., *2180*
Lotter, V., *1753*, *1803*, *1927.5*
Lourie, C. H., *0852*
Lourie, R. S., *0268*, *0314*, *0556*, *0557*, *0745*, *0891*, *0893*, *1597*, *1601*, *1636*, *1682*, *2129*, *2999*, *3476*
Lovaas, O. I., *2015*, *2016*

Love, L. R., *3978*
Lovell, K., *2398*
Lovibond, S. H., *2456*
Lovitt, T. C., *2894*, *3007*
Lowery, V. E., *2923*
Lowrey, L. G., *0005*, *0008*, *0015*, *0028*, *0029*, *0036*
Luborsky, L. B., *3758*
Lucas, A. R., *0623*, *0689*, *0949*, *1044*, *2919*, *3000*, *4174*
Lucas, J., *1903*
Ludwig, E. G., *3832*
Luke, J. A., *0622*
Lunceford, J. L., *1216*
Lunde, D. T., *0218*
Lundell, F. W., *1036*
Luparello, T. J., *0850*, *0851*, *0852*
Luria, Z., *3992*, *4116*
Lurie, H. L., *0031*
Lurie, O. R., *2630.2*, *3898*
Lustman, S. L., *0208*, *0783*, *2386*
Lyman, M. S., *2600*
Lynch, M. J., *0975*
Lynn, D. B., *0832*, *0835*
Lyons, H. A., *0850*, *0851*
Lytton, H., *0135*

Maas, H., *2371*
Maberly, A., *4150*
MacCarthy, D., *1091*
Maccoby, E. E., *0178*, *0317*, *0460*, *2352*
Macdonald, N., *0865*
Macfarlane, J. W., *3907*, *4095*
Macgregor, H., *4093*
MacGregor, R., *2635*, *2760*
Machover, S., *2757*
Macht, L. B., *3816*
Mack, I., *1128*
Mackay, J., *2546*
Mackeith, S. A., *3178*
Mackey, R. A., *3603*
Mackie, J., *3921*
Macklin, D. B., *0441*, *2324*, *3461*
Maclay, I., *2559*
MacLennan, B. W., *2818*
Macmillan, A. M., *0441*, *2324*
MacMillan, M. B., *0006*

Mendelson, N., *1022*
Menkes, J. H., *2953*
Menkes, M. M., *2953*
Menlove, F. L., *4039*
Menolascino, F. J., *1746, 1782,*
  1797, 1894, 2100, 2163, 2170,
  2177, 2188, 2191, 2192, 2239,
  3957
Mensh, I. N., *3713, 3951, 3959*
Mental Health Law Project,
  2130.2
Menzer, D., *2086*
Mercer, J. R., *2158.1, 3331.4*
Mercer, M. E., *3576*
Mercer, R. D., *0878*
Merklin, L., *3694*
Merleau-Ponty, M., *4181*
Messinger, S. L., *2713*
Metcalf, D. R., *0099.1, 0237*
Meyer, E., *0998*
Meyer, L. R., *1843*
Meyer, M., *3452*
Meyerowitz, S., *0918*
Meyers, D. I., *1914*
Michael, C. M., *2564, 4129*
Michael, S. T., *3462*
Michaux, M. H., *2970*
Middleman, R., *3040*
Middleton, R., *2354*
Midelfort, C. F., *2661*
Midtown Manhattan Study, *2322,*
  3262, 3462
Miezio, S., *2816*
Miklich, D., *0847*
Miksztal, M. W., *2920*
Millar, G., *2557*
Millar, T. P., *0973*
Miller, A. A., *3711, 3745,*
  3746
Miller, A. D., *2319.1*
Miller, B. M., *1938*
Miller, D., *1446.6*
Miller, D. R., *2689*
Miller, E., *0080, 2477, 3929*
Miller, F. T., *1860.3*
Miller, H., *0807, 0808, 0854*
Miller, H. C., *3032*
Miller, K. S., *3245*
Miller, L., *0136, 3292*
Miller, L. C., *4118, 4129.4*

Miller, M. B., *1706*
Miller, M. H., *3687*
Miller, N., *3684*
Miller, P. R., *3794*
Miller, S., *3700*
Miller, S. C., *2873*
Millican, F. K., *0556, 0557,*
  0891, 0893
Millichap, J. G., *1035, 2948,*
  2956, 3008
Millman, I. K., *1352*
Mills, C. W., *1278*
Mills, R. C., *4029.2*
Milman, D. H., *0924, 0992*
Milman, L., *0829.1, 0872.1*
Milne, D. C., *2783*
Milner, A. D., *0722*
Milowe, I. D., *1601, 2200, 3476*
Milstein, V., *2951*
Minde, K., *1022, 1029, 1031,*
  2957, 4152
Minde, K. K., *2584, 2904, 3551*
Minuchin, P., *0363*
Minuchin, S., *0829.1, 0829.2,*
  0872.1, 1515, 2361, 2504, 2531,
  2532, 2536, 2540.1, 2664, 2668,
  2677.2, 2677.3, 2679, 3321,
  3639, 4123
Mira, M., *2589*
Mishler, E. G., *2661.1, 2707*
Mitchell, K. M., *4129.6*
Mitchell, P., *2002.2*
Mitchell, S., *3892, 3897, 3923*
Mitchell, W. E., *2726*
Mittelmann, B., *0295, 0544*
Mittler, P., *0172, 2099*
Mizushima, K., *3938*
Mnookin, R. H., *4046.5*
Modell, A., *1830*
Moffat, P. J., *3234.1*
Mohr, G. J., *0787, 0806, 0955,*
  0977
Molish, H. B., *0037*
Molling, P. A., *2908, 2922, 2933*
Moloney, J. C., *1087, 1865*
Monashkin, I., *3969*
Money, J., *0723, 0739*
Money, J. W., *0738*
Money-Kyrle, R. E., *1828*
Monk, M. A., *0332, 0333, 0546,*

Risley, T. R., *2898.5*
Ritvo, E. R., *0066.4, 0619,
1766, 1768, 1785, 1793,
1877, 1878, 3924.6*
Ritvo, S., *0711, 1369*
Ritz, M., *3924.6*
Rivlin, L. G., *4233*
Rizzo, A. E., *2798*
Roach, J. L., *4023*
Robbins, L. C., *0255, 4057*
Robbins, M. D., *4194, 4195,
4196*
Robbins, P. R., *3513*
Roberts, A., *1998*
Roberts, B. H., *2630*
Roberts, G. E., *1902*
Roberts, J., *0363.1, 3888*
Roberts, L. M., *3304*
Roberts, N. S., *3494*
Roberts, R. H., *1031.5*
Robertson, J., *0316, 1094,
3230, 3377*
Robertson, N. C., *3911*
Robertson, R. E., *4158*
Robey, J. S., *0235*
Robin, M., *0956*
Robins, E., *0715*
Robins, L. N., *2332, 2574,
2575, 3464.1, 4142*
Robinson, D. B., *1495*
Robinson, H. B., *2218, 2242*
Robinson, J., *3779*
Robinson, J. F., *3020, 3120,
3176, 3231*
Robinson, M. E., *0843*
Robinson, N. M., *2218*
Robison, O. L., *2771*
Robson, K. S., *0270, 0271*
Rochlin, G., *0554, 2066*
Rock, N. L., *0598*
Rockberger, H., *2843*
Rodrigue, E., *1828*
Rodriguez, A., *2048.1, 2565,
2965*
Rodriguez, M., *2565*
Rodriguez-Torres, R., *0924,
0992*
Roe, A., *4201, 4206*
Roeske, N., *4037.5*
Roff, M., *2575, 3464.1, 4143*

Rogawski, A. S., *3535*
Rogeness, G. A., *3306.2*
Rogers, C. R., *2395, 2556*
Rogers, M., *2518, 4011*
Rogers, W. J. B., *2937*
Rolland, R. S., *1534, 2533.2*
Rollins, M., *0826*
Rollins, N., *0476.1, 2472,
2661.6*
Roman, P. M., *2338*
Rondell, F. R., *3180*
Rose, J. A., *3214*
Rose, S. D., *2761.2*
Rosen, B. C., *2268*
Rosen, B. M., *4018, 4019*
Rosen, E., *4209*
Rosen, H., *3780*
Rosen, J. N., *2122*
Rosenbaum, C. P., *3795*
Rosenbaum, M., *0792, 2766, 2825,
2835, 2837, 2850, 2878, 3733*
Rosenberg, B. G., *4222*
Rosenberg, C. M., *0692*
Rosenberg, I., *0214.2*
Rosenberg, R. M., *1511*
Rosenberger, L., *1262*
Rosenblatt, B., *0496, 1237*
Rosenblatt, J. S., *0210*
Rosenblith, J. F., *0112*
Rosenblum, A. H., *0986*
Rosenblum, G., *3333*
Rosenblum, L. A., *0272.1*
Rosenblum, S., *2941*
Rosenblum, W., *4198*
Rosenbluth, D., *0576, 2156*
Rosenfeld, E., *3865, 4112*
Rosenfeld, J. M., *3236, 3914*
Rosenfeld, R., *1048.7*
Rosenfeld, S. K., *0633, 0634*
Rosengren, W., *0198*
Rosengren, W. R., *2374*
Rosenhan, D. L., *3648*
Rosenheim, M. K., *3331.5*
Rosenthal, A. J., *2541, 2551,
2602*
Rosenthal, H. R., *3625*
Rosenthal, M. J., *0954*
Rosenthal, P. A., *2533.2*
Rosenthal, R., *3833*
Rosenzweig, M. R., *0060*

Stambler, M., *1899.1*
Standish, C., *2086*
Stanley, E. J., *1435*
Stanton, A. H., *3071, 3232,*
  3644, 3645, 3646, 3647, 3649,
  3651, 3653, 3665
Stark, G., *0756*
Stark, M. H., *0892, 2168*
Stark, S., *4256*
Starr, P., *2695*
Staub, E. M., *1092, 3472*
Staver, N., *1313, 1333, 1354*
Stedman, J. M., *2676*
Steele, B. F., *1575, 1611*
Steele, R., *1897.2, 2661.2,*
  4158.2
Stehbens, J. A., *2455*
Stein, A., *2835*
Stein, A. H., *1279.1*
Stein, H., *0870*
Stein, J., *1446.7*
Stein, M., *0849, 3615*
Stein, M. K., *4203*
Stein, M. L., *0894*
Stein, S., *3511*
Stein, Z., *2219*
Steinhauer, P. D., *3894*
Steisel, I. M., *2376*
Stemmer, C. J., *1024, 1631*
Stennett, R. G., *3405, 3890*
Stephens, C. A., *0975*
Stern, A., *3202*
Stern, E., *0253*
Stern, R., *1062*
Sternbach, R. A., *3494.1*
Stevens, D. A., *2950*
Stevens, H. A., *2224, 2244*
Stevens, J. R., *2951*
Stevens, M., *1095*
Stevenson, H. W., *0063, 0109,*
  0179, 2282
Stevenson, O., *0254*
Steward, A. H., *3395*
Stewart, B., *1450.1*
Stewart, E. C., *2282*
Stewart, K. K., *3088*
Stewart, M. A., *1015, 1020.1,*
  1025, 1031.6, 3982
Stewart, R. H., *2772*
Stewart, R. S., *1343*

Stickler, G. B., *2136*
Stierlin, H., *0353.1, 1399.1*
Stillman, R., *3795*
Stoch, M. B., *3258*
Stocking, M., *1085.1*
Stoddard, F. J., *3314.4*
Stoffer, D. L., *4134*
Stollak, G. E., *2586*
Stoller, F. H., *2745*
Stoller, R. J., *0567, 0727,*
  0728, 0731, 0733, 0740, 0740.1,
  0740.4
Stolorow, R. D., *0709*
Stone, C. L., *2284*
Stone, H. K., *3690, 3723*
Stone, L. J., *0233.1*
Stone, W. E., *0922*
Stonehill, E., *0898*
Stotland, E., *2281*
Stott, D. H., *2158, 2572, 3944,*
  4015, 4043
Stouffer, G. A. W., *3919*
Stout, I. W., *0138, 3968*
Stover, L., *2591, 2593, 3989,*
  4121
Straight, B., *2811, 3161*
Stranahan, M., *3162*
Strang, R., *1318*
Straus, R., *1395.2, 1395.3,*
  1395.4, 3924.2
Strauss, A. A., *3019*
Strauss, A. L., *1176*
Strauss, M., *3816*
Street, E., *4100*
Stretch, J. J., *3274*
Strickland, R. G., *0285.2*
Strickler, M., *3622*
Stringer, E. A., *1685*
Stringer, L. A., *2606, 3590,*
  4041
Strother, C. R., *1020.3*
Stunkard, A. J., *0900, 0901,*
  0911, 0912.1
Sturge, B., *4150*
Sturgis, L. H., *2956*
Sturtevant, W. C., *2310*
Stutte, H., *1752.1*
Subotnik, L., *2503*
Succop, R. A., *0827, 0978*
Sucgang, R. C., *3128*

Winokur, G., *0730*
Winsberg, B. G., *0800.4, 1783,*
3015.2, 4129.7
Winter, W. D., *2678*
Wisdom, J. O., *0650*
Wise, L. J., *3080*
Witkin, H. A., *0115*
Witmer, H. L., *0017, 1304,*
2406, 3400
Witmer, L., *1716*
Wittkower, E. D., *0989, 2038*
Wodinsky, A., *3589*
Woerner, M. G., *1755*
Wohl, M. G., *3391*
Wohl, T., *2875*
Wohl, T. H., *2805*
Wohlwill, J. F., *4015.1*
Wolberg, L. R., *3714*
Wold, P., *0829.3*
Wolf, A. W. M., *1164*
Wolf, E. G., *1789, 1995,*
4072.1
Wolf, K. M., *0638, 1587, 2059*
Wolf, M. G., *4042*
Wolf, M. M., *2885*
Wolf, S. G., *3837*
Wolfensberger, W., *2170, 2193,*
2194, 2195, 2196
Wolfenstein, C. M., *4063*
Wolfenstein, M., *0350*
Wolff, E., *1117*
Wolff, H. G., *0900, 1925*
Wolff, P., *1783*
Wolff, P. H., *0055, 0203,*
0259, 1014, 2390
Wolff, S., *0549, 0750, 0841,*
0999, 3941, 3984, 3986
Wolins, M., *0327*
Wolking, W. D., *3983*
Wollersheim, J. P., *2003, 2510*
Wolman, B. B., *2825, 3363,*
4177
Wolman, H. M., *1104*
Wolman, M. B., *2946*
Wolman, R. N., *4149*
Wolman, S. R., *1860.3*
Wolpe, J., *2506.1*
Wolpert, E. A., *0649, 2082,*
2475
Wolters, W. H. G., *1193, 2458*

Woltmann, A. G., *2394*
Womack, M., *2005*
Wood, A. C., *2376*
Wood, H. P., *3712, 3741*
Woodmansey, A. C., *3722*
Woodruff, R., *0717*
Woods, H. B., *3779*
Woods, S. M., *3696*
Woodward, K. F., *2184*
Woody, R. H., *4058*
Woodyard, E. R., *2144*
Wooldridge, R. L., *2892*
Woolley, L. F., *0651*
Worby, C. M., *3742*
Worden, F. G., *1726, 3813*
Work, H. H., *3822*
World Health Organization,
0749, 1049, 3375
Seminar on Standardization of
Psychiatric Diagnosis, Classi-
fication and Mental Statistics,
3928
Worsfold, V. L., *3331.6*
Wortis, H., *0277, 0555, 0890*
Wortis, J., *2246*
Wright, A. L., *2980*
Wright, B., *3107, 3189, 3672*
Wright, C. R., *3491*
Wright, D. M., *1927.2*
Wright, H. F., *0354*
Wright, J. C., *3421*
Wright, L., *4129.6*
Wright, S. W., *2923*
Wyatt, R. J., *1860.2*
Wyden, P., *2731*
Wynne, L. C., *3994*
Wysocki, A. C., *1748, 3940*
Wysocki, B. A., *1748, 3940*

Yager, J., *3730.3*
Yahalom, I., *1852,*
Yalom, I. D., *0218, 2751, 2836,*
2838, 2852, 2859, 2863, 2874,
2880, 4178
Yamamoto, J., *1413.1*
Yamamoto, K., *4228*
Yando, R., *4103.1*
Yang, E., *1897.2, 4006.6*
Yap, P. M., *0448, 0451*
Yarnell, H., *0624, 0628*